# Instructor Resources—Redefined!

## INTRODUCING
### *Pearson Nursing Class Preparation Resources*

- **New and Unique! Correlation to Today's Nursing Standards!**
  - Correlation guides link book and supplement content to nursing standards such as the *2010 ANA Scope and Standards of Practice, QSEN, National Patient Safety Goals, AACN Essentials of Baccalaureate Education* and more!

- **New and Unique! Pearson Nursing Lecture Series**
  - Highly visual, fully narrated and animated, these short lectures focus on topics that are traditionally difficult to teach and difficult for students to grasp
  - All lectures accompanied by case studies and classroom response questions for greater interactivity within even the largest classroom
  - Useful as lecture tools, remediation material, homework assignments and more!

- **Additional instructor resources!**
  - Find assets such as **videos, animations, lecture starters, classroom and clinical activities** and more!
  - **Add selected resources** to presentations that can be shown online or exported to PowerPoint™ or HTML pages
  - Organized by topic and **fully searchable** by type and keyword
  - **Upload your own resources** to keep everything in one place
  - **Rate resources** and view other instructor ratings!

## • Pearson Nursing My Test
- Even **more** accessible with both pencil and paper and online delivery options
- **All New!** Approximately 30% of questions now in alternate-item format!
- **Complete rationales** for both correct and incorrect answers mapped to learning outcomes

## Book-specific resources also available to instructors including:
- Instructor's Manual and Resource Guide organized by learning outcome
- Comprehensive PowerPoint™ presentations integrating lecture notes and images
- Image library
- Classroom Response Questions
- Online course management systems complete with instructor tools and student activities

## REAL NURSING SIMULATIONS
- 25 simulation scenarios that span the nursing curriculum

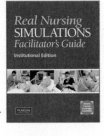

- Consistent format includes learning objectives, case flow, set-up instructions, debriefing questions and more!
- Companion online course cartridge with student pre-and post-simulation activities, videos, skill checklists and reflective discussion questions

# BRIEF CONTENTS

# Leadership and Management for Nurses

## *Core Competencies for Quality Care*

## Second Edition

**Anita Finkelman, RN, MSN**

*Faculty*
*Bouvé College of Health Sciences, School of Nursing,*
*Northeastern University*

**Pearson**
Boston   Columbus   Indianapolis   New York   San Francisco   Upper Saddle River
Amsterdam   Cape Town   Dubai   London   Madrid   Milan   Munich   Paris   Montréal   Toronto
Delhi   Mexico City   São Paulo   Sydney   Hong Kong   Seoul   Singapore   Taipei   Tokyo

Cataloging-in-Publication data on file with the Library of Congress.

**Publisher:** Julie Levin Alexander
**Publisher's Assistant:** Regina Bruno
**Executive Acquisitions Editor:** Pamela Fuller
**Development Editor:** Elisabeth Garofalo
**Editorial Assistant:** Cynthia Gates
**Managing Production Editor:** Patrick Walsh
**Production Liaison:** Cathy O'Connell
**Production Editor:** GEX Publishing Services
**Manufacturing Manager:** Ilene Sanford
**Art Director:** Kristine Carney
**Cover Designer:** Rachael Cronin
**Interior Designer:** Black Horse Designs
**Art Editor:** Patricia Gutierrez
**Director of Marketing:** David Gesell
**Marketing Manager:** Phoenix Harvery
**Marketing Specialist:** Michael Sirinides
**Digital Media Product Manager:** Travis Moses-Westphal
**Media Project Manager:** Rachel Collett
**Composition:** GEX Publishing Services
**Printer/Binder:** Courier/Kendallville
**Cover Printer:** LeHigh Phoenix Color/Hagerstown
**Cover Image:** Hospital reception: David Joel/Photodisc/Getty
Images. Female nurse working at a computer in hospital
setting: Phil Cantor/SuperStock, Inc.

Notice: Care has been taken to confirm the accuracy of information presented in this book. The authors, editors, and the publisher, however, cannot accept any responsibility for errors or omissions or for consequences from application of the information in this book and make no warranty, express or implied, with respect to its contents.

The authors and publisher have exerted every effort to ensure that drug selections and dosages set forth in this text are in accord with current recommendations and practice at time of publication. However, in view of ongoing research, changes in government regulations, and the constant flow of information relating to drug therapy and drug reactions, the reader is urged to check the package inserts of all drugs for any change in indications of dosage and for added warnings and precautions. This is particularly important when the recommended agent is a new and/or infrequently employed drug.

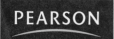

www.pearsonhighered.com

V011
10 9 8
ISBN-10: 0-13-213771-2
ISBN-13: 978-0-13-213771-3

To Fred, Shoshannah, and Deborah, my family. Nothing happens without their support and guidance.

Anita Finkelman, MSN, RN is a faculty member at Bouvé College of Health Sciences School of Nursing, Northeastern University. Her past positions include assistant professor of nursing at University of Oklahoma (OU) College of Nursing where she taught undergraduate and graduate nursing research online, was course coordinator of undergraduate nursing research, was awarded a VANA program grant to develop a special undergraduate long-term experience at the VA and develop a summer internship and a post-graduate nurse residency program. She has managed several projects to migrate nursing curriculum to distance learning. At the University of Cincinnati she served as director of undergraduate curriculum and as associate professor/clinical nursing.

Anita's BSN is from TCU, master's degree in psychiatric-mental health nursing from Yale University, and post-master's graduate work in health care policy and administration from George Washington University. Additional health policy work was completed as a fellow of the Health Policy Institute, George Mason University. Her thirty-five plus years of nursing experience includes clinical, educational, and administrative positions and considerable experience developing distance learning programs, development of curriculum and other online products related to simulation learning, and teaching online. As a consultant she works in the area of distance education, curriculum, and teaching strategies. She has authored many books, journal articles, served on editorial boards, and lectured on administration, health policy, continuing education, and psychiatric-mental health nursing, both nationally and internationally, particularly in Israel for Hebrew University Hadassah School of Nursing in Jerusalem and at Ben Gurion University in Beer-Sheva. She has served as a member of the Interdisciplinary Advisory Committee for The Center for Research, Implementation and Dissemination of Evidence-Based Practice at Haifa University, Israel. She serves as a consultant to publishers and health care organizations in areas of distance education and product development. In addition to her *Teaching IOM: Implications of the Institute of Medicine Reports for Nursing Education* (American Nurses Association, 2009, second edition; co-author Carole Kenner) other recent textbook publications include *Professional Nursing Concepts: Competencies for Quality Leadership* (Pearson Education, 2010; co-author Carole Kenner), and *Case Management for Nurses* (Pearson Education, 2011). Her book *Teaching IOM* has been a best seller, and both first and second editions have won awards from the Society for Technical Communication, Washington, DC (2007–2008 and 2010). Anita has presented workshops across the country focusing on this book for nurse educators and staff development.

# THANK YOU

Our heartfelt thanks go out to our colleagues from schools of nursing across the country who gave their time generously to help us create this exciting new edition of our book. We have reaped the benefit of your collective experience as nurses and teachers, and we have made many improvements due to your efforts. Among those who gave us their encouragement and comments include the following:

**Teresa Aprigliano, EdD, RN**
Associate Dean & Professor
Molloy College
Rockville Centre, New York

**Gail Bromley, PhD, RN, CNS**
Associate Dean, Academics
Kent State University
Kent, Ohio

**Candace M. Burns, PhD, ARNP**
Professor
University of South Florida
Tampa, Florida

**Janet Craig, RN, MSN, MBA, DHA**
Assistant Professor
Clemson University
Greenville, South Carolina

**Linda K. Daley, PhD, RN**
Clinical Instructor
The Ohio State University
Columbus, Ohio

**Erlinda N. Dubal, MBA, MA, BSN, RN, BC**
Director: MS Executive Program for Nursing and Healthcare Management
Long Island University
Brooklyn, New York

**Carole Kenner, DNS, RNC-NIC, FAAN**
Dean/Professor School of Nursing;
Associate Dean Bouvé College of Health Sciences
Northeastern University
Boston, Massachusetts

**Pamela Kohlbry, RN, PhD**
Assistant Professor
California State University, San Marcos
San Marcos, California

**Ava S. Miller EdD, RN, AHN-BC**
Associate Professor
The University of Texas at Brownsville
Brownsville, Texas

**Lyn Stankiewicz Murphy, PhD, MBA, MS, RN**
Assistant Professor
University of Maryland
Baltimore, Maryland

**Ann M Popkess, PhD RN**
Instructor
Southern Illinois University
Edwardsville, Illinois

**Melissa Popovich, RN, MSN, CNL**
Clinical Instructor
The Ohio State University
Columbus, Ohio

**Kathleen A. Roberts, RN, DNP**
Assistant Professor
Midwestern State University
Wichita Falls, Texas

**Polly A. Royal DNP, RN-BC**
Clinical Assistant Professor
Purdue University
West Lafayette, Indiana

**Mary S. Tilbury, EdD, RN, CNAA, BC**
Associate Professor
University of Maryland
Baltimore, Maryland

**Nina M. Trocky, DNP, RN, NE-BC, CCRA**
Assistant Professor/Program Director
Clinical Research Management Specialty
University of Maryland
Baltimore, Maryland

**John J. Whitcomb, PhD, RN, CCRN**
Assistant Professor
Clemson University
Clemson, South Carolina

**George A. Zangaro PhD, RN**
Assistant Professor
University of Maryland
Baltimore, Maryland

Health care is undergoing major changes, and the nursing profession plays a major role in health care delivery. An important reason for these changes is the Institute of Medicine (IOM) initiatives to examine and recommend solutions focused on improving care. This second edition uses the IOM quality initiative as its framework particularly the IOM five core health care profession competencies. Nurse leaders and managers need to meet the competencies of

- Provide patient-centered care
- Work in interdisciplinary/interprofessional teams
- Employ evidence-based practice
- Apply quality improvement
- Utilize informatics

There is a great need to improve care in all types of health care settings, and this should be an integral part of leadership and management as well as practice.

Leadership and management are content areas included in all nursing programs for undergraduate and graduate programs. There is a great need to have nurses who are knowledgeable about these topics and able to apply the knowledge to their practice wherever it might be. This text provides opportunities for students to examine critical issues in health care delivery today. Typically nurses do not serve in management positions until they have some clinical experience; however, every nurse serves as a leader in practice as they provide and coordinate patient care, communicate and collaborate with staff and the interprofessional team, and solve problems and make decisions to ensure that patients receive quality, safe care. Nurses are also involved in health care delivery processes on an organizational level such as serving on committees, task forces, and other teams that plan and make decisions for the organization as a whole, and also serve in leadership positions in professional nursing organizations. Every nurse who strives to provide quality, safe care, continues to advocate for patients and their families, and strives to be recognized as a critical member of the health care team needs to demonstrate leadership.

## Organization of This Textbook

This textbook is divided into two sections that focus on basics and then the IOM core competencies. All of the content is based on the need for leadership and improvement of care.

Section I Basic Leadership and Management Concepts This section lays the foundation for effective leadership and management. These concepts are the conceptual base and include leaders and managers, and competencies; health care policy, legal issues and ethics; change and decision making; organizational structure and effective care delivery; and health care financial issues. The last chapter in this section focuses acute care organizations as an example of health care organizations. This content sets the stage for the second section that focuses on critical core competencies.

Section II Core Competencies This section focuses on the Institute of Medicine health care profession core competencies. The eleven chapters in this section emphasize these core competencies and include content related to managing patient-centered care, diversity and disparities, recruitment and retention to meet staffing requirements, consumers, building interprofessional teams, improving teamwork through collaboration, coordination, and conflict resolution, and effective communication. Two chapters focus on health care quality: one chapter is dedicated to policy issues and the second on implementation of quality improvement. The last chapter addresses the fifth competency, informatics. These core competencies relate to practice in all settings but also to effective leadership and management.

## Textbook Features

The textbook features provide students with additional methods to explore and apply leadership and management content.

*Chapter Outline*—Provides an outline of the content to guide reading of the chapter.

*Key Terms*—Identifies the terms that are important in the content. Definitions are provided in the textbook glossary found on the website.

*Learning Outcomes*—Directs your reading and approach to each chapter.

*What's Ahead*—Introduces the chapter's content.

*Evidence for Leadership*—Within the chapter content is an example of evidence that focuses on leadership. This includes a summary of a published article, citation, and questions to consider. You may want to locate the article and read it. Evidence-based practice and evidence-based management are very important in health care today.

*Case Study*—Within the chapter content is a case, which provides a brief scenario and questions.

*Application of Content*—This feature is found at the end of each chapter and allows you to examine and apply the content by using a variety of methods.

*My Hospital Unit*— Before you begin this book and related course, you need to take the first step to engage yourself in this topic. You need to create your own virtual clinical unit. What type of unit would you want to serve as a nurse manager? Within this unit you will reflect on content in each chapter as you build your knowledge of leadership and management in nursing and then apply that knowledge as you apply the Institute of Medicine five health care professions core competencies. You will be the nurse manager on the unit. Once you create the framework for your unit you cannot make changes in the information that describes your unit unless you are doing so in response to a specific learning activity. You have to work within this description just as you would if you were nurse manager on a real unit instead of a virtual unit.

How do you create your own virtual unit? First, you need to put your description in writing. Respond to the following questions as you describe your unit. Use the virtual unit site found on the textbook website to record the work that you do in the role of nurse manager for your unit.

- Name your unit.
- What services are provided in the unit (can be acute care or ambulatory care, e.g., medical [may be sub-specialty such as respiratory], surgical [may be a sub-specialty such as orthopedics], OR, ER, ICU, obstetrics, pediatrics, behavioral health, and so on]?
- What is the size of the unit (number of beds)? What is the size of the hospital (fewer than 100, 100–200, 200–300, more than 300 beds)?
- Is it an urban or rural hospital? Academic-teaching hospital, private, or government owned?
- How long have you been the nurse manager?
- What types of shifts do you have currently (8-, 10-, or 12-hour shifts; mix)?
- What hours/days do you typically work?
- Briefly describe at least four RNs, four UAP, and decide if you have LPNs; if so describe several. In the description give first names and a description of their personalities, and current performance.

- You have a unit secretary. Name the unit secretary and briefly describe personality and current performance.
- You have nursing and medical students on your unit.

You now need to create a floor plan for your unit. Indicate if rooms are single or double and location of work areas. You are now ready to get into textbook content. At the end of each chapter you will be asked to go to your unit on the website and engage in interactive questions and problems that may be occurring in your unit or in your hospital. This will help you to apply the content and examine issues.

*Critical Thinking Questions and Activities*—Provides chapter interactive learning activities.

*Media Links*—Identifies important websites that are related to chapter content.

*References*—Lists the chapter references.

# ACKNOWLEDGMENTS

Projects like this one take time and certainly require support. My family deserves much of the credit for putting up with my endless writing projects. Elizabeth Karle played an important role in helping with the first edition, which is carried over in the second edition. Lisa Gaw assisted with new graphics for the second edition. Elisabeth Garofalo has served as my incredible developmental editor. She is a pleasure to work with and has been very helpful. Pam Fuller, Executive Acquisitions Editor at Pearson, has provided oversight and guidance throughout this project. I thank all of these great experts for their assistance. My students and faculty I have worked with always provide me with issues to think about and to consider in a project like this one.

# CONTENTS

# BASIC LEADERSHIP AND MANAGEMENT CONCEPTS

Section I of this textbook lays the foundation for effective leadership and management. These concepts are the conceptual base including change, leaders and managers, and competencies; health care policy, legal issues, and ethics; change and decision making; organizational structure and effective care delivery; and health care financial issues. The last chapter in this section uses acute care organizations as an example of health care organizations. This content sets the stage for the second section that focuses on critical core competencies.

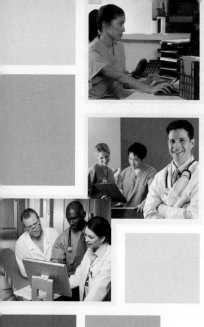

# 1

# Conceptual Base for Leadership and Management

## LEARNING OUTCOMES

Before you begin, take a moment to familiarize yourself with the learning outcomes for this chapter.

- Interpret the implications of change in the health care delivery system on nurse leadership.
- Analyze the key modern leadership theories comparing to older theories.
- Compare and contrast characteristics, roles, and responsibilities of leaders and managers.
- Explain the importance of transformational leadership today and the relationship to the recommendations of the Institute of Medicine.
- Discuss the importance of nurse leadership and its relationship to modern leadership theories.
- Explain the role of the clinical nurse as a leader and why it is important.
- Compare and contrast the leadership and management competencies described by AONE, ANA, and AACN.

## KEY TERMS

- Accountability
- Autocratic
- Empowerment
- Influence

- Leadership
- Management
- Management functions
- Mission statement

- Peter Principle
- Transformational Leader
- Values
- Vision

## WHAT'S AHEAD

In the changing health care environment, nursing needs effective leaders who can understand change and take on opportunities as they arise. Nurses need to recognize that every nurse needs to be a leader—even nurses providing direct care. Sternweiler (1998) presents some interesting ideas that can be applied to success in today's health care environment. Her motto is "be a willow tree." This unusual motto has relevance to many situations in which nurses find themselves today. Her comments focus on clinical nurse specialists, but they also apply to all nurses. The first point she makes is that willow trees have many branches, and many branches are required to extend into all of the different areas in which nurses find themselves today. As nurses begin to consider where they want to begin their practice of nursing, they are soon confronted with many wonderful choices. Many of these opportunities are clearly defined, while others are not, and some have yet to be created. Willow trees also bend gracefully in the wind. This is an effective image of what nurses must do during change, which is a constant phenomenon today. Flexibility leads to more success than rigidity—the branch that refuses to bend often breaks. Willow trees have wide-reaching but shallow root systems. Uprooting deep, entrenched roots is much more painful than having an intricate, but shallow root system. Again, flexibility is the key to success during such a period. Each day brings a new piece of information, a new perspective, a new change, and a new challenge. All this requires nurses who are able to move thoughtfully with the changes. This image of nursing demonstrates that it is an exciting career, not a profession that does not change. Nurse leaders, both formal and informal, need to set the stage for a positive approach to change and act as role models for staff; however, all nurses need to participate in making changes that improve care and the practice of nursing. Some of the key issues facing nurses are the following:

1. The need to work together as a team, made all the more challenging as age differences and cultural diversity enrich the workforce and language and work ethics become more disparate
2. Health care environments in which blame and punishment are practiced, even as those practices are disavowed on the surface, and the need to develop a culture of safety (Institute of Medicine, 1999)
3. Increasing pressure for results and less tolerance for mistakes; burnout, anger, and other negative emotions still have a stronghold in many health care settings
4. The need for greater creativity, collaboration, and learning, coupled with requirements for managers to do more with less
5. The increasing press for successful recruitment and retention of current and future nursing personnel (Robinson-Walker, 2002, p. 148)
6. Increasing occupational stress and violence in the workplace

As leadership and management are explored in this chapter and throughout the text, many perspectives will be presented. Professional nurses need to open themselves up to a variety of ideas in order to arrive at a perspective of health care that enhances care delivery and the practice of nursing. This chapter discusses a variety of leadership and management theories and styles, nurse leadership, effectiveness, and managers. As nurses move through their careers, some nurses will always provide direct care and yet still need to demonstrate leadership; some will decide to move into management positions and yet still need to demonstrate leadership; and then others may move back and forth between direct care and management positions. Being a nurse today requires leadership. "The term 'dispersed leader' has been described as the leadership of the future. This holds that there is not *a* leader, but that there are *many* leaders dispersing the responsibilities of leadership across the organization. Gone are the up/down, top/bottom, superior/subordinate relationships. We must be developing leaders at every level" (Shaw, 2007, p. 26). Shaw notes that the following are important aspects of nursing leadership today, and these aspects will be emphasized in this chapter and across the textbook (2007, pp. 13–18).

- Nurse leaders must have an understanding of the broader health and social system within which nursing functions.
- Nurse leaders must have good external awareness.
- Nurse leaders must be able to use the benefits of technology.
- Nurse leaders must have the ability to contribute to, and help influence, health and public policy.
- Nurse leaders must be able to motivate and encourage others to take positive action.
- Nurse leaders and nursing must be well informed and strategic in their thinking and action.
- Nurse leaders must be able to work with others to achieve common goals.
- Nurse leaders must be able to assess and develop new opportunities for nursing.
- Nurse leaders must be able to adapt and develop new roles and new skills as health systems change.

# Change in the Health Care Delivery System: Implications for Nurse Leadership

As nurses enter the health care environment, they find an environment that seems to be constantly changing. It is easy to become frustrated with this as it is much easier to work when change is limited—one knows what to expect and when. However, the reality is not routine but instead requires health care organizations to cope with changes. Nurses must participate, too. What is meant by these changes that seem so important? Consider the examples of changes found in Box 1-1. Most students have observed many of these changes before they graduate.

This text includes content about all of these topics as they are important in understanding the nurse's role, as well as leadership and management. Chapter 3 specifically focuses on change

---

**BOX 1-1       A RAPIDLY CHANGING HEALTH CARE ENVIRONMENT**

- New medical knowledge and technology
- Greater use of information technology
- Managed care and complex reimbursement system
- Greater use of a variety of settings where care is provided outside of acute care hospitals
- Increase in the uninsured and underinsured
- Greater diversity in patients and health care workforce
- Need to increase use of evidence-based practice
- Role changes (increasing use of unlicensed assistive personnel and others) and implications for nursing roles and functions

- Use of advanced practice nurses, clinical nurse specialists, physician assistants, and hospitalists/intensivists
- Need for greater collaboration and interprofessional education and practice to prepare nurses and other health care professionals to work on interprofessional teams
- Greater importance of the consumer, the patient, and the patient's family
- Lack of health care policy or limited policy development in many areas, such as mental health, the uninsured, prescriptions for the elderly, chronic illness, and changing population demographics

and decision making. Porter-O'Grady closes his discussion on health care change by suggesting that, "Without engaging and embracing the issues around a new emerging foundation for nursing practice in the 21st century, it is quite possible that nurses will fail to find a meaningful place in the 21st century health service" (Porter-O'Grady, 2001, p. 186). This could be viewed as a pessimistic viewpoint, but it can also be viewed as a challenge to all nurses. Response will require leadership from all nurses. To be successful in today's health care delivery system, a leader needs to actively pursue collaboration with peers and other health care professionals as well as reach outside of health care (for example, to consumers, local businesses, and local governmental agencies). Collaboration as described by the American Nurses Association (ANA) requires "recognition of the expertise of others within and outside the profession, and referral to those other providers when appropriate" (2003, p. 8). Collaboration requires that nurses work across professional boundaries, which has been difficult for nurses. They need to work with physicians, social workers, pharmacists, physical therapists, admission staff, and many more. The meaning of collaboration implies the ability to be flexible, listen to others, include others, share information and ideas, work toward the best solution to a problem, and most of all to be comfortable in the collaborative environment. Nurses encounter many opportunities to collaborate every day. As theories of leadership and management are discussed and applied in this chapter's content, it is important to remember that collaboration is a key characteristic of effective leaders and managers. Collaboration is discussed in more detail in Chapter 12; however, collaboration is a critical component of effective leadership.

# Leadership and Management Theories and Styles

This section discusses modern **leadership** and **management** theories and styles. These theories and styles affect health care leaders and nurse leaders who work in all types of health care settings. One should not get the impression that only those who hold the highest nursing management position or other high management positions in health care organizations are necessarily nurse leaders. Nurse leaders do not even have to be in formal "management positions" with a management title. There are many more nurses who are in lower level "management positions," and if they demonstrate leadership competencies, they are considered nurse leaders (for example, nurse managers, charge nurses, team leaders, and others). All are important to the profession and to health care delivery. As leadership theories and styles are discussed in this chapter, it is noted that one can be a manager and yet not be a leader because to be a leader the manager must also demonstrate leadership qualities and competencies. Some staff members are informal leaders and do not hold formal leadership positions. In the end, leadership competencies are something that every nurse should strive to reach. To accomplish this, nurses need to have an understanding of relevant leadership and management theories and styles.

## An Historical Perspective of Leadership Theories

There are many leadership theories and styles that have affected management and care delivery in health care organizations; however, it is important to understand some aspects of the history of leadership and the effects that some of the past theories and styles have had on modern theories. Typically, the theories of the past emphasized control, competition, and getting the job done. Creativity was not a critical part of past leadership theories. Leadership theories and styles have changed over time; some still apply and some do not, and some of them have been developed into modern theories. An historical review of the stages of leadership theory development indicates that there are four stages, which are highlighted in Box 1-2.

It is still possible to find leaders in health care organizations that use the theories that were developed in the first three stages; for example, there are still organizations that use the autocratic and bureaucratic approach to leadership and management as described in Box 1-3, though these theories are not considered to be as effective in the current health care delivery system.

The modern or current leadership theories and styles have their base in earlier theories, but they have been developed as the needs of organizations changed requiring different types of leaders and managers. Box 1-4 highlights the key theories and styles that are discussed in this section.

## BOX 1-2    A REVIEW OF THE STAGES OF LEADERSHIP THEORY DEVELOPMENT

### STAGE I *LEADER TRAITS*

Emphasized up to the late 1940s. The theories tried to determine what personal qualities and characteristics were demonstrated by leaders. An important assumption with this approach was the belief that leaders were born rather than made. Many qualities and characteristics were examined during this time, and the conclusions served as the basis for other theories.

### STAGE II *LEADERSHIP STYLES*

Began in the late 1940s and continued until the late 1960s. The emphasis was on training leaders, which was different from the earlier stage in which the emphasis was on the selection of leaders who innately had the required qualities. A critical concern was how to determine if someone was a leader prior to putting the person into a leadership position.

### STAGE III *FOCUSED ON CONTINGENCY APPROACH*

Began in the late 1960s and continued through the early 1980s. This approach examined all the situational factors surrounding leadership that might affect the effectiveness of different leadership approaches. What is happening in the environment and organization that might affect the leader?

### STAGE IV *NEW LEADERSHIP APPROACHES*

Began in the early 1980s and continues today. This stage is the focus in this text. Transformational Leadership, Charismatic Leadership, and Visionary Leadership, as well as others, have become more and more acceptable. There is increased interest in organizational culture and its effect on leadership as well as leadership's effect on organizational culture (Bryman, 2001).

DEMING'S THEORY    "The magic of Deming's management of leadership system is that it creates opportunities for management and staff to interact often. Personal interaction has the greatest potential for creating trust because it increases the likelihood of effective communication" (Crow, 2002, p. 10). Group work or teamwork and team ownership of work are the focus in this theory. Despite the fact that Deming's approach has been successful in some U.S. businesses, it

## BOX 1-3    WHAT IS AUTOCRATIC, BUREAUCRATIC, AND LAISSEZ-FAIRE LEADERSHIP?

### WHAT IS . . .

**Autocratic (authoritarian, directive)** The leader makes decisions for the group and may do this by "simply issuing detailed orders and expecting them to be carried out automatically" (Curtin, 2001, p. 238). The leader assumes people are externally motivated and incapable of independent decision making. External motivators might be salary and benefits or job security. Today, this style is most effective in emergencies (e.g., a fire on the unit or a cardiac arrest), when clear direction is required from one person. It is not as effective for long-term use.

**Bureaucratic** The bureaucratic style is directly related to the autocratic style as the leader also presumes the group is externally motivated. The leader relies on organizational rules and policies, takes an inflexible approach, and gives directions, expecting them to be followed.

**Laissez-faire (nondirective, permissive, ultraliberal)** The leader assumes the group is internally motivated by recognition, achievement, increased responsibility, and so on and needs autonomy and self-regulation. The leader uses a "hands-off" approach. This leadership style is directly opposite of autocratic and bureaucratic leadership as the leader allows staff members to do as they please rather than telling them exactly what they must do. Sometimes this style can be too detached, resulting in no leadership and floundering staff. When staff on a patient care unit feels there is no real leadership or guidance, the nurse manager is probably using laissez-faire leadership, though the manager may not actually realize this is the approach.

---

| BOX 1-4 | SELECT MODERN LEADERSHIP THEORIES AND STYLES |
|---|---|

- *Deming's theory*
  Groups and teams
- *Drucker's theory*
  Modern management; participatory management; leadership learned
- *Contingency theory*
  Situation changes affect leadership
- *Management Grid theory*
  Five styles ranging from little interest in production and people to maximum interest in production and people
- *Connective Leadership theory*
  Caring, inter-connectedness, collaboration

- *Emotional Intelligence theory*
  Feelings and self-awareness; emotional competence
- *Chaos or Quantum theory*
  New possibilities with change; potential always present; linking experiences and change
- *Knowledge Management theory*
  Importance of knowledge; knowledge worker asset to organizations
- *Transformational Leadership theory*
  Motivating followers; participatory leadership; moral agency; high recognition of staff

---

has had less of an immediate impact on health care organizations. Health care organizations still feature much centralized control, with upper management making many of the decisions rather than staff participation. There are, however, an increasing number of health care organizations that are slowly recognizing the value of staff participation. Later leadership and management theories included the need for greater staff participation.

DRUCKER'S THEORY   Peter Drucker is considered to be the father of modern management (Porter-O'Grady & Finnegan, 1984). His view of management stimulated the shift toward the realization of the importance of participatory organizations, which is similar to Deming's approach. Drucker felt that staff should participate in as much of the planning and establishment of goals and decision making as possible. Individual autonomy is a critical part of this theory of management. Drucker believed that when staff participated in the core functions of management the organization would be more effective. For example, staff nurses should provide input into planning and changes that might be necessary on the unit, and nurse managers should seek out staff members' ideas and ask them to assist with planning. Drucker's theory includes the assumption that leadership can be learned. Leaders are not born, but rather staff can be nurtured to gain greater leadership competency. This approach offers more opportunity to develop leaders and is important to nursing. Including leadership and management content in undergraduate education indicates that the nursing profession values leadership and recognizes the need to develop leadership and management competencies in students.

CONTINGENCY THEORY   In 1967, Fiedler developed the Contingency theory by focusing on the situational variables that affect the leader–member relationship, task structure, and position power (Fiedler, 1967; Huber, 2010).

1. The leader–member relationship variable describes the type and quality of the leader's personal relationships with the followers. This variable is affected by the amount of confidence and loyalty followers have in their leader (Grohar-Murray & DiCroce, 2003).
2. The task structure, the number of correct solutions to a given situational dilemma, focuses on the level of structure found in the group's task.
3. Position power, which addresses the power or amount of organizational support that the leader receives from the organization as a part of the position the leader holds, is critical to success.

Using these three major variables, Fiedler arrived at a number of variable combinations and identified which combinations were advantageous and which were disadvantageous to the organization and its leadership. He concluded that the best type of situation occurs when there are positive leader–member relations, high task structure, and high position power. Groups do change, which then changes the situational variables. Leadership, which is contingent on these variables, then must also change. This might also be called situational leadership. With the leader taking into account the changes in the situation this is not a static approach to leadership.

**MANAGEMENT GRID THEORY**  Another approach to understanding leadership is the Management Grid Model (Blake & Mouton, 1964; Blake & McCanse, 1991). This model identifies five styles of leadership.

1. **Impoverished leadership.**  In this style the leader has limited interest in production or people. Work requirements are established at a minimum level.
2. **Country club leadership.**  This type of leader has an interest in people, and staff describes the leader as friendly and outgoing. Productivity, however, is not a major concern.
3. **Authority–obedience leadership.**  This type focuses on efficiency and getting the job done. This includes providing a work environment in which staff can be productive, but the leader has less concern for staff members as people.
4. **Organizational man.**  Focuses on balancing the necessity to accomplish the task with maintaining morale.
5. **Team leadership.**  This type of leader is very concerned about productivity and about the staff, morale, and satisfaction.

**CONNECTIVE LEADERSHIP THEORY**  Connective Leadership theory focuses on caring. Interconnectedness is a key element in health care today with the increasing emphasis on the continuum of services to meet the needs of patients and communities across the age span and different delivery settings. In this particular approach to leadership, the leader needs to promote collaboration and teamwork within the medical organization and among other organizations in the community. It recognizes that many groups exist within an organization and outside an organization that can affect leadership style. Connecting to others—individuals, groups, and organizations—leads to greater success. This viewpoint of leadership is incorporated in many of the current modern theories.

**EMOTIONAL INTELLIGENCE THEORY**  As leadership theory has moved toward considering the leader–follower relationship, theories have focused more and more on feelings and self-awareness, such as Goleman's theory of Emotional Intelligence (EI). Emotional competence is "a learning capability based on emotional intelligence that results in outstanding performance at work" (Goleman, 1998, p. 24; Bradberry & Greaves, 2003). Emotional competencies are learning abilities or job skills that can be learned. A person has the potential to develop the necessary skills or required competencies (Goleman, 2001). This relates back to other theories that have been discussed that assume people can learn to be more effective leaders. Goleman identifies domains or dimensions that are important to Emotional Intelligence, which he calls *clusters*. Within each cluster there are identified competencies, which are highlighted in Box 1-5.

It might seem that all of these competencies stand alone; however, Goleman notes that they occur in groups, which is why they are described as clusters. Each competency is on a continuum in that an individual may perform the competency at different levels. Nurses may demonstrate leadership and management competencies anywhere on the continuum. It takes time and support to learn about leadership. At some point an individual competency may reach what is called a "tipping point," which is when the individual excels in the competency (Goleman, 2001). For example, a team leader seems to have it all together—the team is functioning well; feedback is routinely given to team members by the team leader; team members are very active in planning and are able to speak up when they have concerns; team members support one another and feel the team leader will support the team; communication is clear—the work seems to flow.

BOX 1-5    EI: CLUSTERS OF COMPETENCIES

## THE SELF-AWARENESS CLUSTER

Understanding feelings and applying accurate self-assessment. Leaders recognize their own feelings and how they affect others and their performance. Self-assessment is important so that the leader can identify strengths and limitations. Leaders with these competencies try to find ways to improve, seek feedback, and actively learn from past experience. Self-confidence is a critical element in this cluster. It is easy to see how understanding oneself and using this information to improve oneself can lead to greater self-confidence.

## THE SELF-MANAGEMENT CLUSTER

Managing internal emotions, impulses, and resources. This cluster includes six competencies:

1. *Emotional self-control.* Most people have probably encountered persons who were in positions of authority and yet not able to handle their own emotions. Usually these leaders are described as ineffective leaders. Emotional self-control does not mean that the leader never expresses emotions but rather that the leader often expresses emotions appropriately.
2. *Trustworthiness.* "This competence translates into letting others know one's values and principles, intentions and feelings, and acting in ways that are consistent with them. Trustworthy individuals are forthright about their own mistakes and confront others about their lapses" (Goleman, 1998, p. 34).
3. *Conscientiousness.* This competency is demonstrated when the leader is careful, self-disciplined, and ensures that responsibilities are met.
4. *Adaptability.* This is a competence that really makes a difference in leaders today. Leaders with this competence are open to new ideas, search out challenges and opportunities, and use them to move forward. This is the leader who "thinks outside the box" and for whom a risk is not a barrier to moving forward.
5. *Achievement drive.* This is "an optimistic striving to continually improve performance" (Goleman, 1998, p. 35).
6. *Initiative.* People who take initiative act before they are found in situations where they may be forced to act. They are a step ahead at all times and seem to seek out opportunities before others are aware of them.

More nurse leaders who have these competencies are needed—leaders who can analyze a situation and create opportunities for nurses to expand their roles, improve staff roles, and develop leadership competencies, which will also improve patient care.

## THE SOCIAL AWARENESS CLUSTER

The focus is on reading people and groups accurately and includes three competencies.

1. *Empathy* or being aware of others' feelings, needs, and concerns. Self-awareness is required for successful empathy. Understanding oneself comes before understanding of others.
2. *Service orientation.* This is "the ability to identify a client's or a customer's often unstated needs and concerns and then match them to products or services" (Goleman, 2001, p. 36).
3. *Organizational awareness.* The leader is able to identify group feelings and organizational needs, which helps the leader develop coalitions and network. If a leader does not understand the feelings of others or their needs, it is difficult to get staff to work for the leader and the organization.

## RELATIONSHIP MANAGEMENT CLUSTER

This cluster focuses on inducing desirable responses and includes eight competencies.

1. *Developing others.* The leader knows when staff is ready for further development.
2. *Influence.* This is the ability of a leader to persuade others.
3. *Communication.* For leaders to be effective they need to have communication competence, the ability to communicate emotions and facts, listen, share information, and encourage sharing of information. In today's world information is a driving force in many work activities.
4. *Conflict management.* It is not easy to learn how to manage conflict, but leaders with Emotional Intelligence must develop this competence to be successful. Conflict management requires negotiation and the ability to see outside the box.
5. *Visionary leadership.* This is the leader who can develop a vision and includes staff in the vision for success.
6. *Change catalyst.* Leaders with Emotional Intelligence must see change as an opportunity, recognize barriers to change and remove them whenever possible, challenge

the status quo, and involve as many of the staff as possible in the change process.

7. *Building bonds.* This competence assists the leader in finding ways to make connections with others, build trust, and recognize the importance of relationships.

8. *Collaboration and teamwork.* This competence depends on many of the earlier competencies that have been identified.

How does Emotional Intelligence leadership affect the organization's performance? This is an important question as there is no reason to continue with a leadership approach if it is not having a positive effect on the organization's staff and work. "The evidence suggests that emotionally intelligent leadership is key to creating a working climate that nurtures its employees and encourages them to do their best with enthusiasm, in turn this pays off in improved business performance" (Goleman, 2001, p. 40). Applying EI to leadership style requires that the leader demonstrate the EI competencies of self-confidence, empathy, change catalyst, and visionary leadership. "For jobs of all kinds, emotional intelligence is twice as important as a person's intelligence quotient and technical skills combined" (Strickland, 2000, p. 112). How smart a nurse is will not be as important as whether or not the nurse has, or is able to develop, critical EI competencies as a leader. Much has been discussed about the positive aspects of EI leadership theory; however, caution needs to be exercised in connecting or applying Emotional Intelligence theory to workplace success even though it is very popular today (Vitello-Cicciu, 2002). New nurses typically need to develop at least some of the social and emotional competencies needed for effective performance in today's health care environment, and some new nurses demonstrate some of these competencies at the time of graduation. It still has not been proven that EI or the presence of emotional intelligence in leadership is a strong predictor of success. Instruments to measure Emotional Intelligence have been developed, but many of these instruments have been found to be less effective than had been hoped (Vitello-Cicciu, 2002). Many of the instruments are self-assessment measures, which sometimes leads those who use them to respond in ways to impress others or what would be expected responses. There is no doubt that nursing, as a "people-oriented" profession, is a profession in which emotional issues and responses are critical. It is also important for nurses to understand and manage their own emotions in an effective way. In the work that the American Organization of Nurse Executives (AONE) has done on nurse executive competencies it has been noted that "today, relational or 'people' skills may be more important for nurse leaders to develop than technical skills. One set of relational skills that nursing faculty may want to foster in their students falls under the rubric of emotional intelligence, the ability to recognize and understand emotions, and the awareness to skillfully manage one's own, emotions and relationships with others" (Corning, 2002; Bradberry & Greaves, 2003; as cited in Harris, et al., 2006, p. 438). Nurse leadership is challenged to "create the climate for satisfied staff, patients, and their loved ones and diminish the degree of emotional labor which may cause burnout of nursing staff" (Vitello-Cicciu, 2002, p. 208). "Effective leadership is one of the most elusive keys to organizational success and yet it is the key ingredient to making any organization work. Leadership is also changing in nature" (Snow, 2001, p. 440). Those who support EI recognize that Emotionally Intelligent nurse leaders will bring the following to health care organizations.

1. Improved performance of nursing personnel
2. Improved retention of top talent
3. Improved teamwork among nurses
4. Increased motivation by team members
5. Enhanced innovation in the nursing group
6. Enhanced use of time and resources
7. Restored trust between nurses and their leaders (Snow, 2001, p. 443)

The outcome should be more satisfied patients, nurses, physicians, and families and a work environment that provides the best for all concerned—quality care, safe care, effective work environment, retention of staff, and an environment of improvement.

**CHAOS OR QUANTUM THEORY**    Porter-O'Grady (2007) suggests that health care organizations have focused their organization and leadership on approaches that have not recognized that all things are interdependent. Leaders need to a change to a quantum thinking approach—recognizing that the "relatedness of processes, actions, behaviors, and functions" (Porter-O'Grady, 2007, p. 22). Health care organizations in the past were able to rely on orderliness, following policies without considering options, viewing problems as having limited solutions, and creating clear lines of who reports to whom. This describes Newtonian thinking, which is no longer the reality in health care organizations. Problems and their solutions are not always clear, risk taking may be required, and mistakes will be made. Many factors affect how work is done and whether or not work processes need to be altered unexpectedly. Policies may not always be easily applied. Because of past experiences, health care managers have become quite good in using control, and many managers use it in such a way that staff does not complain about it but rather just accepts it. Neither of these approaches will result in positive outcomes in today's complex, changing environment where rigid approaches are not successful in the long run. The relationship between people and management has also changed in the Quantum Age. As systems have become much more important, it is recognized that new forms of leadership are required. Creativity and health care worker knowledge are critical to the organization's success. Teams and partnerships continue to have a major impact on the organizational work. We may not be able to provide a detailed description of the future and need to "incorporate the vagaries of complexity and chaos into the process of anticipating and planning for the future" (Porter-O'Grady, 2007, p. 23). **Accountability** needs to be in the hands of those doing the work, where there is more expertise. This is supported further by participative leadership, which is an important part of current leadership theories. All of these factors are integral parts of the Quantum Age. To accomplish many of the needed changes in a health care organization's "chaos," a major role of the leader is to help staff adjust to new roles and strategies. What are some guidelines that leaders might use to address these new roles and strategies?

1. Leaders should not predict the future as no one really knows what the future may be.
2. Leaders need to be very sensitive to indicators of change and must respond when required.
3. The manager or leader should translate information so that it can be used to produce outcomes. With the increasing amount of information today, there is a critical need for analysis of information, which is related to the next theory, Knowledge Management (Porter-O'Grady, 1999, p. 39).

KNOWLEDGE MANAGEMENT THEORY    Sorrells-Jones (1999) noted that the emphasis on the knowledge worker, knowledge-intense organizations, interprofessional collaboration, and accountability found in the Information Age provides nurses with opportunities to improve and expand their practice. Knowledge work is a combination of routine and non-routine knowledge-based work. Routine work (e.g., providing immunizations or other routine interventions or procedures) may require specialized knowledge that includes some level of predictability with anticipated probable outcomes. Non-routine knowledge work is full of exceptions, lacks predictability, requires interpretation and judgment, and may not be fully understood (e.g., altering care based on assessment data). Learning is an important component of knowledge work (Sorrells-Jones, 1999). Drucker (1993, 1994) first used the term *knowledge worker* when he described a person who works with both his or her hands and with theoretical knowledge. A knowledge-intense business organization is one in which 40% or more of the workers are knowledge workers (Sorrell-Jones, 1999). In this type of organization staff are the organization's knowledge assets or intellectual capital. Health care organizations meet the criteria for this type of organization. As will be discussed in later chapters, critical thinking, clinical reasoning and judgment, and evidence-based practice and evidence-based management are important in today's organizations—focusing on the need for knowledge that can be applied to improve care. This new age of knowledge growth requires workers who use information to produce knowledge, solve problems, and meet organizational goals (Weaver, 2001). Nurses should be viewed as knowledge workers, not laborers (Drucker, 1993). Today, a person's title is *not* the most important element; rather, it is the person's expertise in knowledge that is the critical element. As noted in EI theory; however, some staff members have "too much college, too little kindergarten" (Weaver, 2001, p. 82). This means that these staff may have expertise and knowledge, but they lack the insight that allows them to appreciate the impact of their behavior on other individuals or effective interpersonal skills. The latter represents a lack of "kindergarten skills" (for example, a sense of fair play, commitment to collaboration, willingness to share the limelight, and a growing sense of self that considers one's strengths and weaknesses). In addition, these skills are critical for the development of team effectiveness. It may not always be easy to clearly predict what may be the result of problem solving, which means that a person or team must be willing to take risks (Weaver, 2001). It is important to remember that when staff takes a risk during decision making there is some probability of loss. Therefore, the risk taker must work to decrease this probability (Milstead, 2004). It is, however, not always possible to have time to assess a situation to its fullest nor is it always possible to recognize all possible solutions to a problem. These factors can make risk taking difficult but should not eliminate the need for taking risks in some situations. What does the manager in a knowledge-work environment do when the manager is no longer expected to tell staff what to do? This new manager brings people together with different knowledge bases in order to reach the most effective performance. The focus is on developing the most effective teams, leading change initiatives, coaching teams, providing performance expectations, helping knowledge workers (e.g., RNs) and knowledge work teams (e.g., care team) self-regulate themselves, teaching the team to use systematic decision making, and encouraging an attitude of continuous improvement (Mohrman & Mohrman, 1997). Knowledge-based managers must be leaders who are facilitators and integrators. They support diverse team members who work toward reaching a common goal. No single staff member can know everything that is required for practice today, and so the interprofessional team becomes the focus as emphasized by the Institute of Medicine core health care professions competencies. Important goals today are the development of staff to maximize team member efficiency. Team members should be viewed as assets; they are valuable to the team and the organization. A major goal is the following: It is important to decrease the time that team members spend doing functions and tasks that are not as important or, if they are professionals, functions that are not critical professional tasks. Examples of these are (a) RNs transporting patients, (b) RNs completing paperwork that does not require professional competencies, and (c) RNs searching for equipment or needed supplies, often called "hunting and gathering."

TRANSFORMATIONAL LEADERSHIP THEORY    There are two major types of leaders, the Transactional Leader and the **Transformational Leader** (Curtin, 2001). The first, the Transactional Leader, is the most common type of leader found in health care organizations today, though this is changing in many health care organizations to Transformational Leadership, which is much more applicable in today's dynamic health care system. Some leaders may use both types of leadership depending on their needs. "The transforming leader looks for potential motives in followers, seeks to satisfy the needs and engages the full person of the followers. The result of transforming leadership is a relationship of mutual stimulation and elevation that converts followers into leaders and leaders into moral agents" (Curtin, 2001, p. 239). In addition, Burns emphasizes the importance of morals and ethics, which is particularly relevant to leaders who are also members of a profession that must meet professional ethical codes (Curtin & Falherty, 1993, p. 64).

1. *What is Transformational Leadership?* Transformational Leadership is a theory that focuses on the need for leaders who are willing to embrace change, reward staff, guide staff in understanding its role within the organization and the importance of the organization or a positive work environment, and work toward developing a self-aware staff that is able to take risks to improve. This does not mean that the Transformational Leader is not concerned with the critical organizational functions that are required to get the work done that are emphasized in Transactional Leadership; however, the Transformational Leader begins with a vision. What is meant by a **vision**? A vision is a view of the organization in the future. What could the organization be? A **mission statement**, supporting the vision, describes the organization's purpose and the current position of the organization. Why is it so important to have a vision? The vision allows the organization, its leaders or managers and staff, to look into the future, based on reasonable facts and experience, and to use this vision to become involved in opportunities to improve.

2. *Why did Transformational Leadership develop?* The key reason for the development of Transformational Leadership is change (Sullivan, 1998). "Transformational leadership has been suggested in the literature as a leadership model that best fits with the changing health care environment" (Bass & Avolio, 1997; as cited in Ohman, 1999, p. 16; Medley & Larochelle, 1985). As the health care system began to experience extreme and frequent

change, it found that its leadership styles were not working in the chaotic changing atmosphere. To cope, organizations needed the skills and knowledge of a greater number of the staff. The leader also needed to be ahead of the change as much as possible. This required vision, creativity, and new leadership styles that empower staff. These leaders typically exhibit both Transformational and Transactional Leadership; however, transformational is usually predominant (Bass, 1998; Dunham-Taylor, 2000). Transformational leadership is the leadership style recommended by the IOM in its report *Leadership by Example* (2003). As has been discussed, the characteristics described as part of Transformational Leadership are also found in EI, Chaos theory, and Knowledge Management theories.

3. *What are the qualities of a Transformational Leader?* Qualities that have been identified in Transformational Leaders are self-confidence, self-direction, honesty, energy, loyalty, commitment, and the ability to develop and implement a vision. **Empowerment** is an important component of Transformational Leadership. Effective nursing Transformational Leadership is influenced by three factors: individual consideration, charisma, and intellectual simulation (McDanie & Wolf, 1992). The more power the leader gives to staff, the more power the leader will gain (Fullan, Lando, Johansen, Reyes, & Szaloczy, 1998). The Transformational Leader who has these qualities can lead staff during times of creative development but also can ensure that operational issues are handled, making sure the work is done effectively. "This is different from a Transactional Leader who emphasizes primarily the "functions in a caretaker role and is focused on day-to-day operations. Such leaders survey their followers' needs and set goals for them based on what can be expected from the followers" (Huber, 2010, p. 17).

4. *Is Transformational Leadership always successful in all organizations?* Transformational leadership is not always successful. When it fails, it is usually related to one of the errors that are highlighted in Box 1-6 (Kotter, 1995).

A CONCLUSION: EFFECTIVE LEADERSHIP   It is not easy to describe effective leadership. There is certainly no magic formula that will guarantee effective leadership. As noted in the previous discussion of leadership theories and styles, effective leaders have vision, influence, and power. The vision of the future guides the leader in making day-to-day decisions. Leaders use **influence**, which is the informal strategy of cooperation combined with formal authority of a position to develop trust. The leader needs to be persuasive and use productive communication. Power enables the leader to influence others, and by doing this, the leader can change staff attitudes and behavior, hopefully moving toward meeting expected outcomes. **Values**, the importance that is attached to something that guides action, are more important today in understanding effective leadership. An example of the impact of values is found in health care organizations that focus on the bottom line, cutting costs with little concern about the effect this has on the quality of care. This communicates a particular value to their staff, patients, and community. Health care organizations, however, that communicate the importance of a caring environment where the highest quality care is provided to individual patients are communicating a different value. Leaders of these two types of organizations are actively involved in communicating critical values, though very different ones. The leader in the first type of organization focuses more on financial issues and is less willing to listen to staff concerns about the quality of care unless it has a major impact on costs. The leader in the second type of organization is more willing to look at the total care picture, listen to staff, and look for opportunities to improve care, but does not forget the need to consistently monitor costs.

## BOX 1-6   TRANSFORMATIONAL LEADERSHIP ERRORS

- Lack of a sense of urgency
- Lack of a guiding coalition
- Lack of a vision
- Lack of communication about the vision

- Lack of removals of barriers to the vision
- Lack of systematic planning
- Declaring a victory too soon
- Lack of recognition of organization culture

## APPLYING EVIDENCE-BASED PRACTICE

### Evidence for Effective Leadership and Management

**Citation:** Gowen, C., Henagan, S. & McFadden, K. (2009). Knowledge management as a mediator for the efficacy of transformational leadership and quality management initiatives in U.S. health care. *Health Care Management Review, 34*(9), 129–140.

**Overview:** This exploratory study included a survey of 350 hospitals across the United States with a 59% response rate. The study examined the efficacy of transformational leadership, knowledge management, and quality management—looking at the influence of each of these approaches on one another since they are often implemented in the same organizations. The results indicate that transformational leadership and quality management improve knowledge management; transformational leadership is fully mediated by knowledge responsiveness; and quality management is partially mediated by knowledge responsiveness for their effects on organizational performance. The researchers recommend that further research be conducted to examine the relationship and impact of these three approaches.

**Application:** With greater emphasis on transformational leadership today this study has important implications. As noted in this chapter, knowledge management is also important in today's health care organizations. With the increasing emphasis on quality through the Institute of Medicine reports, which are also mentioned in this study, we need to better understand whether or not a combination approach will yield positive or negative outcomes. The study does not indicate that knowledge management should replace transformational leadership or even quality management, but a combination may have positive benefits for organizational performance.

**Questions:**

1. *Compare and contrast transformational leadership, knowledge management, and quality management.*

2. *Why would you think that these three approaches would benefit one another—have a positive impact on the organization performance when combined together?*

3. *How is knowledge management important to patient outcomes?*

Understanding a leader's values is critical to understanding how that leader might function in an organization and how the organization's values might mesh or collide with the leader's values, which has an impact on the effectiveness of leadership.

## Leaders and Managers: A Comparison

Leadership and management are not the same. It is important to understand how these concepts compare and recognize that the goal is really to have managers who are also leaders. The key **management functions** are

- Planning
- Organizing
- Leading
- Controlling

There is no doubt, however, that leadership plays a critical role in management. In fact, a successful manager exhibits leadership qualities. The key difference between managers and leaders is that managers typically focus on managing or maintaining equilibrium, whereas leaders are focused more on change. Most people think of management as a particular position in an organization, and this is true. Leadership, however, does not require a specific position. Nursing requires management, but nursing also needs leadership. What are some examples of the differences between a leader and a manager? What does it mean for a person to inspire others as a leader? The leader communicates to staff the importance of staff contributions and recognizes staff members' successes. In doing so, the staff member is motivated to continue to improve and to be effective. Leaders are also persuasive in that they are able to convince others to make changes and to improve. Through the leader's influence care can be improved, and the work situation can become more productive. Leaders ask questions, take risks, and are challenged by change. In contrast, managers are typically less able to handle unstable or non-routine situations. Managers who develop leadership competencies are more effective and handle non-routine situations better. With a greater understanding of leadership, it is important to consider how leaders and managers are compared and contrasted. "There is a profound difference—a chasm—between leaders and managers. A good manager does things right. A leader does the right thing" (Bennis & Goldsmith, 1997, p. 4). The following descriptions provide examples of some of the differences.

- Leaders conquer the context always going on around them; managers surrender to it.
- Leaders assess reality, identify critical factors, and use analysis; managers accept the truth from others with few questions.
- Leaders focus on effectiveness; managers focus on efficiency.
- Leaders focus on what and why; managers focus on how.
- Leaders innovate and initiate; managers copy and keep the status quo.
- Leaders empower, compel others with their creative vision, and translate that vision into action; managers are less concerned with empowerment and vision.
- The manager administers; the leader innovates.
- The manager is a copy; the leader is an original.
- The manager maintains; the leader develops.
- The manager accepts reality; the leader investigates it.
- The manager focuses on systems and structure; the leader focuses on people.
- The manager relies on control; the leader inspires trust.
- The manager has a short-range view; the leader has a long-range perspective.
- The manager asks how and when; the leader asks what and why.
- The manager has his or her eye always on the bottom line; the leader has his or her eye on the horizon.
- The manager imitates; the leader originates.
- The manager accepts the status quo; the leader challenges it.
- The manager is a classic good soldier; the leader is his or her own person (Bennis & Goldsmith, 1997, pp. 4, 9–10).

Leaders gain their authority from their ability to influence others to get the work done; because of this, anyone has the potential to be a leader. A manager's authority comes from the manager's position in the organization, such as a team leader, nurse manager, assistant director of nursing, or vice president of nursing. There is no doubt that managers are different in not only what they do but also in how they do their work, staff roles, and authority. Since the main goal of leadership is to guide and facilitate staff to achieve its best, leaders cannot ignore quality and practice improvement (Heller, 1999). To be successful as a leader, leaders commit to lifelong learning and improvement. They also encourage staff members to pursue lifelong learning goals and serve as coaches and mentors. This should help to reach the goal of improving care. Flexibility is a key factor in leadership. This is demonstrated when leaders must plan and respond to problems as well as work with others to achieve goals. This requires knowledge. What are the key leadership roles?

1. **Expert.** An expert has an in-depth understanding of a particular topic or function. An expert will strive toward the best performance.
2. **Administrator.** The leader makes sure that the organization, unit, or service operates effectively. In this role, the leader looks for ways to improve efficiency and provides the framework for practice, such as policies and procedures, guidelines, values, systems, and other necessary rules, to get the job done.
3. **People person.** In this role the leader ensures that the staff has the training and education to meet the performance requirements. In addition, the leader strives to provide a work environment in which the staff feels comfortable to share information and opinions and is willing to work as a group.

4. **Strategist or planning for the future.** The leader also takes on the role of change agent. In this role the leader strives to make the most of change to improve the organization, even taking risks to accomplish effective change.

If one rereads these descriptions of the roles, "manager" could be substituted for "leader" *if* the manager demonstrated leadership qualities. In comparison, with the management focus on planning, organizing, staffing, directing, and controlling, management is different from leadership. "This view of management, as an orderly set of processes suited to orderly organizations, supported by Kotter's (2004) view of management as process focusing on systems to produce goods and services efficiently" (Shaw, 2007, p. 28). An overlap of management and leadership is found in the need for broad-perspective decision making, communication, and motivation of followers. Even management is changing, as managers today need management skills that

- Change focus from process to outcomes
- Align role to information infrastructure rather than functional performance
- Focus on team results rather than individual performance
- Manage data complexes rather than individual events
- Facilitate resources that then direct work
- Transfer skill-sets rather than make decisions for staff
- Develop staff self-direction rather than giving direction
- Focus on obtaining value rather than simply finding costs
- Focus on consumer-driven structure rather than provider-based system
- Construct horizontal relationships rather than maintain vertical control mechanisms
- Facilitate equity-based partnerships rather than control individual behaviors (Porter-O'Grady, 1999, p. 40)

It is easy to assume that leaders can do it all. This is a myth. There are other myths about leadership, some of which are described in Box 1-7.

What are some differences between the nurse manager and the nurse leader (Laurent, 2000)? Registered nurses are clearly trained to manage patient care. The term *management* is used frequently in nursing. "Nursing managers are successful because of one word, control. Managers control their environment, things can be controlled, and patient care is manipulated or managed. In this process nurses learn about crisis management or how to re-establish control" (Laureant, 2000, p. 84). This has worked to nursing's benefit; however, the first step in moving from a nurse manager to a nurse manager who is also a leader is to give up some of this control. This is not always easy for new nurse managers to do, and many experienced nurse managers also have problems giving up control and allowing staff to participate more in decision making and planning.

| BOX 1-7 | MYTHS ABOUT LEADERSHIP |
|---|---|

There are many popular myths about leadership. Goffee and Jones (2000) identified some of these myths.

- *Everyone can be a leader.* This is not true. Everyone may have the potential to be a leader; however, the person needs to develop certain leadership competencies such as self-knowledge or authenticity to be a leader.
- *Leaders deliver business results.* They do not always deliver the desired outcomes.

- *People who get to the top are leaders.* This is not true as many people in management are not leaders and have limited leadership qualities. A manager may or may not also demonstrate leadership qualities and competencies.
- *Leaders are great coaches.* They are not always great coaches, as leaders cannot always share important technical skills while at the same time inspire staff.

### Who Is a Nurse Leader?

To develop a fuller understanding of nurse leadership and the need to "step outside the box," it is important to have an appreciation of the following:

1. Where nursing leadership came from
2. Where nursing leadership is today
3. How nursing might be affected by leadership and management theories and styles

The manager's job is to accomplish the work of the organization. This is true regardless of the type of organization such as acute care hospital, home care agency, long-term care organization, clinic, and so on. Manager roles and functions vary with the type of organization and the level of management. Typically, management is viewed from three levels: first-level, middle-level, and upper-level managers. First-level managers focus on managing the work of non-managerial staff or on the day-to-day activities of a specific work group. Examples of first-level managers are unit nurse managers and charge nurses. Middle-level managers focus on supervising several first-level managers. An example of middle-level manager is a director of surgical services or women's health. These managers also serve as liaisons between first-level managers and upper-level managers. The upper-level managers are responsible for establishing goals and strategic plans for the organization. They are the organization's executives and top administrators. Examples of upper-level managers are a chief nurse executive (CNE), vice president of patient services, chief executive officer (CEO), chief operating officer (COO), and medical director. Not all organizations have all three levels. There are also nurses who hold positions that are not usually considered to be managers and yet require effective leadership competencies to meet their required functions. Examples are clinical nurse specialist (CNS); advanced practice nurse (APN), who may work in any setting including acute care; clinical nurse leader (CNL); and doctor of nursing practice (DNP). These positions will be discussed later in this text.

What is the historical development of the "nurse leader" in health care organizations (Ulrich, 2001)? The nurse leader in acute care settings was first called the director of nursing (DON). The DON focused on nursing care in hospitals and had limited interaction with hospital administration about planning. The DON typically had little idea about the budget and did not seem particularly interested in it. These positions were held for many years with very low turnover rates. Early on few of these nurses had advanced degrees. In the late 1970s and early 1980s, as the DON's power began to increase, some hospitals began to change the DON title to vice president of nursing, but the focus was still on nursing. In these cases, more of these nurses had advanced degrees. Slowly, this nurse leader began to interact more with hospital administration and to assume more responsibility for the nursing department's planning and budget. The next step in title changes was the move to vice president of patient services, which in some organizations is called the chief nursing officer (CNO). This was a significant change as it recognized that the nurse leader had the ability to have an impact on broader patient care issues, not just nursing. This nurse leader is responsible for nursing care, other clinical delivery services, and sometimes covers support services such as medical records. Health care organizations continue to vary in their views of the nurse leader. The last example of a vice president for patient services is not found in every acute care setting, but it is increasing. In addition, more nurses are now moving into overall administration positions in health care settings such as acute care hospitals, home care, long-term care, and ambulatory care. When nurses hold the positions of chief executive officer (CEO) or chief operating officer (COO), they have reached the point where they oversee the entire health care organization. How did this happen? Some nurse leaders have clearly demonstrated to health care organizations that they can handle these responsibilities. In addition, many of the values that are important to nursing have become more important in health care in general (e.g., caring, respect for the patient, and identification and evaluation of outcomes). When nurses move into these higher positions they bring these values with them; however, to be successful these nurses also need to be competent in all of the administrative tasks that are involved in these high-level positions. "Leadership and care management are the principal strategies used by nurses in the nursing administration advanced practice specialty role" (Harris et al., 2006, p. 437). Appendix A describes the American Organization of Nurse Executives competencies illustrating how this position requires leadership and management competencies.

## Preparation and Development of Nurse Managers

THE NURSE MANAGER ROLE     Nurse managers are directly responsible for maintaining standards of care, managing fiscal resources, and developing staff. Some of the titles for this middle management position include "nurse manager," "head nurse," "nursing unit manager," and "nursing or nurse coordinator." Nurse manager responsibilities vary from organization to organization, but the most effective nurse managers recognize the importance of point-of-care leaders (O'Rourke, 2007). Some positions focus more on management and others more on clinical care. "Nurse managers are internal stakeholders who play essential roles in managing change, cultural integration, retention, and direction of staff attitudes toward changing health care structures" (Mathena, 2002, p. 136). Many nurse managers need to be prepared to deal with staff stress, low morale, staff uncertainty, staff turnover, inadequate quality care outcomes, and decreasing budget, all of which are common problems today. Nurse managers who are also leaders are involved in visioning, interprofessional team building, workload and work process analysis, stakeholder analysis, and interactive planning (Mathena, 2002). Critical competencies to accomplish these activities include the following:

- Directing others
- Group management
- Interpersonal sensitivity
- Self-confidence
- Use of influence strategies
- Analytical thinking
- Initiative
- Achievement orientation
- Direct persuasion

O'Rourke has identified the need for role-based nurse managers. "Role-based managers remember why they went into nursing. Role-based managers see their raison d'etre as ensuring that the standard of practice is met every day with every patient. Role-based managers are inspired by the idea that they can help staff to develop into strong, well-prepared professional nurses and work diligently to create an environment supportive of professional practice. They understand that their role is to create more efficient operations and improve practice" (2007, p. 48). These comments and view of the nurse manager strongly supports the IOM's initiative to improve care at all levels and settings.

THE PETER PRINCIPLE     The **Peter Principle** (Peter & Hull, 1969) describes a major leadership and management problem in bureaucratic organizations (Milgram, Spector, & Treger, 1999). The problem occurs when staff members are promoted for doing a good job with their assigned tasks; however, as they climb up the hierarchical ladder, they eventually are promoted to a position for which they are not competent. An example is the staff nurse who provides quality care and is considered to be an expert clinician who is then promoted to a management position. It is assumed that because the nurse is an expert clinician that he or she will be an effective manager. This is not necessarily the case, and even if the nurse has the potential to be an effective manager he or she would still need to develop additional leadership and management competencies. The danger of this type of promotion is that demotion is not something that is done very easily. Typically, the staff member stays in the position though the staff member may be incompetent as a manager and a leader. The reward system in nursing has typically been to reward good clinical staff with a management position, which has led to problems and is an example of the Peter Principle. Nursing really needs to reward clinical expertise in manner that retains nurses in direct care positions.

**NURSE MANAGEMENT DEVELOPMENT**　　Hill (1993) conducted long-term surveys of new managers in businesses and was able to identify many needs and concerns of the new managers that can also be applied to nursing today. The most difficult task for these new managers was developing interpersonal skills. Many of the current theories that have been discussed, such as EI, Knowledge Management, and Transformational Leadership, emphasize the importance of interpersonal skills. Development of self-awareness and personal growth are clearly the most challenging experience for staff nurses who move into a manager role. How do managers change? Typically, they learn slowly over time, and they are not always aware of what they are learning. Most managers seem to learn on the job with limited formal training or education in management; however, formal training and education in management makes the transition to the position much easier. This is just as true in health care organizations as it is in other types of businesses. In one study of nurse managers the managers felt that they needed further education to develop financial management competency and technical skills such as data analysis (Mathena, 2002). Even though nurse managers recognized the importance of communication skills they did not rank it as a high competency. The health care environment with its increased interest in reducing health care costs is probably a major reason for identifying the need for more financial information by managers, who are typically responsible for their unit's budget. There is no doubt that nurse managers who have an understanding of budgets and costs will be more effective. Management development is a long-term self-learning process, as was noted in Hill's study of business managers. As the manager learns, it is important for the manager to receive feedback and guidance. "Adopting attitudes and a psychological perspective consistent with their new role can be even more demanding" (Hill, 1993, p. 155). A manager needs to actively use introspection, which requires much adaptation. New managers often have many misconceptions about management and about themselves. The most important guideline for leadership success is the importance of using self-learning. Having access to peers for discussion and feedback assists the manager when new tasks and responsibilities are learned. New managers need mentors and coaches. Ideally, the new manager's supervisor should form a relationship with the new manager that encourages feedback and open discussion. The supervisor may need to reach out first to the new manager, as it may be difficult for the new manager to ask for help. When managers gain interpersonal judgment this increases self-confidence and self-assurance. They are then more able to delegate and give up some control. To do this, new managers need to learn how to listen before making rapid decisions and consider factors that affect decisions and delegation. New managers often first adopt a hands-on **autocratic** approach to management because they want to influence results. When they do this, they appear to be very directive. However, despite the fact that they really are directive, when new managers are asked to describe their management style, they typically describe it as consultative rather than authoritative. Over time new managers discover the limits of their formal authority. They may give staff directions, but that does not mean staff will follow them. It is at this point that the manager learns about the need for persuasion. When managers finally learn that staff that can offer its own reactions and input into decisions are motivated, then managers experience greater success. Hill also identified concerns that new managers have about the process of administration. Managers often define "administration as routine communication activities such as paperwork and exchange of information. . . Their administrative responsibilities seemed to be constraints that interfered with their autonomy and stole precious time for more important responsibilities" (Hill, 1993, p. 24). Nurse managers also often experience this concern when they try to do their jobs and examine quality of care and requests from higher management (administration) that demand certain responses. They must work with multiple disruptions, which is probably different from the managers that Hill followed. Interprofessional issues also make the management process more complex. Nurse managers work in complex health care environments just as the managers in Hill's study worked in complex organizations. To accomplish effective management and leadership, managers need to remember that actions speak louder than words. Managers need to establish a culture of high standards and openness, and empower or share power with their staff.

## *CASE STUDY*

### *Leadership Style: How Do You Decide?*

A nurse, who has been working at a hospital for 6 years on the orthopedic unit, has been chosen for the nurse manager position. She wanted the position, but she is now concerned about how she will handle it. A nurse manager from another unit will mentor her in the nurse manager role. As the orientation takes place the new nurse manger begins to assess the different leadership styles that are used. What she notices most is that the nurse manager she is shadowing usually tells staff what to do and that there are morale issues on her unit. She hears staff talking behind the back of the nurse manager about how they don't trust her, and they hold back on information. They receive very little feedback, and when it is given, it is usually negative feedback. A staff nurse comments, "We never know what is going on." The new nurse manager is having lunch with her mentor, and she asks her how she should approach this new position. The response is, "Just do what comes naturally." The new nurse manager is dissatisfied with this approach.

### Questions:

1. Do you think the new nurse manager's response is normal or abnormal? Why?
2. Based on the information that is provided, what type of leadership style is the mentor using? If you were the nurse manager, how would you have responded to the nurse?
3. If you were the new nurse manager, select the leadership style you would use, describe it and the related leadership theory, and why you chose it.

### Nurse Manager Competencies: Overview and Views from Nursing Professional Organizations

As has been discussed, the best managers are also leaders, and it is a challenge to be both. It is easy to get stuck in management functions and forget the leading aspect of the process. Key skills and competencies that assist managers to be effective managers *and* leaders are

- Critical thinking—Verbs that can be used to describe the critical thinking skills required for managers are evaluate, select, analyze, utilize, consider, align, proactive, plan, think, recognize, and predict. All of these are active verbs. Critical thinking requires an active stance rather than a passive one (Child, Lingle, & Watson, 2001).
- Ability to guide staff in using clinical reasoning and judgment
- Communication skills
- Networking
- Managing resources (e.g., budgeting, staffing)
- Enhancing employee performance (e.g., mentoring)
- Team-building
- Evaluating effectiveness and efficiency
- Delegating
- Clinical and organizational expertise
- Flexibility
- Collaboration (multidisciplinary)
- Coordination
- Outcome oriented
- Problem solving
- Evaluation and analysis

In fact, these skills are important for every RN, and this is one reason why this content is important for all nursing students. It is easy to say, "I am not going to be a manager," but many management skills as well as leadership skills are required in the daily practice of every RN. Box 1-8 describes the role characteristics of the nurse with unit-based or service-line-based authority.

| BOX 1-8 | ROLE CHARACTERISTICS OF THE NURSE WITH UNIT-BASED OR SERVICE-LINE-BASED AUTHORITY |

- Promoting care delivery with respect for individuals' rights and preferences;
- Participating in nursing and organizational policy formulation and decision-making involving staff, such as in shared governance;
- Accepting organizational accountability for services provided to recipients;
- Evaluating the quality and appropriateness of health care
- Coordinating nursing care with other healthcare disciplines, and assisting integrating services across the continuum of health care;
- Participating in the recruitment, selection, retention of personnel, including staff representative of the population diversity;
- Assessing impact of plans and strategies to address such issues as
    - Ethnic, cultural, and diversity changes in the population
    - Political and social influences
    - Financial and economic issues
    - The aging of society and demographic trends
    - Ethical issues related to health care;
- Assuming oversight for staffing, and scheduling personnel considering scope of practice, competencies, patient needs, and complexity of care;

- Proving appropriate orientation for new staff, and providing individual feedback on staff development and progress;
- Encouraging staff members to attain education, credentialing, and continuing professional development;
- Evaluating performance of personnel in a fair and transparent manner;
- Developing, implementing, and monitoring the budget for their defined area(s) for responsibility;
- Participating in and involving the nursing staff in evaluative research activities to promote evidence-based practice;
- Facilitating educational experience for nursing and other students;
- Encouraging shared accountability for professional practice;
- Advocating for a work environment that minimizes work-related illness and injury;
- Reporting any injuries or safety hazards, and taking corrective action as quickly as possible;
- Providing an open forum of communication with staff, allowing them ample opportunities to discuss issues and seek guidance; and
- Understanding and complying with state and federal laws concerning the healthcare services and practice they manage, and complying with the all facility regulations and policies.

Source: American Nurses Association. (2009). *Nursing administration: Scope and standards of practice*. Silver Springs, MD. (pp. 16–18). Reprinted with permission. All rights reserved.

A key job of a manager is to make sure that the staff understands instructions and that these instructions are carried out effectively. In doing this, the manager is exercising authority. The manager establishes an environment in which the staff understands that it is acceptable to identify problems and to speak out when his or her performance has not been as effective as possible. Staff members should not fear that they will be reprimanded and should feel that they can trust their manager rather than be concerned about negative outcomes (Institute of Medicine, 1999).

CARING AND TRUST   Managers who are leaders need to care for their staff. What does this mean? This means that the manager listens to staff, recognizes when staff needs special support and guidance, and takes time to respond to the staff. There are times when staff lacks confidence, and it is then the role of the manager to help increase staff confidence. To accomplish this, the manager may provide positive feedback and guidance or provide additional educational opportunities to develop new competencies. Giving staff recognition for positive performance develops staff confidence. It may be simply recognizing a staff member with a kind word and comment. When errors occur, and they do, a manager who is also a leader does not punish staff but uses the error as an opportunity for improvement and assess the impact of the system on the error. This approach is discussed further in Chapters 16 and 17. Managers also need to be able to admit failure themselves, and in doing so, act as role models for staff by demonstrating that managers also need to improve. The effective manager will be seen as a leader, inspire excellence, and motivate others to excellence, all of which relate to earlier theories discussed such as Emotional Intelligence, Connective Leadership, Transformational Leadership, and so on. There are four critical qualities that are important in developing trust: competence, congruity, constancy, and caring. In today's health care environment, the complex work environment may be tense; staff may be tired; morale may be low; and work requirements may have increased. Leaders must constantly foster trust by demonstrating loyalty and supporting staff. Staff members need to feel that they can share their feedback, whether positive or negative, and not feel threatened when they disagree with the manager or for their creative ideas. How does a manager develop trust? First, the manager needs to have competence, hopefully leadership competencies. How does staff recognize when a person is a leader? Usually, staff will say that it has a feeling that the manager is able to accomplish what is supposed to be accomplished. It describes a manager as a person of integrity. Staff members want their manager to be on their side and do not want to be left alone when things get difficult at work. This is particularly important when there is conflict. Managers who make promises to staff need to keep the promises. If the manager cannot keep a promise, staff should be given a timely, clear explanation. In addition, managers need to demonstrate to their staff that they trust that staff performance will be effective. Most people have likely experienced relationships in which trust was not present. Typically, these relationships involve situations where the person's actions and words did not mesh. If this becomes a pattern, then trust never develops or is destroyed. It is then very difficult to regain trust. Managers must be honest and play fair with their staff. Consistency is critical in any leadership position and is also related to caring and trust. When authority is exercised it must be consistent in order to develop staff respect for the manager. If staff feels that some staff are given extra credit, rarely receive criticism when it is deserved, or is assigned less work, staff will feel uncomfortable with the manager and resentment will build (Heller, 1999). Distrust will develop. In these situations staff will not respect the manager, and this will affect work outcomes and patient care.

## Leadership in Community Health

Is leadership in the community different from leadership in other health care settings? As the level of health care delivered in the community increases, nurse leadership will need to become more effective in this setting, and today, more nurses are needed to assist in developing leadership within the community. By 2020 the United States is expected to need 250,000 additional public health professionals (*Orlando Business Journal*, 2008). Nurses who function in the community should not take over the leadership and direct the community but rather should facilitate the building of community leadership by providing their expertise and guidance to empower the community. To do this nurses need the following skills: "capacity to create negotiated partnerships and shared responsibility and accountability as they work with other professions and members of the community; capacity to create new order by seeing relationships between unrelated parts and can anticipate and plan for the future . . . to approach the situation with an open mind and improvise inadequate reaction requires a different set of skills. It is based on the knowledge that there are multiple ways to address the situation and that the best solution resides within the problem itself" (Koerner, 2000, pp. 16–17). Community health nursing has become more important in nursing. Community leadership should not be ignored in this setting; however, nurses may need to consider new and different competencies for this environment. There is also no doubt that, despite the many exciting new opportunities, the U.S. health care delivery system has major problems, and this text discusses many of them. The IOM (2001) suggests that a major reason for the chaotic health care delivery system is that the system has lost its focus on what is truly important to the people it serves, the patients. The emphasis on the five health professions core competencies indicates the need to have a common base from which all health care professions practice (Institute of Medicine, 2003). In addition, the health care system requires greater health care consumer participation, which is also emphasized in the core competency to provide patient-centered care. Wolf (2000) describes a key transformational model of care that has four components that can be applied to any type of health care organization. The components of this model are highlighted in Box 1-9. This model can be helpful in integrating the health care system as well as developing and maintaining an organization's cultural identity and its leaders and staff.

## The Image of Nursing

The image of nursing is an important aspect of nursing leadership. How nurses are viewed affects if they may be seen as possible leaders and whether or not nurses can be more effective. A *New York Times* article (Villarosa, 2001, May 22) on the image of nursing noted that national polls consistently confirm that nursing is viewed as one of the most trusted professions; however, the image of the profession is not that positive. A survey of schoolchildren indicated that they saw nursing as a "scary, stressful, low-status job, terrible hours, and an ugly uniform" (Villarosa, 2001, May 22, p. D7). Nursing's image has suffered over the past few years (Vestal, 2002). One reason for this is that consumers do not really have a complete or accurate view of the roles that nurses play throughout the health care system. "However, the side of nursing that involves human caring and making a difference in people's lives was not part of the story. If the image of nursing continues to be one that detracts from our ability to recruit new professionals, then we have to work on our stories that go out to the public" (Vestal, 2002, p. 4). Nursing still must contend with the fact that it is primarily a women's profession. There have been many media stories about how difficult the job is and how the work environment is stressful with staff shortages. As people who might consider the profession are listening to these messages, they do have an effect on the recruitment of potential students. More needs to be done to ensure that there is a more consistent message. Johnson and Johnson partnered with nursing to develop some excellent television ads that demonstrate positive qualities of nursing as a career choice (Gordon & Nelson, 2005). The first series emphasized the caring aspects of nursing and second a broader view of the profession. This is an important goal—to make sure that nurses see their choice of nursing as a lifetime commitment to a career and that nurses have a sense of pride in their profession, and then communicate this to the public, especially to groups who might consider it as a possible profession to enter. The message needs to be clear and accurate to really be effective and some are recommending that there be a move away from "the 'virtue script' toward a knowledge-based identify for nurses" (Gordon & Nelson, 2005, p. 62). Leadership can play an important role here. Nursing needs to emphasize how nurses can be, and in many cases are, leaders in the health care environment. Leadership is a critical component of the profession. The ANA's *Nursing's Agenda*

---

| BOX 1-9 | TRANSFORMATIONAL MODEL OF CARE |
| --- | --- |

1. The *first component of the model is a professional practice component*, which focuses on deliberate critical thinking, negotiation, and decision making. In this process, individual needs of patients, professional recommendations, and effective resource management are considered. It is important that each health care discipline consider its practice and what elements of its practice are critical for patient outcomes. Wolf identifies four concepts that are important to this component: Transformational Leadership, care delivery systems, professional growth, and collaborative practice.

2. The *second component focuses on process*, which includes the processes that each health care professional group uses in its practice (for example, the nursing process). However, it is important that nurses as well as other health care professionals continually evaluate routines of care to determine if they continue to be necessary. As is done in nursing, it is important for other health care professionals to consider the patient as a partner in the care development process.

3. The *third component is the primary outcome*, and here the emphasis is on the relationship of patients to the process and outcome of care delivery.

4. The *fourth component focuses on identifying strategic outcomes related to the organization*, such as the ability to adapt to change, compete financially, and so on. Wolf also identifies strategic outcomes related to the profession which are professional organization, education, research, and professional publications.

*for Change* (2002) identifies a major goal related to public relations/communications and nursing: "Nursing's pivotal role in health care will be demonstrated on a regular basis to various publics outside of the profession" (p. 14). This is not easy to accomplish, but it is a critical goal. The Center for Nursing Advocacy was founded in 2001 to address the nursing shortage problem; however, it has focused more and more on the image of nursing as a component of the problem. It assesses and identifies media examples that support a positive or a negative nursing image through its Golden Lamp Awards. The Center also works to change how nursing is portrayed in the media.

Uniforms have resurfaced as an issue in nursing, mostly related to image. A recurring issue is the white uniform and its value (Tobin, 2006). Has the move to a variety of uniforms, most of which are scrub clothes of different colors, hurt the professional image of nursing? Is it clear who is the RN other then reading a name tag that might be too small to read well? Tobin also notes that maybe this is also disguising the nursing shortage. Patients and families see a lot of staff and yet do not have an idea about professional nursing coverage or lack of it. When on the job nurses need to project a professional image, whether in uniform or street clothes.

## Making a Difference: Increasing Nurse Leaders

How do nurses become leaders? "Nurse leaders do not just appear. It is a professional responsibility for all of us to become leaders and to mentor future leaders" (Anderson, 2000, p. 47). Nursing education should take advantage of leadership opportunities. The first step is to make a commitment to lifelong learning. As students enter clinical practice and then their careers, they will be confronted with change. Leaders use change as opportunities for learning. Becoming involved in professional organizations is also an important part of developing leadership. This may begin with participation in the National Student Nurses Association (NSNA), Sigma Theta Tau (STTI), the nursing honor society that has an invitation membership based on scholastic and leadership criteria, or other campus organizations. The NSNA Leadership U provides opportunities for student recognition for leadership and management skills they develop in NSNA activities. The website provides leadership resources and other information for students. Mentoring is also part of leadership. Some nursing programs have mentoring programs so that students can help one another. Networking, which can be helpful, can begin as a student. It is important to remember that faculty, peers, and nurses in the clinical settings, as well as nurses who might be met outside of school or clinical practice, may at some point be important individuals in a nurse's career. Through networking, connections are made to assist a nurse throughout the nurse's career. There are not enough nurses to fill all of the nurse leadership positions that are available today. Some nurses will eventually move into formal management positions, and others will apply leadership skills in non-management positions and in professional activities such as professional nursing organizations. Nursing must find a way to increase the pool of potential nurse leaders. Some solutions to this problem include (a) develop clinical/career ladders for nursing managers, (b) define goals and competency-based outcomes to direct manager growth and development within organizations and within the profession, (c) provide mentorship, and (d) develop a system for identifying novice to expert among nurse leaders (Coughlin, 2002). Clinical ladders are used in many health care organizations to recognize performance and competencies. Typically, a new nurse enters the organization at the lowest level and then must meet specific criteria and competencies to move "up the ladder" to different clinical levels. Leadership is included in the criteria and competencies, (e.g., membership on committees, chair of committees, development of unit-based materials such as patient education or a change in a policy or procedure, mentoring new nurses, preceptor for nursing students, implementing evidence-based practice, or developing research). "The American Organization of Nurse Executives (AONE), professional association for nurse executives and nurse leaders, is committed to identifying and adopting evidence-based management practices. AONE believes that nursing leadership plays an extremely important role in creating the work environments that attract and keep nurses and that current management practices are not uniformly successful" (Watson, 2004, p. 207). As organizations and the nursing profession consider the best methods for leadership development, there are guidelines that should not be forgotten. Leaders need to "exemplify leadership, not formulas; demonstrate empowerment by developing, not ruling followers; learn to provide leadership opportunities for others, all the while learning to coach. Leaders need nurses to expand their own definitions of themselves and their role" (Ferguson & Brindle, 2000, p. 5). The majority of nurses will never be in a formal management position. So why is there all of this interest in leadership and management? "Is there a magic formula to resuscitate today's management? Perhaps, but formula or not, the antidote for today's management dilemma is leadership" (Stahl, 1998, p. 7). It is important to recognize that leadership skills are not only required for those in high positions in nursing. "In today's increasingly less hierarchical and more lateral organizational structures, leadership is not about position of authority, as much as it is a role of influence. Staff nurses can and must lead through teamwork, the development of better practices, through the development of centrality in communication networks, and in contributing to the strategic management of the units and departments. The leadership role and task is pivotal, not peripheral to the success of health care facilities" (Ferguson & Brindle, 2000, p. 5). Ferguson's comments about leadership are very important and continue to be important. In May of 2003, the American Association of Colleges of Nursing (AACN) published a white paper, *The Role of the Clinical Nurse Leader* (2003). The position of the AACN is that leadership is very important in nursing. This position is supported in recent Institute of Medicine reports related to the quality and safety of health care in which nurses are described as leaders and important in making a difference in the quality and safety of health care (Finkelman & Kenner, 2009). There needs, however, to be greater recognition that leadership is required for all nursing positions. To meet this need for nursing leaders, the AACN recognizes the need to incorporate more leadership development in undergraduate and graduate programs. This decision is based on 10 assumptions about the health care delivery system and nursing.

1. Practice is at the systems level. Nurses must practice in all types of settings and are accountable for care outcomes of clinical populations (e.g., mothers in labor population, patients in a clinic, children in a community).
2. Population-level care outcomes are the measure of quality practice. Performance will be measured by clinical and cost outcomes.
3. Practice guidelines are based on evidence.
4. Client-centered practice is intra- and interprofessional.
5. Information will maximize self-care and client decision making.
6. Nursing assessment is the basis for theory and knowledge development.
7. Good fiscal stewardship is a condition of quality care.
8. Social justice is an essential nursing value.
9. Communication technology will facilitate the continuity and comprehensiveness of care.
10. The CNL must assume guardianship for the nursing profession (American Association of Colleges of Nursing, 2003, pp. 5–9).

These assumptions are clearly related to current leadership and management theories and styles that have been discussed in this chapter and will be emphasized throughout the text. The role of nurse leader is critical for patients, their families, and the delivery system as a whole. Nurses have really been in this role for a very long time. Some were more prepared than others for it, and now it is important to recognize that every nurse needs to develop leadership qualities and competencies, whether or not they are in a formal management position.

# APPLYING LEADERSHIP AND MANAGEMENT

## MY HOSPITAL UNIT

In the text introduction you were asked to create a description your own unit. You will be the nurse manager on this unit. You will revisit your unit at the end of each chapter. Decisions you make in each chapter will need to be considered when subsequent decisions are made. For this chapter, you enter your unit and consider the following. As the nurse manager of this unit what type of leadership do you want to use? How would you demonstrate this in day-to-day activities? Write a position description for your position as nurse manager that reflects your philosophy of leadership and management. How would you develop staff leadership? Use the content in this chapter and information found in the appendix. Use the virtual unit site found on the textbook website (www.nursing.pearsonhighered.com) to record the work that you do in the role of nurse manager for your unit.

## Critical Thinking Questions and Activities

1. Select a nurse manager in one of your clinical sites. Ask the nurse manager the following questions: (1) What made the nurse manager want to become a nurse manager? (2) What are the key management skills that the manager uses? (3) Ask the nurse manager to compare and contrast the differences between a nurse manager and a nurse leader. Share your data with your classmates and compare and contrast with their data.
2. Working in small teams review the white paper on *The Role of the Clinical Nurse Leader* found at http://www.aacn.nche.edu/Publications/WhitePapers/ClinicalNurseLeader.htm. Consider the points in this paper and develop a survey that you might distribute to nurses to determine how this new role relates to nursing practice. Try out the survey with nurses who work in a variety of settings with different years of experience. What results did you get? Analyze the results.
3. As you gain more clinical experience in school and after graduation, observe how others lead and manage. Make a conscious effort each week in clinical to observe leadership and management. Begin a blog with your classmates in this course to share your observations. Do not include staff names, patient names, or name of organization for privacy reasons. Explore issues or questions that intrigue you.
4. In your own words, compare and contrast the role of the nurse executive and the nurse manager. How do you think the role of the nurse team leader might be different?
5. Select a time when you had to take the leadership role. This could be current role or one from the past. Considering the content in this chapter analyze how you thought you demonstrated leadership or could have improved your leadership.

## Media Links

- **URL: http://www.nursingadvocacy.org**
  Center for Nursing Advocacy
  Information on the image of nursing

- **URL: http://www.nsnaleadershipu.org/nsnalu/**
  National Student Nurses Association: Leadership U
  Leadership for students

- **URL: http://www.aacn.nche.edu/Media/shortageresource.htm**
  American Association of Colleges of Nursing
  Nursing shortage resources, fact sheets, and reports
  **http://www.aacn.nche.edu/Publications/WhitePapers/ClinicalNurseLeader.htm**
  Paper on the role of the clinical nurse leader

- **URL: http://www.aone.org**
  The American Organization of Nurse Executives
  A leadership organization for nurses in leadership roles
- **URL: http://nursequest.com/**
  NurseQuest
  An excellent resource for nurse leaders
- **URL: http://www.cnl.org/**
  The Center for Nursing Leadership
  The website for nurse leaders and nurses who see themselves as leaders
- **URL: http://www.mapnp.org/library/ldrship/ldrship.htm#anchor508500**
  Separating "Leading" from "Managing" Can Be Destructive
  Read this article to see why leadership and management, although different, cannot exist without each other.
- **URL: http://www.mapnp.org/library/ldrship/ldrship.htm#anchor508500**
  Introduction to Management
  **http://www.mapnp.org/library/mng_thry/mng_thry.htm**
  Reading this article will help you understand management and the skills required to carry functions of management.
- **URL: http://cgean.org/cert.php**
  Links about Nursing Administration and Management Certification
  AONE-Certified Nurse Manager and Leader
- **URL: http://www.nursecredentialing.org/NurseSpecialties/ NurseExecutiveAdvanced.aspx**
  AACN- Nurse Executive, Advanced
- **URL: http://www.nursingsociety.org/Career/CareerMap/Pages/nursing_orgs.aspx**
  Nursing specialty organizations (provides links to most major nursing organizations)

**Pearson Nursing Student Resources**
Find additional review materials at
**nursing.pearsonhighered.com**
Prepare for success with additional NCLEX®-style practice questions, interactive assignments and activities, Web links, animations and videos, and more!

# References

American Association of Colleges of Nursing. (2008). *The essentials of baccalaureate education for professional nursing practice*. Washington, DC: Author.

American Association of Colleges of Nursing. (2003, May). *White paper on the role of the clinical nurse leader*. Retrieved June 16, 2003, from http://www.aacn.nche.edu/CNL/Index.htm

American Nurses Association et al. (2002). *Nursing's agenda for change*. Retrieved May 16, 2002, from http://www.nursingworld.org/default.aspx

Anderson, C. (2000). The critical path to leadership development: A student perspective. *Imprint, 47*(4), 47–48.

Bass, B. (1998). *Leadership and performance beyond expectations*. New York: Free Press.

Bass, B., & Avolio, B. (1997). *Transformational leadership development: Manual for multifactor leadership questionnaire*. Palo Alto, CA: Consulting Psychologists Press.

Bennis, W., & Goldsmith, J. (1997). *Learning to lead: A workbook on becoming a leader*. Reading, MA: Perseus Books.

Blake, R. & Mouton, J. (1964). *The managerial grid*. Houston: Gulf Publishing.

Blake, R. & McCanse, A. (1991). *Leadership dilemmas—Grid solutions*. Houston: Gulf Publishing.

Bradberry, T. & Greaves, J. (2003). *The emotional intelligence quickbook: Everything you need to know*. San Diego, CA: TalentSmart.

Burns, J. (1985). *Leadership*. New York: Harper Collins.

Child, R., Lingle, G., & Watson, P. (2001). Managing diversity in the environment of care. *Seminars for Nurse Managers, 9*(2), 102–110.

Corning, S. (2002). Profiling and developing nursing leaders. *Journal of Nursing Administration, 32*, 373–375.

Coughlin, C. (2002). Saving nursing management. *Journal of Nursing Administration, 32*(4), 178–179.

Crow, G. (2002). The relationship between trust, social capital, and organizational success. *Nursing Administration Quarterly, 26*(3), 1–11.

Curtin, L. (2001). Guest editorial: EQ is more important now than ever before. *Seminars for Nurse Managers, 9*(4), 203–205.

Curtin, L., & Falherty, M. (1993). *Nursing ethics: Theories and pragmatics.* Upper Saddle River, NJ: Prentice Hall.

Deming, W. (1986). *Out of crisis.* Boston: MIT Press.

Drucker, P. (1994). The age of social transformation. *Atlantic Monthly, 274*(5), 53–80.

Drucker, P. (1993). *Post-capitalistic society.* NY: Harper Business Publications.

Dunham-Taylor, J. (2000). Nurse executive transformational leadership found in participative organizations. *Journal of Nursing Administration, 30*(5), 241–250.

Finkelman, A. & Kenner, C. (2009). *Teaching IOM: Implications of the Institute of Medicine Reports for nursing education.* Silver Springs, MD: American Nurses Association.

Ferguson, S., & Brindle, M. (2000). Nursing leadership: Vision and the reality. *Nursing Spectrum, 10*(21DC), 5.

Fiedler, F. (1967). *A theory of leadership effectiveness.* New York: McGraw-Hill.

Fullan, C., Lando, A., Johansen, M., Reyes, A., & Szaloczy, D. (1988). The triad of empowerment: Leadership, environment, and professional traits. *Nursing Economics, 16*(5), 254–257.

Goleman, D. (1998). *Working with emotional intelligence.* New York: Bantam Books.

Goleman, D. (2001). An EI theory of performance. In C. Cherniss & D. Goleman (Eds.), *The emotionally intelligent workplace* (pp. 27–44). San Francisco: Jossey-Bass.

Gordon, S. & Nelson, S. (2005). An end to angels. *AJN, 105*(5), 62–69.

Grohar-Murray, M., & DiCroce, H. (2003). *Leadership and management in nursing* (3rd ed.). Upper Saddle River, NJ: Pearson Education.

Harris, K. et al. (2006). Future nursing administration graduate curricula, Part I. *JONA, 36*(10), 435–440.

Hammer, M. (1997). The soul of the new organization. In F. Hesselbein, M. Goldsmith, & R. Beckhard (Eds.), *The organization of the future* (pp. 27–31). San Francisco: Jossey-Bass.

Heller, R. (1999). *Learning to lead.* New York: DK Publishing, Inc.

Hill, L. (1993). *Becoming a manager: How new managers master the challenges of leadership.* New York: Penguin Books.

Huber, D. (2010). *Leadership and nursing care management.* Philadelphia: W.B. Saunders Company.

Huber, D. (2000). *Leadership and nursing care management.* Philadelphia: W.B. Saunders Company.

Institute of Medicine. (2003). *Leadership by example.* Washington, DC: National Academies Press.

Institute of Medicine. (2001). *Crossing the quality chasm.* Washington, DC: National Academies Press.

Institute of Medicine. (1999). *To err is human.* Washington, DC: National Academies Press.

Koerner, J. (2000). Nightingale II: Nursing leaders remembering community. *Nursing Administration Quarterly, 24*(2), 13–18.

Kotter, J. (1995). Leading change: Why transformation efforts fail. *Harvard Business Review, 73*(3), 59–67.

Kotter, J. (2004). From leaders to leadership: Managing change. *Journal of Leadership and Organizational Studies, 10*(4), 114.

Laurent, C. (2000). A nursing theory for nursing leadership. *Journal of Nursing Management, 8*(2), 83.

Mathena, K. (2002). Nursing manager leadership skills. *Journal of Nursing Administration, 32*(3), 136–142.

McDaniel, C. & Wolf, G. (1992). Transformational leadership in nursing service: A test of theory. *Journal of Nursing Administration, 22*(2), 60–65.

Medley, F., & Larochelle, D. (1995). Transformational Leadership and job satisfaction. *Nursing Management, 26,* 64JJ–64LL, 64NN.

Milgram, L., Spector, A., & Treger, M. (1999). *Managing smart.* Houston, TX: Cashman Dudley.

Milstead, J. (2004). Challenging five traditional leadership principles. *Policy, Politics, & Nursing Pratice, 5*(1), 5–9.

Mohrman, S., & Mohrman, A. (1997). *Designing and leading team-based organizations.* San Francisco: Jossey-Bass.

Ohman, K. (1999). Nurse manager leadership. *Journal of Nursing Administration, 29*(12), 16, 21.

*Orlando Business Journal.* (2008, February 29). 250,000 more health care workers needed by 2020. Retrieved from http://www.bizjournals.com/orlando/stories/2008/02/25/daily37.html

O'Rourke, M (2007). Role-based nurse managers: A linchpin to practice excellence. *Nurse Leader, August,* 44–48, 53.

Peter, L., & Hull, R. (1969). *The Peter Principle: Why things go wrong.* New York: William Morrow.

Porter-O'Grady, T. (2001). Profound change: 21st century nursing. *Nursing Outlook, 49*(4), 182–186.

Porter-O'Grady, T., & Finnegan, S. (1984). *Shared governance for nursing: A creative approach to professional accountability.* Gaithersburg, MD: Aspen Publishers Inc.

Porter-O'Grady, T. & Malloch, K. (2007). *Quantum leadership. A resource for health care innovation.* (2nd ed.). Boston: Jones and Barlett Publishers.

Robinson-Walker, C. (2002). Guest editorial: Coaching culture. *Seminars for Nurse Managers, 10*(3), 148–149.

Shaw, S. (2007). *Nursing leadership.* Oxford, UK: International Council of Nurses; Blackwell Publishing.

Snow, J. (2001). Looking beyond nursing for clues to effective leadership. *Journal of Nursing Administration, 31*(9), 440–443.

Sorrells-Jones, J. (1999). The role of the chief nurse executive in the knowledge-intense organization of the future. *Nursing Administration Quarterly, 23*(3), 17–25.

Stahl, D. (1998). Leadership in these changing times. *Nursing Management, 29*(4), 16–18.

Sternweiler, V. (1998). Career journeys: How to be a successful conical nurse specialist—be a willow tree. *Advanced Practice Nursing, 3*(4), 31–33.

Strickland, D. (2000). Emotional Intelligence: The most potent factor in the success equation. *Journal of Nursing Administration, 30*(3), 112–117.

Sullivan, T. (1998). Transformational leadership. In T. Sullivan (Ed.), *Collaboration: A health care imperative* (pp. 467–497). New York: McGraw-Hill.

Tobin, S. (2006). How do you look? *American Nurse Today, October,* 37, 39.

Ulrich, B. (2001). Successfully managing multigenerational workforces. *Seminars for Nurse Managers, 9*(3), 147–153.

Villarosa, L. (2001, May 21). Working to burnish nursing's image. *New York Times,* D7.

Vestal, K. (2002, July). The big picture. *Newsweek,* p. 4.

Vitello-Cicciu, J. (2002). Exploring Emotional Intelligence: Implications for nursing leaders. *Journal of Nursing Administration, 32*(4), 203–210.

Watson, C. (2004). Evidence-based management practices. *Journal of Nursing Administration, 34*(5), 207–209.

Weaver, D. (2001). Transdisciplinary teams: Very important leadership stuff. *Seminars for Nurse Managers, 9*(2), 79–84.

Wolf, G. (2000). Vision 2000: The transformation of professional practice. *Nursing Administration Quarterly, 24*(2), 45–51.

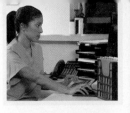

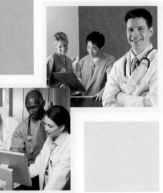

# 2

# Health Care Policy, Legal Issues, and Ethics in Health Care Delivery

## CHAPTER OUTLINE

## LEARNING OUTCOMES

Before you begin, take a moment to familiarize yourself with the learning outcomes for this chapter.

- Explain why nurses should be involved in health care policy.
- Compare and contrast private and public policy.
- Apply the policy-making process.
- Critique the health care reform legislation of 2010 and the provisions that are relevant to nursing.
- Discuss how nurses can be involved in the policy-making process.
- Explain how federal and state laws can affect health care.
- Explain how malpractice and negligence relates to nursing practice.

- Apply ethical decision making to management situations.
- Analyze the impact of health care fraud on the health care system.
- Examine how nurses can become involved in reducing health care fraud and cope with ethical dilemmas presented by fraud.

## KEY TERMS

- Anti-managed care legislation
- Assault
- Autonomy
- Battery
- Beneficence
- Civil law
- Common law
- Consent
- Consent implied by law
- Cost-benefit analysis
- Criminal law
- Disparity
- Doctrine of *res ipsa loquitor*

- Do-not-resuscitate (DNR) directive
- Durable power of attorney (medical power of attorney)
- Ethics
- Informed consent
- Justice
- Law
- Living wills
- Lobbyists
- Malpractice
- Mandated benefits
- Medical-industrial complex
- Negligence

- Nonmalfeasance
- Policy
- Policy criteria
- Policy-making process
- Political process
- Private policy
- Provider protection initiatives
- Public policy
- Resource allocation
- *Respondeat superior* (vicarious liability)
- Veracity
- Whistleblowers

## WHAT'S AHEAD

Nurses in one medical center, who recognized the need for change and the roles of nurses in the change process, made the following statement: "To preserve the quality of care while becoming cost competitive, and to strengthen nurses as integral players in this evolving market, we must become a part of the solution—for our patients, ourselves, and the institutions in which we practice. Our goal is to improve the quality of care provided by nurses, increase both job and patient satisfaction, and strengthen our institution's position in a highly competitive market" (Nokleby et al., 1998, p. 34). This viewpoint continues to be critical today and is even supported more by the Institute of Medicine *Quality Chasm* series of reports on health care. When nurses assume a leadership role in policy development, this better ensures that both nurses' and patients' needs are included in critical health care policies, legislation, and regulation, all of which are directly connected to ethical decision making in the health care environment. This chapter presents content about health care policy and legal and ethical issues. These three topics are interrelated. Policy has both ethical and legal ramifications, and both can be a factor in policy development and implementation. Nurses need to understand policy development, ethics, and legal concerns while they provide care and when they are in leadership roles.

## Health Care Policy

Why is health policy relevant to nurses? "Nurses are aware that today's health care system is in trouble and in need of change. The experiences of many nurses practicing in the real world of health care are motivating them to take on some form of an advocacy role in order to influence change in policies, laws, or regulations that govern the larger health care system. This type of advocacy necessitates stepping beyond their own practice setting and into the less familiar world of policy and politics, a world in which many nurses do not feel prepared to participate effectively (Abood, 2007, p. 3). Nurses should not avoid active participation in health policy and pretend it has nothing to do with nursing. An isolationist approach is never helpful, and for nursing it may actually be a destructive approach. The "changing and unpredictable work environment, coupled with the lack of understanding of broader healthcare policy and finance issues, places nurses in a profoundly disorienting dilemma—How can one be a good nurse amidst increasing technology, decreasing lengths of stays, shifting care from hospitals to ambulatory and home settings, increasing regulations, and shrinking resources? Typically, many nurses respond by taking issues

**FIGURE 2-1  Why is health care policy relevant to nurses?**

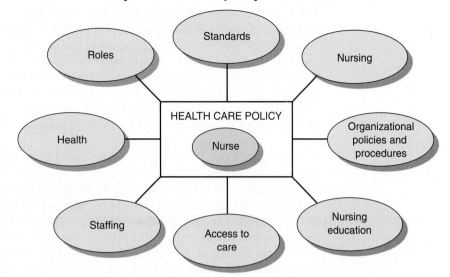

personally, becoming defensive, and 'digging in their heels.' As a result, their perspective narrows instead of broadens; it becomes 'us' versus 'them' (administrators, managers, and regulators)" (Dingel-Stewart & LaCoste, 2004, p. 214). Nurses practice in the health care environment, and health policy and its effects on health care services and the profession are part of that practice. Health policy impacts changes that affect nursing practice, education, staffing, roles, and responsibilities. Legislation and regulation on the state and federal levels affect nursing practice daily. In order to become active participants in the health care environment and the changes that are inevitable, nurses as leaders must become involved in policy development at the local, state, and national levels. Health care policy is critical because it determines what health care services are provided, who provides the services, and who can receive services, reimbursement, quality care, improvements, and requirements. Nurses have always been concerned about consumers. This concern for and understanding of consumers and their needs is an important component of successful policy development. As patient advocates, this is an ideal time to take a leadership position to protect patient rights, ensure that patient needs are met, and ensure that the profession of nursing retains its strength. Figure 2-1 provides a view of the importance of health policy to nurses.

This section of the chapter focuses on health care policy. Policy and how it is developed are addressed to provide background for the specific policy issues that are discussed. There are many health care policies that could be discussed, so those included are only some of the possibilities. Legislation is also discussed in this section because it plays a critical role in health policy. Box 2-1 provides a list of the critical issues found in the rapidly changing health care environment that either become health policy issues or are related to policies.

| BOX 2-1 | THE CHANGING HEALTH CARE ENVIRONMENT: CRITICAL ISSUES |
|---|---|

- Changing practice patterns and the physician
- Cultural diversity
- Federal and state governments
- Growth of advanced practice nursing
- Diagnosis-related groups
- Health care consumerism
- Health care organization mergers and acquisitions
- Health care role changes
- Immigration
- Legislation

- Third-party health care reimbursement
- Medical–industrial complex: Privatization and corporate health care
- Managed competition
- Minority health
- Move from acute care to primary care
- Quality care
- Health care reform
- Restructuring and reengineering of health care organizations
- Uninsured and underinsured

## Key Health Care Policy Issues

There are many important health care issues. Later in this chapter there is a discussion about the health care reform legislation signed into law in 2010, a significant change in health care. The following examples are discussed here: increasing cost of health care, disparity in health care delivery, commercialization of health care, and consumers. Solutions for these issues are typically related to policies. The most significant health policy change in last few decades is the health policy reform legislation passed in 2010: Patient Protection and Affordable Care Act (P.L. 11-148) and Health Care and Education Reconciliation Act (P.L. 111-152). Comments about laws are found in several of the text chapters, and a summary of some of the provisions is found in Appendix B.

INCREASING COST OF HEALTH CARE    "The United States operates a health care system that is unique among nations. It is the most expensive of systems, outstripping by over half the health care expenditures of any other country. By many technical standards, U.S. medical care is the best in the world, but leaders in the field declared in 1997 at a national round table that there is an 'urgent need to improve health care quality'" (Broder, 1997, p. 1). In 2008, Senator Daschle took this perspective a step further and stated, "We like to boast that we have the highest standard of living in the world, and yet at the dawn of the twenty-first century we are the only industrialized nation that does not guarantee necessary health care to all of its citizens" (p. 3). This view has been further supported by the Institute of Medicine (IOM) reports describing the U.S. health care system (1999; 2003):

- The American health care delivery system is in need of fundamental change. (p. 1)
- Health care today harms too frequently and routinely fails to deliver its potential benefits. (p. 1)
- The performance of the health care delivery system varies considerably. (p. 3)
- The health care system as currently structured does not, as a whole, make the best use of its resources. (p. 3)
- What is perhaps most disturbing is the absence of real progress toward restructuring health care systems to address both quality and cost concerns, or toward applying advances in information technology to improve administrative and clinical processes. (p. 3)
- Health care today is plagued today by a serious quality gap. (p. 35) (Institute of Medicine, 2001)

In conclusion the IOM notes that "needed new infrastructures will challenge today's health care leaders—both clinical leaders and management. The necessary environmental changes will require the interest and commitment of payers, health plans, government officials, and regulatory bodies. New skills will require new approaches by professional educators. The 21st-century health care system envisioned by the committee—providing care that is evidence-based, patient-centered, and systems-oriented—also implies new roles and responsibilities for patients and families" (Institute of Medicine, 2001, p. 20). Chapter 16 includes more content about these critical reports.

The U.S. and global economic problems of 2008–2010 had a major negative impact on health care, though the system and insurance coverage were already major problems. In a survey of Americans conducted February 2009, the news was not positive (Henry J. Kaiser Family Foundation, 2009). More than half of Americans (slightly more than 53%) indicated that they limited their medical care due to cost in the past year. The results indicate that there was grave concern about affordability and accessibility of health care when needed. Many people were relying more on over-the-counter drugs rather than visiting physician (35%), and 34% were not keeping dental appointments. Twenty-one percent were not filling prescriptions, and 15% were cutting pills in half or skipping doses. Nineteen percent experienced major financial problems due to medical care that could not be put off. The survey also addressed the respondents' view of health care reform. The focus seems to be more on getting help with costs of health care and getting coverage for those who do not have coverage rather than on improving the quality of care. Given that there is considerable concern about the quality of care as noted in recent Institute of Medicine reports it is important to keep this part of the equation in mind. A dysfunctional health care system costs more money than a functional system that provides quality care with less errors and complications.

The health care industry is a large, complex industry whose financing is influenced by many factors, particularly social expectation, economic trends, technological developments, political factors, and in the last few years the U.S. economy has been the most critical factor. Financial issues affect all aspects of the provision of care, settings, and services, such as inpatient care, ambulatory care, home care, primary care, long-term care, public health, pharmaceutical, medical supplies, medical transportation, medical technology, medical research, and so on. Compared with other countries, the United States has the most expensive health care system though it has the highest living standard and economic status. Rising medical costs have driven many of the changes in health care in the last few decades. What are some of the common causes of increasing health care costs that have had an impact for a number of years (McIntosh, 2002)? As insurance coverage expanded, it became available to more people. There was little incentive not to use health insurance coverage when the patient was required to pay limited out-of-pocket expenses. This, however, changed as employers and insurers recognized that this system led to overuse, and eventually the expansion, of managed care. In the past, health care professionals often paid limited attention to the costs of care (e.g., ordering tests and procedures, using supplies, extending hospital stays) and were not concerned about the relationship of treatment appropriateness and costs. Technological advancement has had both a positive and negative impact. Clearly, these advancements have led to more effective diagnostic approaches and treatment; however, advancements also increase costs. The development of new equipment, procedures, and drugs is expensive, and these costs are passed on to the customer or the employer who covers some of the insurance costs and the consumer (patient). The increasing use of prescription drugs and their costs are difficult problems that are increasing. New drugs usually mean improved treatment, but there is a cost. Whether or not it is a reasonable cost is a critical question. Defensive medicine, which is making medical decisions in order to protect oneself from lawsuits (for example, ordering diagnostic tests to make sure nothing is missed), also affects health care costs. Cost-containment and cost-effectiveness efforts have been tried for many years, some with more success than others. This will undoubtedly continue, and it is important for nurses to understand the problems and possible solutions so that they can participate actively in resolving cost issues. The increasing costs and limited access to health care have led to major problems with the number of uninsured and underinsured in this country, estimated in 2009 to be 46 million (Cover the Uninsured, 2009). In 2003 a national effort began to focus on this critical problem called "Cover the Uninsured Week." Universal health coverage is still not a reality for this country. The health care reform legislation of 2010, however, will have an impact over the number of uninsured with the goal of reducing the number by 32 million by 2014, but it is not universal health care coverage. Everyone will be required to have insurance or pay a fee for not having coverage. Medicaid eligibility will increase thereby increasing its enrollment.

DISPARITY IN HEALTH CARE DELIVERY     **Disparity** in health care delivery is certainly related to the number of uninsured and underinsured, but it is also more than this. The Institute of Medicine report, *Unequal Treatment: Confronting Racial and Ethnic Disparities in Health Care* (2002), addressed factors that might provide causes of disparities in health care. The report indicates that bias, prejudice, and stereotyping on the part of health care providers might be major factors in explaining differences in care. In addition, the report identified clinical uncertainty as an important factor. This was described as any degree of uncertainty a physician may have relative to the patient's condition, which leads the physician to depend on inferences: "The doctor can therefore be viewed as operating with prior beliefs about the likelihood of patients' conditions, 'priors' that will be different according to age, gender, socioeconomic status, and race or ethnicity. When these 'priors' are considered alongside information gathered in a clinical encounter, both influence medical decisions" (Institute of Medicine, 2002, p. 3). Disparities were particularly found in cancer, cardiovascular disease, HIV/AIDS, diabetes, and mental illness.

What can be done to improve the problem? Health care reform legislation of 2010 requires greater monitoring of health disparities with analysis of trends and strategies to address; however, there also needs to be more cross-cultural education for health care professionals to improve awareness of how cultural and social factors affect health care, which should focus on attitudes, knowledge, and skills. Nursing education has included more content and learning experiences related to cross-cultural issues. There also needs to be greater standardization of data collection to gain more understanding of the problem. Nurses need to be leaders in providing direction for this data collection as these are data that affect their practice. A third strategy that needs consideration is the development of policies that look at the entire health care system to decrease fragmentation in the delivery system and education of health care professionals. Fragmented delivery affects nursing care (for example, patients may be more acutely ill when admitted to a hospital or when they come to a clinic because previous care was not coordinated effectively). Chapter 8 includes additional content on culture, diversity, and disparities in health care.

COMMERCIALIZATION OF HEALTH CARE    Since 1994, the United States has struggled for some time to determine the best way to "achieve reasonably equitable distribution of health care, without losing control of total spending on health care, and without suffocating the delivery system with controls and regulations that inhibit technical progress" (Reinhardt, 1994, p. 106). This struggle continues today. Most industrialized countries have chosen to focus on equitable distribution of health care by providing universal coverage; however, the United States continues to vacillate between equity and innovative dynamism. The result has been one of limited success on both sides. A definite result of this struggle has been the development of the **medical–industrial complex**. Health care has changed from a social good to a product. Health care delivery has become commercialized, and health care professionals, such as hospitals and physicians, have turned more toward business techniques, using multiple methods such as advertising and tighter control of costs to survive. The rapid growth in hospitals and other types of health care facilities has at times put pressure on all providers to find patients. This pressure has led to economic problems, increasing costs, and new health care delivery approaches. Not all of these factors have been negative as some changes have resulted in improvement with better management and increased focus on community care. In most communities competition is high among all types of health care organizations. After the Clinton effort to reform health care failed, most of the major changes or reform occurred in the private section, though these changes were modest and did not address the growing number of uninsured. It is, however, the private sector focus that set the stage for the rapid growth of managed care and the tremendous change experienced by the health care delivery system. As managed care expanded, it experienced more criticism. Inevitably, blame became an issue. Many questions arose as managed care became more complex. Who started managed care? Who wanted it? Was it the employers, who experienced accelerating health care costs for their employees? Was it the government, who also experienced this cost acceleration? Was it the consumer, who wanted better access to care and also decreased personal costs? What did the provider want? What were these groups willing to give up? What was managed care supposed to be? These questions have not been easy to answer as the health care system turned more to business methods and managed care. The fact is that the health care delivery system is very complex, with many players, and there is no easy solution for the problem of increasing health care costs. Additional content on health care financing and managed care is found in Chapter 5.

CONSUMERS    There is no doubt that consumers have been greatly troubled by many of the changes that have occurred in the health care delivery system. Of particular concern to consumers are:

- Increasing access problems
- Increasing costs
- Decreasing quality
- Confusion over the role of third-party payers
- Caregiver competence and ethics
- Impersonal care
- Decreased communication

Consumers can no longer rely on having the same physician to care for them over time. Communities are finding that their local hospitals are merging, disappearing, or being purchased by large for-profit health care corporations. Hospitals often lose their community identification with these changes. Many consumers lost their trust in the health care system and its providers, physicians, nurses, and the like. During these changes managed care was very influential. The last few years have revealed a backlash against managed care with **anti-managed care legislation**, which was targeted to reduce managed care control over health care processes and decisions. The media played an important role in getting the word out about managed care and consumer concerns. Congress focused on issues of health care consumer rights, and cases related to managed care found their way to the U.S. Supreme Court. Employers even felt the backlash from their employees, who requested more health care plan options and insisted on their right to choose their own health care providers. This does not mean that managed care was eliminated, but rather that it has changed over the years. It has also had an impact on all types of health care insurers that have adopted many of the managed care approaches to health care coverage. Recent legislative activity has finally addressed the growing concern of prescription coverage for seniors, and yet even before the legislation was passed there were criticisms about the proposed coverage (for example, the amount of out-of-pocket costs seniors would still have to pay). It is clear that consumers are playing a greater role in health care policy and that this will continue. Health care reform legislation of 2010 also addressed Part D of Medicare (prescription coverage) by further reducing the cost to Medicare beneficiaries over time. Chapter 10 discusses health care consumerism in more detail. This is a topic that nurses need to be aware of since nurses often assume the role of patient advocate.

## The Policy-Making Process

A **policy** is a course of action that affects a large number of people, and it is stimulated by a need (Bodenheimer & Grumbach, 1998). Policies may include a mixture of laws, regulations, interpretations, court decisions, and other information relevant to the policy content. What is the purpose of health care policy? It can answer questions such as:

- What health care services are reimbursed?
- What is the reimbursement for a particular health care service?
- Who can obtain reimbursement for a service?
- How are health care resources allocated?
- Who is eligible for specific health care services?
- Who may provide a service?
- What are the educational requirements and competencies required for specific health care professionals?
- Who pays for health care services?

These are all critical questions in today's health care environment, and they demonstrate the impact that policy has on health care delivery. Why are these questions important for nurses? Input from health care professionals is important during the policy-making process. Health care professionals have expertise that may affect policy outcome, and nursing practice is often directly affected by health care policy.

PUBLIC AND PRIVATE POLICY    Despite the active involvement of these organizations and others in the United States, the federal government is the major influence on the financing, structure, and delivery of health care services. One might conclude that because of the federal government's major role the United States would have an overall health care policy. This, however, is not the case, and this is a problem. The lack of a coordinated federal and state view of health care delivery often results in different, sometimes conflictual, approaches to health problems. For example, the purposes of some health care policies are not always easy to understand (Bodenheimer & Grumbach, 1998). Some policies are poorly written and designed. Others are purposely vague so that many groups can feel they are represented by the policy. Not everyone will be a winner with every policy. This is particularly important to understand with health care policy. Some groups are represented and receive the services they need, and in the same policy, others are denied services due to lack of funds, resources, and the like.

Box 2-2 identifies some of the key federal government departments and agencies that participate actively in developing public policy in an effort to address these complex issues, and Figure 2-2 describes the U.S. Department of Health and Human Services.

There are two categories of policies: private and public. **Private policy** is health care policy that is developed by either health care organizations or a profession, such as nursing. Some examples of organizations that participate in health care policy development are identified in Box 2-3.

<table>
<tr><td>BOX 2-2</td><td>IMPORTANT FEDERAL GOVERNMENT DEPARTMENTS AND AGENCIES</td></tr>
</table>

- Agency for Healthcare Quality and Research (AHCQR)
- Center for Medicare and Medicaid Services (CMS)
- Centers for Disease Control and Prevention (CDC)
- Consumer Product Safety Commission (CPSC)

- Department of Health and Human Services (DHHS)
- Food and Drug Administration (FDA)
- National Institute of Occupational Safety and Health (NIOSH)
- National Institutes of Health (NIH)
- Occupational Safety and Health Administration (OSHA)
- Veteran's Administration (VA)

**FIGURE 2-2   U.S. Department of Health and Human Services.**

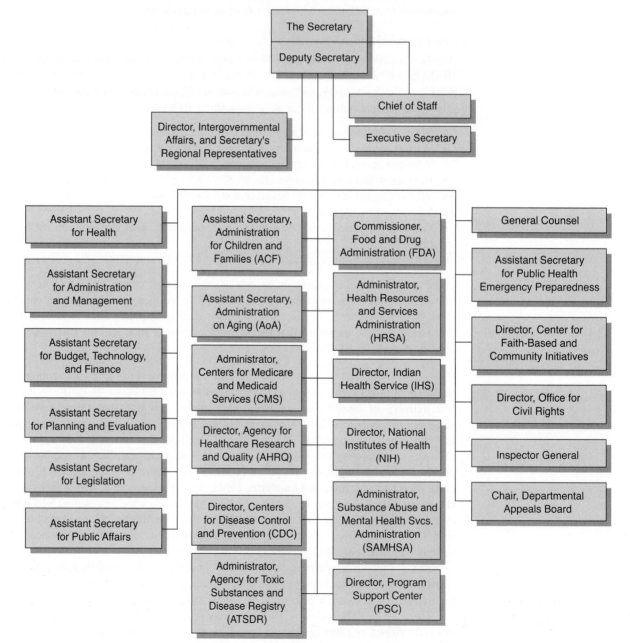

**Public policy** should reflect the needs of the public, but politics influence and shape many policies, sometimes to the detriment of the policy. "The unacceptable options are that you cannot ask people to reduce their own quality of care so more people will have care; you cannot displace them from private coverage to enter a government program; and you cannot ask them to voluntarily go into a government program if it's less generous than the private coverage they already have" (Toner, 1999, p. A1). "There are two main types of public policies: (1) regulatory policies (e.g., registered nurse (RN) licensure that regulates practice) and (2) allocative policies, which involve money distribution. Allocative policies provide benefits for some at the expense of others to ensure that certain public objectives are met" (Finkelman & Kenner, 2010, p. 173). It is difficult to develop public policy because there are often conflicts that must be considered. It is also impossible to meet all needs for all people. This means that choices will be made, and this is where politics have an effect. Deals will be made. Compromises are required. **Cost-benefit analysis** is used to determine the costs and benefits of the various alternatives and then to select the best choice. Figure 2-3 describes several types of public policies that are relevant to health care policy.

The **policy-making process** should be very familiar to nurses because it is the problem-solving process, similar to the nursing process. The policy process steps are described in Figure 2-4.

To begin this process it is critical to assess the problems in order to arrive at the best solution. Part of this assessment must include the impact the policy might have "on people, the economy, the environment, technology, and the health care system as a whole" (Ferguson, 2001, p. 547). **Policy criteria** are identified during the policy-making process to be used as policy issues are analyzed. Today, typical criteria used in the development of health care policy are

- Cost-benefit analysis
- Efficiency
- Equity

Generally, people think of policy as providing the greatest good for the greatest number of people, but not all policies do this. Political feasibility must be considered when policies are developed because it can make the difference between a successful policy and a failed one. If a policy is developed and legislation is proposed that supports the policy but there is limited political support for it, the policy and its legislation will never be accepted. Today, outcomes have become a more important consideration in policy development. Outcome delivery analysis allows for more informed decision-making. Reasons for this interest continue to be

1. Payers are demanding information about the results of care delivery.
2. Outcomes are an integral part of accreditation.
3. Consumers have a right to know about outcomes.
4. Regulatory agencies demand information about outcomes.
5. Outcomes represent the basic reason for providing care (Jones, Jennings, Moritz, & Moss, 1997, p. 261).

| BOX 2-3 | EXAMPLES OF ORGANIZATIONS IMPORTANT TO THE HEALTH CARE DELIVERY SYSTEM |
|---|---|

- National Association of Children's Hospitals and Related Institutions (NACHRI)
- American Academy of Hospice and Palliative Medicine (AAHPM)
- American Association of Homes and Services for the Aging (AAHSA)
- American Association of Retired Persons (AARP)
- American Home Care Association (AHCA)
- American Hospital Association (AHA)
- American Nurses Association (ANA)
- Nursing Specialty Organizations
- American Public Health Association (APHA)
- Disease-focused organizations; for example, Arthritis Foundation (AF), American Diabetes Association (ADA)
- Joint Commission on the Accreditation of Healthcare Organizations (Joint Commission)
- National Association of Private Psychiatric Hospitals (NAPPH)
- National Association of Public Hospitals (NAPH)
- National Committee on Quality Assurance (NCQA)
- National Health Council (NHC)

**FIGURE 2-3   Types of public policy.**

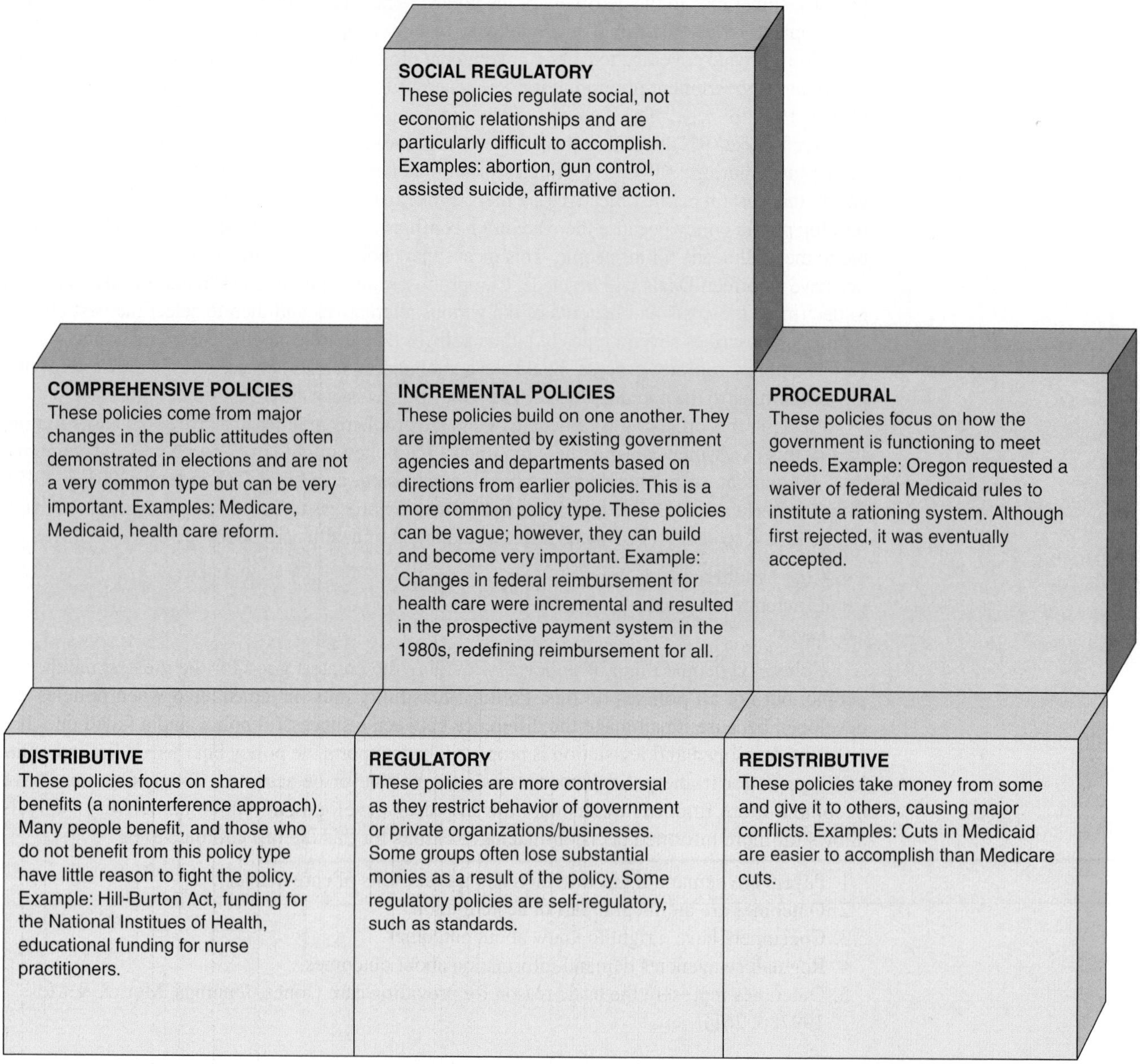

**SOCIAL REGULATORY**
These policies regulate social, not economic relationships and are particularly difficult to accomplish. Examples: abortion, gun control, assisted suicide, affirmative action.

**COMPREHENSIVE POLICIES**
These policies come from major changes in the public attitudes often demonstrated in elections and are not a very common type but can be very important. Examples: Medicare, Medicaid, health care reform.

**INCREMENTAL POLICIES**
These policies build on one another. They are implemented by existing government agencies and departments based on directions from earlier policies. This is a more common policy type. These policies can be vague; however, they can build and become very important. Example: Changes in federal reimbursement for health care were incremental and resulted in the prospective payment system in the 1980s, redefining reimbursement for all.

**PROCEDURAL**
These policies focus on how the government is functioning to meet needs. Example: Oregon requested a waiver of federal Medicaid rules to institute a rationing system. Although first rejected, it was eventually accepted.

**DISTRIBUTIVE**
These policies focus on shared benefits (a noninterference approach). Many people benefit, and those who do not benefit from this policy type have little reason to fight the policy. Example: Hill-Burton Act, funding for the National Institues of Health, educational funding for nurse practitioners.

**REGULATORY**
These policies are more controversial as they restrict behavior of government or private organizations/businesses. Some groups often lose substantial monies as a result of the policy. Some regulatory policies are self-regulatory, such as standards.

**REDISTRIBUTIVE**
These policies take money from some and give it to others, causing major conflicts. Examples: Cuts in Medicaid are easier to accomplish than Medicare cuts.

Outcome data are then used to assist in the development of health care policy by either improving policy, deleting policy or by creating new policies. With the increasing concern about the quality of care outcomes are even more important to better understanding current care delivery (Institute of Medicine, 2001).

## The Political Process

Since most health policy comes through the legislative process, politics cannot be ignored. "Generally, health policies influence groups and organizations. Health policies express decisions made by legislators and regulators or other judicial and governmental entities" (Ferguson, 2001, p. 547). Nurses get involved in the **political process**, often at the local and state levels, to provide input in the direction that health policy will take; how it will be implemented; and how best to evaluate the results or outcomes. Nurses need to understand the process and the system so that they can influence these decisions. More nurses have assumed

**FIGURE 2-4    The policy-making process.**

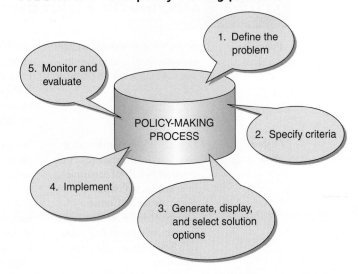

leadership roles in policy making by holding elected public offices in state legislatures and Congress and holding positions in many government agencies. This gives nursing more voice in policy making at all levels. Lobbying is another important tool. Coalition building helps nurses join together with other groups that have similar interests. This increases opportunity to demonstrate strength in numbers and better clarify nursing perspectives about health care and about the nursing profession. Networking and collaboration require some compromises. The end result should be as effective as possible. All of this is related to leadership and the skills of communication, planning and decision-making, collaboration, responding to change effectively, and encouraging participation of nurses on all levels. Recognizing the importance of political feasibility requires that political factors need to be factored into the consideration of the review of possible solutions to policy issues and also included in the selection of the recommended solutions. Selecting a solution that does not have a chance of succeeding due to politics is not helpful and only leads to frustration. When legislation is enacted, the next step is to develop rules or regulations that guide implementation of the law or the policy. As policy is implemented, it should be monitored, which may lead to additional changes. This entire process is cyclical in that evaluation data lead to other policies or reshaping of current policy. The process is also dynamic as it is affected by many factors throughout the process. Table 2-1 describes this process.

## Health Care Policy and Nursing

As changes occur in the health care environment, health care policy, legislation, regulation, and ethics, it is important for nurses to understand and participate in the legislative process and consider how policy may affect ethical decision-making. Active involvement of nurses in all of these areas must occur at the local, state, and federal levels. What are some examples of issues that have affected nursing?

1. An example of a policy issue that offered nursing many opportunities and substantial risks is the development of managed care in health care reimbursement. Nurses recognize that there are aspects of managed care that demonstrate positive changes in health care delivery, such as preventive services and a greater emphasis on the continuum of care rather than episodic care. Nurses are also confronted with staffing shortages, shortened hospital stays, increasing patient acuity both in the hospital and in the community, less staff, and a complex reimbursement system. These changes have made it difficult for nurses and other health care professionals to deliver what they believe is quality care.

| TABLE 2-1 | APPLYING THE POLICY DEVELOPMENT PROCESS | |
|---|---|---|
| Policy issue develops | Senator learns about consumer concern about a health issue and has staff work on the issue. | Staffing levels in acute care hospitals are affecting the quality and safety of care. Examples of errors and lack of quality are provided from various hospitals that have led to patient deaths and to complications that have extended the need for treatment. |
| Gather data about issue | Legislative staff gathers data about the issue; some data may come from federal departments or agencies, which act as resources for legislative activity. Criteria are developed to evaluate the data (e.g., cost, efficiency, equity, and political feasibility). | Testimony may be provided from experts, patients, insurers, hospitals, nurses, physicians, and so on. Data related to errors, quality, and access will be used to further understand the problem. Data about enrollment and graduation rates in nursing schools would be important to obtain. Costs would be critical to obtain related to lack of staff: costs for the hospitals, insurers, employers, and patients (consumers). |
| Coalition building | Senator will form coalitions to back the legislation with other Senators, Congressmen, and stakeholders. | Stakeholders that would be interested in this problem and solution would be health care professionals and their organizations (nurses, physicians), American Hospital Association, insurers, employers, consumer groups, nurse educators, and others. Building a coalition from these groups would help to get the bill passed. |
| Identify possible solutions | Apply cost-benefit analysis of data to determine possible solutions; testimony from experts, lobbyists input and pressure; arrive at list of possible solutions. | Cost data would be used to help assess cost-benefit for each of the possible solutions. Some examples of solutions might be: do nothing, require every hospital to have a specific number of staff, require hospitals to use a patient classification system or require that every hospital use the same system, require minimum ratios, and many others. |
| Select a solution | Federal (or state) written law will probably repeat some of the activities described as part of "identify possible solutions" to gather more data or clarify. Coalition building also continues throughout the process. | For this example, requiring a minimum ratio is selected as the solution. (This does not indicate that it is the best solution but is just used for an example in this scenario.) A law is drafted by the Senator based on information gathered during the first phases of the process. The Senator will need to gain additional support in the Senate and then in the House of Representatives to get the law supported by a Representative(s). The law will wind its way through the legislative process. |
| Implement policy | Rules and regulations are developed; staff receives feedback on rules and regulations; and implement rules and regulations to apply the law. | DHHS develops draft of rules and regulations that will be used to implement the law. Professional organizations respond to them by providing feedback. The American Hospital Association submits criticisms. Rules and regulations are revised and may be posted for additional comments. By specific date, rules and regulations are effective and required by law. Hospitals will have to get this information and make appropriate changes to meet requirements (e.g., increase staffing or alter ratios, recruit more staff, and so on). |

| TABLE 2-1 | APPLYING THE POLICY DEVELOPMENT PROCESS (CONTINUED) | |
|---|---|---|
| Monitor outcomes: evaluation | Federal department or agency responsible for implementation develops evaluation plan and monitors outcomes. The department may have to report to Congress at specific times, and may recommend and implement changes as long as within framework of the law. Otherwise, the department will need to recommend legislative changes (new law or amendments to law). | Outcomes analysis is ongoing. What are the outcomes of the plan to establish a minimum staffing ratio? Are hospitals able to meet the requirement deadlines? If not, what are the barriers? Can the barriers be addressed and how? |

2. Understanding health policy and its implications for leadership and management is a journey through the health care delivery system, its players, its successes and its limitations, and its future. If there is acceptance that the health care environment is a dynamic, changing environment, critical questions to consider are what will be the role of the nurse in this process and what will be the end product? The new health care environment demands that providers take responsibility for whole populations. The focus is not just on curing patients but also preventing illness and providing care across the health care continuum. High-quality care must be provided in all types of settings and by all providers, and it must be cost-effective. Health care professionals need to develop new skills, competencies, and attitudes toward their work in order to reinvent their professional culture. Nursing has recognized this change by including more content about community health in nursing education.

3. The increase in direct reimbursement for care provided by advanced practice nurses is an excellent example of the impact of legislation and government on nursing practice. Over time this reimbursement has expanded.

4. The federal government continues to provide additional funding for nursing education, something that is a major concern each year as the federal budget is developed. State legislation has also had a major impact on nursing practice. This legislation offers many opportunities to pilot new programs in education and delivery. Health Resources Services Administration (HRSA) offers funding for grants to trial new education and practice approaches such as academic/clinical partnerships, nurse residency programs, and programs to increased diversity in the nursing profession, and scholarship and loan opportunities.

5. An example of a health policy change that has had a major impact on health care delivery in California was the passage of legislation that requires California hospitals to meet fixed nurse–patient ratios (Purdum, 1999). This policy is affecting health policy in other states and on the federal level, as similar legislation is considered. Health care issues that are affected by nursing, and few are not, require nursing input if nursing is to remain a viable health care profession in the health care environment.

How do nurses participate in health care policy development? Active participation in nursing organizations gives every nurse a voice, as nursing organizations are often represented on committees that develop health care policy or provide input (for example, the President's Advisory Commission on Consumer Protection and Quality in the Health Care Industry, 1996–1998, and the recent Institute of Medicine reports on quality health care). Chapter 16 includes additional information on these topics. Nursing organizations use **lobbyists** to make regular contact with elected officials, both state and federal, in order to influence policy development. In fact, some of these lobbyists are nurses. Each year, the American Nurses Association (ANA) identifies key issues that it will focus on as it lobbies Congress. Typical issues include: nurse staffing plans and ratios, mandatory overtime, nurse education incentives and funding, needlestick protection, advanced practice Medicaid reimbursement, whistleblower protection, ergonomics, nursing workforce data, latex allergies, continued competence, unlicensed assistive personnel, violence in the workplace, and immigration and the nursing workforce. These issues have a direct impact on practice. Individual nurses are encouraged to contact their own elected representatives by mail, e-mail, or telephone and provide them with important information about nursing and health care needs in their communities. Nursing expertise has been very beneficial to policy makers, but if nurses do not speak out, they will not be recognized for their expertise.

An example of how nursing expertise can be used to assist policy development occurred when the president of the ANA testified before a Senate committee about the relationship between staffing decisions and patient safety (Gross & Reed, 1999). This testimony was related to the release of the government-initiated report, *To Err Is Human. Building a Safer Health System* (Institute of Medicine, 1999), which has evolved into a major health care issue today (Finkelman & Kenner, 2009). There are many examples of nurses representing many nursing organizations by providing testimony on the local, state, and federal levels. Understanding consumer needs and acting as the patient's advocate have been important elements of nursing for a long time. Nurses can help consumers understand health care policy, legislation, regulation, and their effect on health care delivery. There should be no doubt that every nurse has a role to play. It may be in writing a letter to a member of Congress, calling a senator, attending a nursing organization meeting, providing expert testimony, serving on a local or state health care planning committee, or participating in other types of activities to influence policy development.

IMPORTANCE OF COLLABORATION IN HEALTH CARE POLICY    Concern over health care changes, policy, and reimbursement has even brought nurses and physicians closer as they work collaboratively for a common goal: better-quality care. Nurses and physicians need to do much more of this to solve problems such as staff cutbacks, quality issues, patients' rights, and ethical concerns.

An example of collaboration between nursing and other organizations is ANA's project with Johnson & Johnson to developed several media campaigns to address the need for more nurses. Nurses recognize the need to further develop the image of nursing and that combining communication skills, consumer education, and media expertise will help to improve the image. Sometimes this will mean collaborating with others such as physicians and other health care professions to initiate a broader media impact that affects the profession's image as a member of the interprofessional team, and at other times, it will mean focusing just on nursing and what nurses can do. Collaboration is required as health care professionals participate in health care changes. New ways to support collaboration need to be created (Institute of Medicine, 2003; Finkelman & Kenner, 2009).

## Legislation: Impact on Health Care Delivery and Policy

What is important health care legislation, both federal and state, and how has this legislation affected health care delivery? Legislation is a part of health policy and also has a direct impact on legal and ethical issues in health care delivery. Legislation occurs at all three government levels: federal, state, and local. Most health care legislation is found at the federal and state levels, so these two levels will be the focus in this chapter. Nurses should, however, be aware of relevant local legislation that might be passed by cities or counties.

FEDERAL LEVEL    The federal legislative process is clearly defined and is important to nursing. The American Nurses Association (ANA) website includes a description of the process so that it can be used by nurses as they become involved in policy development. The political action component of the ANA is very active in influencing health policy and monitoring legislation. Other nursing organizations are also involved such as the American Organization of Nurse Executives (AONE), the National League for Nursing (NLN), the American Association of Colleges of Nursing (AACN), and nursing specialty organizations. When legislation is signed into law, the work is not done. Most legislation establishes or modifies federal or state programs. When this occurs, the administrative responsibility of a federal or state law becomes the responsibility of a federal or state agency, program, or department. An example is the Department of Health and Human Services (DHHS), the Centers for Medicare and Medicaid Services (CMS), which is responsible for implementation of Medicare and Medicaid laws. Before a law is implemented, regulations are developed. Regulations are critical because they describe how the law will be implemented. The regulations can make a difference in the law's success. In the federal arena, draft regulations are published in the *Federal Register*, which makes the regulations available for public comment. In some cases, public hearings are held to discuss the regulations. When health care legislation and its regulations are important to nurses, representatives from nursing organizations often comment on regulation drafts. In addition, nurses may have participated earlier in the health care policy development, such as by providing expert testimony to Congressional committees, lobbying efforts, and so forth. Regulations can affect staffing, health care organization policies and procedures, access to care, and other delivery issues. All comments about regulations are considered, and then the agency/program/department releases the final regulations. This occurs at least 30 days prior to the effective date of application. After that date, the law and its regulations are in effect. Understanding the history of critical health care legislation, relationships between laws, and their effect on the delivery system is very important for all health care professionals who hope to participate in future health care policy development and implementation. There is no doubt that remaining current with federal legislation can be a time-consuming activity, which is why nursing organizations have lobbyists who follow legislation and provide input, as well as political action committees (PACs), to influence the policy making and election processes. There are many more options that could be explored. As nurses enter practice, laws relevant to their practice should be understood. With access to the Internet, it is easier to keep current with health care legislation.

What are the critical federal legislation and regulation actions related to health care delivery in the United States? The two pieces of legislation and their amendments that have had the most impact on the health and welfare system in the United States are the Social Security Act of 1935 and the Public Health Act of 1944. The changes and additions to these laws demonstrate the long-term effect that laws can have on society. Passing legislation should not be taken lightly because it may not be easy to reverse and has a major impact on citizens/consumers. Accountability and responsibility are critical components of the legislative process.

STATE LEVEL    States play an active role in health care policy, legislation, and regulation. Generally, they are involved in financing, delivery of services, and oversight of insurance. The latter has become very important as managed care developed and had an impact on all types of health care insurance. There are five typical health care areas in which the states have major input.

1. **Public health and safety.**   States are responsible for protecting public welfare, including services related to such areas as prevention and treatment of communicable diseases, monitoring of environmental health conditions, harm from violence, and workplace accidents.
2. **Provision of indigent care.**   Most state constitutions require that the state, either alone or with local governments, provide health care to those who cannot pay for it. This is usually done through state or local government-run facilities and the Medicaid program. This care changes as health care policy, delivery, and reimbursement change.
3. **Purchase care.**   Many states have been changing from providers of health care to purchasers of care. This is particularly relevant for the Medicaid program and for state public employees for whom the state provides insurance coverage. This requires that states monitor the care they that purchase.
4. **Regulation.**   States are responsible for licensing and/or credentialing facilities and professionals to ensure quality and for regulating insurers. Through this process states get involved in regulation of health care services issues such as quality improvement, utilization review, solvency, benefits, marketing, access to services, provider contracting, rating, grievances and appeals, organizational structure, reporting, consumer concerns, and confidentiality. These activities demonstrate the major role that states have in the regulation of insurers.
5. **Resource allocation.**   Historically, states have not been responsible for funding of medical and nursing education because this has been in federal hands; however, some states have become more involved in funding issues for nursing education due to the increasing concern about the nursing shortage problem at the state level. States are involved in identifying state health care delivery needs (e.g., number of health care professionals that a state needs to graduate to meet state health care needs). Some states still assist in funding some public health care facilities. Due to the California legislation in 2002 that directed the California state health department to develop staffing guidelines, many other states have now considered doing something similar, which means the states will be more involved in health resource allocation. This is a good example of how legislation passed in one state can have impact on other states and what they might consider legislative issues.

States have their own process for developing, passing, and implementing their laws and procedures related to its regulation process, although this process is usually similar to the federal process. Nurses need to understand their own state process and participate when content is relevant to nursing. Nurses are usually even more involved in the process at the state level than at the federal level. The state nurses' association is often the major player. State activities are more accessible to nurses for lobbying, support of candidates, involvement in committees, and personal contact with legislators. Often nurses feel less intimidated by the state level than the federal level. As noted earlier, Table 2-1 provides a description of the relationship between the policy process and the legislative process.

## Health Care Reform

Early in the Obama administration significant steps were taken to begin to address the crisis in health care, for example (The White House, 2009):

- The President signed the Children's Health Insurance Reauthorization Act on February 4, 2009, which provides quality health care to 11 million children—4 million who were previously uninsured.
- The President's American Recovery and Reinvestment Act protects health coverage for 7 million Americans who lose their jobs through a 65 percent COBRA subsidy to make coverage affordable.
- The Recovery Act also invests $19 billion in computerized medical records that will help to reduce costs and improve quality while ensuring patients' privacy.
- The Recovery Act also provides
  - $1 billion for prevention and wellness to improve America's health and help to reduce health care costs
  - $1.1 billion for comparative effectiveness research that will give doctors objective information about which treatments work and which do not
  - $500 million for health workforce to help train the next generation of doctors and nurses

The Obama Administration's 2009 health care reform approach initiative goals included (The White House, 2009):

- Reduce long-term growth of health care costs for businesses and government
- Protect families from bankruptcy or debt because of health care costs
- Guarantee choice of doctors and health plans
- Invest in prevention and wellness
- Improve patient safety and quality of care
- Assure affordable, quality health coverage for all Americans
- Maintain coverage when you change or lose your job
- End barriers to coverage for people with pre-existing medical conditions

The Patient Protection and Affordable Care Act became law on March 23, 2010 (P.L. 111-148) and then the Health Care and Education Reconciliation Act of 2010 became law on March 30, 2010 (P.L. 111-152). The latter law reconciled some concerns with the Senate version, which became P.L. 111-148. Public Law 111-148 has numerous provisions covering a broad range of issues from health reimbursement, delivery, research, delivery models, and practice. This is significant legislation; however, there is always the potential that over time the law will be changed—this is part of the political process. The law will be implemented over a number of years with some provisions not implemented until 2018 (*Washington Post*, 2010). Appendix B provides a summary of some of the new law's provisions, and content about reimbursement is found in Chapter 5, though many chapters include comments about this new law and its impact on health care delivery.

The American Nurses Association's press release following the signing of the health care reform legislation stated, "'ANA strongly believes that this law is a significant victory for the patients we serve. They'll have greater protection against losing or being denied health insurance coverage, and they'll have better access to primary care and the wellness and prevention programs that will keep them healthier,' said ANA President Rebecca M. Patton, MSN, RN, CNOR. 'However, we recognize that the debate over reform is not over. We are committed to helping nurses and the public understand how this change affects their lives, and will continue our work to build an affordable health care system that meets the needs of everyone.' Heading into the 2008 elections, ANA, the nation's largest nursing organization, published *Health System Reform Agenda*, an update of principles first disseminated in the early 1990s that defines health care as a basic human right and calls for guaranteed access to high-quality, affordable health care for everyone. Registered nurses nationwide have heeded the call since the election to try to make the promise of universal health coverage a reality by contacting members of Congress, testifying at hearings, sharing personal stories, participating in high-profile press conferences, attending rallies and events, and joining ANA's health care reform team" (American Nurses Association, 2010, p. 1).

# Legal Issues and Nursing

Each nurse confronts legal issues daily in practice, although often it may not be obvious. Administering medication, restraining patients, protecting patients from falls or observing a patient on suicide precautions all have a legal component. Documentation is critical to any legal issue that may arise in the clinical setting. The statement "if it isn't documented it didn't happen" is highly relevant to any malpractice suit. What do nurses need to know about the legal issues? They certainly do not have to be attorneys, and they should seek the advice of an attorney whenever they are involved in a serious legal issue. Some issues, however, bear some review so that nurses have a basic understanding of the critical issues. Prior to reviewing these issues, it is important to distinguish the difference between law and ethics. **Law** is the formal organization of societal values that are demonstrated through laws that are passed and then implemented on the local, state, and federal level, and in some cases, even internationally. **Ethics** focuses on what ought to be done in relation to what is done. This section also discusses some aspects of ethics in relation to health care delivery in a later section. Understanding legal issues is important for any nurse in practice and for nurses who are leaders.

## Basic Legal Terminology

Laws are developed and implemented through organizations within society. State legislatures or the Congress, as well as state and local governments, develop these laws. They are then implemented by state and federal law enforcement agencies or other agencies such as the state board of nursing. There are several types of laws.

1. **Common laws** are rules and principles that were derived from past legal decisions that were developed in England and then brought to the United States.
2. **Criminal law** concerns offenses against the general public, and response is directed at deterrence, punishment, and/or rehabilitation of the person who committed the crime. Examples of behavior or actions that relate to this law would be murder, robbery, and rape. Criminal law can also apply to health care situations as it covers assault and battery, which can occur in the health care setting.
3. **Civil law** concerns the rights of individuals, and remedies typically involve payment of money or some type of compensation. An area of civil law that most concerns nurses is tort law as it includes negligence, personal injury, and medical malpractice.

The following provides information about basic legal terms that are important for the nurse to understand.

1. Negligence and malpractice are terms that are not uncommon for nurses to hear. What is the difference between malpractice and negligence?
   - "**Negligence** is a general term that denotes conduct lacking in due care. Thus, negligence equates with carelessness. . . . **Malpractice** is a more specific term and looks at a professional standard of care as well as the professional status of the caregiver . . . the failure of a professional person to act in accordance with the prevailing professional standards or failure to foresee consequences that a professional person, having the necessary skills and education, should foresee" (Guido, 2001, p. 79). Negligence is the failure to act as an ordinary prudent person would under similar circumstances. This is based on that person's education and training.
   - The standard in negligence is average level of care. A variety of sources for standards exist (for example, expert witness testimony, accreditation requirements, publications by experts, clinical practice guidelines or pathways, statutes and regulations, advertising

for services, contracts, and professional standards). To prove negligence there are four elements that must be met, which are described in Box 2-4.

- Damages or injuries may be physical, emotional, loss of job, loss of present and/or future earnings, disfigurement, disability, pain and suffering, loss of enjoyment of life, and so on.

- Negligence can be unintentional (when no harm was intended) or intentional (for example, invasion of privacy or false imprisonment are examples of intentional acts, although these are rare in health care). Both of types of negligence can occur in health care when a patient's privacy is not maintained or when a patient is held against his/her wishes without legitimate medical reasons.

- The elements that must be met for malpractice are the same as those for negligence with the emphasis on what would be expected from a professional. Some of the examples of potential risks for nurses are failure to adequately assess, monitor, and communicate, failure to act as the patient's advocate (for example, not providing patient education to a patient who has diabetes), or failure to protect a patient when the patient is suicidal or when at risk for falls. Every nurse needs to consider these risks when care is provided or when holding management positions.

- As noted earlier there are certain elements that must be proved by the plaintiff; however, there is an exception, which is called the **doctrine of** *res ipsa loquitor*, which means that the "thing speaks for itself." This rule of evidence indicates that although one may not be able to prove that an individual did something to cause harm or injury, because there is harm or injury, the negligence can be inferred.

- A question that often comes up with nurses is who is responsible for negligence: the nurse or the nurse's employer? *Respondeat superior* is the doctrine that says the employer may also be responsible if the nurse was functioning in the employee role at the time of the negligence in a situation where the employer controlled the nurse (Guido, 2001). This means that both the health care organization and the nurse could be sued. This is also referred to as **vicarious liability**, which extends liability.

- Other terms of interest are assault and battery, although many nurses may not see how these apply to nursing care. **Assault** does not require physical contact, but only that the patient fears harmful contact may occur. There has to be some consideration given to timing and the fear that results, as one could not call a threat that happens several days earlier assault. **Battery** requires actual physical contact. Both of these are considered intentional torts. They are good reasons for obtaining informed consent from patients before procedures are performed, which could be assault or battery if the patient does not consent.

2. Consumer rights issues have become more and more important in health care. Consent, living wills, durable powers of attorney, and assisted suicide are some of these issues.
   - **Consent** "may be either oral, implied by law, or apparent" (Guido, 2001, p. 109). This can be as simple as the patient orally consenting to being touched by a nurse, and in this case, there is no risk of battery.
   - **Consent implied by law** is consent that may occur in emergency situations when, even though the patient may not be able to provide consent for emergency treatment, emergency treatment can be given. The following elements must be met to be consent implied by law: "(1) An immediate decision is made to prevent loss of life or limb; (2) The person is incapable of giving or denying consent; (3) There is no reason to believe that consent would not be given if the patient were capable of such; and (4) A reasonable person in the same or similar circumstances would give consent" (Guido, 2001, p. 109).

---

### BOX 2-4    ELEMENTS OF NEGLIGENCE

1. There was a duty owed to the patient.
2. There was a breach of duty or standard by the health care professional.

3. There was harm caused by the breach of duty or standard.
4. The person (plaintiff) experienced damages or injuries.

- **Informed consent** "mandates to the physician or independent health care practitioner the separate legal duty to disclose needed material facts in terms that patients can reasonably understand so that they can make an informed choice" (Guido, 2001, p. 129). It is an interactive process in that the practitioner is required to tell the patient who will perform the procedure or treatment, discuss available alternatives to the recommended treatment, and identify possible harm in language the patient can understand. Patients must be informed that they have the right to refuse treatment. If there is no informed consent, the practitioner is at risk for negligence. Informed consent can be given orally or in writing, and it can also be implied by the patient's behavior, or as noted earlier, in emergency situations it can be presumed. The physician or the independent practitioner is accountable for obtaining informed consent. So where does this leave the nurse who is not an advanced practice nurse functioning as an independent practitioner? The nurse is not accountable for obtaining the consent for every nursing action, as most routine nursing interventions are implied or there is oral consent (for example, the patient agrees to take the medication). The critical elements for the nurse are to "continually communicate with the patient, explaining procedures, and obtaining the patient's permission. What it also means is that the patient's refusal to allow a certain procedure must be respected" (Guido, 2001, p. 135). A nurse is not required to obtain informed consent for medical procedures for which the nurse is not the primary provider. Guido (2001) provides an example of a surgical patient and the nurse's responsibility for postoperative teaching that is begun before surgery. The best approach is for the nurse to wait until the patient's physician explains the procedure and obtains informed consent and then to begin patient teaching. Some hospitals and other types of health care organizations may prohibit nurses from obtaining written consent for specific procedures that are provided by other providers. It is important for each nurse to know about these prohibitions and to follow them. Physicians may legally delegate getting informed consent to a nurse; however, if a problem occurs the physician is still at risk. In this situation the nurse is also at risk (Guido, 2001).
- Informed consent for human research is very important. Many nurses participate in research in a variety of settings such as hospitals, clinics, and research institutes. The key elements of consent for research include:
  1. Nature, purpose, procedures, drugs, or devices involved
  2. Identification of any experimental procedures
  3. Potential benefits, risks, and discomforts to participant
  4. Alternative treatments
  5. Confidentiality of research records
  6. Compensation if injury occurs
  7. Persons to contact about rights, and what to do if research results in an injury
  8. A statement indicating that research is voluntary and that withdrawal does not incur penalty (Karigan, 2001, p. 30)
- **Living wills** "are directives from competent individuals to medical personnel and family members regarding the treatment they wish to receive when they can no longer make the decision for themselves" (Guido, 2001, p. 152). If a person is competent, a living will serves no purpose as the person can speak for himself. Several important points about living wills should be noted. Living wills are usually not very specific. Health care providers are not required by law to follow the living will, and there is no legal protection for the health care provider against civil or criminal liability.
- The **durable power of attorney (medical power of attorney)** is another method that an individual can use to determine the type of care the individual wants. A competent person may appoint a surrogate (often several are identified in priority order) to make health care decisions for that person when the person is not able to do so. This addresses some of the limitations with the living will since it identifies a person who is actually making the decisions for the patient. Typically, individuals select someone that they trust will carry out their directives and are discussed while the individual is competent to do so. The surrogate does not have to be a family member, although it is highly advisable that persons inform their family about these documents and decisions prior to needing them.

- The Patient Self-Determination Act of 1990 was initiated to address issues about patient decisions (Guido, 2001). Health care providers must now ask patients if they have living wills, durable powers of attorney, or advance directives. The goal of this law is to make individuals more aware of their rights and the importance of making informed decisions hopefully give some consideration of costs of care. Nurses must follow their organization's policies and procedures related to any of these issues. A recent study on advance directives indicates that these directives are effective (Silveira, Kim, & Langa, 2010). In this study of 3,746 participants, 92.7% of those with living wills were more likely to want limited or comfort care. Those with living wills 83.2% who wanted limited care and 97.1% who requested comfort care received the care that that they requested. Participants with a durable power of attorney were less likely to die in a hospital or receive all care possible compared to those with no durable power of attorney.
- A **do-not-resuscitate (DNR) directive** is another form of advance directive that patients may request when they receive care. The physician may be implementing advance directives when writing a DNR order, but DNR orders can be written without an advance directive. Family members should also be consulted to prevent increasing family stress and possible legal actions. Health care organizations have policies and procedures to follow when patients request DNR, and these should be followed. If the patient is able, there should be some discussion between the physician and patient about the decision. Families are included if the patient agrees. There are specific intervals designated for reevaluation of the decisions. With all of these issues related to treatment it is critical that nurses contribute by assessing the patient and communicating effectively with the patient, family, and physician. End-of-life decisions are not easy to discuss. The nurse is often in a position to discuss these critical issues; however, the physician should also be involved in the process. What happens if a patient's preferences are disregarded (Habel, 2001)? The nurse should contact the organization's ethics committee, which many health care organizations have. In doing this, the nurse acts as the patient's advocate. The nurse, of course, needs to be aware of state laws and requirements related to these serious decisions. If there is no ethics committee or procedure, then the nurse should contact nursing management, though nursing management should also be contacted if there is a referral to the ethics committee.
- Assisted suicide is another patient rights issue that has become more important; however, this one is much more complex. States typically have laws related to this popular topic in the media. The American Nurses Association opposes any nursing participation in assisted suicide, as this would violate the ANA *Code for Nurses* (2008). Any concerns about potential assisted suicide should be reported to management staff and to the organization's ethics committee.

In conclusion, "nurses have an ethical and legal obligation to provide safe patient care, to maintain competency, and to identify those situations where the provision of safe care is jeopardized. Without a doubt, malpractice is a preventable problem" (Morris, 2002, p. 16). How can lawsuits be prevented, as many occur even when quality care was provided? Why do patients sue health care providers (Mock, 2001)? Many patients who sue are angry with one or more of their health care providers, perhaps about not being told what they needed to know, lack of respect, lack of privacy, or they may feel that they received substandard care. It is very important to understand the patient's perception as this helps explain why a lawsuit has been filed. Effective communication must be part of the relationship. Effective leadership is also critical—understanding and applying legal principles while providing care and guiding others as they provide care such as unlicensed assistive personnel (UAPs) and licensed practical nurses (LPNs) or other team members. Keys to success are connecting with the patient, appreciating the patient's situation, responding to the patient's needs, and empowering the patient (Mock, 2001).

### Patient Privacy: The Law Expands

"It has been foundational, at least since Hippocrates, that patients have a right to have personal medical information kept private. . . . The chief public-policy rationale is that patients are unlikely to disclose intimate details that are necessary for their proper medical care to their physicians unless they trust their physicians to keep that information secret" (Annas, 2003, p. 1486). Regulations about patient privacy were added to Health Insurance Portability and Accountability Act of 1996 (HIPAA) and went into effect in April, 2003. This established the first comprehensive federal standards for medical privacy related to the medical record or any identifiable information about the patient (Pear, 2002, August, p. A1). Each nurse needs to be aware of and follow the policies and procedures related to oral, written, or electronic patient identifiable data set up by the health care organization regarding issues where the nurse practices; however, there are some key areas that are affected by these new privacy regulations.

- Patients must be informed of their privacy rights.
- Patients must be informed as to who will see their records and for what purpose.
- Patients have the right to inspect and obtain a copy of their medical records. (There are some exceptions to this that each organization should make clear to staff.)
- Valid authorization to release health information must contain certain information, such as a copy of the signed authorization given to the patient, in understandable language, and how the patient may revoke authorization.
- Although information may be used for research purposes to assess outbreak of a disease, all individual identifiable data must be removed.
- Personal data may not be used for marketing (for example, pharmacies may not share this information with others for this purpose).

These privacy standards are complex and require health care organizations to make changes in how they manage information. They also require that staff are trained and updated about the changes. The standards give patients more control while at the same time make providers more accountable for keeping information private. This is federal law, but if a state has more rigorous privacy requirements then the state requirements would have to be followed.

## Ethics: Impact on Decision Making, Planning, and Practice

Ethics is interwoven throughout health care policy development, implementation, and legal issues that arise during the delivery of health care. Nurses cannot avoid ethical issues and need to understand ethical decision making. Leadership competencies are related to ethics; for example, decision making often includes ethical issues. Implementing health policies may require consideration of ethics. "Ethics refers to a standardized code or guide to behaviors. Morals are learned through growth and development, whereas ethics typically is learned through a more organized system, such as a standardized ethics code developed by a professional group" (Finkelman & Kenner, 2010, p. 196) such as the *Guide to the Code of Ethics* (Fowler, 2008).

### Ethical Decision Making

"An ethical dilemma is a difficult moral problem that involves two or more mutually exclusive, morally correct courses of action. Health care organizations are frequently confronted with two key questions: "What is fair?" and "What is the right and just thing to do?" (Koloroutis & Thorstenson, 1999, p. 13). These are not easy questions to answer, and each situation is different. Organizations need to integrate an ethical framework into their daily operations and require leaders to lead by example. It is important to recognize that "articulated values have no meaning or use if they are not demonstrated in the lives of organizational members" (Koloroutis & Thorstenson, 1999, p. 16). Individual nurses and other health care providers must also deal with these critical questions when confronted with ethical issues.

Four primary principles, as described in Figure 2-5, are used to make ethical decisions: autonomy, beneficence, justice, and veracity (Chally & Loriz, 1998).

1. **Autonomy** is a principle that has always been important to nurses. Patients have the right to determine their own rights.
2. The second ethical principle is **beneficence**, or doing something good. Nurses are to inflict no harm and to safeguard the patient.

**FIGURE 2-5   Ethical decision making.**

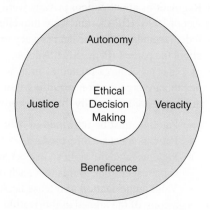

3. Patients should also be treated fairly or with **justice**. This, of course, is a problem when decisions are made that determine which patients will receive treatment.
4. The fourth primary principle is **veracity**. Truth telling is critical for effective patient communication and developing trust with the patient. Informed consent is one example of a potential ethical problem that may be affected by veracity. If incomplete information is not shared with a patient, then veracity has not been met.

As has been discussed, professional organizations play an important role in policy making and legislation at the local, state, and federal levels, but they are also important in defining professional standards and ethics. The ANA's *Code for Nurses with Interpretive Statements* (2008) is the primary resource for nursing ethical guidance as noted in Provision Nine of the *Code*: "The profession of nursing, as represented by associations and their members, is responsible for articulating nursing values, for maintaining the integrity of the profession and its practice, and for shaping social policy" (Fowler, 2008, p. 121). All provisions in the *Code* are described in Box 2-5.

## Professional Ethics

Professional ethics applies to both nursing management and clinical issues. Several nursing studies have been conducted about nursing ethics. A study conducted in 1994, but still relevant today, asked nurse administrators to identify decisions that had represented ethical dilemmas for them. The following were considered important in rank order, with the first decision occurring most frequently:

1. Staffing levels and mix situations
2. Developing/maintaining standards of care
3. Allocating/rationing of scarce resources
4. Incompetent physicians
5. Demotion/termination of employees
6. Employee relations
7. Incompetent nurses
8. Selection/hiring of employees
9. Treatment versus non-treatment
10. Promotion of employees
11. Diversification of services
12. Downsizing services
13. Access to care for the indigent
14. Marketing/advertising services
15. Labor negotiations with nurses (Borawski, 1995, p. 61)

These issues indicate that nurses struggle with many situations that place them in an ethical dilemma (e.g., what to do and how to do it right). Today, these issues continue to present ethical dilemmas for nurses as practitioners and leaders.

| **BOX 2-5** | **CODE OF ETHICS FOR NURSES** |
|---|---|

**PROVISION 1**

The nurse, in all professional relationships, practices with compassion and respect for the inherent dignity, worth, and uniqueness of every individual, unrestricted by considerations of social or economic status, personal attributes, or the nature of health problems.

**PROVISION 2**

The nurse's primary commitment is to the patient, whether an individual, family, group, or community.

**PROVISION 3**

The nurse promotes, advocates for, and strives to protect the health, safety, and rights of the patient.

**PROVISION 4**

The nurse is responsible and accountable for individual nursing practice and determines the appropriate delegation of tasks consistent with the nurse's obligation to provide optimum patient care.

**PROVISION 5**

The nurse owes the same duties to self as to others, including the responsibility to preserve integrity and safety, to maintain competence, and to continue personal and professional growth.

**PROVISION 6**

The nurse participates in establishing, maintaining, and improving health care environments and conditions of employment conducive to the provision of quality health care and consistent with the values of the profession through individual and collective action.

**PROVISION 7**

The nurse participates in the advancement of the profession through contributions to practice, education, administration, and knowledge development.

**PROVISION 8**

The nurse collaborates with other health professionals and the public in promoting community, national, and international efforts to meet health needs.

**PROVISION 9**

The profession of nursing, as represented by associations and their members, is responsible for articulating nursing values, for maintaining the integrity of the profession and its practice, and for shaping social policy.

Source: Fowler, M. (Ed.). (2008). *Guide to the Code for Nurses. Interpretation and Application.* Silver Springs, MD: American Nurses Association. Reprinted with permission.

## Making Complaints to the Board of Nursing

Each state board of nursing has the responsibility to protect the public health in its state. Nurses who are licensed in a state can and should make complaints to the board when they are concerned about patient health and safety. In the late 1980s and early 1990s, Texas experienced major psychiatric health care fraud and abuse problems in some for-profit psychiatric hospitals, which is discussed in more detail later in this section. Some psychiatric nurses said they contacted their board and did not receive assistance (Mohr, 1996; 1997). Boards of nursing must be responsive, or they will find that nurses will not bother to contact them.

Leadership is required of all nurses, even those on boards of nursing. A leader is able to confront difficult issues and take risks, which is what the nurses did who reported problems. All nurses should be knowledgeable about their state's practice act and use this law and its related rules and regulations as a guide in making decisions about issues and complaints to the board. If nurses have any concerns about legal issues and personal professional liability, consulting an attorney is also recommended. Boards of nursing have a specific process for reviewing complaints and deadlines that must be met. During the investigation period, boards do not reveal the source of a complaint. State boards of nursing should be contacted for information about each state's reporting process.

## Health Care Reimbursement and Ethics

The medical industry struggles with medical and business ethical issues daily, and nurses are also confronting more and more ethical dilemmas due to these struggles. Managed care has had a major impact on health care delivery and reimbursement, with health care organizations and providers facing conflicts between financial incentives and the insurer's mission (or potential ethical duty) to provide appropriate care. The truth of the matter is that all types of non-governmental insurers including managed care organizations (MCOs) are businesses. It is recognized that some insurers are better than others, and this must imply that some type of standard has been used to compare one with the other to arrive at this conclusion. Are there standards? Can conflicts between business ethics and medical ethics within the same organization be resolved? Health care professionals want to apply medical ethics to MCOs because some MCOs deliver medical care in addition to provide traditional reimbursement for care, for example health maintenance organizations (HMOs). Many people view medical care as being a different product from other business "products." Do the same ethical obligations that apply to health care professionals also apply to insurers? Business ethics that promote fair competition—people are free to make voluntary choices to buy or sell goods or services—do not fully apply to the health care insurance business. Patients are not always free to choose their insurance or their provider, or they may have limits placed on these decisions by their employers. Investor-owned (for-profit) insurers have a very important relationship with their stockholders, who expect a financial return on their investment in the insurance business, and the same is true of investor-owned healthcare provider organizations (e.g., hospitals, clinics, home care agencies, long-term care facilities). These organizations will always experience conflicts between their business needs to control costs to meet their budgetary requirements and their contractual obligations to provide health care services to the purchasers of their services, typically the employer who contracts for employee health benefits and their stockholders.

The relationship between the insurer and the patient/enrollee is a contractual one. The insurer is responsible only for meeting the requirements of the health plan contract, and there is no requirement that all contracts must be the same. There is inequality in insurer contracts and benefits, and this is not considered to be an ethical problem. Lack of choice is a common complaint about managed care plans; however, the very nature of managed care denies choice: "If care is managed, then, by definition, the patient is not free to choose what care he or she gets. . . . The purpose of managing care is to eliminate choices that are wasteful, harmful, or too expensive" (Mariner, 1995, p. 236). Choice comes into play in the patient/enrollee's decision to join a health plan, and even that is limited by the employer's selection of plans. Patients rarely have complete information about the plan when they join, and many do not really become interested in these details until they need services. The ideal would be the patient/enrollee who reviews each health plan option, including all of the details related to benefits, providers, outcome data, and the like, and decides on the best plan based on the individual's and his or her dependents' health status and needs. Choice is more operable in this scenario, but this rarely occurs.

If one could identify ethical standards for insurers, these standards would include insurer accountability for the scope and quality of the patient care delivered, fairness, honesty, truthfulness, respect for persons, and justice. These standards, however, may be difficult to meet. For example, allocation of resources may conflict with many of these standards. If an insurer must ensure that all of its enrollees receive care, there will be decisions to make that will be unfair or unjust for some enrollees, but fair and just for others. Patient satisfaction is directly affected by decisions that the insurer makes, and sometimes insurers make decisions that dissatisfy enrollees but meet the insurer's financial goals. The insurer makes a choice and decides what will bring it the most benefit; however, this is a delicate decision because patient satisfaction is also very important to insurer survival. Too much patient dissatisfaction can lead to the loss of employer health contracts. Additional content on reimbursement is found in Chapter 5.

## CASE STUDY

### Risky Staff Performance and Ineffective Management

As nurse manager of a behavioral health unit in an acute care hospital, you are responsible for the overall management and quality of care provided on a 30-bed inpatient unit with an average length of stay of 4 days. Staffing is short, and you have four new nurses with limited or no mental health experience. Last night a patient was injured during a restraint procedure. You are reviewing the incident report in your office and decide to review restraint data for the last three months. You are shocked when you see that restraints have increased by 15%, and that one nurse has been involved in 75% of these restraints regardless of the shift she worked. This is a new employee of 4 months. You then review the medical records for these patients and find that documentation of the incidents is not complete; there is little re-evaluation of the patient as required; and basic patient needs were not met effectively. You then talk to several staff members who have worked with the nurse during the shifts when the restraints occurred. They describe the nurse as "difficult," "demanding," and has "limited tolerance for negative patient behavior." She does not include staff in decision making such as decisions to restrain a patient. This all concerns you so next you look at her personnel file. The nurse had 6 months of previous mental health experience and 2 years of acute care medical nursing experience. You notice that she should have had two to three completed reference checks, but only one is in the file and that one is vague. You are overwhelmed with what you have uncovered.

### Questions:

1. What do you think about this nurse manager and how she has handled quality improvement issues, personnel issues, and overall decision making on her unit?
2. What are the legal and ethical issues related to the care this staff nurse has provided?
3. How should the nurse manager respond to this nurse and to the multiple problems she has?
4. After this experience what does the nurse manager need to do to improve her own management competency long term?

---

## Health Care Rationing

Health care rationing does occur in the U.S. health care delivery system, though it is not a formalized rationing system. Actually, there was a time when rationing was more the norm, but the patient played a critical role. Prior to health insurance, patients served as their own gatekeepers. As patients were financially responsible for their own care, they rationed services for themselves and their families, aided by a physician with whom they shared strong community, and often personal ties. These physicians realized that any care provided beyond the financial means of the patient was, and would probably remain, uncompensated care (Randall, 1994). An example of current rationing is the organ donation programs that allocate organs to patients based on identified criteria. Another example was Oregon's rationing system for Medicaid patients. This system prioritized diagnoses that would receive health care reimbursement; however, the system experienced problems. No other state has developed a rationing system similar to Oregon's.

Resource allocation is a more acceptable term for rationing. Resource allocation is necessary and inevitable in some form due to excessive health care costs and limited resources. The key question is how it should be done. Bedside rationing occurs when the individual physician declines to administer beneficial treatments because of costs that will be incurred by the insurer or services the insurer will not cover, preferably in consultation with the patient and patient's family (Hall & Berenson, 1998). Is this preferable to having a rationing or resource allocation system that is centralized and bureaucratic with many rules? Is this more equitable, impartial, visible, and predictable? These are difficult questions for which there is no perfect answer. When this is applied to insurers the view changes because managed care reimbursement focuses on the needs of the population, which is different than the traditional fee-for-service insurance plans; however, the population is only the insurer members. Insurers are generally not concerned with the greater good of the entire community, but only with decisions that affect their members. This is a major ethical dilemma that will continue to be present in the health care system.

## Health Care Fraud and Abuse

Over the past two decades health care has experienced major problems with fraud and abuse, and these have implications for nursing. Health care fraud and abuse includes legal and ethical elements that need to be considered. Nurses have also been involved in these fraud and abuse cases. It is important that nurses are aware of these situations and their outcomes, and that they consider implications for individual nurses and the profession as a whole.

In the mid-1990s as health care organizations (HCOs) changed to corporate models it was noted that "the transformation of our health care system is having several perverse effects. It is producing corporate conglomerates with billions of dollars in assets that compensate their executives as grandly as basketball players. These conglomerates are battling to control physicians in many locations and because they have cash and monopolistic power, they often succeed" (Kassirer, 1995, p. 50). At a U.S. Congressional committee meeting in 1994, the health care fraud problem was described in the following manner: "An effective antifraud program will be crucial to curing the health care crisis. Fraud is a cancer, spreading rapidly throughout our health care system. Unless we do something about fraud, and waste, and abuse we will never, never get health care costs under control. The General Accounting Office (GAO) estimates that 10% of our total health care expenditures, both public and private, are lost to fraud and abuse" (U.S. House of Representatives, 1994, p. 1). Health care fraud has been defined by the National Health Care Anti-Fraud Association (NHCAA) as "the intentional deception or misrepresentation that an individual or entity makes when the misrepresentation could result in some unauthorized benefit to the individual, or the entity or to some other third party" (Coppola, 1997, p. 46). Health care fraud and abuse have been particularly problematic in psychiatric care, large health care corporations, and more recently in long-term care and home care.

WHISTLEBLOWING    The False Claims Act (FCA) was passed during the Civil War to award citizens who exposed fraud against the government; however, it became a more useful law after it was amended in 1982. This is the federal law that protects whistle blowers—those who expose federal fraud. Health care fraud, as is true of most fraud, is very difficult to prove. Having people on the inside of the organization who are willing to share information is often critical to successfully prove fraud. If a nurse decides to file a suit and report fraud and the government decides to intervene in the nurse's case, the nurse is entitled to a percentage of the government's ultimate recovery. If the government does not intervene with the nurse's case, and the nurse continues with the case, the nurse is entitled to larger percentage of the recovery. Needless to say, this is quite an incentive; however, it is not easy to report an employer. Employees have concerns about retaliation, and there is no doubt that this is a highly stressful, long, drawn-out process. There are protections for employees who act as **whistleblowers** for example if the employee is fired, demoted, or discriminated against for these actions, he or she can bring a claim against the employer for unlawful retaliation. The employee would be entitled to both job reinstatement and twice the amount of lost back pay. The FCA, however, applies only to federal cases. When an employee reports fraud, the employee must be the original source of the knowledge. An employee cannot obtain the information from a publicly disclosed source, such as a newspaper or government report, and then report it.

In 2010 a major whistleblowing case occurred that involved two nurses in Texas (Lowes, 2010); however, there was dispute if this was whistleblowing or employees just doing their job. This term may no longer be relevant when staff report concerns about quality, which should be an expectation. In this particular case in Texas two nurses at a hospital reported a physician to the medical board. They were concerned about safe practice. The advantage to whistleblowing is it legally shields someone who reports, but in this case the nurses were charged with misuse of information. The sheriff in the town was a close friend of the physician. One of the charges against one nurse was dropped, and the second went to trial, receiving a not guilty verdict. The fact that this occurred when the nurses were doing what is expected from a licensed health care professional—to advocate for patient safety—is disturbing. As is discussed in more detail in Chapters 16 and 17, health care organizations need a culture of safety where the staff feels safe reporting quality concerns. There is no need for more of blame culture, where fear drives decisions rather than patient advocacy. The Health Insurance Portability and Accountability Act of 1996 (HIPAA) established a program to identify and prosecute health care fraud. This program is called Health Care Fraud and Abuse Control Program (HCFAC). "During FY 2007, the Federal Government won or negotiated approximately $1.8 billion in judgments and settlements, and it attained additional administrative impositions in health care fraud cases and proceedings. The Medicare Trust Fund received transfers of approximately $797 million during this period as a result of these efforts, as well as those of preceding years, in addition to $266 million in Federal Medicaid money similarly transferred separately to the Treasury as a result of these efforts. The HCFAC account has returned over $11.2 billion to the Medicare Trust Fund since the inception of the Program in 1997" (U.S. Department of Health and Human Services and Department of Justice, 2008, p. 1). This type of expenditure increases U.S. health care costs.

Not all who are accused of fraud and abuse are guilty. The complex, ever-changing regulations make it very difficult for organizations and their staff to keep current; consequently, it is easy to make an honest error. This is not fraud because fraud requires intention to do wrong. Calling this fraud can be a serious problem. A fraud accusation affects an organization's and its providers' reputation, and it is often difficult to erase this when an honest error is finally recognized. The number of fraud and abuse cases has increased in the last few years, and much of this increase is due to greater efforts to discover fraud and abuse, with Congress allocating more funds to combat health care fraud and abuse.

**EXAMPLE: HEALTH CARE FRAUD AND ABUSE IN PSYCHIATRIC HOSPITALS**   There is no doubt that corporate health care fraud has increased in the last 15 years. The psychiatric health care fraud and abuse of the 1980s and 1990s provides a view of what can happen when a system confronts the care versus the bottom-line dilemma and chooses the bottom line (Mohr, 1996; 1997). During this time period, health care corporations, particularly investor-owned chains that provided psychiatric services, increased throughout the country. New hospitals were built, and hospitals were rapidly bought and sold. What happened in these hospitals? Patients were charged for care they did not receive. Patient records indicated that inappropriate care was provided, such as a large number of medications that could not have been administered in one day without causing detrimental effects, which indicated that the medications had not actually been administered. Patients, however, were charged for multiple doses that never were administered. Fraudulent submissions of insurance claims were common. Patient abuse occurred when

- Patients were admitted when they did not need to be hospitalized.
- Parents were told that their children were seriously ill when they were not.
- Patients were given medications that they did not need.
- Teenagers were abducted and admitted to the hospital.
- Patients were restrained unnecessarily and for long periods of time.
- Patients were denied their rights.
- Patients experienced verbal abuse.

These examples are only a few of the many abuses and examples of fraud from this scandal. The Federal Bureau of Investigation (FBI) conducted raids on hospitals to confiscate records and shut down computers to prevent purging of records (Rundle, 1993). After reviewing congressional testimony, it is easy to wonder if the examples are from the late 19th century rather than the end of the 20th century (U.S. House of Representatives, 1992, 1993; U.S. Senate, 1992). Texas State Senator Michael J. Moncrief stated in one of these meetings, "In Texas, we have uncovered some of the most elaborate, aggressive, creative, deceptive, immoral, and illegal schemes being used to fill empty hospital beds with insured and paying patients" (U.S. House of Representatives, 1992, p. 7). Clearly, these health care organizations were focusing on business, using questionable business ethics, and had little concern for health care professional ethics such as the *Code for Nurses* and physician ethics.

What happened to health care professionals in these hospitals? Some staff members spoke out, including nurses and physicians, but it was not uncommon for them to be threatened with job loss or to actually lose their jobs. There were threats of blacklisting and reports of false claims against employees such as use of illegal drugs to licensing boards; verbal abuse and ostracism; and other types of threats to prevent employees from reporting fraud and abuse (Mohr, 1996, 1997). Why would someone continue to work in this environment? In some cases, reporting problems to the board of nursing or state agencies did not get timely responses. Others experienced extreme stress, fear, and emotional and physical problems. In other situations, nurses felt that if they stayed and worked in the situation they might be able to help the patients who were abused, even though this typically did not happen. There were some nurses who did speak out but found it extremely stressful and painful. This example of psychiatric fraud and abuse demonstrates how easy it is for some health care organizations and individual professionals to cross the line and ignore ethical behavior. This is certainly not a positive example of what can happen when ethics are left behind, but much can be learned from it.

**EXAMPLE: OPERATION RESTORE TRUST**   In the late 1990s, other major health care corporations, such as Columbia/ HCA, experienced major fraud and abuse problems (Eichenwald, 1997; 1998; U.S. Department of Health and Human Services and U.S. Department of Justice, 2009). Federal investigations found widespread fraud, overcharges, and substandard care. The elderly are a vulnerable group in the United States, as are those with mental illness. Naturally, the vulnerable are most prone to experience the impact of fraud and abuse. When Medicare fraud and abuse occurs, the federal government can become involved because Medicare is a federal program. The psychiatric problems were exposed when patients who received Civilian Health and Medical Program of the Uniform Services (CHAMPUS) coverage, the federal program for military dependents, were abused or experienced fraud. The federal government could then become involved and use all of its related agencies such as the FBI and the General Accounting Office in the investigation. The home care Medicare fraud led to the development of a program to monitor and correct these problems called Operation Restore Trust. This program has been a burden for many home care agencies, particularly for those who have not committed fraud but made honest mistakes; however, the government is determined to correct health care fraud and abuse. This abuse continues with estimates that there is a $60 billion a year crime. There is a website used to try to get consumers and providers to report abuse. The website is in the Media Links at the end of the chapter.

## Organizational Ethics

Many health care organizations have followed other types of businesses in creating processes to address ethical concerns. Why all this interest in corporate ethics? Certainly, one could cite the increasing examples of health care fraud as previously discussed as one reason, but probably even more important was the creation of new federal sentencing guidelines in 1991. Fines were reduced for white-collar crimes if a business could demonstrate that it has a comprehensive ethics program. The Center for Medicare and Medicaid Services (CMS) established conditions of participation for providers who provide services to Medicare and Medicaid beneficiaries. The Office of Inspector General (OIG) of the Department of Health and Human Services is responsible for enforcing these rules. "In 1999, the OIG issued a model corporate compliance program for hospitals" (Bartis & Sullivan, 2002, p. 67). Since few if any hospitals do not receive these government reimbursements, most hospitals must comply. Due to these changes, health care corporate compliance committees are now more common. The quality and commitment of compliance ethics programs must, however, be monitored. Monitoring can easily be another paper process that might look good in theory but does not truly reflect the organization's culture and the behavior of its employees. Organizations must ensure that behaviors change. Some of these organizations also have ethics officers. What is their authority and how can they really effect change? These are critical questions that should be asked by organizations. It is not easy to change organizational culture, and it takes time. Is there a true commitment to improve, or is this being done to put the organization in a better legal position in case there are problems? What are some of the activities of these compliance programs?

An example of a nursing corporate compliance program is a program developed at Hartford Hospital in Connecticut, which identified five steps that needed to be taken in the program:

1. Identification of high-risk areas
2. Development of plans and tools that support the process for monitoring and measuring compliance with the high-risk areas
3. Implementation of the program
4. Education
5. Compliance related to auditing and monitoring (Bartis & Sullivan, 2002, p. 68)

The high-risk areas that this organization identified, which might vary from one organization to another, were licensure and credentialing with current and appropriate licensure, scope of practice that is consistent with the state nurse practice act, compliance with hospital policies and procedures, and documentation.

Employee education is an important compliance activity that affects compliance outcomes. Topics that might be covered include the organization's mission and values, code of conduct, compliance plan, roles and responsibilities of the compliance officer, compliance with laws and regulations, conflicts of interests, financial and accounting records, fraud and abuse, professional standards and codes of ethics, confidentiality of patient information and organization information, physician relations, patient rights, respect and concern for others, and anti-trust issues. Some of these topics are not applicable to all staff. For example, not all staff needs an understanding of financial and accounting records. All staff does, however, need to know the procedure for reporting their concerns about ethical issues in a manner that protects them form employer retaliation. Staff may see the compliance program as just another "change" that will have little impact on the organization, culture, or staff behaviors. This staff attitude needs to be addressed by the organization if the organization plans to truly change its organizational culture and commit itself to a more ethical work environment. Organizational leaders must be role models for all of the staff, and they need to

## APPLYING EVIDENCE-BASED PRACTICE

### Evidence for Effective Leadership and Management

**Citation:** Rathert, C. & Fleming, D. (2008). Hospital ethical climate and teamwork in acute care. The moderating role of leaders. *Health Care Management REVIEW*, October–December, 323–331.

**Overview:** The researchers of this study "propose that the health care organization's ethical climate has an important impact on the social and professional interactions of care team members, which in turn influence team processes and patient and team member outcomes" (p. 324). This cross-sectional research study examined acute care staff's perceptions of how the work environment, a benevolent ethical climate, and continuous quality improvement leadership influence teamwork and identified approaches to improve teamwork. The setting for the study was a 500-bed hospital. The sample included mostly RNs with a 42% return rate of the survey (306 surveys). Teamwork was measured using the Agency for Healthcare Research and Quality Patient Safety Culture survey. The benevolent climate was measured using validated measures. The study concludes that when staff perceive the ethical climate to be benevolent, they were significantly more likely to say that teamwork was better. Continuous quality improvement (CQI) leadership styles moderated the relationship between the ethical climate and teamwork unit. Team leaders who exhibit behaviors that emphasize CQI, such as listening to frontline staff ideas, talking to team members before making changes, and facilitating communication across professional boundaries, can help facilitate improved teamwork.

**Application:** Typically, when staff consider ethics, they think of individual ethics; however, from an organizational perspective ethics is more than this. It can have an impact on how staff works together and consequently on patient outcomes, as noted in this study. Greater exploration of the role of ethics in organizations is needed: how it works and what it impacts. This study describes benevolent climates as "the work context supports staff members who make decisions that might benefit patients or the care team as opposed to themselves. Such climates support staff in looking out for each other, encourage members to be concerned about how decisions and actions affect patients and the community, and promote a focus on doing the 'right' thing for the patient and society" (p. 325).

**Questions:**

1. *Why is ethics important in health care organizations?*
2. *Describe how you think the ethical approach and teamwork are related. Provide three specific examples to support your description.*
3. *If you were a nurse manager how would you promote a benevolent climate on the unit?*

know what is right or wrong and then do the right thing. It is not uncommon for managers to deal with several ethical issues at one time, all of which affect decision making.

### Nurses Coping with Ethical Dilemmas

Nurses have responsibilities related to ethics, including maintaining knowledge of the professional *Code for Nurses* (2008), recognition of personal values, understanding of the decision-making process and its application to nursing practice, recognition and understanding of the importance of policy and legal issues, and the ability to be assertive. As nurses confront ethical dilemmas, there are decision-making traps that continue to be important and need to be avoided (Wocial, 1996):

- Prematurely reaching a decision
- Overconfidence in your own judgment
- Failing to follow a system
- Inability to recognize the effect of your own personal value system
- Inability to recognize the conflict between what is best for the patient and what is best for the organization (p. 155)

Curtin (1995) advocates "putting decisions through the 'stink test.' If it smells, rethink your priorities" (p. 101). This can be an effective test because it recognizes the importance of each individual's perspective on decisions; however, it is also important to understand and recognize opposite viewpoints.

The goal is to reach a balance between the extremes, and this is not easy to accomplish. Decision making in the health care environment requires recognition of different viewpoints and compromises. This is also true for all ethical dilemmas. Wallace and Pekel (2001) developed an ethical checklist for staff to use as they assess an ethical situation—questions to ask oneself. These questions included the following:

- **Relevant information test.** Have I/we obtained as much information as possible to make an informed decision and action plan for this situation?
- **Involvement test.** Have I/we involved all who have a right to have input and/or to be involved in making this decision and action plan?
- **Consequence test.** Have I/we anticipated and attempted to accommodate for the consequences of this decision and action plan on any who are significantly affected by it?
- **Fairness test.** If I/we were assigned to take the place of any one of the stakeholders in this situation, would I/we perceive this decision and action plan to be essentially fair, given all of the circumstances?
- **Enduring values test.** Does this decision and action plan uphold my/our priority enduring values that are relevant to this situation?
- **Universality test.** Would I/we want this decision and action plan to become a universal law applicable to all similar situations, even to myself/ourselves (p. 29)?

Strategies that are used by some health care organizations to cope with ethical dilemmas are ethics committees and nursing ethics groups. Ethics committees provide opportunities for interprofessional staff to discuss ethical dilemmas that staff experience in the organization. The committee is advisory. As is true with all discussions of ethics, there is no perfect answer. Typical issues that are discussed by these committees are: do-not-resuscitate policies, patient self-determination, brain-death protocols, informed consent, euthanasia, and patient competency. Issues related to managed care and reimbursement and clinical decision making have also become more common topics. Ethical dilemmas such as these can lead to staff frustration and do affect the delivery of patient care.

Nursing ethics groups provide forums for discussion about nursing ethics. One problem that occurs is nurses are not always comfortable discussing their ethical dilemmas in institutional ethics committees (Otto, 2000). Nurses who participate in nursing ethics committees gain knowledge and skills that are required for ethical decision making. These nurses are then better prepared to participate in interprofessional ethics committees and to make their own ethical decisions.

"A political ethical conflict occurs when what one is told to do (either covertly or overtly) by those having more power in the organization or what one feels compelled to do by the organization is in conflict with one's ethical belief structure" (Brosnan & Roper, 1997, p. 42). This is demonstrated daily today in health care as nurse managers and other staff confront conflicts between financial issues and care. What is best for patients and what is best for the organization are not always the same. These can be tough choices. A health care organization is a political one, and leaders need to be aware of the political environment. Nurse managers and staff must consider beneficence, which is "the obligation to benefit one's institution and those it serves" (Brosnan & Roper, 1997, p. 42). However, should the team agree with the institution without thought of what this agreement means and the ethics involved? Nurses must consider **non-malfeasance**, to do no harm to the institution or those it serves. This obligation also relates to the employees. Respect for persons, another key principle, is also important when staff makes decisions that affect patients but also when managers make decisions that affect staff. Managers have to ensure that procedures are followed; however, when this is done, it needs to be done respectfully (for example, when staff is told that mistakes have been made). Justice, or treating others fairly and impartially, is a frequent dilemma for managers. Staff need to be approached in an impartial manner with fairness. Truth telling is the obligation to be truthful or honest in decisions and approaches to others. Utility is also important, and this focuses on "maximizing the greatest good when decisions are made" (Brosnan & Roper, 1997, p. 43). Staff confronts ethical issues daily; however, "The leader's actions may be 'the single most important factor in fostering corporate behavior of a high ethical standard,' but surveys rank an ethics policy as very important, too" (Dessler, 2002, p. 50).

# APPLYING LEADERSHIP AND MANAGEMENT

## MY HOSPITAL UNIT

It is time to return to your unit. You may wonder how you would apply this content on health policy to your unit today. Search for information about current health policy issues. You might examine current health care issues that your state legislature is considering; search Government Affairs section of the ANA website; and review newspapers and Internet for current health policy issues. Select one topic and examine it. How would you apply this topic and the information to the work you do as a nurse manager on your unit? Be as specific as possible. Why is it important for you as a nurse manager to keep current with health policy issues? Use the virtual unit site found on the textbook website to record the work that you do in the role of nurse manager for your unit.

## Critical Thinking Questions and Activities

1. Visit the American Nurses Association site on health care policy at http://www .nursingworld.org/MainMenuCategories/HealthcareandPolicyIssues.aspx. What are the current policy issues addressed? How might you apply them to nursing leadership and management?
2. Visit the American Nurses Association site on Government Affairs at http://www .nursingworld.org/MainMenuCategories/ANAPoliticalPower.aspx. What information is available? How might you use this information? Examine a current health policy issue. Discuss with your classmates.
3. Visit the American Nurses Association site at http://www.nursingworld.org and search for "ethics." What information is available? How might a nurse manager use this information? Discuss with your classmates.
4. How would you support the statement, "Nurses need to be aware of and involved in health policy development"?
5. Examine the issue of patient privacy and how it applies to management of a unit.
6. How are the ethical principles of beneficence and justice related to health care reimbursement policy?
7. Review Appendix B, which describes some of the provisions of the health care reform law of 2010. Discuss the law in small teams and its potential impact on health care delivery and nursing.

## Media Links

**URL: http://www.dhhs.gov**
U. S. Department of Health and Human Services
- **URL: http://www.pbs.org/moyers/journal/07312009/profile.html**
Profits before Patients. July 31, 2009. PBS. View video and/or read information.
- **URL: http://www.cms.gov**
Centers for Medicare and Medicaid Services
- **URL: http://www.ahrq.gov**
Agency for Healthcare Research and Quality
- **URL: http://www.hrsa.gov**
Health Resources and Services Administration

- **URL: http://www.nursingworld.org**
  American Nurses Association
- **URL: http://www.aacn.nche.edu/**
  American Association of Colleges of Nursing
- **URL: http://www.nln.org**
  National League for Nursing
- **URL: http://www.aone.org**
  American Organization of Nurse Executives
- **URL: http://www.stopmedicarefraud.gov/**
  U.S. Department of Health and Human Services and U.S. Department of Justice. Stop Medicare Fraud

**Pearson Nursing Student Resources**

Find additional review materials at
**nursing.pearsonhighered.com**

Prepare for success with additional NCLEX®-style practice questions, interactive assignments and activities, Web links, animations and videos, and more!

# References

Abood, S. (2007). Influencing healthcare in the legislative arena. *The Online Journal of Issues in Nursing, 12*(1), 3.

American Nurses Association. (1994). *Position statement on assisted suicide.* Washington, DC: Author.

American Nurses Association. (1998, January–February). Mass. nurses, docs spark health care revolution. *American Nurse, 30*(1), 6.

American Nurses Association. (March 30, 2010). Press Release: ANA's Nurses' Efforts Pay off in Historic Health Care Bill Signing. Silver Spring, MD: Author.

Annas, G. (2003). HIPAA regulations—A new era of medical-record privacy? *The New England Journal of Medicine, 348*(15), 1486–1490.

Bartis, J., & Sullivan, T. (2002). Developing a nursing corporate compliance program. *JONA's Healthcare Law, Ethics, and Regulation, 4*(3), 67–77.

Bodenheimer, T., & Grumbach, K. (1998). *Understanding health policy: A clinical approach* (2nd ed.). Stamford, CT: Appleton & Lange.

Borawski, D. (1995). Ethical dilemmas for nurse administrators. *Journal of Nursing Administration, 25*(7/8), 60–62.

Broder, P. (1997, October 26). Health care: The problems persist. *Washington Post*, p. A1.

Brosnan, J., & Roper, J. (1997). The reality of political ethical conflicts: Nurse manager dilemmas. *Journal of Nursing Administration, 27*(9), 42–46.

Chally, P., & Loriz, L. (1998). Decision making in practice: A practical model for resolving the types of ethical dilemmas you face daily. *American Journal of Nursing, 98*(6), 17–20.

Coppola, M. (1997, March–April). Identifying and reducing health care fraud in managed care. *Group Practice Journal* (3), 46.

Cover the Uninsured. (2009). Current Data. Retrieved July 8, 2009, from http://covertheuninsured.org/

Curtin, L. (1995). Ethics in management: Creating an ethical organization. *Nursing Management, 26*(9), 96–101.

Dessler, G. (2002). *Management.* Upper Saddle River, NJ: Prentice Hall.

Dingel-Stewart, S. & LaCoste, J. (2004). Light at the end of the tunnel. A vision of empowered nursing profession across the continuum of care. *Nursing Administrative Quarterly, 28*(3), 212–216.

Eichenwald, K. (1997, November 4). Reshaping the culture at Columbia/HCA. *New York Times*, p. C2.

Eichenwald, K. (1998, February 14). Columbia/HCA fraud case may be widened, U.S. says. *New York Times*, p. B2.

Ferguson, S. (2001). An activist looks at nursing's role in health policy development. *JOGNN, 30*(5), 546–551.

Finkelman, A. & Kenner, C. (2009). *Teaching IOM: Implications of the Institute of Medicine reports for nursing education.* Silver Springs, MD: American Nurses Association.

Finkelman, A. & Kenner, C. (2010). *Professional nursing concepts. Competencies for quality leadership.* Boston: Jones and Bartlett.

Fowler, M. (Ed). (2008). *Guide to the code for nurses. Interpretation and application.* Silver Springs, MD: American Nurses Association.

Gross, L., & Reed, S. (1999). ANA calls for medicine reform. *American Journal of Nursing, 99*(11), 50, 52.

Guido, G. (2001). *Legal and ethical issues in nursing* (3rd ed.). Upper Saddle River, NJ: Prentice Hall.

Hall, M., & Berenson, R. (1998). Ethical practice in managed care: A dose of realism. *Annals of Internal Medicine, 128*(5), 396–402.

Henry J. Kaiser Family Foundation. (2009). News Release. Retrieved February 27, 2009, from http://www.kff.org/kaiserpolls/posr022509pkg.cfm

Institute of Medicine. (1999). *To err is human: Building a safer health system.* Washington, DC: National Academies Press.

Institute of Medicine. (2001). *Crossing the quality chasm.* Washington, DC: National Academies Press.

Institute of Medicine. (2002). *Unequal treatment: Confronting racial and ethnic disparities in health care.* Washington, DC: National Academies Press.

Institute of Medicine. (2003). *Health professions education.* Washington, DC: National Academies Press.

Jones, K., Jennings, B., Moritz, P., & Moss, M. (1997). Policy issues associated with analyzing outcomes of care. *Image: Journal of Nursing Scholarship, 29*(3), 261–267.

Karigan, M. (2001). Ethics in clinical research. *American Journal of Nursing, 101*(9), 26–31.

Kassirer, J. (1995). Managed care and the morality of the marketplace. *New England Journal of Medicine, 333*(1), 50–52.

Kilborn, P. (1998, March 22). Looking back at Jackson Hole. *New York Times,* pp. A1, A5.

Kilborn, P. (1999, January 3). Oregon falters on a new path to health care. *New York Times,* pp. A1, A16.

Koloroutis, M., & Thorstenson, T. (1999). An ethics framework for organizational change. *Nursing Administration Quarterly, 23*(2), 9–18.

Lowes, R. (March 3, 2010). Whistleblowing nurses case highlights need for more open quality of care culture. *Medscape Medical News.* Retrieved June 6, 2010, from http://www.medscape.com.

Mariner, W. (1995). Business vs. medical ethics: Conflicting standards for managed care. *Journal of Law, Medicine and Ethics, 23*(3), 236–246.

McIntosh, M. (2002). The cost of health care to Americans. *JONA's Healthcare Law, Ethics, and Regulation, 4*(3), 79–89.

Mock, K. (2001). Keep lawsuits at bay with compassionate care. *RN, 64*(5), 83–84, 86.

Mohr, W. (1996). Dirty hands: The underside of marketplace health care. *Advances in Nursing Science, 19*(1), 28–37.

Mohr, W. (1997). Outcomes of corporate greed. *Image: Journal of Nursing Scholarship, 29*(1), 39–45.

Morris, K. (2002, September). Issues and answers. *Ohio Nurses Review, 77*(9), 16.

Nokleby, E., et al. (1998). Managed care: The value you bring. *American Journal of Nursing, 98*(6), 34–39.

Otto, S. (2000). A nurse's lifeline. A nursing ethics committee offers the chance to review and learn from ethical dilemmas. *American Journal of Nursing, 100*(12), 57–59.

Pear, R. (2002, August 10). Bush rolls back rules on privacy of medical data. *New York Times,* pp. A1, A8.

Purdum, T. (1999). California to set level of staffing for nursing care. *New York Times,* pp. A1, A21.

Randall, V. (1994). Impact of managed care on ethic answers and underserved populations. *Journal of Health Care Poor Underserved, 5*(3), 224–236.

Reinhardt, E. (1994). Managed competition in health care reform: Just another American dream or the perfect solution. *Journal of Law, Medicine and Ethics, 22*(2), 106–120.

Rundle, R. (1993, August 27). National medical facilities raided by U.S. agents. *Wall Street Journal,* pp. A1, A4.

Silveira, M., Kim, S., & Langa, K. (2010). Advance directives and outcomes of surrogate decision making before death. *New England Journal of Medicine, 362*(13), 1211–1218.

The White House. (February, 2009). Health Reform. Retrieved May 10, 2009, from http://www.whitehouse.gov

Toner, R. (1999, June 16). Drug coverage dominates fight brewing on Medicare. *New York Times,* pp. A1, A22.

U.S. Department of Health and Human Services and the Department of Justice Health Care Fraud and Abuse Control Program. (2008). *Annual Report for FY 2007.*

U.S. Department of Health and Human Services and U.S. Department of Justice. (2009). Stop Medicare Fraud. Retrieved November 30, 2009, from http://www.stopmedicarefraud.gov/

U.S. House of Representatives. (1992, April 28). *The profits of misery: How inpatient psychiatric treatment bilks the system and betrays our trust. Hearing before the Select Committee on Children, Youth and Families, One Hundred Second Congress, Second Session.* Washington, DC: U.S. Government Printing Office.

U.S. House of Representatives. (1994, July 19). *Deceit that sickens America: Health care fraud and its innocent victims. Hearings before the Subcommittee on Crime and Criminal Justice of the Committee on the Judiciary House of Representatives, One Hundred and Third Congress, Second Session.* Washington, DC: U.S. Government Printing Office.

U.S. Senate. (1992, July 28). *Hearing before the Committee on the Judiciary United States Senate, Senate Bill 2652, One Hundred Second Congress, Second Session.* Washington, DC: U.S. Government Printing Office.

Wallace, D., & Pekel, J. (2001). *Complete guide to ethics management: An ethics booklet for managers.* McNamara, CO: Fulcrum Group.

*Washington Post.* (2010). Landmark. The inside story of America's new healthcare law and what it means for us all. Washington, D.C.: Author.

Wocial, L. (1996). Achieving collaboration in ethical decision making: Strategies for nurses in clinical practice. *Dimensions of Critical Care Nursing, 15*(3), 150–15.

# 3

# Change and Decision Making

## CHAPTER OUTLINE

## LEARNING OUTCOMES

Before you begin, take a moment to familiarize yourself with the learning outcomes for this chapter.

- Discuss critical nursing issues related to reengineering, redesigning, re-regulating, rightsizing, and restructuring.
- Explain why the concept of change is important in the health care environment and to nursing leadership and management.
- Assess the external trends and factors that impact nursing practice and health care organizations.
- Compare and contrast two key change theories.
- Apply eight key steps in the change process.
- Analyze the issue of resistance to change and strategies for overcoming this.
- Develop strategies to improve responses to change.
- Apply the decision-making process.
- Critique the keys to successful planning.
- Distinguish between strategic and project planning.

## KEY TERMS

- Change
- Clinical judgment
- Clinical reasoning
- Compacts
- Critical thinking
- Decisive decision making
- Decision-making process
- Dichotomous thinking
- Empathy
- Empower/empowerment
- External policy
- Facilitators
- Flexible decision making
- Force-field analysis
- Hierarchic decision making
- Integrative decision making

- Internal policy
- Intuitive decision makers
- Moving stage
- Mutual recognition
- Non-programmed decisions
- Planning
- Policy planning
- Proactive planning
- Programmed decisions
- Project planning
- Quinn's theory of change
- Readiness for change
- Reciprocity
- Redesigning
- Reengineering
- Refreezing stage

- Regulations
- Re-regulating professional practice
- Resistance
- Restraining forces
- Restructuring nursing education
- Rightsizing
- Sensory overload
- Strategic planning
- Systematic decision makers
- Team decision making
- Unfreezing stage
- Vision
- Work redesign
- Workaround

## WHAT'S AHEAD

The health care delivery system is not a static system as it experiences changes daily and in some cases hourly. Staff members tend to think that leaders and managers will save the day by helping them cope with the ever-changing health care environment, maybe making it disappear; however, nurse leaders and managers also struggle to cope with change and to help staff. What does this mean? Nurses at all levels must make a commitment to the change process and take active roles in the process. Change that comes from and is totally managed by a manager will not be successful today. Staff members who pull back and wait for the manager to make the difference will also find that changes will continue to occur but without their input. "Understanding change and its potential landmines are important to be successful today, but we must also recognize the benefits of change, though we often complain about it. Change can invigorate us. If we had no change, there would be no need for critical thinking. After a time we would know all of the answers or approaches to expected problems. I am sure after a time we would also find this to be a rather boring environment in which to work, though for most of us it would be comfortable initially. Complacency and isolationism can be very destructive landmines" (Finkelman, 2001, p. 195). This chapter focuses on change and decision making in organizations. What are the critical change and decision-making processes, and how does change impact staff, health care organizations, and their decisions? It is difficult to separate change from decisions as responding to change requires that decisions are made, some minor, some more important and complex. Nurses participate in the change process and make decisions wherever they practice.

# The Five "Rs": Change and Decision Making in Action

The health care delivery system has been adjusting to changes in reimbursement, staff shortages, budget cuts, technology, role changes, and much more, all of which have had a major impact on nursing. Change has driven the need for the five "Rs," which particularly affect health care organizations, nursing education, and nursing practice. The five "Rs" are as follows:

1. Reengineering/redesigning/restructuring the health care organization
2. Redesigning the workforce
3. Re-regulating professional practice
4. Rightsizing the workforce
5. Restructuring nursing education

Each one of the five Rs is about change and requires decision making on the part of the organization and its staff. Understanding their historical and in some cases current impact provides an introduction to the importance of change and decision making for nurses.

## Reengineering/Redesigning/Restructuring the Health Care Organization

**Reengineering** was used in many health care organizations for a number of years, and though not used currently, it had an influence on the current status of many organizations. The Institute of Medicine discusses the impact that reengineering has had on nursing in its report on nursing (2004). Other terms used to describe this process are restructuring and **redesigning**. This process represents more than a minor organizational change—it was a reinvention or recreation of processes, work, and systems. The IOM discusses reengineering in health care and notes that the goal was to make patient care processes more efficient (2004). Often reengineering was not easy for nurses to accept as the process sometimes resulted in radical changes in how nursing was practiced, and thus nurses were reluctant to participate. To actively participate in reengineering, nurses needed to understand their own work and be willing to explore improving their practice.

Nurses experienced what was described as reengineering when the major focus was actually only on reducing full-time equivalents (FTEs), primarily nursing, developing or reducing services, or decreasing length-of-stay. This was usually done with limited nursing input. Varied reengineering strategies were used. An important strategy for nursing is the growing emphasis on patient-centered care, a combination of reengineering and work redesign. The goals are to improve patient and customer satisfaction, quality of care, and cost reduction. The use of the term patient-centered care is important in the Institute of Medicine reports on health care quality and is one of the five core health care professions core competencies. The idea of arranging work around the patient rather than specialized departments has great potential for providing an opportunity to deliver nursing care that meets patient needs; however, this has not been easy to accomplish. The Institute of Medicine reports (2003; 2004) now consistently emphasize patient-centered care. Though the reports emphasize quality IOM also includes efficiency and design of work. It takes time and commitment and requires significant change in the organization to provide patient-centered care. Over many years, patient care has been delivered in hospitals with the number of departments increasing and more and more staff interacting with the patient. Specialization has led to problems of poor communication, complex processes, increased paperwork, poor collaboration, and error. How would a hospital become more patient-centered? What redesign would be necessary? What role would nurses play? These are critical examples of decisions that must be made as planning is done to make major changes in health care organizations. Whenever health care organizations undergo major redesign retrospective evaluation needs to occur to assess the outcomes.

The new initiative Transforming Care at the Bedside (TCAB), which was influenced by the Institute of Medicine report *Keeping Patients Safe* (2004) and the Institute of Health Improvement, has had an impact on organizations in which TCAB is used. This initiative is discussed further in Chapter 17. The focus is again on quality but also the design of work to improve quality care. TCAB uses the change approach called Deep Dive, which is discussed later in this chapter. With this initiative small pilots are begun in hospitals to make needed changes and actively uses nurses in the process. This is an example of current approaches to reengineering care, but it is important to understand the history of the use of reengineering as it had a major impact on how nurses practice today in hospitals.

## Redesigning the Workforce

Demands that managed care placed on clinical settings to increase productivity and patient and customer satisfaction, and at the same time provide lower cost quality care, pressured nurse executives and managers to institute **work redesign**. With the nursing shortage, the need for work redesign is even more important. Improved efficiency that results in more effective practice with less staff is critical. This has led to the development of, and changes in, inpatient care delivery models, such as the use of patient-centered care and changing staff mix and thus altering the number of RNs, unlicensed assistive personnel (UAP), and licensed practical nurses (LPNs/LVN) and changing responsibilities. The effectiveness of these changes varies. Traditional nursing roles and activities need to be assessed, and then often rejected in order to change to more effective roles that allow for more innovative approaches. Nurses need to provide supportive data to demonstrate the impact that their own roles and activities have on efficiency, improved care, and patient outcomes. The problem, however, is that there are many perspectives on nursing work redesign. Determining the best way to design how staff works together to provide quality, safe care that includes patients is the key issue. Some hospitals have introduced the new role of the Clinical Nurse Leader (CNL), which is discussed in Chapters 4 and 6; however, the introduction of a new role needs to be planned. New roles impact current roles and cause problems if not thought through carefully.

When health care organizations confront the need to make changes in responsibilities, functions, and tasks in the delivery system, the most common reasons have been due to concerns about costs, productivity, and outcomes. Work redesign is used to address these concerns; however, there are other factors that need to be considered. Nurses are responsible for ensuring a baseline level of performance. If UAP are used, nurses need to ensure that training and supervision are provided to the UAP to ensure patient safety and quality care. Content from Chapter 14 on delegation applies to this issue. The nursing profession must also be careful about new delivery models or how staff is organized to provide care (for example, the use of teams), as discussed in Chapter 4. There needs to be more research to validate the outcomes of these models so that evidence-based management (EBM) can be implemented more effectively. The bottom line is nursing needs data to support these delivery changes.

Are models effective? If not, why? What can be done to make them more effective? Should the model be used? Under what circumstances is the model effective or ineffective? Nurses should be asking these questions and not waiting for others to do so. Nurses should also be directly responsible for finding the answers, analyzing the results, and making decisions about changes that need to be made.

Professional nursing organizations need to look at methods of examining best practices such as the Magnet Recognition Program and to utilize evidence-based management and evidence-based practice. This program, which is discussed in more detail in Chapter 6, identifies health care organizations that are providing excellent nursing care and have work environments that support professional nursing.

## Re-Regulating Professional Practice

Why is **re-regulating professional practice** an important change issue today? Nurses have discovered that many of the changes that are taking place in health care, such as the use of telehealth, workforce mobility, and mergers (or several health care organizations forming one organization, which may then have parts of the organization in different states), are affecting licensure. Today many nurses are providing care across state lines and in situations in which the patient is in a different state from the one in which the nurse is licensed and located, particularly near state borders, which makes access easier. The use of telenursing is also growing, which allows for greater opportunities to provide nursing care over distances using telecommunication technology and other technology. This type of care is considered to be within the practice of nursing, even if it is not "hands-on care" or direct care. In addition, restructuring of health care has led to an increase in multistate health care systems, and this has affected how nurses are employed and where they work.

In 2006 the National Council of State Boards of Nursing (NCSBN) began a long-term initiative to develop an evidence-based regulatory model for transitioning new nurses to practice (National Council of State Boards of Nursing, 2010). In 2010 the NCSBN began the process of developing pilots. This model would require new nurses to take and pass the nursing board exam (NCLEX) after graduation in order to practice in state of choice, obtain employment and complete a transition program of a minimum of 6 months and preferably participate in ongoing support program for an additional 6 months. At the end of first year of licensure the nurse would need to provide documentation to the state board of nursing that the transition program has been completed. The transition program is based on the five IOM health care professions core competencies. Though this change in regulation was in process in 2010, and it is important to note that the NCSBN cannot dictate change in individual state practice acts. This change in regulation would have to be made on an individual state basis. The model does accept other nurse residencies; however, these residencies would have to meet the basic criteria of the NCSBN model. This is a good example of how regulation might change and also how regulation is integrated with practice.

In order to understand the recent proposed changes in regulation, it is important to understand how regulation is applied. The purpose of practice regulation is to ensure public safety. Boards of nursing, which regulate nursing practice, began in the early 1900s (Hutcherson & Williamson, 1999). The right of states to regulate practice is based on the Tenth Amendment of the U.S. Constitution, the states' rights amendment. This amendment provides *each state* with the right to regulate nursing practice within its own state but not within other states. This is why nurses who move from one state to another to work must obtain licensure in the new state. **Reciprocity** or the right to practice is primarily based on national board scores; however, the nurse must still apply for an RN licensure in the state, meet individual state requirements such as continuing education, and pay state fees. Due to changes in health care, boards of nursing and nursing organizations have been discussing changes that need to be made in the regulation of nursing practice nationally. The dilemma is that licensure remains state-based and yet state lines may no longer bind nursing practice. Various options were considered by the National Council of State Boards of Nursing (NCSBN) to resolve this dilemma, but the option selected to address this licensure problem is **mutual recognition**. The implementation of this type of licensure requires an interstate compact, which is an agreement between two or more states, entered into for the purpose of addressing a problem that transcends state lines. **Compacts** are created when two or more states enact identical statutes establishing and defining the compact and its role. The result is the creation of both state law and an enforceable contract with other states that adopt the compact. Not all states have made decisions to make this change and collaborate with adjacent states about RN licensure, but there is a trend to move in this direction. Information about current states participating in mutual recognition can be found on individual state boards of nursing websites and at the National Council for State Boards of Nursing (NCSBN) website and individual state board of nursing websites.

## Rightsizing the Workforce

**Rightsizing** and downsizing are terms that cause nurses to shudder, as they suggest that the health care organization might reduce staff. During times of downsizing hospitals decreased their staff and beds, and then they had to reverse these decisions as needs rose. This has not been easy to accomplish since there is a nursing shortage now with fewer numbers able to get into nursing programs. The number of applications has increased, but wait lists have grown at the same time. "Almost 40 percent of all qualified applications to basic RN programs were turned away in 2008–2009" (National League for Nursing, May 13, 2010). The economic crisis of 2009–2010 has had a major impact on this problem, increasing the number applying. In addition, hospital acuity remains high requiring greater number of competent staff. Chapter 9 discusses staffing issues in more detail.

Rightsizing focuses on how much staff is required to do the job, and this has never been easy to predict or accomplish. Budget plays a major role. Since education for health care professionals takes time, it is important to try to predict future needs. The goal is to determine how many health care professionals need to be educated to meet the needs and ensure that there will be jobs for them when they complete their education and training. It is clear that there are not enough nurses now, and the predictions for the future are also bleak. Many more nurses will be needed to fill future empty positions as baby boomers retire from nursing (Buerhaus, Staiger, & Auerbach, 2009). The shortage has undergone fluctuations such as during the economic crisis of 2009–2010 more nurses returned to practice and there was an increase in number of applicants to nursing programs. Some areas of the country found that they no longer had a severe shortage and new graduates had a difficult time getting a position due to the return of nurses who had not practiced and the impact of nurses not taking early retirement because they needed more income. However, this does not eliminate the concern of the number of nurses who will be retiring soon and the need for replacement. Approaching the problem only from the point-of-view of getting the "right" number of nurses is not a helpful approach. Since it will probably not be possible to get the number of nurses desired, other strategies will be needed to change how nursing care is provided to reduce the number of nurses required.

## Restructuring Nursing Education

When **restructuring nursing education** is discussed there are two critical focus areas. The first is academic education, and the second is continuing education for nurses who are practicing. Nursing education must make curriculum changes in order to prepare nurses who meet today's and tomorrow's health care needs and needs to work more collaboratively with practice partners (Finkelman & Kenner, 2007). Several recent reports emphasize the need for change and improvement such as the IOM report *Health Professions Education* (2003) and the newest Carnegie Foundation study of nursing education, *Educating Nurses: A Call for Radical Transformation* (Benner, Sutphen, Leonard, & Day, 2010). Beverly Malone, chief executive officer for the National League of Nursing, comments on the nursing report (Benner, Sutphen, Leonard, & Day, 2010): "This book represents a call to arms, a call for nursing educators and programs to step up in our preparation of nurses. This book will incite controversy, wonderful debate, and dialogue among nurses and others" (Benner, Sutphen, Leonard, & Day, 2010, back cover). The report is all about change: Change in the delivery of health care and the practice of nursing that drives critical need for change in nursing education. The IOM report emphasizes need for change and five core competencies that all health care professions should meet. These five core competencies are also emphasized in the newest edition of the *Essentials of Baccalaureate Education for Professional Nursing Practice* (American Association of Colleges of Nursing, 2008).

The importance of the consumer as a significant player in the health care environment, emphasizing patient-centered care, must be part of this preparation; however, this is not new to nursing education as nursing has always emphasized the importance of the patient's role. Understanding the interplay of values, motivations, and incentives of the major players or stakeholders in health care including insurers, providers, purchasers of health care, and consumers, helps nurses understand the health care culture in which they practice. Stakeholders sometimes have competing interests that affect decisions. Health care markets continue to change, which means nurses at all levels need to be aware of these changes and also know how to react positively to change, and in many cases to even anticipate it. Understanding the reasons health care delivery has become more business oriented and knowing its effect on nursing practice is also important. Today, there is a greater emphasis on service, innovation, cost-effectiveness, and customer service. To be successful in the more business-oriented health care environment, nurses need to be flexible. Nurses do need to have some understanding of the impact of costs on care and recognize that nurses have a fiscal responsibility or should be active in trying to reduce costs whenever it is possible. Lack of understanding about this responsibility is no longer an acceptable reason for not participating in reducing costs. All nurses need to be prepared to be leaders as well as team members, and restructuring education needs to provide content and learning experiences that assist students in developing leadership competencies.

The second area of concern about nursing education is the need for continuing education. All nurses need to be lifelong learners. Practice should be based on current knowledge. Not only is current information needed, but there also needs to be opportunities to understand and apply the knowledge.

The education needs of both groups, practicing nurses and nursing students, must be met to ensure that nurses are able to practice and participate actively in the change process within the health care delivery system, as well as make decisions. Several important factors related to nursing are important in understanding the changing health care environment.

1. Demographic trends are a very important issue related to workforce needs. Racial distribution and gender disparity in the nursing profession are problems. Another fact related to the future of health care delivery is the aging of the nursing workforce. Who will replace nurses as large numbers retire?

2. Another issue is the changing demand for nursing services, something that continues to be very difficult to determine. The present nursing shortage is the number one topic in nursing today. The shortage has had a major impact on the effectiveness of the entire health care delivery system. Roles and responsibilities have to be considered as needs and demands for nursing services are analyzed.

3. The shifting nursing employment settings are a critical topic in both education and practice. Patients are sicker in the hospital, requiring complex care, and more and more care is provided outside the hospital and in the community. How are nurses prepared to meet both the needs of the acute care patient and the patient in the community?

4. The separation of nursing education and practice has provided many advantages for developing university-based nursing education, but it has caused problems for employers who want a more clearly articulated continuum of education and practice. Employers have become more involved in identifying minimum competencies for employment.

5. The changing nursing workforce competencies require that nurses possess **critical thinking** skills, independent clinical reasoning and judgment, management and organizational skills, leadership abilities, technological understanding, informatics, quality improvement, and the ability to practice in a variety of settings using evidence-based practice (Institute of Medicine, 2003). Nurses, not just nurse managers, need to be able to manage and coordinate personnel, services, data, and resources. They also need to demonstrate leadership.

6. There is a need for greater integration of research and nursing practice. Isolating education and research from the clinical setting is not helpful to nursing practice. Evidence-based practice (EBP) is having an important impact on the application of research findings in practice as well as the use of standards, clinical guidelines, and clinical pathways. Evidence-based management is also critical. Evidence-based practice and management are discussed in more detail in Chapter 15.

# The Concept of Change

**Change** is something that occurs that makes a difference. Change has become the normal state for all health care providers, but what is being changed? In general, everything; however, the important examples of change are related to an organization's structure, roles and responsibilities, communication methods and systems, policies and standards, culture, leadership and management approaches, and competencies and attitudes. In fact, before one change is completed there seems to be another one waiting in the wings to come on center stage. Some changes even come together, forcing staff and management to juggle multiple changes at one time. Change can be viewed from three interrelated perspectives as described in Figure 3-1 (Fisher, 1996).

Change disturbs the equilibrium, and so there also needs to be an effort to learn how to work in an environment whose equilibrium is frequently out of balance. Every staff member and nurse manager needs to understand his or her own personal response to change, both effective and ineffective responses. One concern is there are organizations or units in organizations that feel stability and security are more important than looking forward to the opportunities that are offered by the change process. In these organizations, staff feels frustration as it struggles with change that will inevitably occur and yet experience a leadership that says, "We want things to stay the same."

FIGURE 3-1 Interrelated perspectives.

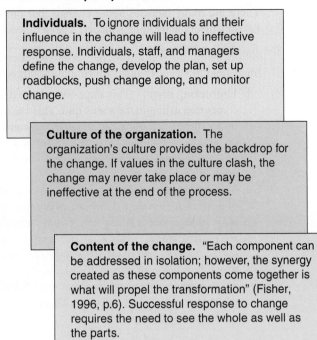

**Individuals.** To ignore individuals and their influence in the change will lead to ineffective response. Individuals, staff, and managers define the change, develop the plan, set up roadblocks, push change along, and monitor change.

**Culture of the organization.** The organization's culture provides the backdrop for the change. If values in the culture clash, the change may never take place or may be ineffective at the end of the process.

**Content of the change.** "Each component can be addressed in isolation; however, the synergy created as these components come together is what will propel the transformation" (Fisher, 1996, p.6). Successful response to change requires the need to see the whole as well as the parts.

So why bother with change if it causes so much stress and problems? External factors outside the health care organization are a key driver in the need for change. Some changes are actually made so that the organization can survive. Many health care organizations today function from day-to-day, and in the long term they may close or merge with other health care organizations. Nurses work daily in environments where external factors have an impact on what they do and on their ability to influence the health care delivery system. Each nurse has opportunities to be a change agent, but these opportunities are driven by and affected by many critical external factors. Box 3-1 identifies examples of these external factors that may affect change in health care delivery.

| BOX 3-1 | EXTERNAL FACTORS THAT AFFECT CHANGE |
| --- | --- |

- Local, state, and federal government: policy, laws, and regulations
- Technology
- Economics
- Reimbursement
- Competition
- Providers
- Managed care
- Providers of all types
- Medicare and Medicaid
- Demographics
- Nurse Practice Acts
- Health care professional organizations
- Health care professional standards
- Accreditation of health care organizations
- Malpractice issues
- Community culture
- Nurse recruitment and retention
- Community support of health care organizations
- Labor unions
- Research
- Local businesses
- Access to care
- Nursing education
- Marketing
- The uninsured and underinsured
- Pharmaceutical industry
- Consumers and consumer organizations
- Information technology
- Social service agencies
- Health status of the community
- Media and image
- Patient rights, privacy, and confidentiality
- Disasters and response

## Examples of Change Theory

There are many theories about change, but only two theories are discussed in this chapter: Lewin's theory and Quinn's theory, a newer theory.

LEWIN'S FORCE-FIELD MODEL OF CHANGE   Lewin proposed a change theory that he called a force-field model of change, which includes three stages (Lewin, 1947).

1. **Unfreezing stage.**   This stage focuses on developing problem awareness and decreasing forces that maintain the status quo. This includes the recognition of a problem and whether or not there is a feeling that the problem can be improved. Examples of methods that might be used to promote unfreezing are interview results, surveys, or meetings in which there is an open discussion of relevant issues. The result should be a better understanding of the issue or problem.
2. **Moving stage.**   In this stage the issue or problem is clearly identified, and goals and objectives are developed. Strategies are developed and implemented. This is the working stage of the process where new values, attitudes, and behaviors are promoted.
3. **Refreezing stage.**   This stage occurs when the change is incorporated into the work environment and its processes. This stage may take some time as it is easy to slip back to the way things were, so during this phase, the goal is to prevent a return to the past. In today's health care environment, organizations typically experience refreezing for one change while beginning another change. This is something that was not as critical when Lewin developed his theory.

FORCE-FIELD ANALYSIS   The theory of **force-field analysis** is used to improve the change process. In this analysis the manager (change agent) and staff identify the driving forces or factors that will help to move the situation in the direction of the anticipated change or the desired outcome. To be effective this should be a collaborative process between the manager and staff. If the manager identifies these forces and analyzes them without staff input, the analysis may not be as effective. Frequently staff is able to identify factors that might make a strategy more effective. Examples of driving forces are increasing staff, increasing staff time to provide direct care, decreasing costs, or increased availability of expertise. The focus should be on increasing acceptance of the change.

**Restraining forces** or forces that may keep the change from occurring should not, however, be ignored. What might be a restraining force? Examples are staffing concerns, increased safety risks, or decreasing quality. These factors may be anything that prevents change from moving forward. After the driving and restraining forces are identified, there are three possible approaches that might be used to cope with driving and restraining forces, which are described in Figure 3-2:

1. Increase the number or strength of the driving forces
2. Decrease the number or strength of the restraining forces
3. A combination of both

It is easy to apply these approaches in health care, but it does require information about the organization, staff, processes, and the change issue or problem. It is also important to include the informal processes such as the grapevine and informal leaders who may or may not be supportive. This information must be carefully analyzed using each of the approaches described in Lewin's theory.

Rogers' theory (2003) focused on change as being more complex than how Lewin described change. This led to the term "diffusion of innovations," meaning that when a new idea is adopted or an innovation occurs there are consequences. These consequences need to be considered.

QUINN'S THEORY OF CHANGE   When an organization experiences change it usually faces a major dilemma of a "slow death" or "deep change" (Quinn, 1996, 2000). When does "slow death" occur? If an organization finds it is more comfortable accepting the status quo and not changing, "slow death" occurs. This is demonstrated when staff experiences burnout, lacks energy, or feels hopeless or trapped. Staff is seen as pulling back and running around doing insignificant things. "'Slow death' exists when self-interests triumph over collective responsibilities" (Pesut, 2001, p. 118). There is no vision or clear description of the future for the organization.

**FIGURE 3-2 Force-field analysis.**

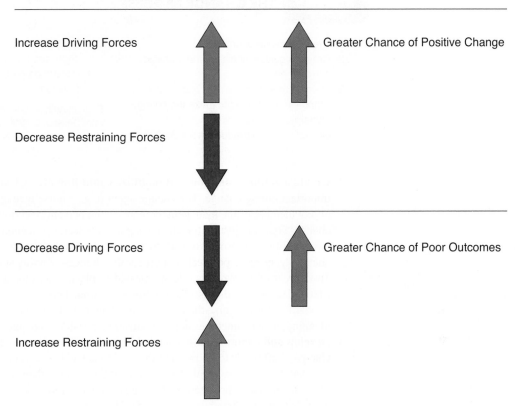

Increase Driving Forces

Greater Chance of Positive Change

Decrease Restraining Forces

Decrease Driving Forces

Greater Chance of Poor Outcomes

Increase Restraining Forces

How do organizations and their leaders typically cope with "slow death"? The first method is probably obvious: they resign themselves to the situation. The second method is to try to find a way around the problem or a way out, hoping that the "slow death" will not cause a major problem. These two methods are not positive responses and usually make the situation worse as the organization will not adapt when it is needed. The last coping method is the positive approach of engaging in "deep change." This is the method that a Transformational Leader would take. Deep change requires that the need for change is understood and accepted and that adjustments are made in the organization to respond to the need. Transformation change leads to strategic change—improving the vision, change structure and culture (Robbins & Davidhizar, 2007). Empowers others and makes changes in the power structure. **Quinn's theory of change** is an approach that is easily applied with current leadership theories discussed in Chapter 1 such as Transformational Leadership and Emotional Intelligence.

## The Process of Change

The literature discusses many approaches to change. Dessler (2002) describes one of these in his eight-step process for leading organizational change that is helpful in understanding the key elements of the change process. When the eight steps of the change process are experienced, change can occur at all levels of the organization (for example, within a unit or division, at one location such as a community clinic, or throughout the entire organization). Regardless of where or how much of the organization is affected, **resistance** and acceptance will be experienced. The following steps, which are highlighted in Box 3-2, provide some description about what happens during the process and also applies to Lewin's theory of change.

1. **Create a sense of urgency.** Applying unfreezing means that staff needs to be motivated to make the changes. "Urgency does more than overcome employees' traditional reasons for resisting change: It can also jar them out of their complacency" (Dessler, 2002, p. 302). Staff needs to feel that change is required. This impacts motivation to make change successful. If, however, change occurs too fast, the organization and its staff may not be able to respond effectively, and this may affect other organizational functions.

| BOX 3-2 | THE CHANGE PROCESS |
|---------|--------------------|

1. Create a sense of urgency
2. Create a guiding coalition and mobilize commitment
3. Develop and communicate a shared vision
4. Empower employees to make the change
5. Generate short-term wins
6. Consolidate and produce more change
7. Anchor the new ways of doing things in the organizational culture
8. Monitor progress and adjust the vision as required

Source: Author created summarization of content from Dessler, G. (2002). *Management*, pp. 302–306. Upper Saddle River, NJ: Prentice Hall.

2. **Create a guiding coalition and mobilize commitment.**   Clearly, the change agent is important during change. The change agent (e.g., a nurse manager, team leader, staff nurse, or any member of the management team) is the person(s) who works to bring about the change. Focusing just on the change agent, however, is not enough. It is important to also have coalitions or groups of staff that can help push the change forward. This means the change agent seeks political support for the change—gaining staff support and agreement. Task forces often play this role and provide a place to develop a shared understanding. Many ideas will be discussed, and this is exciting. This process also helps bring "staff onboard"—to recognize the need for the change. If, however, the discussion never gets to planning, it can sometimes act as a barrier or resistor to change.

3. **Develop and communicate a shared vision.**   The **vision** provides direction for the change. Staff needs to know what that vision is and how it relates to them. After they agree on what the outcome should be—a view of the future—then specific objectives need to be identified to reach the outcome. Change agents need to keep the vision simple and real, and it needs to mean something to the staff. Sharing the vision with staff members so that they can understand and participate actively requires multiple methods, forums, and repetition to ensure that all staff members gain an understanding.

4. **Empower employees to make the change.**   Major changes in an organization require empowerment of staff members so that they can actively participate in all phases. To **empower** or **empowerment** is to enable to act so that when staff feel empowered they are then more committed to the change and buy into it. This process involves an interrelationship of authority resources, timely and accurate information, and accountability. It is at this time that barriers, such as resistances, are dealt with in order to move the change process along.

5. **Generate short-term wins.**   If a change process only focuses on the long-term results, management and staff will lose steam somewhere along the way. Change takes time, but people need to feel that they are moving along. Identifying short-term, measureable goals or outcomes and then evaluating when they are met will help management and staff members feel that they can make it to the end point and they can see that some progress has been made but are also important to effective evaluation. These short-term wins do much to build morale and a sense of success. They act as benchmarks that keep the change process on target.

6. **Consolidate and produce more change.**   It is at this point that complacency can return. Staff may feel that things really are fine and nothing more needs to be done. When short-term goals are met and recognized, this helps staff to recognize that there is movement, hopefully positive movement, toward the goal. Staff members may need to be reminded that some changes take time. A typical problem that is encountered with change is how to keep it going. Many managers and staff seem to be able to recognize a need for change, plan for change, and even implement change with greater ease than maintaining the change. There is a greater risk of slowing down the change process at this point, almost as if all involved say, "Okay we did it. What's next?" If this occurs, then the final goal(s) will not be met. Stopping too soon often is the reason staff feels that the organization never seems to make changes effectively—it never completes anything.

7. **Anchor the new ways of doing things in the organizational culture.**   Shared values are important in every organization. As change occurs, there may need to be changes in these values so that there is a match between the change and the organizational culture. One

example of values is recognition of the importance of staff involvement in decisions, diversity, and management that respects the employee. Changing values must be done carefully and only when absolutely necessary. This can cause stress as management and staff may feel insecure when values are challenged, but this can be worked through with recognition of new shared values. For example, if an organization wants more staff input and will use this feedback, but this approach has not been valued in the past, staff may be unsure about this change in values. Some may wonder why managers are now interested in what they have to say. Some may doubt that the change will actually happen. Management will need to take the time to explain why they now value staff input, and then managers at all levels will have to demonstrate that they mean it. It is important, however, to recognize that not all changes require changes in values.

8. **Monitor progress and adjust the vision as required.** Evaluation should not be ignored. The measurable goals or outcomes developed earlier in the process are now used to measure success. Were the goals met? Changes that organizations and their staff undergo are not written in stone. As has been noted in this chapter, change is constant now, so getting too settled is not a good idea. Organizations not only have to be concerned with future change, but they also need to monitor each change process. Adjustment may be needed, and if so, it needs to take place as soon as possible. Staff will become very discouraged if this does not occur. The inability to adjust can do considerable damage to morale, recruitment and retention, productivity, and quality of care and impact staff willingness to participate in other change experiences.

READINESS FOR CHANGE **Readiness for change** means that management and staff are willing to take on the challenge of change and to invest in the effort. At this time they are ready to begin the work of change. Not all staff will be ready at the same time, and some will never be ready. Readiness is affected by trust, the relationship between staff and management, fear and concern about what might be lost, staff experience, seriousness of the change, past history with both personal and work related change, effectiveness of communication, staff and management commitment to the organization, and the planning process or lack of a process. Assessment of readiness for change might include the following questions (Free Management Library, 2009):

- Does the change-management approach suggest what organizational development activities should be used now, for example, the method of strategic management might suggest that a SWOT analysis be done; strategic goals established along with the action plans for each goal; and then implementation of the action plans, which are closely monitored?
- Is the selected activity most likely to address or solve the problems or achieve the goals?
- Does the nature of the activity match the culture of the organization?
- Do the change agent(s) and key members of the organization have the ability to conduct the activity?
- Does the activity require more time to conduct than the time available in which to address the problem or goal?
- Does the organization have the resources that are necessary to conduct the activity, considering resources such as funding, attention, and time from people and facilities?

Many barriers and facilitators that affect the change process can be found in any organization. Some of the typical barriers are as follows:

- Staff members are too focused on their own specialty and not able to see beyond it—they are focusing on parts and unable to see the whole, which often results in isolationism and territoriality.
- When managers overdirect, overobserve, or overreport, staff will not be innovative. In this case staff members feel they will be taken care of by the manager.
- When staff or managers say, "This is the way things have always been done," "They'll never accept it," or "We can't"—they see no need to respond positively to change.
- Policies and procedures can be barriers if they prevent staff from approaching change in a creative way.
- Clear measurable goals or outcomes were not developed resulting in ineffective evaluation of outcomes.

Clearly, some policies and procedures must be followed; however, if they interfere with the consideration of alternative options in the change process then they act as barriers, such as the following examples.

- Managers and staff with hidden agendas or motives are barriers.
- Criticizing staff when they make suggestions and identifying them as troublemakers when the appropriate response should be rewarding staff who challenge and question ideas, thereby contributing new ideas.
- Organizational inertia or organizations that just do not seem to be changing or keeping up with current trends act as a barrier to effective organizations.
- Budgetary constraints can act as a barrier. If there is not enough money to make changes, this can be deadly for the organization.
- Bureaucratic organizations set up too much "red tape" and thus limit creativity. There are too many steps and staff to consult to get something accomplished.
- **Sensory overload** occurs when staff has just experienced too much change in a short period of time acts as a barrier. Staff needs a break to recoup.
- Fear of failure will be a barrier if one cannot get over the fear and move on. This limits risk taking, which is necessary for successful responses to change.
- The complexity of a needed change may make it difficult to initiate change that requires major planning. Initiating a response to change may require funding, excessive staff time, additional staff, and so on.
- Change means there needs to be a willingness to alter direction. When a change decision is viewed as written in stone, this then acts as a barrier (Fisher, 1996; Gebelein et al., 2000).

**Facilitators** for change are committed change agents and also situations, factors, and behaviors that can reduce or eliminate barriers to change (Fisher, 1996). These facilitators make it possible to make a change. Managers who use self-reflection to understand behavior and how the behaviors affect the organization's response to change are more effective facilitators of change. They are visible and accessible, and thus better able to lead the staff. The staff members can easily communicate with their manager to express their reactions and ideas. Getting teams involved in the change process facilitates change. Staff members who feel that they can participate in this process and have some freedom to act will improve the change process to reach a more effective outcome. Few situations are so clear that there is only one approach. Recognizing this acts as a facilitator. "When organizations are rigid and job descriptions are defined too precisely, little room for flexibility and shifting of responsibility is possible" (Fisher, 1996, p. 56). Wiggle room that allows for flexibility helps organizations to develop creative approaches to change.

**Empathy** is a critical key to readiness for change, and when it is present there is a greater chance of reaching a successful outcome (Kirkpatrick, 2001). It is related to effective communication and participation, which are always important. What is empathy? Empathy occurs when one is able to put oneself in the shoes of another person. It is empathy that helps in the understanding of acceptance, resistance, or a mixed reaction to change. With this information, concerns can be better addressed, and hopefully, the change process will go more smoothly. If managers and staff take time to get to know one another, this will improve empathy. Then there will be some ability to anticipate how one another might respond. "Communication means to create understanding" (Kirkpatrick, 2001, p. 58). This is more than just sending and receiving information. Staff needs to understand the "why," "what," and "how" about the change. Change cannot really be successful without inclusion of some empathy and effective communication.

Participation from all staff involved also improves communication and the final outcomes. Participatory management/leadership sometimes is viewed as the miracle that will solve all problems. Just get the staff involved, and the task is accomplished. It does not work this way. Participation must be managed and used carefully. It is also means staff must have responsibility and accountability. Timing and clear direction must also be part of the process. An important factor is how much management really believes that staff participation is critical to success. Lip-service acceptance of the need for staff participation will only be more destructive leading to distrust between staff and management. Staff will know when management is asking for participation because it is "the thing to do" rather than from a deep-seated belief that this is the best approach. Empathy clearly affects readiness for change since understanding, which is improved with empathy, is required for readiness.

**RESISTANCE TO CHANGE**   Most managers and staff have experienced forced change, change that appeared to be useless, as well as times when it would just be better to have things stay the way they were, protecting the status quo. Staff resistance to change places major roadblocks to success and progress. Why might staff or even managers be resistant to a change? Typically, change means someone has to give up something or make some adaptation, and this is stressful. Along with the stress, the person may not be able to see the benefits and no one points the way to the positive aspects of the change. The person is concerned about

1. his/her *fears and biases* due to lack of understanding;
2. *perceptual issues* when the person cannot appreciate the situation around the change;
3. *economic threat*, which may lead to job change, job loss, decreased salary, and lack of promotion; and
4. *social threat* when the social structure of the organization changes.

Resistance to change is inevitable and can be experienced by managers, staff, the organization as a whole or parts of it, the community outside the organization, and by consumers. Most people do not like disequilibrium because it makes them feel uncomfortable. Resistance to change is often the first response to disequilibrium. With the need for change occurring rapidly today, there is less time for adjustment though staff does need time to do this. When there is little time for adjustment, resistance can be greater. What are some of the typical reasons for manager and staff resistance that need to be considered before a change is instituted?

- Staff or managers see no need for a change and feel that the way things are done is fine, which is the effect of habit and inertia.
- Staff or managers see the need for change as a personal criticism.
- Staff or managers feel that the organization is constantly changing and do not feel a sense of stability anywhere in the organization.
- Staff and a new nurse manager or new team leader may not have had enough time to develop the relationship that is critical to successful response to change.
- Staff or manager may have developed a negative attitude toward his or her manager/supervisor, the nursing department, or the organization and view all changes negatively.
- Staff does not respect the nurse manager, or the nurse manager does not respect the staff and is unable to be objective.
- Staff does not hear about a change directly from the manager but rather as secondhand information.
- When staff or managers have a negative attitude toward the organization, this results in a negative attitude toward change.
- The change will add to work, and thus it is viewed as a burden.
- Staff or manager may feel that the change may cause more problems than it solves.
- Staff or manager may fear the unknown and the loss of predictability.
- Administration or management may not have admitted that some past decisions related to change were inadequate.
- Change that is directed rather than participatory tends to experience more resistance (Kirkpatrick, 2001).

Though all of these are possible reasons for resistance, the most common reason for resistance is lack of staff input and participation. Sometimes it is difficult to identify the reasons for resistance; however, it is important to try and identify these reasons. If this can be done, strategies can then be taken to prevent them or to decrease their impact, such as by applying Lewin's theory to decrease the barriers and increase the facilitators.

Loss plays a role in resistance to change and should be included in the assessment of resistance. Loss is a natural experience with change. What is loss? Examples of loss that staff may experience are old ways of doing things, old job responsibilities, a manager or staff person who may leave his or her job, or old structure. Staff needs to grieve these losses and then move on. Some staff members do this with greater ease than others. Grieving requires (a) recognition of the loss, (b) letting go, and (c) moving on. Some of the common losses that those who resist change are concerned about when change is introduced include the following:

- **Security.**   Staff members may lose their jobs.
- **Money.**   Staff may experience a decrease in salary, overtime, benefits, travel expenses, education expenses, or budget level.
- **Pride and satisfaction.**   Job redesign may mean that the job is less prestigious or less interesting.
- **Friends and important contacts.**   Change may bring an alteration in staff interactions on the job.
- **Freedom.**   Freedom may lead to changes in the ability to function independently or the assignment of a new manager who does not allow as much freedom.
- **Responsibility.**   The level of responsibility may decrease or it could increase, leading to a loss of competency in the job.
- **Authority.**   Power and authority over others may change or be lost with reorganization.
- **Good working conditions.**   Staff may experience a change in space, location, sharing more with others, work hours, and so on.
- **Status.**   Staff may fear reduction to a low level or less recognized position (Kirkpatrick, 2001, pp. 20–21).

Management and staff can experience any of these losses. These possible losses will be on their minds as change occurs. It is natural for staff to want to protect what is valuable, and this can then become a resistance to change.

Is there value to this resistance to change? Yes, there can be value to resistance as it can force management or the change agent to clarify the need for change and then develop a plan with a clearer statement of purpose. Those who question change may be providing valuable information of flaws that can be solved before more serious errors are made. Resistance may indicate that the communication process has not worked in getting a clear message across, and this should not be ignored. Sometimes resistance is used against those who are resistant. Staff members who are resistant may be identified as non-team players. This approach can be very destructive, as it sets a tone of clamping down on those who offer a different point of view. Resistance should be viewed as a motivator to make the message clearer and to use input from others. Further assessment is then required to improve the plan and clearly state the outcomes.

A critical factor in coping with resistance to change is the long-term relationship that exists between management and staff. If this relationship has been positive, with trust and open communication, then resistance can usually be handled effectively. If this relationship does not exist, then coping with resistance will be more difficult. As was discussed in Chapter 1, managers must spend time on building and maintaining staff relationships as this will be the key to success. Managers who demonstrate leadership competence will understand the need to respond in the following way: "I need to stop and listen."

Since some resistance should be expected, planning for resistance needs to be included whenever change is occurring. First, staff needs to understand why change is needed—the vision for change, advantages and disadvantages, how it might adversely affect staff, how change relates to competitive needs, and the financial benefits. Losses may occur, and this potential requires open discussion. Alliances need to be formed to gain political support for the change. What is political support? This is when one person supports another because that person feels a personal allegiance and will support the person's ideas. When leaders allow staff to openly discuss concerns without fear or punitive actions, resistance can be dealt with openly. Clearly, data that can be provided to support the need and direction for change are very important. It may be necessary to stop doing what is being done and take a step back. Resistance needs to be viewed as an honest friend or a cue. Allowing others to tell their story or express their concerns will help make resistance a positive experience rather than a barrier to success. When children cross the street they are taught to, "Stop, look, and listen." This is what needs to be done when resistance occurs.

ACCEPTANCE OF CHANGE    After this discussion of resistance to change, it is easy to assume that all staff resist change, but this is not true. What is different about situations that are accepted and in some cases welcomed (Kirkpatrick, 2001)? There is no doubt that when a situation is very bad staff tends to welcome change, hoping it will improve a dysfunctional situation. What about the situations that are not so extreme? The key issue in acceptance is not what might be lost, but rather what will be gained. This is where the focus should be, though concerns about what might be lost should not be ignored. These gains are related to the loss factors, but they focus on the positive. Staff members feel they will be more secure in their jobs and more of their skills will be used. There may be an increase in money through salary, benefits, and other incentive changes. There may be an improved overall budget. Someone may receive a promotion or a new manager may be assigned who may give staff more authority. Status and prestige may improve with more space, special responsibilities, or a new location. Job responsibilities may change and improve. Better working conditions may be gained with new equipment, work schedule, or better workspace. Self-satisfaction in the job or the work environment may occur. Staff members may find themselves in work situations that provide them with better personal contacts or social relationships. The change may require less time and effort to get the job done because work will be more efficient. In conclusion, there may also be some staff members who have mixed reactions to change—some resistance with some acceptance. How an individual identifies or predicts what will be gained and what will be lost are critical factors in directing the individual's response to change—whether it is resistance, acceptance, or somewhere in-between.

WHERE TO BEGIN WHEN CONFRONTED WITH CHANGE    There are internal and external key factors that influence how an organization responds to change (for example, a change in policy, regulations and accreditation, organization, and financial issues). Each of these factors needs to be considered.

1. **Internal and external policies.**    It is important to understand how change affects and is affected by **internal** and **external policies** before actions are taken. Are there health policies such as state or federal laws that would affect a decision about the need for a decision? External policies may seem to be disconnected but really provide required direction (for example, a state's nurse practice act describes what RNs may do). Internal policies are those that exist within an organization. Clearly, internal policies might be changed and may again be changed to adapt to a situation; however, what is the policy's present status? An example is the increased use of UAP, which has caused much concern in nursing. If a hospital wants to increase the use of UAP in the organization, what does the hospital policy say about the UAP's present role, and how does this role relate to the change the hospital wants to make? What does the state board of nursing say about the UAP role and responsibilities? Internal and external policies must be reviewed and met when changes are made. Changes in external policy require political advocacy.

2. **Regulations and accreditation.**    **Regulations** are very important. They describe how laws are to be implemented, and they are developed by governmental agencies after legislative bodies pass laws, as in the previous example regarding boards of nursing that develop regulations relating to nurse practice acts. Another example is the U.S. Department of Health and Human Services (DHHS), which develops regulations for specific laws passed by Congress (for example, when laws about Medicare are passed there still needs to be rules set up to address implementation of the law, which are much more detailed than the law). Standards and accreditation also have an impact on change (for example, nursing standards of care and the standards developed by the Joint Commission that are used when health care organizations are evaluated for accreditation).

3. **Organization.**    Organizational issues, such as the organization's vision statement of how it views itself in the future; structure (departments, who reports to whom); size, roles, and functions of staff and administration; communication; morale and culture; willingness to change; financial status; quality improvement; and the organization's position and relationship with the community are all key to understanding the organization, how it will respond to change, and what needs to change. For example, if a health care organization is experiencing low staff morale as well as having financial problems, it will have problems responding to a need to

change its documentation system. Staff will probably not be eager to make changes, and there may be limited funds to develop a new system. In addition, consideration of the organizational structure from the microsystem, mesosystem, and macrosystem perspectives is important in improving care and function across the organization during times of change (Godfrey, Melin, Muething, Batalden, Nelson, 2008). The microsystem level looks at the organization from "inside out," at the unit level where direct care work is done. The mesosystem level focuses on "creating the conditions" leading to organizational performance improvement, for example helping staff be successful, identifying and getting resources staff need, and develop measures to track improvement. The macrosystem views the organization from "outside in," setting vision for micro and mesosytems, leadership and management support, and so on across the organization for the organization as a whole.

4. **Financial issues.**   Costs can never be ignored, and during change responses may be costly. Change may actually be driven by increased cost. For example, a hospital may decide to eliminate its obstetrical service because it is not getting enough admissions and is in competition with another hospital that has a large obstetrical service. In an uncertain health care industry, two things are facts. First, regardless of the decision maker (government, managed care organizations/insurers, businesses, health care organizations), cost constraints will continue to tighten. Second, as data become more available and more reliable, data will increasingly be used in decision making. Data will drive how care is delivered by driving improvement opportunities and how the organization competes with other health care organizations.

Along with the consideration of influences on the organization, an organization needs to include total quality improvement in the change process. In doing this, the organization's leaders create a plan for excellence and better ensure implementation of the plan. Quality improvement is discussed in more detail in Chapters 16 and 17.

Strategies to respond to change are very important throughout the change process. To adjust to change, nurses need to develop their mental flexibility, which is the ability to consider new information and a broad range of alternatives (Gebelein et al., 2000). When a nurse uses mental flexibility, the nurse listens to others and avoids snap judgments. This is an attitude of "yes and . . ." rather than "yes, but. . . ." This nurse will ask others who are trusted for honest feedback, develop personal creativity, and will improve coping with change through these acts. How can coping with change be improved? Examples of guidelines are found in Box 3-3 (Gebelein et al., 2000; Marrelli, 2004).

THE CHANGE AGENT   During the change process, the change agent, who may be a nurse executive, nurse manager, nurse team leader, staff nurse, and so on, has four major leadership functions: charismatic, enabling, instrumental, and missionary. There is no doubt that leadership is one of the most critical factors affecting change, particularly major changes, in a health care organization. It can make a difference in whether or not the change process will be effective. Transformational leadership has a positive effect on the change process.

1. The charismatic change agent is an envisioning leader who can describe the vision, set high expectations, and is a role model for staff. In this process the change agent needs to energize others and be excited and stimulated about the potential opportunity.
2. As an enabling change agent, the change agent expresses personal views, empathizes, and lets others know that they can do it.
3. Change agents need to also demonstrate instrumental leadership, which is the management component of leadership referred to as Transactional Leadership, by providing staff members with resources they need to do their jobs (funds, appropriate staff levels, supplies and equipment, and so on).
4. As a missionary change agent, the change agent shares and clearly communicates the vision that is required to meet the goals (Dessler, 2002, p. 307).

Like their staff, managers must cope with frequent changes. It is important for staff to understand the manager's response to change as it affects staff involvement. The major role of the manager is to implement change as directed from upper level administration or management.

## BOX 3-3　GUIDELINES FOR COPING WITH CHANGE

- During the creatively stage, give up critical judgment; avoid using, "It won't work."
- Instead of asking, "Why?" ask, "Why not?"
- Use a multidisciplinary group to develop responses to change needs.
- Expect that resistance to change is a fact, but approach it as a problem, not a character flaw.
- Talk, talk, talk to get the ideas flowing. Be challenged by opposite points-of-view. Try taking the opposite point-of-view and defend it.
- Generate as many options as possible. This will lead to finding the best method of coping with change.
- Do not throw out ideas too quickly. These may be important ideas.
- Join together with the change champions in the organization, those who seem to do well with change.

- View change as a challenge or opportunity for innovation.
- Control is very important as it means that the staff members feel that they can make a difference.
- Commitment is part of a successful response to change.
- Working together and using social support can give staff extra energy and resources.
- Use stress management when stress increases, as it often does during the change process.

Source: Robbins, Stephen P.; Decenzo, David A., *Fundamentals of management: Essential concepts and applications*, 3rd, © 2001. Printed and electronically reproduced by permission of Pearson Education, Inc., Upper Saddle River, New Jersey.

Some managers feel that they must respond positively to all requests even if they disagree with the need or the specific change. Why do they do this? They may be afraid about what might happen to them if they do not agree. They may want to be seen as a loyal manager. If the manager does disagree, the manager may decide to ask why this change is required. The manager may then need to explain why he or she disagrees with the change and make recommendations for other approaches. There are certainly managers who have come to the point where they cannot agree with upper level management directives for change, and if they cannot influence the change process, they may then leave their positions. During these times, stress will be very high, and undoubtedly this will spill over onto the staff.

There are other roles that managers need to take. Change agents do not wait for change—they look for it and embrace it as an opportunity. In addition, a manager may implement some change independently from the total organization, without involvement from those above the manager. These changes usually pertain to the manager's unit or department and do not affect others outside that area. There are fewer and fewer situations that can meet this criterion as collaboration across areas is becoming more important in successful organizations. If the budget is involved, then the manager must carefully consider how to respond and how to involve upper management. It takes courage to initiate change as it involves risk taking, a higher risk than just implementing change that may be directed from above. Staff needs to be involved and understand that the risk taking includes them. The manager may risk altering staff morale, loss of staff, loss of quality care, loss of money from the budget, poor image, and so on. Participation from staff members means they become direct participants, adding their input to the plan. Changes that are implemented when there is a crisis carry with them an even higher risk for success. At this time careful planning may be put aside; the result is then often a haphazard response.

Change agents need to be very effective in initiating adaptive work (figuring out the best way to adapt how work is done and still meet the work demands). Certainly change is stressful for everyone, and yet this cannot be used as a barrier to improvement. Six principles for leading adaptive work include the following.

1. **"Get on the balcony."**　See the context, the environment, or situation for change or create it. This requires seeing the larger picture.
2. **Identify the adaptive challenge.**　How can improvement occur? It is important to clearly identify the issue or problem, or the plan for change will not be effective.

## APPLYING EVIDENCE-BASED PRACTICE
### Evidence for Effective Leadership and Management

**Citation:** Kalisch, B. & Begeny, S. (2010). Preparation of nursing students for change and innovation. *Western Journal of Nursing Research, 32*(2), 157–167.

**Overview:** The critical question that influenced this study was how do we prepare the next generation of nurses who will need to adapt and innovate in the changing health care delivery system? To respond to this question the study examines "the information processing styles of nursing students in baccalaureate programs and also the extent to which the current nursing educational system promotes the development of creativity, an action orientation, and a willingness to change to prepare them for the demands of the health care system" (p. 158). The Organizational Engineering Model is used in this study. This model describes four information processing styles: reactive simulator, logical processor, hypothetical analyzer, and relational innovator. The sample included 271 freshman, sophomores, and seniors in two baccalaureate nursing programs. The study used a validated survey, I-Opt, to determine preference in task completion, change, and directions (performer, conservator, perfector, and changer). The study concludes that schools of nursing recruit students who use the *conservator information style,* which focuses on "outcome certainty and deliberate response" (p. 157). In addition to frequently recruiting *conservator* students, schools of nursing are graduating students who are *conservators,* so the students have not changed their processing style by the time of program completion.

**Application:** Change is critical in clinical practice and in leadership and management. Understanding how nurses respond to change can help to determine if interventions are needed to improve change response. According to this study, though the sample is small and more research is required, nurses do have a problem with their change response. As noted in this study, Benner's nursing education report (2010) also identifies this as a major concern.

### Questions:

1. *How does your typical response to change relate to the styles described in this study?*
2. *Do you think you need to improve in how you respond to change? If so, why and how?*
3. *What recommendations would you give to your nursing program to help students better understand and respond to change? Provide specific examples.*

3. **Regulate the distress caused by adaptive challenge.**   Managers or change agents need to recognize that work and change need to be paced. This requires asking tough questions without getting anxious. Staff needs to have confidence in the change agent; therefore, the change agent needs to remain calm during stress.
4. **Maintain disciplined attention.**   Watch for signs of work avoidance; expose conflict, do not hide it—all these can lead to a source of creativity and learning. It is easy to get distracted so it is important for the change agent to recognize distractions and intervene to prevent them.
5. **Give the work back to the people.**   Distress can lead to passivity and dependency on management—move to getting staff to assume responsibility. Many staff members expect the change agent to take on most of the responsibility. Some of this is from habit when staff members expect the manager to carry the responsibility, and some is because it is easier to say it is someone else's responsibility.
6. **Protect voices of leadership from below.**   Listen to those who identify contradictions, though they seem to upset the status quo. Leadership can come from all levels of the staff, and it needs to be encouraged. Initially, leadership from the staff may not be perfect, but it should be nurtured and encouraged to grow (Heifetz & Laurie, 2001, p. 131).

During the change process, it is also important to consider the impact of the organizational culture. How does the change agent create and sustain the right culture? Change agents demonstrate through their words and actions the critical values. As managers who are change agents manage the environment and work, they also provide a vision for the staff. This is a time when words and actions need to be consistent. It is not a time for conflict or inconsistency. For some changes, the culture also needs to change. This is not easy to do and requires a planned approach. During the change process, staff empowerment becomes important. "Empowering employees means giving employees the authority, tools, and information they need to do their jobs with greater autonomy, as well as the self-confidence required to perform the jobs effectively" (Dessler, 2002, p. 246). This helps to increase motivation. When staff members are empowered they need to know their responsibilities and be given the authority that they need to get the job done. If training or further education is required, then staff needs assistance in getting it. In order to move forward with change, staff needs information, and standards need to be clear.

# A Decision: A Response to Change

"You may notice that the planning process parallels the decision-making process; this makes sense, since developing plans involves deciding today what you'll do tomorrow. Both involve establishing objectives or criteria, developing and analyzing alternatives based on information you obtain, evaluating the alternatives, and then making a choice" (Dessler, 2002, p. 93). This section of the chapter focuses on decision making and planning, which are functions that every nurse uses in the practice of nursing. Any response to change requires decisions, and many of these decisions require careful planning."

**Decision making** is a process that begins with the identification of a problem and ends with the evaluation of the choices and taking a course of action" (Bernard & Walsh, 1990, as cited in Krairiksh & Anthony, 2001, p. 16). Decisions are a means rather than ends. They are used to achieve a goal. When decisions are made, the goal is usually related to both tasks and relationships. Some decisions may focus more on one than the other (Gebelein et al., 2000). Those who make decisions must learn to cope with being right some of the time and also learn to live with imperfect solutions. To make a sound decision, which is what people desire to do, the most important consideration is the criteria that are used to make the decision. Some examples of the criteria that might be used are "(1) Minimally impacts current operations, (2) Helps achieve important priorities, (3) Is consistent with values, (4) Is acceptable to those involved in the decision, (5) Can be implemented with the constraints (time, resources, other priorities), and (6) Considers pros, cons, and risks" (Gebelein et al., 2000, p. 114).

How is decision making related to planning? Nurses actively use decision making in a variety of situations, particularly during planning—patient care planning, planning the work day, and more involved planning for specific projects such as changing documentation or how the unit is organized. "**Planning** is setting goals and deciding on courses of action, developing rules and procedures, developing plans (both for the organization and for those who work for it), and forecasting (predicting or projecting what the future holds for the organization)" (Dessler, 2002, p. 3). During all phases of the planning process, decisions are made. Each day a nurse makes multiple decisions that affect the nurse, the patient, other staff, patient's family, and many others as nursing practice is made up of a series of decisions. "A problem is a discrepancy between a desirable and an actual situation" (Dessler, 2002, p. 68). Decisions are required to resolve this discrepancy. Typically, decision making and problem solving are used interchangeably though decisions do not always focus on problems. Decisions, however, are made when problems are solved. Figure 3-3 describes some of the key reasons for planning.

## Decision Styles

Why is creativity important in the decision-making process? Stepping "outside the box" is mentioned frequently today in all types of organizations. Decision making that routinely results in similar outcomes and does not consider innovative outcomes will not be as effective in the long run. Styles of decision making are affected by creativity or innovation. The common types of styles are unilateral, individual, and authoritarian decision making, all of which focus on one person making

**FIGURE 3-3 Reasons for planning.**

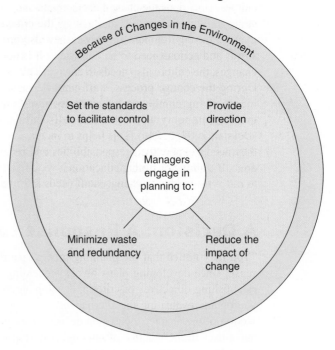

a decision with limited or no input from others. The opposite of this style is participative and consensus decision making. Here the emphasis is on including others in the decision making, even if an individual must make the final decision. The individual, however, who uses this style would pay close attention to feedback from others before making the final decision.

Other decision-making styles that have been described are **decisive**, **integrative**, **hierarchic**, and **flexible** (Milgram, Spector, & Treger, 1999). These styles apply to managers and to staff. The difference in these four styles is in the amount of data that are used to make a decision and the options that are considered.

- The decisive style depends on less data to arrive at one decision.
- The integrative style uses all available data and identifies multiple alternatives.
- The hierarchic style focuses on a large amount of information but arrives at one alternative or solution.
- The flexible style uses a small amount of data while generating multiple alternatives and may change as information is reinterpreted.

It is typical for managers to primarily use one style, though some managers use mixed styles or may switch styles depending upon the situation. For example, as was discussed in Chapter 1 about Contingency Leadership theory, when a situation changes different factors become more important and the manager may change styles to adjust. A nurse manager may encourage staff participation in decisions and allow time for this, but if the unit is suddenly short staffed then the manager may need to step in and make decisions quickly.

Systematic versus intuitive decision styles are two other approaches to decision making. **Systematic decision makers** form their decisions more logically and use a structured approach. **Intuitive decision makers** are at the other end of the spectrum; here the focus is on a trial-and-error approach. They may ignore information and change their alternatives if it does not feel right. This is the "gut" approach. A staff member will say, "I just had a feeling about it." Again, the situation can make a difference. When a nurse has expertise in an area, decisions may appear to be more intuitive because the nurse may feel more confident and can rely more on a "gut feeling," though the decision is probably supported by expertise.

**Team decision making** is another style that is used more today. It focuses on synergy, which is the combination of people's efforts that results in an output which is greater than the sum of the parts. Multiple ideas and experiences come together to form a decision. There are advantages and disadvantages to using team decision making. Advantages clearly focus on the fact that ideas from more than one person tend to improve other ideas and the final decision. As team members discuss an issue, ideas tend to bounce off of each other, which stimulates further ideas. The major disadvantage of using this style is it takes longer to make a decision. Some issues or problems are made worse by team decision making (for example, during an emergency when decisions must be made quickly and clearly so that all can follow them). The need during a crisis is for someone to make a decision and move the process along. Staff members need to know that their ideas are important though they cannot always be used. These ideas or suggestions can be considered after the potential crisis has passed and then be used to improve future decisions. When feedback is not recognized, those giving the feedback will feel left out and wonder why they wasted their time. Managers sometimes think that they use staff feedback and that this should be obvious, but often it is not so obvious to staff. Recognition goes a long way to improve morale, encourage staff to increase participation, and improve group decision making.

Dessler (2002) identifies additional advantages and disadvantages for using team decision making. The generally accepted advantage is "two heads are better than one." This allows for more points of view and develops more acceptance and commitment from those who participate. The result usually is greater effort to make the decision work during implementation. Why would there be disadvantages to team decision making? If the team process is ineffective it may actually shorten or interfere with the decision-making process, which affects the quality of the outcome. There may be greater pressure for consensus when members may not actually agree. Some teams experience dominance by one individual, diluting the effect of group input. Team members can believe so much in their own ideas that they are unable to openly consider other ideas. Team decisions can also take longer, which for some situations may be a disadvantage.

Teams can, of course, be quite successful in making decisions, but decision making does not just happen. There usually must be some guidance or facilitation. Brainstorming requires that all members are clear about what the issue is about and what it is not about. Setting a reasonable time limit pushes staff to move toward a result. Ground rules should make clear that the following are not helpful: (a) digression into details, (b) focusing on reasons about why it will not work or the constraints, and (c) criticism of ideas or evaluation of alternatives (Gebelein et al., 2000). While the team develops ideas, recording them is important so that they are not lost.

There are methods other than brainstorming that also facilitate team decision making, such as idea-generating questions (for example, "If we had enough staff, what would we do?" and "If we had the funding, how would we solve the problem?"). It is helpful to stimulate the team so that the team considers how similar problems were solved in the past, and then the team compares and contrasts the past with the present problem. Taking a different point of view than what would normally be taken may help the team understand the problem or issue from another perspective, which may lead to different alternatives, moving the decision making "out-of-the-box."

## CASE STUDY

### Change: An Opportunity or a Disaster?

A home health agency is undergoing restructuring. This involves changes in staffing, roles and responsibilities, scheduling, and client assignments. As the Director of Nursing (DON) you are responsible for this change. You know it will be challenging. The staff is about 50/50 new and long-term employees. One of your supervisors has openly expressed his concern that these changes will not work. You know that the RNs will have to cover more clients, but you have some flexibility in home health aide assignments. You don't want to lose RNs, but the changes have to be made.

### Questions:

1. How would you use the deep dive process to implement these required changes?
2. Apply the PDSA Cycle to this change initiative. Include barriers and strategies to overcome.
3. Describe an evaluation plan that you will use at 3, 6, and 12 months.

## Plan-Do-Study-Act (PDSA) Cycle

It is important to determine if a change will actually improve the work processes and/or environment and meet the intended goal(s). Too often this is neglected when a change really will have no positive impact or limited impact. The PDSA Cycle is used to test a change (Institute of Improvement, 2009). During Step One (Plan) the objective of the test is stated; predictions are made about what will happen and why; and a plan to test the change is developed. In Step Two (Do) a small test is done with identification of problems encountered and first analysis of data. Step Three (Study) leads more in depth analysis of test data with comparison of predictions to data and summarization. In the last step (Act) the change is revised based on what has been learned from the test. Other tests of the plan may be initiated.

DEEP DIVE PROCESS     The deep dive process is used by the TCAB initiative. It was developed by IDEO (Robert Wood Johnson Foundation, 2009). The TCAB pilots use this process of an in-depth brainstorming session to arrive at methods to improve care at the bedside. The process can be applied to any type of change effort. The deep dive process includes the following:

- Clinical and nonclinical representatives from services and departments meet for a half-day session that focuses on innovation related to a specific issue or theme. Management representatives also attend.
- This session encourages engagement in the issue and brainstorming. Time is needed to really get this involvement. After the deep dive, snorkels may occur on a regular basis. These are shorter brainstorming sessions.
- There should be agendas for the deep dive and snorkel sessions. Agendas should include storytelling. This allows time for individual members to discuss specific process-related work challenges. Asking the question, "What is your pet peeve or what are you worried about the most?" can get to the critical concerns.
- Brainstorming should be directed toward identifying how things might be changed to improve.
- Post all ideas so all can see. Allow time for the ideas to reviewed and expanded or changed.
- Then vote on the changes to determine which ones will be tested, setting priorities.
- Describe how the tests will be conducted and evaluated.

Identify who will lead the process, develop timeline, and share this information with staff who needs to know it.

## Types of Decisions

Are there any major differences in the types of decisions? There are two major types that most staff encounters. The first is the need for **programmed decisions**. These decisions are more repetitive and routine. These decisions take less time and typically are related to a policy or procedure. For example, if a patient leaves the hospital against medical advice (AMA), there is a procedure for an AMA discharge, or if a nurse misses an order for a medication, there is a procedure to follow such as whom to notify, what to document, and so on. Most decisions are of this type, which is a good thing as these take less time. The second type, **non-programmed decisions**, are not so routine, and some may be crises. Situations that require this type of decision require more time, collection of data, critical thinking and analysis, and may require consultation with others. These decisions may be completely new experiences. They require more judgment, or the "cognitive or thinking aspects of the decision-making process" (Dessler, 2002, p. 68).

Another view of the types of decisions considers the focus of the decision (Krairiksh & Anthony, 2001). One type is patient care decisions that nurses make in their practice that affect direct patient care. The second type is decisions about the condition of work. This type affects the work environment, groups of patients, and how work is conducted. Most nurses tend to participate more in the first type of decision, those with direct care implications (Krairiksh & Anthony, 2001). This, however, is changing as nurses become more involved as leaders in the health care delivery system.

## The Decision-Making Process

The **decision-making process** is a dynamic process. The most effective decisions are made in collaboration with others in the organization. Collaboration between nurses and physicians also affects nurses' participation as it provides greater opportunities for nurses to participate. When collaboration is present nurses and physicians share responsibility and hopefully respect one another more. Knowledge, ideas, and skills are shared. This type of relationship can only improve decision making. The key steps in the decision-making process are identified in Figure 3-4.

WORKAROUNDS    A **workaround** is "a rushed, improvised response to a breakdown in a work process, without pausing to analyze and correct the underlying problem" (Finkelman & Kenner, 2009, p. 208). How does this apply to change and decision making? Most hospitals are organized around functions with more ambiguity than clear responsibility. The system naturally breaks down as work is done. When this happens, the typical response is to just find a way to accomplish the task that needs to be done without stopping to analyze why there is a problem and solving the problem. In this situation, which is a workaround, frequently nothing is learned from the experience and thus improvement does not occur. The problem most likely will reoccur because no attempt has really been made to solve it. Spear (2005, p. 82) recommends the following steps to avoid workarounds. The change process is imbedded in these steps.

1. Work is designed as a series of ongoing experiments that immediately reveal problems.
2. Problems are addressed immediately through rapid experimentation.
3. Solutions are disseminated adaptively through collaborative experimentation.
4. People at all levels of the organization are taught to become experimentalists.

NURSING AND CRITICAL THINKING    Nursing has become very complex with change occurring almost daily in nursing management and clinical practice. This complex, changing environment often leads to stress for all levels of staff. Managers and team leaders need to be particularly skilled in coping with stress and embrace opportunities to make change a positive experience for themselves, all staff, and the organization, and to actively use critical thinking. "A more progressive, holistic way to define critical thinking is a commitment to look for the best way, based on the most current research and practice findings; for example, the best strategy to manage pain in a specific person or situation. Critical thinking in nursing means constantly striving to find a better way by focusing on two key questions: What are the outcomes? And how can we do better?" (Alfaro-LeFevre, 2001, p. 26). Those who use critical thinking incorporate the following in their thinking process:

- Reasoning
- Generates and examines questions and problems
- Intuition and feelings
- Weighs, clarifies, and evaluates evidence

Box 3-4 identifies some critical thinking skills. Nurses use critical thinking as they provide direct care, but they also use it as they coordinate care; advocate for the patient; work with other staff to

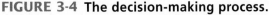

### FIGURE 3-4 The decision-making process.

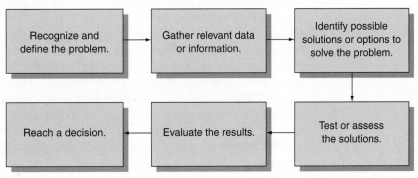

| BOX 3-4 | CRITICAL THINKING SKILLS |
|---------|--------------------------|

- Knowledge, experience, judgment, and evaluation
- Interpretation
- Affective listening
- Application of moral reasoning and values
- Comprehension, application, analysis, and synthesis
- Awareness of self
- Mistakes happen and we learn from them

resolve issues on the unit; ensure that quality, safe care is provided on the unit; and collaborate with others. Nurses who serve on committees and task forces use critical thinking in the work that must be done.

As decision making is experienced, it is easy to slip into **dichotomous thinking**. This should be avoided because when it is used problems and situations are viewed in a polarized manner—things are seen as either "good" or "bad." This approach can lead to ineffective decision making as it limits choices for patients and for other types of decisions that need to be made. Some strategies that can prevent dichotomous thinking and improve critical thinking include the following:

- Replace "I don't know" and "I'm not sure" with "I'll find out."
- Turn errors into opportunities.
- Anticipate questions others might ask.
- Ask, "What if?"
- Look for flaws in one's own thinking, and ask others to identify flaws (Alfaro-LeFevre, 2001, p. 27).

In responding to change critical thinking should be part of problem solving and decision making. It is important, however, to note that critical thinking is not the same as problem solving or decision making. Nurses who develop critical thinking skills will relieve their own stress, solve problems, and make more effective decisions. Table 3-1 compares critical thinking, decision making, and problem solving.

How does one describe a critical thinker? Paul (1995) identifies the following four traits.

1. **Intellectual humility.**   The person is willing to admit what is not known.
2. **Intellectual integrity.**   The person continually evaluates his or her own thinking and is willing to admit when wrong.
3. **Intellectual courage.**   The person is aware of the need to confront ideas fairly, even when negative reactions toward the ideas may be present.
4. **Intellectual empathy.**   The person makes a conscious effort to understand others.

## Clinical Reasoning and Judgment

In the new Carnegie report on nursing education the authors question whether nursing has focused too much on critical thinking, ignoring other aspects of practical reasoning, (Benner, Sutphen, Leonard, & Day, 2010). The report discusses the need to know when to use critical thinking and when to not use it. Critical reflection is also needed so that nurses can ask questions (about an event, patient, and so on) that lead to a new interpretation. "Nurses need multiple ways of thinking, such as clinical reasoning and clinical imagination as well as critical, creative, scientific, and formal critical reasoning. By **clinical reasoning**, we mean the ability to reason as a clinical situation changes, taking into account the context and concerns of the patient and family. When nurses use clinical reasoning they capture the patients' trends and trajectories" (Benner, Sutphen, Leonard, & Day, 2010, p. 85). **Clinical judgment** is needed to determine if published research is relevant for a specific patient and situation and the value of the research. This is evidence-based practice. The report states that "cynicism and excessive doubt, often the by-product of overuse of critical thinking, will not help the nurse draw on appropriate knowledge and act in a particular situation" (pp. 85–86).

| TABLE 3-1 | COMPARISON OF CRITICAL THINKING, DECISION MAKING, AND PROBLEM SOLVING |
|---|---|

### Critical Thinking

Definition: "A process of examining underlying assumptions, interpreting and evaluating arguments, imagining and exploring alternatives, and developing relative criticism for the purpose of reaching a reasoned, justifiable conclusion" (Sullivan & Decker, 2001, p. 151).

- Seeks no single solution.
- Focuses on creativity and innovation.
- Purposeful and constantly reevaluating.
- May be used in both decision making and problem solving.
- Allows the person to "think outside the box" and consider many ideas without prejudice.

### Decision Making

Definition: "A process whereby appropriate alternatives are weighed and one is ultimately selected" (Sullivan & Decker, 2001, p. 153).

- Decisions are made daily by nurses: care decisions, management decisions, professional decisions.
- Decisions may not involve a problem.
- Ideally, critical thinking is used when decisions are made.
- Decisions require a choice between alternatives.

### Problem Solving

Definition: "A process whereby a dilemma is identified and corrected" (Sullivan & Decker, 2001, p. 153).

- A problem is a gap in how things are and how they might be.
- Problem solving requires that the problem is identified or diagnosed.
- There may not be the need to select a correct solution—for example, there may be no response to the problem. This in itself is a form of a decision.
- Resolving a problem may include critical thinking—and the best resolutions include critical thinking.
- Resolving a problem includes many decisions, typically some minor and some major.
- Problem-solving process: define the problem, gather information, analyze the information, develop solutions, make a decision or choose the solution, implement the decision (solution), and evaluate the decision (solution).
- The problem-solving process corresponds to the nursing process.

Source: Sullivan, Eleanor J.; Decker, Philip J.; Jamerson, Pat, *Effective leadership and management in nursing*, 5th, © 2001. Printed and electronically reproduced by permission of Pearson Education, Inc., Upper Saddle River, New Jersey.

**IDENTIFY THE NEED FOR DECISION MAKING: WHAT IS THE PROBLEM?**   After a review of related issues, the need to make a decision should be carefully defined. A solution cannot be found for something that is truly unknown or poorly understood. Clarifying the problem is not always easy. Staff may have different perspectives on the issue. For example, one staff member may think a problem about quality care might be due to low staffing and another may attribute it to lack of appropriate training of unlicensed assistive personnel. The questions found in Box 3-5 should be considered in this step of the process.

After the analysis of the answers to the questions found in Box 3-5, goals need to be established so that all staff knows the direction that is to be taken. Identifying goals is the only way to know if results are met. Who sets the goals? This can vary. The typical situation is the manager of change agents sets the goals, or this is done by higher levels of managers. As discussed throughout this text, however, the more staff is involved the better the decision-making process. Setting goals is part of this process. Team leaders also set goals, and individual staff members also set goals as they do their work. In the end, who sets the goals depends on the issue or problem that is being addressed.

What are some guidelines for setting goals (Milgram, Spector, & Treger, 1999)? Goals need to be reasonable. By evaluating strengths and weaknesses, additional information can be identified to assist in setting realistic goals. Setting goals should not be done in a vacuum. If consideration is not given to external factors that might affect the goals, the goals may not be what should be achieved, may be unreasonable, or may not receive critical support. Throughout the decision-making process, perception is a critical factor. "Perception is the selection and interpretation of information we receive through our senses and the meaning we give to the information" (Dessler, 2002, p. 75). Many factors influence how stimuli are perceived, such as level of participation, past history with decision making, how and what information is shared, who is involved, commitment to the issue or problem, morale and stress level, level of staffing, and so on.

| BOX 3-5 | **IDENTIFYING THE NEED FOR DECISION MAKING: QUESTIONS TO ASK** |
|---------|-----------------------------------------------------------------|

- What is the issue or problem? State the issue or problem in terms of need rather than a solution, using terms that are understood.
- What important, critical facts are known? Describe these as clearly as possible.
- What is unknown? How important is the unknown? Who might know the information or how can it be obtained? Be willing to identify factors that might be negative or different.
- When does the problem occur? When is it absent? Consider days of week, time of day, and factors that might affect timing.
- What is the consequence of the problem or issue? This step should include negative and positive consequences.
- What has been tried in the past to deal with the situation? This may be an action that occurred within the organization or externally considered (literature review, network with others, and so on). What happened as a result of these actions?
- How do people feel about the situation and changes to it?
- What related problems are present? If something changes, what else will likely change as a result of the initial change?
- What assumptions—about people, technology, systems, funding—have been made that might need to be challenged?

Source: Author content and some summarized content from Gebellin, S., et al. (2000). *Successful manager's handbook.* Minneapolis, MN: Personnel Decisions International Corporation; Marrelli, T. (1997). *The nurse manager's guide.* St. Louis, MO: Mosby-Year Book, Inc.

**Proactive planning** helps to improve decision making and decrease stress about decisions that need to be made. This means there must be some anticipation of problems. Those who understand trends, past history, risks, health care policy, and how problems are connected to one another, as well as identify signs that might indicate a need for a response, will be more able to anticipate and begin decision making early rather than later when the problem may be more complicated.

DECISION-MAKING CONDITIONS   When discussing decision-making conditions the first major issue is who is responsible for making the decision. Managers and staff can get themselves into further problems when they take on decisions that are not theirs to make or they do not make decisions they are responsible for making. How does one find out about who is responsible for a decision? Position descriptions should clarify some of this. The immediate supervisor is also an important resource to help clarify this responsibility. During the hiring process and orientation, staff members need clear direction about their responsibilities. If they are confused or unclear about their decision-making responsibilities, they are responsible for asking about this to gain greater clarification. A staff member's comfort level with making decisions is also very important. Staff members who feel uncomfortable may avoid decisions, let others make the decision, execute the decision-making process poorly, or arrive at poor decisions, which only makes them more uncomfortable. Those who work with this staff member will also feel uncomfortable about the decisions that are made, which affects morale, productivity, safety and quality, staff turnover, and the overall working environment.

What are the key reasons for staff discomfort with decision making (Gebelein et al., 2000)? When a person feels that there is a lack of knowledge about the true risk of the alternatives, then discomfort increases. Further data collection and analysis are important at this time. Some staff members are uncomfortable with the possible consequences of risk taking. When this occurs, the staff member might ask, "What is the worst thing that could happen?" It is important to consider impact and strategies to reduce risks. Maybe the person is focusing too much on the negative aspects. Others feel uncomfortable when the risk factors are unknown. Again, there needs to be more data collection, analysis, and talking to others who may help clarify the issue. Others find they are uncomfortable when certain types of decisions must be made such as decisions related to budget, staffing, or termination of personnel. If this is the case, it is important to learn more about these areas and gain some expertise and confidence. Improving decision-making competency is important for all staff and managers. Increasing knowledge, researching to gain more information, and getting additional experience helps to improve decision making. Discussing concerns with colleagues is an important strategy for every nurse to use.

**BARRIERS TO DECISION MAKING**   Barriers to decision making may focus on a variety of factors, and they are similar to barriers to change. Whenever barriers are considered, it is critical to be clear about the barriers that exist within the organization. Examples of typical barriers are dysfunction, poor communication, lack of staff participation, changing organization ownership or administration, inadequate staff, poorly prepared managers, inadequate budget, inadequate staffing levels, policies and procedures, and poor relationships with the community and consumers. There are other barriers that focus more on the individuals who make the decisions. Taking decision-making shortcuts can be an advantage, but this can also be a barrier to success when the shortcut limits data collection, analysis, and the quantity and quality of alternatives that are considered. If description of an issue or problem is really off track, this can act as a barrier. A frequent error in describing an issue or problem occurs when the person unconsciously considers some information to be more important when it is not. Another major barrier is an individual's psychological set, which is a rigid strategy or point-of-view. When a staff member enters the decision-making process with a rigid idea about possible cause(s) or strategies, there is an immediate block to success. Because barriers change they need to be considered throughout the decision-making process.

**DATA COLLECTION**   Data that are collected are determined by the need and the objectives. It is important first to complete the analysis of the issue or problem. What is the issue or problem? This will then direct data collection. It is easy to get carried away with data collection, which can lead to a situation of just collecting data for the sake of collecting it. The first consideration must be existing data. What data are already available, collected for another purpose, but could be used for this new purpose? When existing data are used, it is important to determine if the data meet the specific need. Four common data collection methods used in nursing are described in Box 3-6.

Data are then analyzed to determine the cause, which requires objectivity. It is easy to assume something is the cause and then unconsciously insert this assumption into the analysis of the data collected. Getting different perspectives of the data is also important rather than relying

---

### BOX 3-6   COMMON DATA COLLECTION METHODS: INTERVIEW

**INTERVIEWS**

Interviews can be unstructured or structured. The unstructured interview provides opportunity to gain more detailed information with limited boundaries. Structured interviews, which use a standard form and/or format, are less flexible and collect standardized data. For both types of interviews, after the interviews are conducted, data must be summarized and analyzed, and this can take time.

**OBSERVATION**

Observation is often used when complex data are required. It might be used if a clinic needed data about the flow of work in the clinic. Observation may be used to document what staff were doing, time factors, and impact of the physical layout. This type of observation would require a standard checklist or documentation form for the observers and clear guidelines as to what is to be observed and recorded.

**QUESTIONNAIRE/SURVEY**

This perhaps is the simplest method, and it is used frequently. It can be less expensive to administer. The questionnaire or survey may be used to collect information about facts such as how many staff are working at a particular time or how many patients were assigned particular staff members. Another type of data is procedure performance data. Evaluative data can also be obtained; for example, how does the staff feel about a change in the admission procedure or a change in documentation. Questions can be asked as to whether or not the procedure was followed or does staff feel prepared for the change.

on just one individual or a few. Figure 3-5 provides several examples of tools that can be used in collecting and analyzing data.

SELECTING ALTERNATIVES    For most problems there are multiple alternative solutions that could be used to solve the problem or prevent a problem if that is the goal. It is best to have a number of alternatives from which to select. When the final alternative is selected, it needs to meet the critical criteria that were identified as important for success such as time limitation and resources including staff, space, expertise, and educational level of staff. Alternatives are usually evaluated according to three conditions.

1. Certainty: indicates that there is considerable information about the issue or problem, which indicates a very high probability of meeting the outcome.
2. Uncertainty: indicates there is no knowledge of the probability of success.
3. Risk: indicates that some information is known but not a high level.

To select the third type of alternative is the least secure approach, but this is how most alternatives are selected. Most staff can provide many examples of situations when problems were confronted with the thought that there was a high probability that the alternative selected was going to achieve the goal desired, and yet this did not occur.

Selecting alternatives also requires a reflection on past experience, which provides data about the probability of success as mistakes can teach staff what not to do or which directions usually do not lead to success. In this selection, trading off or compromise often is required. Decision making is a dynamic process, so give and take is part of the process. Organizational and individual values will affect the alternatives selected, and thus it is difficult to avoid ethics when some decisions are made. For example, organ transplants involve a decision-making process, one that is highly structured, and this is certainly a decision process that involves ethical issues.

When alternatives are selected, it is critical to ask if an alternative is practical. Some alternatives are not practical and pursuing them will only increase frustration and cause more problems. Collaborating with others by asking them if they think it is practical and what might be some of the "real" concerns about the selection of the alternative usually improves decisions. There needs to be realistic estimates of resource requirements (staff, supplies and equipment, and so on) during the planning. At this point planning also includes an assessment of staff capabilities (not just staff numbers), and this information relates to the plan and its implementation. If additional capabilities are required, then this needs to be included in the plan (for example, a consultant or an expert to teach staff new computer skills so that a new computerized physician order system can be implemented that will affect how nurses review orders). Timelines are identified for all of the activities in the plan so specific steps and accountabilities for staff can be identified. Throughout the process it is important to be a step ahead. This can be done by frequently asking "what if" to identify those situations that might arise to block the solution or make strategies or interventions ineffective.

IMPLEMENTING AND SELLING THE DECISION    Selling the decision focuses on decision acceptance. How committed to the decision are those who will be affected by the decision? This is a key question. Earlier in this chapter resistance to change was discussed. This information applies to commitment to decisions. Decisions that meet strong resistance will fail. Those who are needed to move the decision forward need to understand what is behind the decision.

Some decisions require a detailed action plan, but most do not. The key to implementation is timing. When to make the decision and when to implement it are frequently difficult to determine. Procrastination is common in decision making. If a decision is delayed, the typical reasons for this are (a) lack of information, (b) unclear course of action, (c) lack of time for thought, and (d) fear of negative consequences (Gebelein et al., 2000). Each of these reasons has very clear solutions. All relate to getting more information, planning, and developing a clear viewpoint of the issue at hand. Another problem is making impulsive decisions. These decisions lead to more problems. If pressure is felt to make a decision now, then it is best to stop and consider why and what could be done to improve the decision making. It is rarely helpful to make decisions when emotions such as anger are strong. Those who want to jump in too soon should step back and take time to collaborate with others to work through the decision and to write plans down. Time taken to do this will decrease impulsiveness. The plan needs to include specific information as to actions and responsibilities.

### FIGURE 3-5 **Making sense of data: Methods.**

*Cause-and-effect diagram.* This is a diagram that describes a specific process with its causal factors and their consequences. The focus is on improving understanding of possible causes. Another term for this diagram is a *fishbone diagram.*

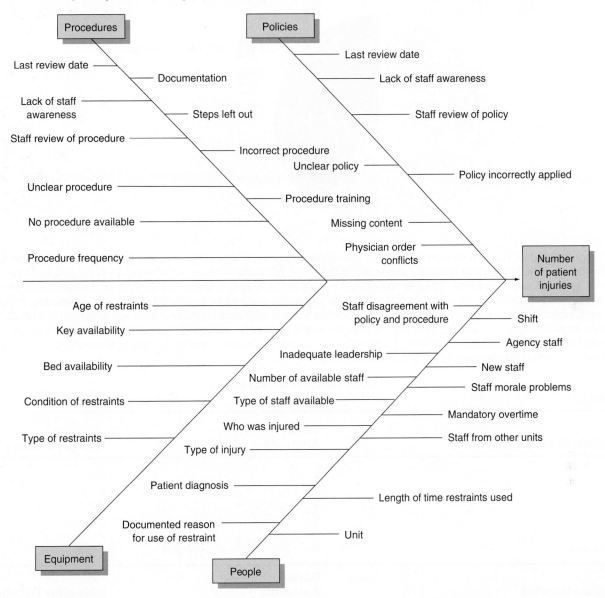

*Pareto chart.* This method may be used after a cause-and-effect diagram is developed in order to identify the causes of primary importance. Data are described according to the frequency of each cause and displayed according to the most frequent and least frequent. This will help to narrow the data so that the data can be used to determine the best action to take.

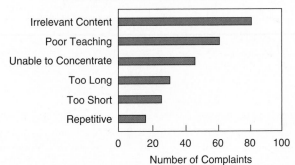

*(continued)*

**FIGURE 3-5 Making sense of data: Methods.** *(continued)*

*Pie chart.* This is another type of graph that provides a description of percentages of the whole. This is a common graph that most have seen.

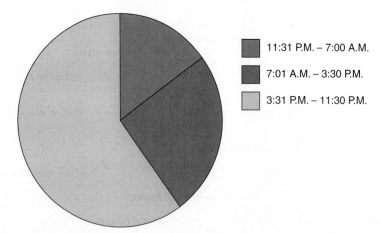

| | |
|---|---|
| ■ (dark gray) | 11:31 P.M. – 7:00 A.M. |
| ■ (darker gray) | 7:01 A.M. – 3:30 P.M. |
| ■ (light gray) | 3:31 P.M. – 11:30 P.M. |

*Cost-benefit analysis.* This is a method that is used to analyze two or more alternatives in order to determine which alternative will bring the greatest rewards or benefits compared with the costs. Cost-effectiveness is the focus. Both tangible and intangible benefits and costs are considered. Tangible costs might include funds, supplies, space, equipment, staff salaries and benefits, loss of staff, orientation costs, recruitment costs, and so on. Intangible costs might include downtime, staff resistance, decrease in morale, increase in errors, and changes in quality. Intangible benefits might include improved morale, improved level of staffing, increase in communication, and so on. Tangible benefits might include an increased number of patients seen or admitted, decrease in length-of-stay or complications, money saved, decrease in incidents, and so on. The cost benefit ratio can then be determined, which is represented by benefits divided by costs.

### COST-BENEFIT ANALYSIS

**Solution:**

| Tangible Costs | Dollar Amounts | Intangible Costs |
|---|---|---|
| ✓ | $ | ✓ |
| ✓ | $ | ✓ |
| ✓ | $ | ✓ |
| ✓ | $ | ✓ |
| | | ✓ |
| Total Costs | $ | |

| Tangible Benefits | Dollar Amounts | Intangible Benefits |
|---|---|---|
| ✓ | $ | ✓ |
| ✓ | $ | ✓ |
| ✓ | $ | ✓ |
| ✓ | $ | ✓ |
| | | ✓ |
| Total Costs | $ | |

$$\text{Cost Benefit Ratio} = \frac{\text{Benefits (}\underline{\quad\quad}\text{)}}{\text{Costs (}\underline{\quad\quad}\text{)}} = \underline{\quad\quad}$$

*Graph.* A graph is used to describe performance over a period of time in an attempt to identify trends. The line graph, used in this example, can describe one or more sets of data. This example describes two sets of data: the number of procedures and the clinical units. Then the data can be compared.

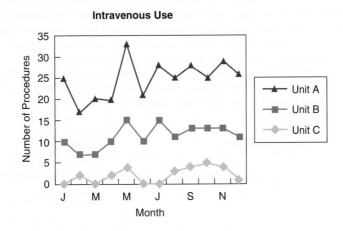

*Flowchart.* This is a type of chart that is helpful when there is a need to describe a decision-making process. The chart should be developed by a group or team who is involved in the process. The flowchart helps all focus on the process rather than just seeing one part or a part that relates to them as individuals. Typically these charts use common symbols, for example, (A) box represents a function, task, or department; (B) a diamond represents a decision; and (C) arrows indicate the flow of information. After the flowchart is developed, it is then easier to identify repetitive steps, unnecessary steps, or other steps that just do not make sense in the process.

*Histogram.* This is a bar graph, which illustrates the frequency distribution of a variable or variables in continuous data.

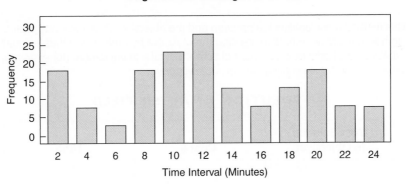

*(continued)*

**FIGURE 3-5 Making sense of data: Methods.** *(continued)*

*WOTS-up.* This is a method that is used to analyze the weaknesses, opportunities, threats, and strengths of a particular situation. Weaknesses focus on internal factors such as lack of management development, qualifications of staff, level of staffing, staff expertise, financial status, marketing efforts, location, quality of services, and so on. Opportunities are the factors that are viewed as positive and have the potential to move the organization forward. Examples are nurse and physician recruitment levels, new programs or services, new markets, population growth, improved technology, new drugs, and new facilities. Threats are serious factors that might hold the organization back such as staff shortage, decreased patient satisfaction, decrease in insured patients, decrease in demand for services, accreditation problems, malpractice litigation, and legislative changes. The fourth category includes the orgnanization's strengths, which might include management style, qualifications and expertise of staff, financial status, increased demand for services, location, and quality of services.

| Weaknesses | Opportunities | Threats | Strengths |
|---|---|---|---|
|  |  |  |  |

*Solution analysis grid.* This method first identifies the problem and the objective. Then each suggested alternative to resolve the problem is analyzed as to how it might contribute to meeting the objective by ranking whether it would have a high, medium, or low contribution; cost in dollars; timeframe or the amount of time it will take to implement (for example, short range, long range, or immediate); and feasibility. The latter is simply a "yes"or "no" response.

**SOLUTION ANALYSIS FIELD**

| Alternative Solution | Cost Solution to Objectives | Cost $ | Time | Feasibility |
|---|---|---|---|---|
|  |  |  |  |  |

EVALUATING RESULTS    Evaluating results of decisions is never easy. By the time one thinks this should be done, another change, decision, and plan are in process. However, neglecting evaluation has long-term consequences. The quality of a decision depends heavily on the goals selected and the strategies used to achieve them. Evaluation is thus intricately tied to the beginning, the middle, and the end of the decision-making process. In addition, evaluation itself does not just happen at the end of the process, but rather needs to be incorporated in all of the steps. This provides valuable data about when approaches need adjustment to prevent the situation from becoming too complex.

Those who were involved in decision making should be involved in the evaluation. This does require objectivity. Staff that buy into a plan may be more reluctant to say it needs adjusting or has failed. For one reason, it probably means more change and stress; however, if this is not done, greater stress can also be expected. The following are some keys for improving decision making and planning that can be used in a variety of situations.

- Take time whenever possible to think through the process, avoiding impulsive decision making
- When appropriate, include others
- Use creative techniques
- Listen and consider ideas from others
- Stay open to ideas and perspectives, even those that are very different
- Challenge self and develop new thinking skills: critical thinking, conceptual thinking, creative thinking, and intuitive thinking
- Recognize the broad implications of issues
- Identify relationships
- Balance short-term and long-term priorities (Gebelein et al., 2000, p. 213)

## Planning

Why is it important to plan? If organizations or staff members go off without a plan or map, will they get to their goals or their destination? An analogy would be traveling to an unknown place without a map. Getting lost increases stress, takes time, may increase expenses, and may interfere with reaching the destination, which is the goal. Most nurses have worked in situations where there were no goals, or the goals were unclear or kept a secret. This is not a great way to work. What if patients were cared for without a plan? How would staff know if outcomes were met? How organized would the care be? How would staff know its responsibilities? Crisis management seems to be more the norm in health care organizations. It is certainly important to learn how to deal with crises, but a better approach, whenever possible, is to plan, both short range and long range. Leaders do not have the luxury of saying, "I don't have time to plan." Organizations cannot afford not to.

When there is recognition that change is needed, particularly one that is fairly major, the planning process goes into action. A plan is a picture of a future vision, ideally painted by a group or team. Planning includes multiple decisions and is directly affected by change. Planning is the pivotal step in the process of getting there. There are three types of planning:

1. **Policy planning.**    This planning focuses on changing the value system or laws and regulations. It is health planning in its broadest concept.
2. **Strategic planning.**    This is the planning that an organization does when it considers long-term issues and goals. It includes planning that is done by the organization's components, such as its departments or services. The organization looks at its vision and its organizational assessment data, and then asks where are the gaps? What would it take to get there? A typical result is the organization's plan for the next 5 years.
3. **Project planning.**    This planning focuses on operational matters in the organization. Examples include a plan to change documentation such as introduce an electronic medical

record (EMR), introduce a new admission procedure or new service, or change staff roles. Project planning must take into account strategic plans so that there is no conflict, and project plans should help the organization reach strategic goals. For example, if one of an organization's strategic goals is to develop the use of interprofessional teams in all departments and units, a project plan that focuses on training staff would need to be developed by staff education.

## Summary Issue: Critical Thinking and the Nurse Manager

What happens if a nurse manager does not use critical thinking? Typically the nurse manager will respond in an automatic, reactive manner when problems arise. Opportunities for change and improvement will be lost (Zori & Morrison, 2009). As was discussed in Chapter 1 the nurse manager has multiple responsibilities and must constantly deal with change. While this is done the nurse manager needs to ensure that there is a positive work environment; goals are met; patients' needs are met with positive outcomes; improvement is a major goal; and that the unit operations run smoothly. Each of these functions is difficult to achieve, and combining them makes it even more difficult. "The development of critical thinking is seen as an antecedent to effective functioning in the manager role. Critical thinking can have a powerful influence on the decision making and problem solving that nurse managers are faced with on a daily basis. The skills that typify critical thinking include analysis, evaluation, inference, and deductive and inductive reasoning" (Facione, Facione, & Sanchez, 1994 as cited in Zori & Morrison, 2009, p. 75). Some methods that nurse managers use to improve their critical thinking are

- Keep a reflective journal, which provides time to consider critical incidents and develops analysis, synthesis, judgment, and creativity (Profetta-McGrath, 2005).
- Use an online chat group that includes other nurse managers. Discuss critical incidents and share different perspectives (Zori & Morrison, 2009).
- Create a journal club with other nurse managers to read and discuss current literature on leadership, management, evidence-based practice and evidence-based management, and other relevant topics (Profetta-McGrath, 2005).
- Use concept mapping when developing a new procedure, process or analyzing an incident. Concept mapping includes graphic diagrams, charts, diagrams, and pictorial representation that is useful in illustrating how ideas are linked (Toofany, 2008).

Porter-O'Grady and Malloch (2007) discuss the need for nurse leaders and manager to use critical questioning. "The purpose of critical questioning, or asking for significant information, is to check individual perceptions of an issue or situation and render it more manageable" (p. 187). The following are examples of critical thinking questions (p. 189).

- Can you tell me your understanding of the situation?
- Why is this important to you? To others? To the organization?
- Is the situation you are describing related to a technical issue, a systems issue, or a people-related issue?
- What do you need to know to make a decision on this issue?
- Do you think others have made false assumptions about this situation?
- Who else cares about this issue as much as you do?
- This sounds very rational. What do people believe about it?
- This sounds very emotional. What do people feel about it?
- What are the choices in the situation?
- Can you propose a solution?

Using methods such as the ones described, nurse managers can develop their own critical thinking and also help their staff to develop critical thinking by acting as a role model and working with staff individually and in groups to use critical thinking effectively and also to understand the need for clinical reasoning and judgment in the practice.

# APPLYING LEADERSHIP AND MANAGEMENT

## MY HOSPITAL UNIT

As the nurse manager on your unit you are confronted daily with new changes that come from above or within your unit. Sometimes you wonder if there will be "normalcy" when you do not have to deal with a new policy, form, new staff, change in budget, and so on. Today, you are sitting at your desk after attending report, and you know that some changes need to be made. You may select any issue that is of interest to you that you might want to change as nurse manager. Describe the issue or problem and then develop a detailed plan using change process and content from this chapter to guide you. Ask a classmate to critique your plan for change, and critique your classmates' nurse manager plans for their units. After you get the critique, revise the plan where you feel it needs revision using the feedback you get. What have you learned from critiquing someone else's plan? Use the virtual unit site found on the textbook website to record the work that you do in the role of nurse manager for your unit.

## Critical Thinking Questions and Activities

1. How do you feel about change? How do you react to change? What do you think you might improve so that you might (1) be a more effective change agent and (2) better handle change made by others that impact you?
2. Team decision making is more and more common in health care today, particularly with the emphasis on interprofessional teamwork. There are many group techniques that can be used to improve team decision making. Nominal Group Technique (NGT) is one type of team decision making. Try using this technique in a small group. Follow these steps: Individuals in the team first present their own ideas without interacting with the group by stating the viewpoint on a topic. The group is then presented with a question related to the topic. Each member writes down his or her own response to the question. The responses are then presented one at a time for clarification. This phase is time-limited. Then all members rank the responses separately, and the ratings are shared and summarized.
3. Several examples of methods that might be used to analyze data are described in Figure 3-5. Find examples of these methods in the literature or in you clinical setting. Do the methods help to provide a picture of the data?
4. Divide into small teams. Change can be approached in a variety of ways; however, for this exercise you are asked to use Lewin's force-field model of change, described in this chapter. The team should identify something that it would like to change in your nursing program or it could be in this course. Select something that is not too complex. Now, clearly state what you want to change and then apply Lewin's model. Describe what you would do in each of the stages of the model. All teams should then share their proposed changes.
5. Visit the TCAB website at http://www.rwjf.org/qualityequality/product.jsp?id=30051. Review the sections describing Transform Care at the Bedside. See pull-down menu for the Table of Contents. There is content, PowerPoint presentations, and videos on the content. How does this content about TCAB relate to content in this chapter?

## Media Links

- **URL: http://changingminds.org/disciplines/change_management/planning_change/planning_change.htm**

  Changing Minds.org

- **URL: http://managementhelp.org/org_chng/org_chng.htm#anchor70003**
  Free Management Library: Organizational Change and Development
- **URL: http://www.ihi.org/IHI/Topics/Improvement/ImprovementMethods/ HowToImprove/testingchanges.htm**
  Institute for Health Improvement: Plan, Do, Study, Act (PDSA)
- **URL: http://www.ihi.org/IHI/Topics/Improvement/ImprovementMethods/ HowToImprove/testingchanges.htm**
  Institute of Health Improvement: Testing Changes
- **URL: http://www.rwjf.org/qualityequality/product.jsp?id=30070&parentid= 30060&grparentid=30051**
  Foundation for Critical Thinking
- **URL: http://www.ncrel.org/sdrs/areas/issues/educatrs/leadrshp/le5spark.htm\**
  Thirteen Tips for Managing Change
- **URL: http://www.managementhelp.org/mgmnt/orgchnge.htm**
  Basic Content for Organizational Change
- **URL: http://www.holberton.com/sol_vol-3-no17.html**
  Initiating Change. The Leader's Biggest Challenge
- **URL: https://www.ncsbn.org/index.htm**
  National Council of State Boards of Nursing.
- **URL: http://dms.dartmouth.edu/cms/materials/worksheets/ nolan_chagne_concepts.doc**
  Change Concepts

# References

Alfaro-LeFevre, R. (2001). Improving your ability to think critically. *Nursing Spectrum Metro Edition,* (March), 25–30.

American Association of Colleges of Nursing. (2008). *Essentials of baccalaureate education for professional nursing practice.* Washington, DC: Author.

Buerhaus, P., Staiger, D., & Auerbach, D. (2009). *The future of the nursing workforce in the United States. Data, trends, and implications.* Boston: Jones and Bartlett Publishers.

Benner, P., Sutphen, M., Leonard, V., & Day, L. (2009). *Educating nurses: A call for radical transformation.* San Francisco: Jossey-Bass.

Carney, M. (2002). The management of change: Using a model to evaluate the change process. *Seminars for Nurse Managers, 10*(3), 206–211.

Dessler, G. (2002). *Management.* Upper Saddle River, NJ: Prentice Hall.

Facione, N., Facione, P., & Sanchez, C. (1994). Critical thinking disposition as a measure of competent clinical judgment. The development of the California Critical Thinking Disposition Inventory. *Journal of Nursing Education, 33*(8), 345–350.

Finkelman, A. (2001). *Managed care: A nursing perspective.* Upper Saddle River, NJ: Prentice Hall.

Finkelman, A. & Kenner, C. (2007). Why should nurse leaders care about the status of nursing education. *Nurse Leader, 5*(6), 23–27.

Finkelman, A. & Kenner, C. (2009). *Teaching IOM: Implications of the institute of medicine reports for nursing education.* Silver Springs, MD: American Nurses Association.

Fisher, M. (1996). *Redesigning the nursing organization.* Albany, NY: Delmar Publishers.

Free Management Library. (2009). Organizational change and development. Retrieved November 1, 2009, from http://managementhelp.org/org_chng/org_chng .htm#anchor7003

Gadfrey, M., Melin, C., Muething, S., Batalden, P. & Nelson, E. (2008). Clinical Microsystems, Part 3. Transformation of two hospitals using microsystem, mesosystem, and macrosystem strategies. *The Joint Commission Journal on Quality and Patient Safety, 34*(10), 591–603.

Hammer, M., & Champy, J. (1993). *Reengineering the corporation: A manifesto for business revolution.* New York: Harper Business.

Heifetz, R., & Laurie, D. (2001). The work of leadership. *Harvard Business Review, 79*(12), 9–18.

Hutcherson, C., & Williamson, S. (May 31, 1999). Nursing regulation for the new millennium: The mutual recognition model. *Online Journal of Issues in Nursing*. Retrieved July 16, 1999, from http://www.nursingworld.org/ojin/topic9/topic9_2.htm

Institute of Health Improvement. (2009). Testing changes. Retrieved November 1, 2009, from http://www.ihi.org/IHI/Topics/Improvement/ImprovementMethods/HowToImprove/testingchanges.htm

Institute of Medicine. (2003). *Health profession education*. Washington, DC: National Academies Press.

Institute of Medicine. (2004). *Keeping patients safe*. Washington, DC: National Academies Press.

Kirkpatrick, D. (2001). *Managing change effectively*. Boston: Butterworth-Heinemann.

Krairiksh, M., & Anthony, M. (2001). Benefits and outcomes of staff nurses' participation in decision-making. *Journal of Nursing Administration, 31*(1), 16–23.

Lewin, K. (1947). Group and social change. In T. Newcomb and E. Hartely (Eds.), *Readings in social psychology*. New York: Holt, Rinehart & Winston.

Marrelli, T. (2004). *The nurse manager's guide*. St. Louis, MO: Mosby-Year Book, Inc.

Milgram, L., Spector, A., & Treger, M. (1999). *Managing smart*. Houston, TX: Cashman Dudley.

National Council of State Boards of Nursing. (2010). Transition to practice model. Retrieved May 25, 2010, from https://www.ncsbn.org/1603.htm

National League for Nursing. (May 23, 2010). Findings latest NLN annual survey of schools of nursing administered October through December 2009 confirm reported trends. Retrieved May 25, 2010, from http://www.nln.org

Paul, R. (1995). *Critical thinking: How to prepare students for a rapidly changing world*. Santa Rosa, CA: Midwest Publishing.

Pesut, D. (2001). Deep change. *Nursing Outlook, 49*(3), 118.

Porter-O'Grady, T. & Malloch, K. (2007). *Quantum leadership. A resource for health care innovation*. (2nd ed). Boston: Jones and Bartlett Publishers.

Profetto-McGrath, J. (2005). Critical thinking and evidence-based practice. *Journal of Professional Nursing, 21*(6), 364–371.

Quinn, R. (1996). *Deep change: Discovering the leader within*. San Francisco: Jossey-Bass.

Quinn, R. (2000). *Change the world: How ordinary people can accomplish extraordinary results*. San Francisco: Jossey-Bass.

Robert Wood Johnson Foundation. (2009). The Transforming Care at the Bedside (TCAB) Toolkit: Chapter 7 Deep Dive and Snorkel. Retrieved December 13, 2009, from http://www.rwjf.org/qualityequality/product.jsp?id=30070&parentid=30060&grparentid=30051

Robbins, B. & Davidhizar, R. (2007). Transformational leadership in health care today. *The Health Care Manager, 26*(3), 234–239.

Rogers, E. (2003). *Diffusion of innovations* (5th ed.). New York: Free Press.

Spear, S. (2005, September). Fixing health care from the inside, today. *Harvard Business Review*, 78-91.

Toofany, S. (2008). Critical thinking among nurses. *Nursing Management/UK, 14*(9), 28–31.

Zori, S. & Morrison, B. (2009). Critical thinking in nurse managers. *Nursing Economics, 27*(2), 75–79.

demands. Change drives the need for adaptation. Efficiency, which is the ratio of input to output, focuses on the amount of effort that is required to reach an outcome. Efficiency and productivity go hand-in-hand. Stakeholders (anyone who is affected by the organization's decisions and services including employees) are very important, particularly in open systems. Thus, it is important to pay attention to stakeholder satisfaction by evaluating key player satisfaction. Who are the key players or stakeholders in the health care system? The customer, third-party payer, providers, and the consumer are the stakeholders.

**INTEGRATED DELIVERY SYSTEM**    An **integrated delivery system** is an organizational structure that became very popular in the 1990s and was thought to reduce costs. The development of this type of system is typically motivated by reimbursement changes and managed care. This system focuses on a continuum of care, provides a cost-efficient approach, and focuses on providing care to patients in the most appropriate setting (Spitzer, 2001). Integration can either be horizontal, vertical, or both.

- **Horizontal integration** merges several organizations doing the same type of work (for example, several acute care hospitals join together to form a horizontal health care organization). This can offer communities major advantages—reducing duplicate services, increasing quality as experts and expert services are developed, and can reduce health are costs. These systems are complicated and difficult to manage. The organizations (or in the previous example, the hospitals that form one organization) may not be close to one another, which causes problems for coordination, collaboration, and communication. Distance between the various system components can make management more complicated. Horizontal integration has not always resulted in one seamless organization, but rather several organizations with a loose connection. This occurs when there is a limited unified identity and commitment to the larger organization. "When corporations merge, certain things usually result: a snappy new name, a single person running the show, consolidated departments. A big production is made of uniting the partners culturally and financially just as in a marriage. Except when the partners are hospitals" (Steinhauer, 2001, p. A1). It is not so simple to accomplish this type of merger and develop one organization out of several. Different competencies are required to manage a horizontal system as compared to a vertical system, and this difference is often neglected. Several organizations come together to form an integrated system, but there is limited change in leadership and management approaches. A major force that pushed health care organizations to become more integrated was the growth of managed care organizations (MCOs). Organizations are trying to better meet the third-party payers including MCO demands and outcomes required by managed care approach to reimbursement.
- An organization that uses **vertical integration** is one that covers the continuum of care (for example, it might include an acute care hospital, a home care agency, a long-term care facility, a rehabilitation center, and an ambulatory care center). Diversification is one of the advantages of moving to vertical integration, which may provide more financial opportunities for the organization. As the organization has multiple services or products (e.g., wellness, prevention, acute and chronic care, disease management and rehabilitation, ambulatory care, long-term care, home care, and hospice care), there are increased opportunities to gain more reimbursement for services and thus increase revenues, or money that comes into the organization.

Regardless of the type of structure, vertical or horizontal, integrated systems need to have leaders who feel committed to all of the elements of the organization; use quantitative and qualitative innovation; are concerned with processes; use decentralized leadership; and design, support, and enhance organizational systems that drive performance (Spitzer, 2001). There has been criticism that the integrated delivery approach may not provide the best of services. Can one organization, the integrated organization, be an expert in all areas? What happens to individual entities that come together to form the integrated organization? Will they lose their strengths as they compete within the new organization (Campbell, Schmitz, & Waller, 1998)? These questions are still important today. Over time some of these organizations have been more effective than others.

SERVICE-LINE ORGANIZATION   The **service-line organization** groups activities according to product or service, such as women's health, emergency and urgent care, behavioral health care, and health and wellness. As an organization changes into a service-line structure, then the big question that arises is how to maintain a unified nursing presence within the organization and yet still experience benefits from this structure (Fitzpatrick, McElroy, & DeWoody, 2001). "Organizing nursing as a discipline into clusters for like areas of practice enhances the development of documentation tools, preprinted care plans, and orientation plans" (Fitzpatrick, McElroy, & DeWoody, 2001, p. 25). Interprofessional planning, which is emphasized more and more including in the Institute of Medicine reports (2003), enhances collaboration because it is easier to identify core health care provider groups that should be included; for example, if planning for behavioral health services, then behavioral health (psychiatric-mental health) nursing staff, psychiatrists, psychologists, social workers, and other mental health staff, would be involved. Even though an organization is structured around services/products there still needs to be some standardized features that continue to apply to all services/products. Position descriptions would have some content that is standardized along with specific content related to the service/product. Another example is some documentation forms might apply across all service areas, but there probably would still need to be some specialized documentation needs such as for the emergency department or for mental health.

But what happens to the centralized functions such as the nursing department in a service-line organization? Fitzpatrick, McElroy, and DeWoody (2001) describe these functions in one organization that changed to product or service lines as follows.

- Vice presidents, who were either physicians or nurses, directed the service lines. These vice presidents were responsible for fiscal management, marketing, physician relationships, quality of care, and growth of the service, and also assumed line accountability for the nursing units or other departments that were associated with the service.
- Administrative responsibilities were assigned to the chief nursing executive, who was responsible and accountable for the centralized cost centers of staff development, patient education, float and per diem pools, and in-house nursing supervisors, which have typically been found in a nursing department. The chief nursing executive was responsible for the final approval of all centralized nursing policies and procedures and responsible for nursing throughout the organization.
- A centralized director of nursing position coordinated the core elements of the discipline of nursing that support nursing practice. "This position had cross-campus reporting relationships for centralized staffing, house supervisors, employee education services, patient education services, and both campuses' nursing administrative offices" (Fitzpatrick, McElroy, & DeWoody, 2001, p. 25).

It is clear that this structure can be confusing for staff that has worked in more traditional nursing departments. It is even difficult to describe. In this type of structure, management and staff need to learn more about the new structure and how it affects processes, staff, and management relationships. Staff should also be asked for input as the organization adapts to these changes.

The service-line type of organization has become more common in health care. What are the advantages and disadvantages to this organization of the product/service-line approach to an organization's structure and process? The advantages are as follows:

- A single manager or director is responsible for ensuring that the service/product outcomes are reached. This means that from the beginning to the end of the service, all parts of the process are overseen, which should result in less fragmentation of care. With the increased concerns about health care delivery dysfunction and need for patient-centered care with interprofessional teams, this type of organization may be more effective in meeting these critical goals. Responses to problems that interfere with care should be timelier. If behavioral health is the service line, then all aspects that the organization provides from crisis intervention, inpatient to aftercare would be included in the service line (e.g., outpatient clinic, inpatient units, behavioral health emergency services, partial hospitalization, home care, and vocational therapy).

- Performance can more easily be judged. Responsibility can also be more clearly defined, which can be a problem in performance evaluation. This may motivate staff to improve. An example related to the behavioral health service would be when a patient is discharged and then rehospitalized within a time period that is considered inappropriate. The patient's entire treatment process can be evaluated and then strategies can be developed within the service line instead of having to go to several different departments. A service line usually prevents one department from placing blame on another department (for example, the outpatient clinic blaming the inpatient unit). When they are both part of the same service line, this is more difficult to do. They would all participate together in planning and decision making and accept responsibility for ensuring that patients receive care in the service rather than respond as separate departments, and all participate in evaluation and quality improvement.
- The director may be more motivated when the entire service is under the director's control.
- Responsibility for giving continuous, undivided attention to the product or service leads to more sensitivity for the unique needs of the focus population that the service addresses (patient-centered). Interprofessional staff develop a better view of how all parts of treatment offered within the service relate to one another, can develop relationships with staff across treatment focus areas, and during evaluation staff can focus more on clearly analyzing problems rather than denying their responsibilities.

The disadvantages are as follows:

- There is duplication of effort, which may reduce efficiency.
- Some services may become isolated from other services and their staff. Increased communication about activities of the various service lines exists, which can result in confusion and overload of information.
- Organization-wide identity and commitment may be compromised as the service lines are emphasized (Dessler, 2002, pp. 137–139).

Disadvantages can be limited if steps are taken early on to recognize these as potential problems and then staff responds proactively. For example, the organization as a whole can determine functions that cross all service lines (such as pharmacy) and decide the most effective way to ensure that resources that are needed in all the service lines are met.

## Structure and Process: Parts of Organizational Theory

STRUCTURE    Typically, a description of an organization includes information about their **structure** and **process**. Why is it important to understand this? As organizational theories developed, they tended to focus on one of these aspects of organization, although some focus on both. Staff in organizations find that the organization's structure (what does the organization look like) and the process (how things are done) become important. For example, if a nurse does not understand to whom he or she reports, this can be a problem (structure), or if the nurse does not understand the communication process for reporting an error (process), this can lead to problems. What are the aspects of structure and process that are important to understand?

First, how does staff find out about an organization's structure? The best place to begin is with the organizational chart for the entire organization and the charts for its components, such as divisions and units. The organizational chart is the best visual of the organization structure, providing titles of key positions and how they relate to one another. It provides a visual of the chain of command, centralization/decentralization approach, departments, and span of control. It is important that this chart is updated as changes are made in the organizational structure. When assessing an organization's structure, it is important to remember that each organization has a formal and an informal aspect. How are these aspects demonstrated in an organization? The organization's organizational chart describes the formal positions and hierarchy; however, this does not reflect the informal structure. Staff members who are leaders even if they do not hold a formal title in the hierarchy would not be identified in the structure described in the organization chart nor would information about which managers are more powerful, although they all have the same authority due to their position as manager. A traditional structure uses vertical relationships or the chain of command that identifies to whom specific positions report. The view of organizational structure has been changing for many organizations as they move to greater emphasis on horizontal organization. Elements of the structure, which are highlighted in Box 4-2, that are important to consider are as follows:

- **Vertical structure.** Establishes line authority and uses centralized decision making. This is the type of structure found in bureaucratic organizations, with staff reporting "up the line" through the organization.
- **Horizontal structure.** Departmentalization related to functions that uses decentralized decision making. Typically, a horizontal organization uses "a structure organized around customer-oriented processes (products/service lines), eliminates functional departments, and spreads functional specialists throughout the key process teams" (Dessler, 2002, p. 170).
- **Line authority or the chain of command.** A more traditional approach to authority in organizations. This description identifies to whom each staff member reports up through the chain of command. For example, in line authority a staff nurse would report to the nurse manager, the nurse manager to the director of the service, the director of the service to the nurse executive, and the nurse executive to the chief executive officer.
- **Staff authority.** Staff that functions in an advisory capacity and cannot force other staff to do something but rather must use influence to make an impact. This can be a difficult position, but it has become more common. Staff authority is less clear because this relationship is advisory. An example is the director of nursing education or staff development in a hospital, who typically has no line authority over the nurse managers but rather a staff relationship. The director can suggest and advise nurse managers to initiate certain educational programs but cannot direct nurse managers to do this. Key skills for success in this type of position are effective communication, negotiation, building collaborative relationships, marketing, evidence-based practice, and leadership. Clinical nurse specialists (CNS) and clinical nurse leaders (CNL) usually hold staff authority positions.
- **Span of control.** Number of people supervised by one person/position. Span of control answers the question of how many staff report to one manager. This is a critical concern in the classical theory of organizations, which emphasizes that there are limits to the number of staff a supervisor can effectively direct. Issues that affect the number of staff are (a) similarity and complexity of the jobs and functions, (b) geographic factors (for example, staff that is spread out in several clinics in a community as compared with staff that works on one unit in a hospital), (c) amount of direction and coordination required, and (d) amount of planning and time required to provide management. More efficient organizations usually have a shorter span of control for their managers.
- **Centralized organizational structures.** Used in health care organizations. A centralized approach focuses tasks and authority in one source.
- **Decentralized organizational structures** spreads tasks and authority out over components of the organization. For example, how is staff education organized in a hospital? In a centralized approach there is a staff development department that is responsible for staff orientation and education throughout the hospital, whereas a decentralized approach gives this responsibility to the divisions or units. In the latter case, there may still be staff that provides some staff development services and also act as consultants to the units. In this case, they typically are also responsible for overall hospital orientation and education/training that is required for all staff, and nurse managers are responsible for their own unit's staff

| BOX 4-2 | ELEMENTS OF ORGANIZATIONAL STRUCTURE |
|---------|---------------------------------------|

- Vertical structure
- Horizontal structure
- Line authority or chain of command
- Staff authority
- Span of control
- Centralized or decentralized
- Departmentalization

development. In a decentralized organization the nurse managers then have more independence in the management of their units in comparison to centralized organizations.

- **Departmentalization.** Occurs when divided tasks are grouped. Functional departmentalization focuses on grouping related jobs while territorial departmentalization focuses on grouping jobs according to location within the organization. An example of a functional departmentalization, which is common in health care organizations, is the department of surgery, which might include the preoperative area, operating rooms, and post-anesthesia care unit (PACU). Another example is the obstetrics department composed of labor and delivery, postpartum, nurseries, and the neonatal intensive care unit. In some organizations the clinics for these specialty areas are also included in the department. This is very similar to a product/service-line approach. A different approach is to have all clinics, regardless of specialty, included in one ambulatory care department.

- **Matrix organization.** Structures attempt to balance functional and service or product organizations. Staff belongs to a functional department, such as a nursing department, and to a service or product department, such as women's health. Dual authority is part of this type of structure as staff reports to two managerial systems. Why would this type of structure be used? It facilitates the efficient use of resources; allows for more flexibility during times of change with more timely response and interchange of information vertically and horizontally; encourages greater interprofessional interaction and innovation; improves motivation and commitment as staff has more responsibility for decision making; and it frees managers for greater opportunity to enhance planning (Dessler, 2002; Robbins & Decenzo, 2001).

The informal organization is also very important. This is what works behind the formal organization. Sometimes informal leaders are even more powerful than formal leaders. They can have significant influence on the change process. Informal organization can be found at all levels of a formal organization from the unit to the upper level of the organization. In the ideal situation the formal and the informal organization work together and not against each other.

PROCESS    Organizational process, the second critical descriptor of an organization, focuses on how the organization operates. Particularly important process factors are communication, decision making, policies and procedures, interprofessional teamwork, organization performance and job performance, goal attainment and results, quality improvement, budget, marketing, and future plans. All of these factors are discussed in other chapters. Nurses participate in all of these aspects of organizational process whether they are staff nurses or in management.

The organization's vision, mission statement, and goals and objectives should be included in a review of an organization's process. The **vision** is important in describing the organization's beliefs and values. An organizational philosophy answers the question of "why" for an organization. "The values and principles of an organization set the parameters for decision making and determining what is critical to the organization. Thus, the organizational philosophy becomes the basis for operationalizing the mission of the institution" (Tuck, Harris, & Baliko, 2000, p. 180).

Tuck, Harris, and Baliko (2000) reviewed nursing philosophies that were written after 1982. In this review value statements were classified according to several categories: caring, professionalism, individualism, well-being or health, culture, need fulfillment, and adaptation. The results indicated that caring and individuation remain central concepts of nursing practice. Reimbursement changes such as managed care has major impact on health care organizations, and presents organizations and nurses with new challenges. How can organizations continue to incorporate these key concepts such as caring in their changing organizations? The responsibility for ensuring that values expressed in an organization's nursing philosophy or vision are implemented is the responsibility of the nurse executive. The mission statement clarifies the organization's purpose. It describes what the organization is while the vision describes what the organization wants to be. Goals and objectives identify how the organization plans to meet its vision and mission. The **mission statement** provides a clear description of the organization's goals and objectives, which are influenced by the organization's core values and purpose. All of the staff needs to understand and be committed to the organization's vision, mission, and goals and objectives.

| **BOX 4-3** | **ELEMENTS OF ORGANIZATIONAL PROCESS** |

- Decision making
- Delegation
- Coordination

- Communication
- Evaluation

Vision and mission statements, as well as goals and objectives, all help to define the organizational process—how things work to get the job done. What are other important elements of process? Box 4-3 highlights the key process elements.

- **Decision making.** Decisions are made frequently in all health care organizations: decisions about patient care, how they will be done, how the organization will run, and about the future of the organization. Decision making is a critical element of organizational processes (see Chapter 3).
- **Delegation.** Decisions should be made as close to the task or activity as possible, which has made delegation even more important in today's health care organizations. It is important to remember that delegation does not relinquish the person who is delegating from the responsibility over the task (see Chapter 14).
- **Coordination.** Coordination is the process by which the parts of a process are synchronized or work together. The Institute of Medicine (2003) describes the purpose of coordination is "to establish and support a continuous healing relationship, enabled by an integrated clinical environment and characterized by a proactive delivery of evidence-based care and follow-up" (p. 49) (see Chapter 12).
- **Communication.** As has been discussed in previous chapters and will be discussed in later chapters, communication is part of any organization's processes. Without communication nothing will get done in an organization; in fact, no one would know what to do without communication (see Chapter 13).
- **Evaluation.** Evaluation of the organization's performance and that of individual staff performance assists the organization in determining its needs in the planning process so that goals and objectives can be met. All processes are evaluated in some form, whether it is a formal evaluation or staff concluding that some action was successful on an informal basis (see Chapter 17).

# Health Care Organizations

This section discusses some key factors about the health care delivery system and its organizations. The health care system consists of all the agencies and professionals that are organized to provide health services. The three major purposes of the health care delivery system are to provide (a) health promotion and illness prevention, (b) diagnosis and treatment of illness and injury, and (c) rehabilitation and health restoration. Box 4-4 highlights these purposes.

There are three levels of health care services based on the complexity of the care required.

1. **Primary care** includes health promotion and education, preventive care, early detection, and environmental protection.
2. **Secondary care** focuses on diagnosis and treatment in the primary settings of acute care and emergency care.

| **BOX 4-4** | **HEALTH CARE DELIVERY SYSTEM PURPOSES** |

- Health promotion and illness prevention
- Diagnosis and treatment

- Rehabilitation and health restoration

3. **Tertiary care**, the last level, focuses on long-term care, rehabilitation, and care of the dying. Health care systems are varied in the level of services they provide, and some provide a combination of services (for example, a large medical center might provide acute care, ambulatory care and primary care, emergency services, wellness center, home care, and also own a long-term care facility).

The second part of the health care delivery system is the public or population system, which provides care for the population or community. Both the personal systems, which focus on care for individuals, and the public systems provide a variety of services including health promotion, prevention and early detection of disease, diagnosis and treatment of disease with a focus on cure, rehabilitative-restorative care, and custodial care. Managed care and other reimbursement approaches have had a major effect on both the personal and the public systems as discussed in Chapter 5.

Health care settings can be described by a variety of important characteristics, including the type of services offered, size, location (urban or rural), type of people served, and reimbursement methods. The following are examples of health care settings.

- **Public health** or government departments and agencies (federal, state, or local) funded primarily by taxes and administered by elected or appointed officials. Local health departments develop and carry out programs to meet the health needs of groups within the community and the community as a whole.
- Physician practices/offices (or advance practice nurses' and nurse midwives' offices)
- Primary care
- Ambulatory care centers (e.g., one-day surgery centers, diagnostic centers)
- Clinics, which may be part of a hospital or free-standing, external to hospitals, provide a variety of services
- Occupational health clinics, which provide health services at the worksite
- Community health centers
- School health services, some of which may be full-service clinics
- Emergency
- Urgent care
- Crisis intervention
- Hospitals (acute care)
- Behavioral health/psychiatric hospitals and community mental health centers
- Substance abuse treatment centers (inpatient and outpatient)
- Extended care facilities, which includes skilled nursing (intermediate care) and/or extended-care (long-term care) facilities and may be part of a hospital system or freestanding
- Retirement and assisted-living centers
- Rehabilitation centers
- Home health agencies
- Hospice services, which may be provided in the home, in a hospital-based hospice unit, and/or in a freestanding facility

This list is not complete, but it does provide examples of the more common types of health care settings or organizations.

The U.S. health care system is complex, although it did not begin this way. In the past, care was primarily provided in the home and by visits to physician offices. This gradually developed into a more complex system as the role of hospitals grew. Today, most care still comes through the personal health care system rather than through the public care system. Physician care has typically been delivered in one of the following models:

1. The solo practice of a physician in an office, which continues to be present in some communities, although it is less and less common.
2. The single specialty group model, which consists of physicians in the same specialty who pool expenses, income, and offices.
3. Multispecialty group practice, which provides interaction across specialty areas.

4. The integrated health maintenance model that has prepaid multispecialty physicians.
5. Community health center—developed through federal monies in the 1960s—which addresses broader inputs into health such as education and housing (Finkelman, 2001, p. 189).

However, there have been other changes occurring in physician practice. Due to the increasing cost of running a practice more physicians are giving up their private practices (Harris, 2010). In 2005 more than two-thirds of the medical practices were physician owned, but three years later the number decreased to below 50 percent. Fifty percent of the practices are now owned by hospitals. Where did the physicians go? Some retired, but most took salaried positions. This is leading to major changes in practice and physician-patient relationships. "The decline of private practices may put an end to the kind of enduring and intimate relationships between patients and doctors that have long defined medicine. A patient who chooses a doctor in a private practice is more likely to see that same doctor during each office visit than a patient who chooses a doctor employed by a health system" (Harris, 2010, p. B5). On the plus side patients may benefit from higher quality care and better coordinated care in the new system—records can more easily be shared; specialists more easily accessible, and so on. There has also been an expansion of nurse-managed clinics and nurse practitioner practice settings. The newest IOM report (2011) emphasizes in its recommendations that nurses, particularly advanced practice nurses, need to be more active in providing primary care.

Health care organizations are confronted with many factors that influence how they are structured and how they operate. The following factors have had an impact or continue to have an impact on health care organization structure and processes.

- Problems with access to health care often resulting in disparity
- Increase in health care cost and cost containment to combat increased costs
- Hospital mergers and closings
- Growth of managed care and development of other reimbursement methods
- Shortage of health care providers (e.g., nurses, pharmacists, physicians)
- Increase in the number of uninsured and underinsured
- Improved technologic advances (e.g., computers, organ transplants, extension of life, genetics, telehealth/telemedicine)
- Increased specialization, which may increase fragmentation of care
- Growing consumerism
- Changes in demographics (e.g., single-parent families, immigrant populations, lack of nearby extended family, aging)
- Increase in homeless populations, uninsured, underinsured, and other vulnerable populations
- Increase in availability of drugs, although many are expensive
- Lack of or limited coverage for prescriptions
- Uneven distribution of services (e.g., urban vs. rural areas)
- Lack of clear health policies
- Unequal treatment for some health problems (e.g., mental health services)

## For-Profit and Not-for-Profit Delivery Systems

Two terms that are often used in health care, for-profit and not-for-profit, can be confusing. They are nonetheless important terms as they identify an organization's characteristics that impact many aspects of the health care organization's structure and process. **For-profit health care organizations** have stockholders/shareholders who own stock in the business/organization. The organization is responsible to the stockholders, who expect to make a profit on their investment. If stockholders do not feel that they are making enough money on their investment, they may sell their stocks, and the organization will then have serious financial problems. Stockholders serve as an external control on decisions that are made by the organization. These organizations receive the same type of reimbursement for care as not-for-profit delivery systems, which are called voluntary or public health care organizations. In contrast, the **not-for-profit organization** does not have stockholders to whom it must report. Charitable institutions, government, churches, and typical reimbursement sources, fund not-for-profit health care organizations. Both types of organizations, for-profit and not-for-profit, must still make a profit to survive today. The not-for-profit organization does not share this profit with shareholders, as the for-profit organization does, but rather this type of organization reinvests its profit into its own organization to continue its services and maintain the organization. The for-profit organization, however, also does the same, but it must still share some profit with stockholders. Both financial approaches have direct effects on the organization's vision, mission, goals, budget, management and decision making, use of resources, types of services, relationships with other organizations and the community, and how quickly the organization responds to change that can make a financial impact on the organization. Some for-profit organizations have experienced ethical and legal problems because of their need for financial success, which are discussed in Chapter 5. Nurses need to be aware of their employer's status related to profits. It can affect why and how decisions are made.

## Marketing

**Marketing** is a new area for most nurses, and for many it may arouse negative reactions because nurses may see it as too "business like" and not ethical. Why is it important for nurses to be aware of health care marketing and understand some aspects of it? The marketing process drives major decisions in health care as health care organizations compete with one another for patients and for third-party payer (insurer) contracts. Ineffective marketing may result in a health care organization cutting staff and services if it cannot attract enough patients. The marketing process includes three elements.

1. A determination of what is wanted and needed
2. A method(s) for reaching what is wanted or needed
3. An understanding of the patient, customer, or consumer and the service or need

These elements should sound familiar because they are similar to those described in the nursing process. Like the nursing process, the marketing process is complex. It is dependent on data, interaction between people, problem solving, decision making, and evaluation of results. A **market** is an actual or potential consumer or **customer** who might need a product or service. For example, for a nurse-midwife, a market sector is women in a specific community or geographic area who are of childbearing age. A more specific market would be the women in that community or geographic area who might use the services of a nurse-midwife. This is referred to as segmenting. Factors that help to identify segments of a market are age, sex, diagnosis, past medical treatment, geographics, accessibility, insurance coverage, and economic status. Selling is often confused with marketing, but selling is only one part of the marketing process. Nurses can be very helpful in the marketing process with their consumer skills: the ability to talk with patients, understanding of patient needs, their emphasis on health promotion and disease and illness prevention, understanding of the health care delivery system and the community, and problem-solving skills.

Marketing goals are established by the health care organization (HCO) based on assessment data. The following are examples of goals that might be identified for a community clinic.

- To develop patient services that are accessible
- To increase the number of patients by 5%
- To provide health promotion and disease and illness prevention services
- To request active patient participation in their care (self-management)
- To develop patient education support groups focusing on chronic illness (e.g., asthma, arthritis, hypertension)

As illustrated by these examples of goals, marketing is connected to providing direct patient care services, quality improvement, risk management, utilization review, administration, decision making and planning, performance appraisal, staff development, and community relationships.

THE FOUR Ps OF MARKETING    The four Ps of marketing are product, promotion, price, and place. Box 4-5 highlights these principles.

- Products are the goods or services that meet the customer's needs. For a community clinic this would include physical exams, patient education, immunizations, well-child care, and blood pressure screening.
- Promotion is what is often referred to as advertising. How does the community clinic get the word out about the services or products that are provided? Informing local hospitals about its services and other community agencies to obtain referrals is promotion.

---

**BOX 4-5    THE FOUR Ps OF MARKETING**

- Product
- Promotion

- Price
- Place

---

- Pricing focuses on identifying the cost of a product or service. Much of this is in the hands of third-party payers and the government, which determine their own reimbursement levels; however, if reimbursement does not cover expenses and provide some profit, this is a major problem for the health care organization.
- The fourth P is place or getting the product or service to the consumer. This includes such factors as physical location, hours, wait time for appointments, type of location, accessibility to the facility, transportation, parking, handicap accessibility, and the type of setting, such as its "warmth," easy-to-locate offices, and so on.

THE MARKETING PLAN    The marketing plan is a written description of the organization and what it wants to be in the future. The plan includes a description of the organization (for example, a group of nurse practitioners, an interprofessional group of practitioners, a clinic, hospital, and so on); the environment in which the organization operates, its potential and actual consumers; its competitors; and its plans for the future. Change is inevitable so a marketing plan is never really complete. If the marketing plan does not change, it becomes just another piece of paper. A marketing plan contains five parts, as highlighted in Box 4-6.

1. Situational analysis is sometimes referred to as SWOT—the strengths, weaknesses, opportunities, and threats analysis of the organization. All of these elements are described with relevant data to support the ideas presented. Data from both internal and external environments are included in the analysis.
2. Marketing goals and objectives are identified that are reasonable and specific to the organization. A marketing goal might be to increase the number of patients from a specific geographic area by 20%. If this geographic area had a large number of professional women, single and married, a related objective might be to develop a special woman's health promotion program for women ages 30 to 40. Decisions like this need to be based on data.
3. Marketing strategy considers the marketing mix and the marketing budget. The marketing mix describes the specific combination of the four Ps, focusing on how the combination of product, promotion, price, and place influence consumers to use the organization's services. As the marketing budget is developed, resources are allocated to each service area. For example, the budget identifies the amount of resources that will be allocated to market the health promotion program for women ages 30 to 40.
4. Action plans describe specifically how the marketing goals and objectives will be met. The written plan identifies actions to be taken, responsibilities and accountabilities, and time frames.
5. Evaluation is ongoing. It provides feedback as the plan is implemented and goals are achieved, as well as information that might indicate a need for a change in the plan. Any change must be carefully considered; however, no plan should be so sacred that it cannot be revised (MindTools™, 2010).

The health care reform legislation of 2010 requires that non-profit hospitals conduct a community needs assessment every three years and adopt an implementation plan based on this assessment.

---

**BOX 4-6    MARKETING PLAN**

- Situational Analysis (SWOT)
- Goals and Objectives
- Marketing Mix and Budget

- Action Plans
- Evaluation

## Health Care Providers: The Interprofessional Team

Health care providers can be classified as organizations such as a hospital or a clinic and as individual providers such as an individual nurse or physician. Both types provide care to individuals and groups of patients. There are many different types of health care provider organizations. The typical ones are hospitals, clinics, physician practices, ambulatory care centers, primary care, home health agencies, long-term care facilities, skilled nursing facilities, rehabilitation centers, hospice services, public health departments, school health clinics, birthing centers, ambulatory surgical centers, occupational health clinics, crisis clinics, and any other type of organization that provides care to the community.

The factors discussed earlier that have affected organization structure and process frequently cause these organizations to change. The growth of managed care works has influenced the decease in hospitalization and length of stays and helped to emphasize the need for provider/physician performance. This led to growth in primary care. Due to the push to decrease hospitalization when patients are admitted to hospitals, they are often much more acutely ill, requiring more intensive care. At the same time hospitals are encouraged to discharge patients as soon as possible. These patients then return home still sick and often require care from family members or a home health agency. Home health services and hospice services have also increased. This shifting has had a major impact on physician practices, clinics, hospitals, home health agencies, hospices, and long-term care facilities, and certainly on nursing practice in all of these organizations. At the same time advanced practice nursing has grown, and advanced practice nurses are now found in many of these organizations.

These changes have also had an influence on the use on of hospitalists and intensivists (Wachter & Goldman, 2002; Wachter, 2003; Wachter, 2010). Physicians usually hold these positions, but some hospitals are using nurse practitioners and clinical nurse specialists in these roles. The hospitalist, a generalist, provides medical coverage for hospitalized patients instead of the patient's personal or primary care physician covering the patient. After discharge the patient returns to his or her personal physician. Intensivists cover patients in the intensive care units and have considerable intensive care experience, something that most primary care physicians do not have. The major disadvantage is the patient does not have relationship with the hospitalist or intensivist.

The following provides a brief review of the major types of professional and non-professional members of the health care team.

- *Registered nurse* (**RN**).   This appears to be a simple designation; however, there are different types of educational routes to obtain a license to practice nursing. These include diploma, associate's degree, and baccalaureate degree. In addition, more nurses are obtaining master's degrees though still only a small number get doctorates. These advanced degrees provide them with the opportunity to practice more independently, teach, or to do research. Nurses practice in all types of health settings.
- *Clinical nurse leader* (**CNL**).   This is a new role requiring a master's degree. The American Association of Colleges of Nursing (AACN) states that the CNL is a "provider and manager of care at the point of care to individuals and cohorts. The CNL designs, implements, and evaluates patient care by coordinating, delegating and supervising the care provided by the health care team, including licensed nurses, technicians, and other health professionals" (2007, p. 6).
- *Nurse practitioner* (**NP**) *and clinical nurse specialist* (**CNS**).   Both of these types of nurses obtain education beyond a baccalaureate degree with special content either related to primary care (NP) or acute care (CNS). A nurse practitioner specializes in such areas as adult health, family health, pediatrics, neonatal, gerontology, anesthesia, and psychiatric/mental health/behavioral health nursing. Nurse practitioners may work in clinics, the community, private practice, the home, the hospital, or long-term care facilities—any setting where health care is provided. A CNS typically works in acute care settings. Some hospitals are using CNSs and ANPs as hospitalists.
- *Nurse midwife* (**NM**).   This is a nurse who has completed an additional educational program that focuses on midwifery. Nurse midwives work in all types of settings in which women's health and obstetrical services are provided.

- *Doctor of nursing practice* (**DNP**).   This is the newest nursing degree and is a practice-based doctoral program. The American Association of Colleges of Nursing (AACN) comments about this degree: "Nurses prepared at the doctoral level with a blend of clinical, organization, economic, and leadership skills are most likely to be able to critique nursing and other clinical scientific findings and design programs of care delivery that are locally acceptable, economically feasible, and which significantly impact health care outcomes" (2004, p. 7).

- *Physician* (**MD**).   A physician has a medical degree and typically specializes in a specific area of practice (e.g., internal medicine, surgery, pediatrics, gynecology, etc.). There is a growing physician shortage, just as there is a nursing shortage. In addition, physicians have gravitated to specialty services rather than to primary care often due to financial concerns. Specialty care reimbursement is higher. This shortage in primary care and also the expected growth in patient numbers due to health care reform of 2010 there is greater interest in increasing the number of ANPs who would serve as primary care providers and set-up independent practices.

- *Licensed practical/vocational nurse* (**LPN or LVN**).   Licensed practical/vocational nurses perform some specific nursing functions and play a critical role in providing direct patient care. They have high school degrees and additional training. They work in all types of settings under the direct supervision of a registered nurse. The use of LPN/LVNs varies from state to state.

- *Unlicensed assistive personnel* (**UAP**).   The increased use of UAP on the health care team has caused some controversy in the last few years; however, UAP are critical members of the team. Aides and assistants have been in existence for a long time. Their responsibilities have changed over the years, and today they are providing more direct patient care. They are supervised by registered nurses, who must ensure that they are able to provide safe care to the patient. The home health aide functions fairly independently in the home, usually seeing the patient more than the home care nurse, who supervises the home health aide and makes periodic home visits. The amount of UAP education and training is highly variable, and this has caused some of the concern about what they are able to do and the effect on the quality of care. Further information about UAP and delegation is found in Chapter 14.

- *Registered dietician* (**RD**).   This health care professional assesses the patient's nutritional status related to health status. A registered dietician may work in hospitals, long-term care facilities, clinics, community health areas, and in the home. Another similar health care provider is the nutritionist who has knowledge about nutrition and food in the community setting and recommends healthy diets and provides nutrition counseling and education.

- *Social worker* (**SW**).   Social workers assist patients and their families with problems related to reimbursement, access to care, housing, care in the home, transportation, and other social problems. They may also hold specialized positions as discharge planners and as case managers, particularly in acute care facilities or hospitals; however, they work in all types of settings.

- *Occupational therapist* (**OT**).   Occupational therapists assist patients with impaired functions to reach the patient's maximum level of physical and psychosocial independence. They work in all types of settings.

- *Speech-language pathologist*.   Speech-language pathologists assist patients who need rehabilitative services related to speech and hearing. They work in all types of settings.

- *Physical therapist* (**PT**).   Physical therapists focus on assisting patients who are experiencing musculoskeletal problems with rehabilitation and reaching maximum physical functioning. They work in all types of settings.

- *Pharmacist*.   Pharmacists are concerned with ensuring that patients receive the appropriate medication by preparing and dispensing medications. Pharmacists have become much more involved in patient education about medications and in monitoring and evaluating the effects of medications. They work in all types of settings including the local drug store, where they play a critical role in ensuring safe prescriptions and in providing consumer education.

- ■ *Respiratory therapist* (**RT**).   Respiratory therapists provide care to patients with respiratory illnesses. They use oxygen therapy, intermittent positive pressure respirators, artificial mechanical ventilators, and inhalation therapy.
- ■ *Chiropractor*.   Chiropractors are concerned with improving the function of the patient's nervous system with various treatment modalities (e.g., spinal manipulation, diet, exercise, and massage). Interest in using chiropractors has been increasing as the consumer has become more interested in nontraditional medical interventions.
- ■ *Paramedical technologists*.   Paramedical technologists work in various medical technology areas (for example, radiology, nuclear medicine, and other laboratories) (Finkelman, 2001, pp. 195–196).

Other common providers are physician's assistants (PAs), who diagnose and treat certain diseases and injuries under the direction of a physician, dentists, case managers, and spiritual support persons (chaplains).

Nontraditional health care providers have become more important as consumers have increased their use of alternative or complementary therapies. There is great variation in how these services are accepted by health care professionals. In some communities some of these services can be found within traditional health care organizations, and traditional health care providers are also incorporating the use of alternative therapies into their practice. In other communities there is less integration of these services. Reimbursement for these services is still highly variable. Some of these therapies are massage therapy, herbal therapy, healing touch, energetic healing, acupuncture, acupressure, and so on. Some of the problem areas with these new therapies are limited research to support their effectiveness, limited or lack of formal training and licensure requirements for practitioners, lack of standards, and limited or no reimbursement. The National Institutes of Health (NIH) has established a center, the National Center for Complementary and Alternative Medicine (NCCAM), that focuses on alternative or complementary therapies and now funds research to determine the effectiveness of these therapies. These issues need to be addressed before these therapies and their practitioners will be fully accepted in the health care system.

## Organizational Analysis

After reviewing some of the critical aspects related to organizations in this chapter, how would one go about analyzing an organization to better understand or assess its functioning? The following might be included in this analysis.

- ■ **Integration of vision and mission into organizational structure**   The vision and mission statements are the driving forces behind all decisions, or should be. They provide critical information about the organization's values and philosophy. It is also important to remember that many organizations have beautifully written vision and mission statements and yet never really make them come alive. When an organization is analyzed, the important issue is whether or not the vision and mission match what the organization and its staff actually do.
- ■ **Description of corporate culture, historical determinants**   The culture of a health care organization and its history have a major impact on the way that staff interact, communicate, work as teams, and feel rewarded and recognized or feel neglected. It also affects organization outcomes. The community in which the organization must survive also affects the organization's culture (see Chapter 7).
- ■ **Structural design of the organization**   Organizational structure varies, and structure affects how organizations communicate, work together, and solve problems or do not solve problems, which represent the organization's process. The structure of health care organizations is changing, and some of these efforts are resulting in positive outcomes.
- ■ **Decision-making patterns**   How does the organization handle decision making? This can be highly variable from one organization to another and even within an organization. Some nursing leaders and other organizational leaders have greater skill in this area than other leaders. All organizations need improvement in decision making. Does staff feel that

decisions are handled well? Is there staff input? Is shared governance used and how effective is it? What is the response to accountability? How empowered are the staff?

- **Communication patterns**   Communication runs an organization. How is communication conducted? Who communicates with whom? What are the formal and informal aspects? How successful is communication? How is technology used? Do staff members feel they are listened to when they speak up? How can this be improved? How are interprofessional, intradepartmental, and interdepartmental communication described? How have the communication patterns affected the change process? How does the health care organization communicate with the community and with other health care organizations?

- **Alignment of goals across subsystems**   Integrative systems and multi-organizations are more common organization structures today. Subsystems, whether they be subsystems of a multi-organization with multiple entities (one hospital in a system that has several hospitals) or the subsystems of one organization (departments and services) must be aligned. If goals of the subsystems are not in alignment with overall organizational goals, there will be conflicts, and it will be difficult to determine organization outcomes. This does not, however, mean that subsystems might not propose different goals; however, then subsystems must convince the overall organization that this change is appropriate.

- **Incorporation of quality and safety as a value**   There is no doubt that quality and safety are critical issues today in health care. All health care organizations are involved in quality improvement; however, some are much more successful than others. In analyzing an organization, its quality improvement effort needs to be assessed. When an organization's quality and safety are assessed, much can be learned about the organization's vision and mission, goals and objectives, structure and process, communication, decision making, utilization of resources, and what is really important to the organization. Is the organization using evidence-based practice? The key question is what are its outcomes (see Chapters 16 and 17)?

- **Utilization of human resources**   Clearly, utilization of human resources is critical today. Some organizations are just sitting around worrying about the number of empty positions, but others are quite active in trying to find creative solutions. Understanding human resource needs and planning to meet them is a daily organizational concern (see Chapter 9).

- **Effective financial and information infrastructure planning**   As organizations are analyzed, consideration must be given to their financial status and effective financial planning. Outcomes are always tied to financial issues and cannot be ignored. All health care organizations and providers are struggling with reimbursement issues and how these issues affect practice (see Chapter 5).

- **Information management**   Information within the organization is also a critical component (Institute of Medicine, 2003). What information is available? Who has it? How is it collected? Is it reliable and valid? How is the information used? How has technology impacted the collection and use of information? Is the organization in compliance with legal requirements (e.g., HIPAA)? All are critical questions. Throughout this text there is recognition of information and its importance (see Chapter 18).

- **Organizational responsiveness to change**   Change is a running thread throughout all of the discussions in this text. Organizations that cannot change effectively will struggle, and many will disappear. Change cannot be avoided so the best approach is to learn how to effectively adapt—making sound decisions based on sound evidence and data. This is also provides opportunities for expanding or adapting educational offerings for staff. Health care organizations are at different stages of development in how they respond to change. Analyzing an organization should include an assessment of the organization's response to change. Leaders have a major impact on the organization's ability to change effectively (see Chapter 3).

- **Organizational readiness for the multicultural world**   The United States and most of its communities are finding that they are now multicultural communities. Providers are caring for patients from many different cultures, and this affects their care. Staff that comes from many different cultures is more common, and this impacts the organization's communication, staff relationships, problem solving, decision making, and morale. The United States is

## APPLYING EVIDENCE-BASED PRACTICE

### Evidence for Effective Leadership and Management

**Citation:** Catrambone, C., Johnson, M., Mion, L., & Minnick, A. (2009). The design of adult acute care units in U.S. hospitals. *Journal of Nursing Scholarship, 41*(1), 79–86.

**Overview:** This descriptive study examined the current state of hospital unit design characteristics recommended by the Agency for Healthcare Research and Quality (AHRQ) in 81 adult medical-surgical units and 56 intensive care units in six metropolitan areas. The AHRQ recommends that the following unit design characteristics positively impact patient outcomes: single rooms, work areas for staff that are not a long distance from the bedside, frequent staff hand hygiene stations, certain types of unit configuration, percentage of private rooms, and presence or absence of carpeting. The purpose of this study is to provide a benchmark and to assess nursing environments. Data were collected by observation, measurement, and interviews. The researchers conclude that few of the hospital units met the AHRQ recommendations. Further research is required to expand understanding of these design elements, their interaction, and impact on outcomes.

**Application:** Health care organizations are much more than a description of the organization. They are also physical buildings. Several recommendations in the Institute of Medicine (IOM) report *Keeping Patients Safe. Transforming the Work Environment of Nurses* (2004) pertain to design of work and workspace to prevent and mitigate errors. This study on unit design elements relates to the IOM work, which is referenced in the study. There are many factors and elements that impact the quality of care and design is one of them. Historically nurses typically have had limited input into design of units, but more hospitals are including nursing management and staff nurses in the decision making process when facilities are renovated or new buildings are built. For a long time nurses just had to work within the space they had even if the design did not consider nursing needs; however, more is known today on the impact of space and design on work processes and staff.

**Questions:**

1. *Based on your clinical experience, your clinical experience why is unit structure important to the staff and to patient outcomes? Identify three examples to support your opinion.*
2. *Why do you think it would be important to have standards related to unit structure and environment?*
3. *If you were a patient, what type of unit would you want to be on? Describe it, and explain why this is the type of unit you would prefer.*

---

confronting many critical issues related to access of care and lack of insurance, and much of this has an impact on minority cultures (see Chapter 7).

- **Effective leadership** Effective leadership is critical to the success of any organization. As organizations are analyzed, its leaders should be identified and assessed. What is the leadership style? Does the leadership provide what is needed to help the organization succeed (see Chapter 1)?
- **Assessment of future organizational challenges and opportunities** Future needs should be considered in the assessment of an organization. Is the organization preparing for the future? Does it have a strategic plan? What is included in the plan? Is the plan reasonable? What is the process the organization uses to cope with future organization challenges and opportunities? Are the challenges and opportunities identified?

### Professional Nursing Practice within Nursing Care Models

The American Nurses Association (2004) defines nursing as "the protection, promotion, and optimization of health and abilities, prevention of illness and injury, alleviation of suffering through the diagnosis and treatment of human response, and advocacy in the care of individuals, families, communities, and populations" (p. 7). The American Organization of Nurse Executives (AONE) emphasizes the following with patient population as the central core (2005).

■ The core of nursing is knowledge and caring. (*evidence-based practice and patient-centered care*)
■ Care is user-based. (*patient-centered care*)
■ Knowledge is access-based. (*evidence-based practice*)
■ Knowledge is synthesized. (*evidence-based practice; informatics; quality improvement*)
■ Relationships of care presence-virtual. (*patient-centered care*)
■ Managing the journey (*interprofessional teams*)

The items in italic describe how each of the AONE elements relate to the five IOM core competencies. These are all interrelated. Also all of these elements have been discussed in earlier chapters or will be discussed in later chapters as they are critical aspects of leadership and management. Intertwined within these critical elements is the recognition of the importance of autonomy, responsibility, delegation, and accountability.

"Autonomy in clinical decision making occurs whenever a nurse makes an independent judgment about the presence of a clinical issue and then provides the resolution to nursing care" (Ritter-Teitel, 2002, p. 32). Autonomy requires competence and skills that focus on the nurse–patient relationship. It also means that there needs to be an organized assessment method to determine patient care needs and reassigning staff. Nurses also have the right to consult with others as professionals when they provide or manage care. Autonomy, control, and decision making are related. "Professional practice implies control over the terms of the work but also control over its content and regulation of its standards" (Ritter-Teitel, 2002, p. 33). Nurses who feel that they have autonomy know that they have the right to make decisions in their daily practice and also actively participate in developing organizational policy and change. Staff autonomy, however, does not work in organizations in which leaders are authoritarian and when centralized decision making and control are key characteristics of the organization. This situation will quickly lead to conflict. In addition, the work environment must be conducive to collaboration with physicians and all relevant staff, as is discussed in Chapter 12. "**Responsibility** refers to being entrusted with a particular function" (Ritter-Teitel, 2002, p. 34). A nursing practice model that does not address responsibility will not be effective. Along with this is the need to clearly recognize the importance of delegation. "**Delegation** involves transferring responsibility for the performance of the task from one person to another" (Ritter-Teitel, 2002, p. 34). Delegation is discussed in more detail in Chapter 14. **Accountability** is a term that is typically found in job descriptions and descriptions of organizational structure. In nursing it is particularly important to recognize that "accountability is the acceptance of responsibility for the outcomes of care" (Ritter-Teitel, 2002, p. 34). Nurses need to know that when they provide patient care their work has relevance—it must reach outcomes. Magnet hospitals are discussed in Chapter 6 as examples of organizations that exemplify these characteristics.

The AONE elements and these characteristics, such as accountability, need to be considered when nursing practice models are assessed. Models of care are developed to support or enhance professional practice, and by considering these elements and characteristics the models will be more effective. Within a health care organization, how do nurses provide nursing care? What is a model of care? Are these elements found in the model? "A model of care is a configuration of nursing practice or pattern of delivery" (Ritter-Teitel, 2002, p. 35). Models might also be called nursing or patient care delivery systems. These models have undergone major changes over the last several decades. Nursing practice models have been used to implement resource-intensive strategies with the goal of decreasing expenses and using staff more effectively. These practice models establish organizational frameworks that provide nursing staff opportunities to become more committed to their practice and to be more involved in decision making (Upenieks, 2000, p. 330). A review of multiple nursing care models (Beattle, 2009) indicates that many models have common themes:

■ Elevating the role of nurses and transitioning from caregivers to "care integrators"
■ Taking a team approach to interprofessional care
■ Bridging the continuum of care outside of the primary care facility

- Defining the home as a setting of care
- Targeting high users of health care, especially older adults
- Sharpening focus on the patient, including an active engagement of the patient and his or her family in care planning and delivery, and a greater responsiveness to patient wants and needs
- Leveraging technology
- Improving satisfaction, quality, and coast

Others have identified the following elements that are still relevant today (Brennan, Anthony, Jones, & Kahana, 1998): continuity of care, participation in management, collaboration, leadership, learning environment, nurse's role, staffing communication, specialization, orientation of temporary staff, and team commitment. O'Rourke (2006) believes that building the professional role is important and describes a professional practice model with a professional role development emphasizing self-direction and decision making, evidence-based practice, role-based transfer of knowledge, and role-based provision of care. See Chapter Media Links for access to website describing the O'Rourke model.

**Nursing models** "provide an infrastructure that decreases variation among nurses, the interventions they will choose, and, ultimately, patient outcomes. Conceptual frameworks also differentiate forward thinking organizations from those where nursing has less of a voice" (Kerfoot, et al., 2006, p. 20). Models help to identify and describe nursing care. The IOM emphasis on the five core competencies could be used for a model and as newer models are discussed later it is easy to see how these five competencies are the key elements of health care delivery. Kimball and Joynt (2007) identify key factors driving innovation in health care delivery. These factors are described in Figure 4-2.

## Historical Perspective on Nursing Models

The following is a description of common models, some of which have undergone many changes over the years or are not used anymore, but they have had an impact on newer models. In addition, how models are implemented in an organization can be highly variable.

TOTAL PATIENT CARE/CASE METHOD    In this model, which is the oldest, the registered nurse is responsible for all of the care provided to a patient for a shift. A major disadvantage of this model is the lack of consistency and coordinated care when care is provided in 8-hour segments. This type of care is rarely provided today, except among student nurses who are assigned to

**FIGURE 4-2  What is driving innovation?**

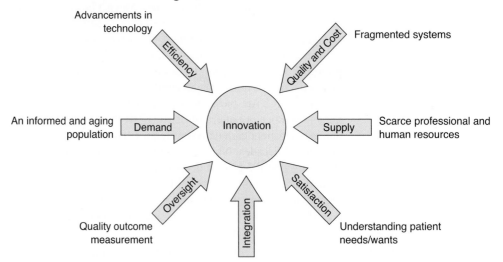

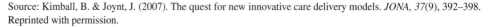

Source: Kimball, B. & Joynt, J. (2007). The quest for new innovative care delivery models. *JONA, 37*(9), 392–398. Reprinted with permission.

provide all of the care for a patient during the hours that they are in clinical. Even in this case, the students frequently do not provide all of the care as they may not be qualified to do this and a staff nurse maintains overall responsibility for the care. Home health agencies use a form of this model when nurses are assigned patients and provide all the required home care; however, even this has been adapted as more home care is provided by a team. An RN may coordinate the care and provide professional nursing services, but a home care aide may provide most of the direct care and other providers such as a physical therapist, dietician, and social worker may be required for specialty care.

FUNCTIONAL NURSING    The model of **functional nursing** is a task-oriented approach, focusing on jobs to be done. When it was more commonly used, it was thought to be more efficient. The nurse in charge assigned the tasks (e.g., one nurse may administer medications for all patients on a unit; an aide may take vital signs for all patients). A disadvantage of this model is the risk of fragmented care. In addition, this type of model also leads to greater staff dissatisfaction with staff feeling they are just grinding out tasks. Individualized care may also be compromised when patient care is provided by different staff members who may or may not be aware of other needs and the care provided by others. This model is not used much now. It can be found in some long-term care facilities and in some behavioral/psychiatric inpatient services, although in a modified form. In the latter situation a registered nurse may be assigned the task of medication administration for the unit, and psychiatric support staff may be assigned such tasks as vital signs and checks of all patients. In this situation, RNs would still be assigned to individual patients to coordinate their care.

TEAM NURSING    **Team nursing**, developed after World War II when there was a severe nursing shortage as well as major changes in medical technology, replaced functional nursing. A nursing team consists of an RN, licensed practical nurses (LPNs), and nurse aides. This team of two or three staff provides total care for a group of patients during an 8- or 12-hour shift. The RN team leader coordinates this care. In this model the RN has a high level of autonomy and assumes the centralized decision-making authority. Although the past approach to team nursing was thought to use decentralized decision making with decisions made closer to the patient, there actually was limited team member collaboration. In addition, these teams tended to communicate only among themselves and not as well with physicians. The team concept or model also focused on tasks rather than patient care as a whole. More current versions of the team model are different from this earlier type. Currently, the team model has been changed to meet changes in organizations and leadership corresponding to the needs for better consistency and continuity of care, as well as collaboration and coordination.

PRIMARY NURSING    In the late 1970s care became more complex, and nurses were dissatisfied with team nursing. In the **primary nursing** model the primary nurse, who can only be an RN, provides direct care for the patient and the family; an associate nurse provides care following the care plan developed by the primary nurse when the primary nurse is not working and assists when the primary nurse is working. The primary nurse needs to be knowledgeable about assigned patients and must maintain a high level of clinical autonomy. When primary nursing was first used and well-accepted it was easier to substitute RNs for other health care providers as cost was not as much of a focus as it is today. When the nursing shortage began to reoccur and salaries increased, implementing primary nursing became more difficult, and health care cost moved to the top of the concerns. There was, however, no research data to support that primary nursing was more expensive than team nursing, but many hospitals nonetheless felt it was (Gardner, 1991; Gardner & Tilbury, 1991; Glandon, Colbert, & Thomason, 1989; Shukla, 1983). Primary nursing is often viewed as a model in which the primary nurse has to do everything, limiting collaborative or team effort, although it does not have to be implemented in this way.

Second-generation primary nursing clarifies some of the issues about this practice model. One of the critical problems with primary nursing was whether or not it required an all-RN staff, which was thought to increase staff costs. The second-generation view of primary nursing noted that the mix of staff is more important than having an all-RN staff. Another concern with primary nursing was a need to develop a clear definition of 24-hour accountability, which was interpreted by some as 24-hour availability. This, of course, is not a reasonable approach, and it really does not apply to primary nursing. When the primary nurse is not working, the associate nurse provides the care. Primary nursing is a responsibility relationship between the nurse and the patient. The primary nurse is not the only caregiver but does have responsibility for planning the care and ensuring that care outcomes are met. Only registered nurses can be primary nurses. This role and the model require RNs who are competent and possess leadership skills. Primary nursing is not used as much today.

CARE AND SERVICE TEAM MODELS   In the 1980s, **care and service team models** began to replace primary nursing. These models are implemented differently in different hospitals, as is true of most of the models. Key elements of these models are empowered staff, interprofessional collaboration, skilled workers, and a case management approach to patient care—all elements related to the more current views of leadership and management (Finkelman, 2011). Care and service teams introduced the different categories of assistive personnel (for example, multiskilled workers, nurse extenders, and UAP). There has been some disagreement as to whether these new staff member roles were complementary or involved substitution of professional nursing care.

COMPLEMENTARY MODELS   **Complementary models** began in 1988 by using nurse extenders, such as a unit assistant, who would be responsible for environmental functions. The nurse would then have more time for direct patient care. Does this reduce costs? Certainly, when nurse positions are changed to nurse extender positions there is some cost reduction; however, some hospitals found that overtime, sick time, and on-call costs rose, particularly with nurse extender staff (Powers, Dickey, & Ford, 1990). Another example is Manthey's (1989) partners-in-practice. Technical assistants signed a partnership agreement to work with an experienced RN. Reduction in costs was initially seen with this model because each partnership could care for the same number of patients as two RNs. Staffing costs, however, continued to increase. Complementary models are not used as much today and have been replaced by substitution models in health care organizations. **Substitution models** tend to use multiskilled technicians to perform select nursing activities. The RNs supervise these activities.

Another approach is **cross-training**. This involves training staff to work in different specialty areas or to perform different tasks. For example, a respiratory therapist may be trained not only to perform typical respiratory therapist tasks but also phlebotomy and basic nursing care. This offers much more flexibility in that staff can fulfill many different needs. They can then be used as staffing adjustments are needed for changes in patient census or acuity. It is critical that this cross-training meet patient needs so that staff will be able to deliver quality, safe care and not feel undue stress while delivering the care. It is also important that state practice act requirements are met, and this is not always easy to accomplish. It requires education staff to provide support, ongoing educational training, and documentation of competencies, as well as management staff who understands which staff members are qualified to move from area to area. Hospitals and other health care organizations are trying to find the best methods for using substitution without compromising quality and safety and yet control costs. As demands change, different models will be required, and nursing leadership to develop these models will be critical.

As with earlier team models, the RN must spend time coordinating care and the work. The focus of the team is on patient-centered care as opposed to the nurse–patient relationship. The Case Management Society of America (CMSA) defines case management as "a collaborative process of assessment planning, facilitation and advocacy for options and services to meet an individual's health needs through communication and available resources to promote quality cost-effective outcomes" (2002, p. 1). Case management is based on the assumption that patients with complex health problems, catastrophic health situations, and high cost medical conditions need assistance in using the health care system effectively and a case manager can help patients with these needs (Finkelman, 2011). Case managers may also work with the teams to achieve outcomes, which increases shared accountability. Case management can be viewed as a nursing model when the case manager is a nurse; however, in some organizations nurses are not used as case managers but rather other health care professionals such as social workers are the case managers. "Case management is not a profession but rather a collaborative and trans-disciplinary practice" (Commission for Case Management Certification, 2009, p. 1). Several health care professional organizations and experts have defined case management; however, there clearly is no universally accepted definition for case management. Case management is used in many different types of settings, and the setting also affects the definition (Finkelman, 2010).

CARE MANAGEMENT MODEL    The **care management model** focuses on the needs of the integrated delivery system. It has many similarities to case management, in that it includes planning, assessment, and coordination of health services. The patient focus, however, is population-based instead of based on an individual patient. The population might be people who live in a specific geographic area, members of a health insurance plan, or could be a specific group with similarities, such as patients with diabetes. The goal is to integrate a continuum of clinical services. Care management is not only concerned with medical care but also health promotion and disease prevention, costs, and use of resources. Case management is often used within the care management model. Typical tools used to facilitate care management are clinical pathways, disease management programs, and benchmarking.

## Newer Nursing Models

INTERDISCIPLINARY PRACTICE MODEL    The **interdisciplinary** or interprofessional practice model is emphasized in the IOM reports on quality improvement by identifying the importance of all health professions meeting the interdisciplinary or interprofessional competency emphasizing the need to work in interprofessional teams "to cooperate, collaborate, communicate, and integrate care in teams to ensure that care is continuous and reliable" (2003, p. 4). These teams include providers from different health care professions and occupations designed to meet the required patient needs. With increasing complex patient care needs this model is better able to address needs and to effectively use a mix of expertise and knowledge to reach patient outcomes. Patient-centered care is the focus. The advantages of using interprofessional teams are as follows (Finkelman & Kenner, 2010, p. 337):

- Decreased fragmentation in a complex care system
- Effective use of multiple expertise (e.g., medicine, nursing, pharmacy, allied health, social work, and so on)
- Decreased utilization of repetitive or duplicate services
- Increased creative or innovative solutions to complex problems
- Increased learning for team members about different roles and responsibilities, communication and coordination, and how to better plan care
- Provides motivation and increased self-esteem in team and individual performance
- Greater sharing of responsibility
- Empowers members to speak up

SYNERGY MODEL OF PATIENT CARE™    This model of care was developed by the American Association of Critical Care Nurses, but it has been applied in all types of nursing units. "Synergy results when the needs and characteristics of a patient, clinical unit, or system are matched with a nurse's competencies" (American Association of Critical Care Nurses, 2009). Patient characteristics incorporated into this model are as follows (American Association of Critical Care Nurses, 2009):

- **Resiliency:** the capacity to return to a restorative level of functioning using compensatory/coping mechanisms; the ability to bounce back quickly after an insult
- **Vulnerability:** susceptibility to actual or potential stressors that may adversely affect patient outcomes

- **Stability:** the ability to maintain a steady-state equilibrium
- **Complexity:** the intricate entanglement of two or more systems (e.g., body, family, therapies)
- **Resource availability:** extent of resources (e.g., technical, fiscal, personal, psychological, and social) the patient/family/community brings to the situation
- **Participation in care:** extent to which patient/family engages in aspects of care
- **Participation in decision making:** extent to which patient/family engages in decision making
- **Predictability:** a characteristic that allows one to expect a certain course of events or course of illness

The Synergy model ties the above patient characteristics with the following nurse competencies (American Association of Critical Care Nurses, 2009).

- **Clinical judgment:** clinical reasoning, which includes clinical decision making, critical thinking, and a global grasp of the situation, coupled with nursing skills acquired through a process of integrating formal and informal experiential knowledge and evidence-based guidelines.
- **Advocacy and moral agency:** working on another's behalf and representing the concerns of the patient/family and nursing staff; serving as a moral agent in identifying and helping to resolve ethical and clinical concerns within and outside the clinical setting.
- **Caring practices:** nursing activities that create a compassionate, supportive, and therapeutic environment for patients and staff, with the aim of promoting comfort and healing and preventing unnecessary suffering. Includes, but is not limited to, vigilance, engagement, and responsiveness of caregivers, including family and health care personnel.
- **Collaboration:** working with others (e.g., patients, families, health care providers) in a way that promotes/encourages each person's contributions toward achieving optimal/realistic patient/family goals. Involves intra- and interprofessional work with colleagues and community.
- **Systems thinking:** body of knowledge and tools that allow the nurse to manage whatever environmental and system resources exist for the patient/family and staff, within or across health care and non–health care systems.
- **Response to diversity:** the sensitivity to recognize, appreciate, and incorporate differences into the provision of care. Differences may include, but are not limited to, cultural differences, spiritual beliefs, gender, race, ethnicity, lifestyle, socioeconomic status, age, and values.
- **Facilitation of learning:** the ability to facilitate learning for patients/families, nursing staff, other members of the health care team, and community. Includes both formal and informal facilitation of learning.
- **Clinical inquiry (innovator/evaluator):** the ongoing process of questioning and evaluating practice and providing informed practice. Creating practice changes through research utilization and experiential learning.

### Primary Care Team

The Primary Care Team (PCT) is a model that emphasizes differentiated nursing practice from a team perspective (Kimball & Joynt, 2007). The team includes an RN care manager, RN or LPN/LVN provider, and clinical assistant. The patient is actively involved in the care process. The team principles are as follows (Kimball & Joynt, 2007. p. 394):

- Every patient deserves an experienced RN.
- Every novice nurse deserves mentoring from an experienced RN.
- Every patient deserves the opportunity to participate in planning of his or her care.
- Every team member is committed to meet the needs of every patient assigned to the team.
- Each PCT member functions within his or her defined scope of practice/experience.

- Work intensity decreases with improved work distribution processes and team support.
- The model of nursing care delivery is an important element in patient safety and patient, staff, and physician satisfaction.

**COLLABORATIVE PATIENT CARE MANAGEMENT MODEL**    The Collaborative Patient Care Management Model is an interprofessional, population-based case management model (Kimball & Joynt, 2007). The model focuses on high risk, high volume, and high cost populations. The team is co-coordinated by a physician and an RN patient care coordinator. The RN leads rounds, and there is an interprofessional plan. This model has been used in acute care and outpatient settings across the continuum of care services.

**TRANSITIONAL CARE MODEL**    This model focuses on providing "comprehensive in-hospital planning, care coordination, and home follow-up for high-risk elders" (Kimball & Joynt, 2007, p. 395). Nurse practitioners lead this model to ensure that the elders receive the care that they need, including post-hospitalization. The model has had a positive impact on decreasing time between readmissions, number of readmissions, and total health care costs. With the increasing number of elders this type of model will become more important.

**PATIENT NAVIGATION**    Patient Navigation is a model that has primarily focused on patients with cancer who are at risk for poor cancer outcomes though other types of patients populations have also benefited from patient navigation (Wells et al., 2008). Clinical nurse leaders often hold the position of nurse navigator. Patient navigation focuses on decreasing barriers to better ensure that patients get the care they need when they need it (Finkelman, 2011). This mode is "an intervention designed to reduce health disparities by addressing specific barriers to obtaining timely, quality health care" (Wells et al., 2008, p. 2010).

**TRANSFORMATIONAL MODEL FOR PROFESSIONAL PRACTICE**    This model integrates patient care services (Beckman Institute for Innovation in Patient Care, 1998 as cited in Wolf, Hayden, & Bradle, 2004). The model has four components: (1) *professional practice*: assessment and activation of professional practice relationships, and support with emphasis on transformational leadership, care delivery system, professional growth, and collaborative practice; (2) *the process component*: engagement in purposeful and deliberate critical thinking, negotiation, and decision-making; (3) *the primary outcome component*: reach targeted outcomes (quality improvement, patient satisfaction, caregiver satisfaction); and (4) *the strategic outcome component*: consumer, organizational, professional health).

**THE QUALITY-CARING MODEL©**    This model emphasizes caring and evidence-based practice with an emphasis on structure-process-outcomes as dimensions of quality care (Duffy & Hoskins, 2003). It addresses concerns about the need to build relationships with patients and families—cooperative, collaborative relationships. This is described as nursing's work rather than a focus on a task oriented biomedical model.

Nursing care delivery models have changed over the years due to economic factors, staffing shortages or excesses, philosophy and goals, nursing research, tasks that need to be accomplished, technology, information management, scientific advancements, and new leadership and organization theories and styles. Some models have disappeared (for example, functional nursing). Another example of a model that is used less often is primary nursing, which was popular in many areas of the country, but is not used as much now, primarily due to costs and the RN shortage. The total patient care or case method, although rarely used, may still be used in critical care settings and home care, although even here there is a movement toward interprofessional care. Why have the changes occurred? Some nursing care can be done by others more cost effectively and still be safe, quality care, and staff are available to do these tasks, such as LPNs/LVNs or UAP. Typically, a hospital will use a combination of models.

## CASE STUDY

### Does a Nursing Model Make a Difference?

As Director of Staff Development in a large university hospital, the Chief Nurse Executive (CNE) has met with you to discuss orientation for student nurses and faculty. The CNE is concerned that students and faculty do not understand the hospital's new nursing model, Synergy model of patient care™. She tells you it is your job to correct this problem. You leave the meeting overwhelmed. This seems like a big responsibility to you. The hospital has many nursing students from three schools of nursing that use its services for practicum. All have to attend a 4-hour orientation to the hospital, which is already overburdened with content. The units have also been struggling with applying the model since it was initiated 6 months ago.

### Questions:

1. Why is it important for the students and faculty to understand the model?
2. How does the nursing model relate to the organization's theory or approach?
3. How would you describe this model? Consider methods and examples.
4. Develop a plan that you will submit to the CNE explaining how you will address this problem. Who might you include in developing the plan and in implementing it?

### Shared Governance

"Governance, or self-regulation, has long been recognized as a privilege given to professions that earn the public trust by demonstrating accountability for their specialized practices" (Maas & Specht, 2001, p. 318). How does this relate to **shared governance**? As a nursing management form, shared governance emphasizes nurses' roles and responsibilities in decision making (Anthony, 2004; Hess, 2004). It thus increases each nurse's influence over the organization, empowering staff and is based on six dimensions of governance.

1. Control over professional practice
2. Influence over organizational resources that support practice
3. Formal authority granted by the organization
4. Committee structures that allow participation in decision making
5. Access to information about the organization
6. Ability to set goals and negotiate conflict

Shared governance can be viewed as a management philosophy, a professional practice model, and an accountability model that focuses on staff involvement in decision making, particularly in decisions that affect their practice. In doing this the model provides staff with autonomy and control over implementation of their practice—legitimizing control over their own practice. Nurses in these organizations usually feel less powerless and are more efficient and accountable.

A critical factor in shared governance is that accountability and responsibility are found in the same person. Accountability should rest in the person who is most likely to be the most effective person to complete the function. For individual staff to be accountable and responsible for a function or task, staff must also have the authority to make sure that the right decisions are made. "Within the professional context, then, the statement that the professional is accountable for his or her practice has meaning only when the necessary authority, which is part of that accountability, is transferred to the individual who assures compliance and who is capable of taking corrective action in the absence of compliance" (Porter-O'Grady & Finnigan, 1984, p. 80).

Shared governance is also a surrogate term for collaboration. "It is an organizational arrangement with a highly participatory staff empowered to function cooperatively with both management and colleagues, and leadership that empowers staff. The organization can be referred to as a learning organization" (Sullivan, 1998, p. 471). Transformational Leadership enhances shared governance. As was discussed in Chapter 1, an important element of leadership is self-awareness, and it is important in shared governance. In this type of organizational arrangement staff members feel committed to the organization and consider themselves to be partners in meeting the goals of the organization. Staff members should not feel that they are working alone, but rather working in teams to meet specific goals (Hess, 2004).

In shared governance nurse managers typically are not directly involved in daily direct patient care, although there are some managers who are still involved in direct care. The typical responsibilities of the nurse manager are staffing, program evaluation, personnel evaluation, coordination, allocation of resources, financial activities, and long-range planning discussed in Chapter 1. If patient care outcomes are not met, it is the responsibility of the nurse providing the care to address this issue. The nurse manager may become involved, but it is the direct care provider who should take the lead. Clinical practice is the responsibility of the practitioners. When clinical problems occur, the nurse who provides direct care must be the one to solve these problems, working with the care team. The main factor in shared governance is that decision making is spread over a larger number of staff and is decentralized. Nurses are accountable for their practice. Health care organizations that use shared governance must have clear communication processes, or the organization will encounter problems and confusion in the decision-making process. Typically, this model leads to greater staff satisfaction with the job and the organization—staff feels empowered (Caramanica, 2004). The key components of shared governance are practice, quality, education, and peer process/governance. How are these accomplished? As with any such change, some organizations change for "real" and others *appear* to change to this model, but in the latter situation very little has really changed in the decision-making process or in actual practice. Shared governance is associated with collaboration, horizontal relationships, and investment and need to be demonstrated in the organization. The change has to be real.

Organizations that use this model have some type of structure that relates to the shared accountability, such as councils, cabinets, committees, or a combination of these groups or teams that make the decisions. The chain of command is not the same as in traditional organizations. In the shared governance model these groups make decisions about policies, procedures, and other aspects of getting the work done. How might shared governance be implemented?

Health care organizations have been working for several years to create leaner and more effective organizations. It is important to recognize that to move toward a shared governance model the organization must take a comprehensive change approach and not an incremental approach. All parts of the organization and all staff must be expected to change. This is very difficult to accomplish, but if shared governance is the goal, it is necessary.

Decentralized decision making is now found in many health care organizations, and it is frequently associated with participative management strategies such as a shared government model. This approach to organizational structure and process is associated with the economy, job satisfaction, and retention. For decentralization to be effective staff must have autonomy to make decisions. All of this is intimately connected with shared governance. It requires staff members who are committed to the organization's values and goals and demonstrate this by working to meet the goals. Magnet hospitals also share these common shared governance characteristics (see Chapter 6). "Whatever the process of changing structure, locus of control, decision processes, and team-based initiatives are called, they are essential to the future of doing health services business. From shared governance to shared leadership, shared decision making, empowerment, point-of-service accountability, or whatever other name might be attached to the dynamic, shared decision making is an essential element of work of reconceptualizing and configuring health care for the future" (Porter-O'Grady, 2001, p. 473).

# APPLYING LEADERSHIP AND MANAGEMENT

## MY HOSPITAL UNIT

Return to your unit. The nursing department has decided that it needs to establish a nursing model. You are on the committee that will lead this initiative. The committee includes three other nurse managers, the CNE, and four staff nurses. Do some research of the nursing literature on nursing models and review content in this chapter to better understand the historical development of nursing models. Select one model that you like and prepare a description and rationale that you would use to convince the committee that this is the best model. This model will be used on all your hospital's patient units, and now you need to decide how you will implement it on your unit. Develop a plan to implement the model. Remember to review content on change because this is a major change. How might this model impact your philosophy of leadership that you developed earlier? For each of the exercises applying content on your unit it is important to build on previous exercises—decisions you made in past chapters. You may find you need to make changes because previous decisions you made do not work well with newer decisions. This is what management and leadership is all about— review, reflection, change, and decisions. Use the virtual unit site found on the textbook website to record the work that you do in the role of nurse manager for your unit.

## Critical Thinking Questions and Activities

1. Visit the website for the American Association of Critical Care Nurses to learn more about their Synergy Model™ of Patient Care (http://www.aacn.org/WD/Certifications/content/ synmodel.pcms?menu=Certification). What do you think about this model?

2. The structure of a health care organization can be highly variable. The chapter content describes some aspects of organization structure. How would you apply this content about the organizational structure? Select a health care organization of any type, although it will probably be easier if you have experience with the organization. Review the organizational chart. Compare and contrast with content in this chapter. What organizational theory applies? Write a brief description of your analysis. You might include information about the types and titles of positions and departments, interrelationships and reporting process, clarity of the chart, complexity of the organization, and types of positions and departments included. Critical aspects are the reporting process and how this is described. Consider vertical and horizontal structure, line of authority, staff authority, span of control, centralized vs. decentralized, departmentalization, and matrix structure. How might the theories discussed in this chapter apply? Write a brief description of your analysis.

3. The processes of a health care organization can be highly variable. The chapter content describes some aspects of organization structure. How would you apply this content about the organizational processes? Select a health care organization of any type, although it will probably be easier if you have experience with the organization. Compare and contrast with content in this chapter. Typical sources of information about an organization's processes are its vision and mission statements and its goals and objectives. You need to try to find information about decision making, delegation, coordination, communication, and evaluation in the organization.

4. There are two links for articles found in *The Journal of Online Issues in Nursing* on shared governance (see Media Links). Additional articles are found in the same site. Select at least one article to read. Summarize the key points. What is your opinion of shared governance?

5. Go to the *Journal of Organizational Behavior* (http://www3.interscience.wiley.com/ journal/4691/home?CRETRY=1&SRETRY=0). Review some of table of contents for issues. What are some of the topics? How do they relate to this chapter's content?

## Media Links

- **URL: http://nccam.nih.gov/**
  National Center for Complementary and Alternative Medicine (NCCAM)
- **URL: http://www.aacn.org/wd/certifications/content/ synmodel.pcms?menu=certification**
  American Association of Critical Care Nurses: Synergy Model™
- **URL: http://www.nursingworld.org/mainmenucategories/anamarketplace/ anaperiodicals/ojin/tableofcontents/volume92004/no1jan04/ sharedgovernancemodels.aspx**
  Read the following article: Anthony, M. (2004). Shared governance models: The theory, practice and evidence. *The Online Journal of Issues in Nursing, 9*(1).
- **URL: http://www.nursingworld.org/mainmenucategories/anamarketplace/ anaperiodicals/ojin/tableofcontents/volume92004/no1jan04/ frombedsidetoboardroom.aspx**
  Read the following article: Hess, G. (2004). From bedside to boardroom—nursing shared governance. *The Online Journal of Issues in Nursing, 9*(1).
- **URL: http://www3.interscience.wiley.com/journal/4691/home?cretry=1&srETRY=0**
  *Journal of Organizational Behavior*
- **URL: http://www.analytictech.com/mb021/orgtheory.htm**
  **O**rganizational theory: determinants of structure
- **URL: http://www.innovativecaremodels.com/**
  Innovative Care Models (site provides examples of models of care)
- **URL: http://www.rolebasedpractice.com/ourservices.html**
  O'Rourke: Role-Based Practice

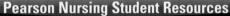
**Pearson Nursing Student Resources**
Find additional review materials at
**nursing.pearsonhighered.com**
Prepare for success with additional NCLEX®-style practice questions,
interactive assignments and activities, Web links, animations and
videos, and more!
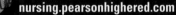

## References

American Association of Colleges of Nursing. (2004). *Position statement on the practice doctorate in nursing.* Retrieved September 8, 2009, from http://www.aacn.nche.edu/DNP/ DNPpositionstatement.htm

American Association of Colleges of Nursing. (2007). *White paper on the education and role of the clinical nurse leader.* Washington, DC: Author.

American Association of Critical Care Nurses. (2009). Synergy™ model for patient care. Retrieved December 28, 2009, from http://www.aacn.org/ WD/Certifications/content/synmodel .pcms?menu=Certification#Nurse.

American Organization of Nurse Executives. (2005). *AONE guiding principles: for the role of the nurse in future patient care delivery.* Retrieved November 11, 2009, from http://www.aone.org/

American Nurses Association. (2004). *Scope and standards of practice.* Silver Springs, MD: Author.

Anthony, M. (2004). Shared Governance models: The theory, practice and evidence. *The Online Journal of Issues in Nursing, 9*(1). Retrieved December 2, 2005, from http://www.nursingworld.org/ MainMenuCategories/ANAMarketplace/ ANAPeriodicals/OJIN/TableofContents/ Volume92004/No1Jan04/ SharedGovernanceModels.aspx

Beattle, L. (2009). New health care delivery models are redefining the role of nurses. Retrieved December 27, 2009, from http://www.nursezone.com/Nursing-News-Events/more-features.aspx?articleId=29442

Buckles-Prince, S. (1997). Shared governance: Sharing power and opportunity. *Journal of Nursing Administration, 27*(3), 28–35.

Caramanica, L. (2004). Shared governance: Hartford hospital's experience. *Online Journal of Issues in Nursing, 9*(1), 1–7. Retrieved on June 3, 2005, from http://www.nursingworld.org/MainMenuCategories/ANAMarketplace/ANAPeriodicals/OJIN.aspx

Case Management Society of America. (CSMA). (2002). *Standards of practice for case management.* Little Rock, AK: Author.

Campbell, C., Schmitz, H., & Waller, L. (1998). *Financial management in a managed care environment.* Albany, NY: Delmar Publishers.

Commission for Case Management Certification. (CCMC). (2009). *Code of Professional Conduct for Case Managers.* Mt. Laurel, NJ: Author.

Crow, G. (2002). The relationship between trust, social capital, and organizational success. *Nursing Administration Quarterly, 26*(3), 1–11.

Dessler, G. (2002). *Management.* Upper Saddle River, NJ: Prentice Hall.

Duffy, J. & Hoskins, L. (2003). The quality-caring model©. *Advances in Nursing Science, 26*(1), 77–88.

Evan, K., et al. (1995). Whole systems shared governance. *Journal of Nursing Administration, 25*(5), 18–27.

Finkelman, A. (2010). The health care system. In M. Nies & M. McEwen (Eds.), *Community/public health nursing* (5th ed., pp. 149–166). Philadelphia: W.B. Saunders Company.

Finkelman, A. & Kenner, C. (2010). *Professional concepts. Competencies for quality leadership.* Boston: Jones and Bartlett Publishers.

Finkelman, A. (2011). *Case management for nurses.* Upper Saddle River, NJ: Pearson. Education, Inc.

Fitzpatrick, M., McElroy, M., & DeWoody, S. (2001). Building a strong nursing organization in a merged service line structure. *Journal of Nursing Administration, 31*(1), 24–32.

Gardner, K. (1991). A summary of findings of a five year comparison study of primary and team nursing. *Nursing Research, 40*(2), 113–117.

Gardner, K., & Tilbury, M. (1991). A longitudinal analysis of primary and team nursing. *Nursing Economics, 9*(2), 97–104.

Glandon, G., Colbert, K., & Thomason, M. (1989). Nursing delivery models and RN mix: Cost implications. *Nursing Management, 20*(5), 30–33.

Harris, G. (2010, March 26). More doctors giving up private clinics. *New York Times,* pp. B1, B5.

Hebbert, E., St. Arnaud, S., & Dharampaul, S. (1994). Nurses' satisfaction with the patient care team. *Canadian Journal of Rehabilitation, 8,* 87–88.

Hess, G. (2004). From bedside to boardroom—nursing shared governance. *The Online Journal of Issues in Nursing, 9*(1) Retrieved from http://www.nursingworld.org/MainMenuCategories/ANAMarketplace/ANAPeriodicals/OJIN/TableofContents/Volume92004/No1Jan04/FromBedsidetoBoardroom.aspx

Institute of Medicine. (2001). *Crossing the quality chasm.* Washington, DC: The National Academies of Medicine.

Institute of Medicine. (2002). *Guidance for the national health care disparities report.* Washington, DC: The National Academies of Medicine.

Institute of Medicine. (2003). *Health care professions education.* Washington, DC: The National Academies of Medicine.

Institute of Medicine. (2011). *The future of nursing: Leading change, advancing health.* Washington, DC: The National Academies Press.

Kimball, B. & Joynt, J. (2007). The quest for new innovative care delivery models. *JONA, 37*(9), 392–398.

Kerfoot, K., et al. (2006). Conceptual models and the nursing organization. Implementing the AACN synergy model for patient care™. *Nurse Leader,* August, 20–26.

Lengacher, C., et al. (1994). Effects of the partners in care practices model on nursing outcomes. *Nursing Economics, 12*(6), 300–307.

Maas, M., & Specht, J. (2001). Shared governance models in nursing: What is shared, who governs, and who benefits. In J. Dochterman & H. Grace (Eds.), *Current issues in nursing* (6th ed., pp. 318–329). St. Louis: Mosby, Inc.

Manthey, M. (1989). Practice partnerships: The newest concept in care delivery. *Journal of Nursing Administration, 19*(2), 33–35.

Mindtools™. (2010). SWOT analysis. Retrieved May 23, 2010, from http://www.mindtools.com/pages/article/newTMC_05.htm

O'Rourke, M. (2006). Beyond rhetoric to role accountability. A practical and professional model of practice. *Nurse Leader,* June, pp. 28–33, 44.

Porter-O'Grady, T., & Finnigan, S. (1984). *Shared governance for nursing.* Gaithersburg, MD: Aspen Publishers Inc.

Porter-O'Grady, T. (2001). Is shared governance still relevant? *JONA, 31*(10), 468–473.

Powers, P., Dickey, D., & Ford, A. (1990). Evaluating RN/co-worker model. *Journal of Nursing Administration, 20*(3), 11–15.

Ritter-Teitel, J. (2002). The impact of restructuring on professional nursing practice. *Journal of Nursing Administration, 32*(1), 31–41.

Robbins, S., & Decenzo, D. (2001). *Fundamentals of management.* Upper Saddle River, NJ: Prentice Hall.

Shukla, R. (1983). All-RN model of care delivery: A cost benefit evaluation. *Inquiry, 20,* 173–184.

Simpson, R. (1999). Changing world, changing systems: Why managed health care demands information technology. *Nursing Administration Quarterly, 23*(2), 86–88.

Spitzer, R. (2001). A case for conceptual competency in an integrated delivery system. *Nursing Administration Quarterly, 25*(4), 79–82.

Steinhauer, J. (2001, March 14). Hospital mergers aren't living happily ever after. *New York Times,* A1, A22.

Sullivan, E. (2004). *Becoming influential.* Upper Saddle River, NJ: Prentice Hall.

Sullivan, T. (1998). Transformational Leadership. In T. Sullivan (Ed.), *Collaboration: A health perspective* (pp. 467–497). New York: McGraw Hill.

Tuck, I., Harris, L. H., & Baliko, B. (2000). Values expressed in philosophies of nursing services. *Journal of Nursing Administration, 30*(4), 180–184.

Wachter, R. (2010). The relationship between hospitalists and primary care physicians. *Annals of Internal Medicine, 152*(7), 474.

Wachter, R. (2003). Intensivist consultation and outcomes in critically ill patients. *JAMA, 289*(8), 986–987.

Wachter, R. & Goldman, L. (2002). The hospitalist movement 5 years later. *JAMA, 287*(4), 487–494.

Wells, K., et al. (2008). Patient navigation: State of the art or is it science. *CANCER, 113*(8), 1999–2010.

Wolf, G., Hayden, M., & Bradle, J. (2004). The transformational model for professional practice. *JONA, 34*(4), 180–187.

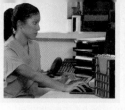

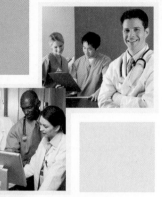

# 5

# Health Care Financial Issues

## LEARNING OUTCOMES

Before you begin, take a moment to familiarize yourself with the learning outcomes for this chapter.

- Distinguish between the macrolevel and microlevel view of health care financial issues.
- Discuss critical issues related to current national health care expenditures.
- Describe the role of the third-party payer.
- Explain how health care insurance is financed and by whom.
- Discuss the importance of the various government benefit programs.
- Discuss how managed care has changed since it began.
- Compare and contrast two examples of managed care models.
- Explain the service strategies used by insurers to control costs and quality.
- Explain the reimbursement strategies used by insurers to control costs and quality.
- Apply the changes found in health care reform of 2010 to reimbursement system for health care services.
- Analyze the budgetary process and its importance to nursing.
- Discuss the importance of productivity.
- Examine strategies to increase nursing participation in cost containment.

## KEY TERMS

- Annual limits
- Authorization
- Benefit plan
- Budget
- Capital budget
- Capitation
- Co-payment/coinsurance
- Cost containment
- Customer
- Deductible
- Diagnosis-related groups (DRGs)
- Discounted fee-for-service
- Exclusions
- Formulary
- Full-time equivalent (FTE)
- Health maintenance organization (HMO)
- Operational budget
- Per diem rate
- Point-of-service (POS)
- Preferred provider organizations (PPOs)
- Premium rate setting
- Primary care provider (PCP)
- Productivity
- Prospective payment
- Prospective payment system (PPS)
- Provider panel
- Resource-based relative value scale (RBRVS)
- Retrospective payment
- Salary and wage budget
- Third-party payer

## WHAT'S AHEAD

An understanding of health care financial issues is important for nurses as they practice in the health care environment and if they assume leadership roles. Financial issues can be viewed from a macro and micro perspective. The macro perspective concerns broad health care expenditures from a national view and reimbursement for health care services. The micro perspective focuses on the financial issues related to individual health care organizations (for example, budgeting). This chapter focuses more on the macro perspective because this perspective must come first, and it is the perspective that most directly affects budgets and all nurses, regardless of their position. This is not to say that the micro perspective is not important or will not be discussed. The basics of micro issues will be discussed; however, extensive details about budgeting and health care organization financing is content that is more appropriate to nurses who are entering management positions where these skills are absolutely critical. The critical need for new nurses is to understand who pays for health care, how this payment is made, and how reimbursement affects health care delivery, which is the macro perspective, and then some essential basics related to budgeting in health care organizations, nurses' role in the process, and how budgets impact nursing care.

# Health Care Financial Issues: The Macrolevel

During nursing's long history, for most of that time nurses showed little interest in financial issues. Nurses were typically unprepared to participate in financial decision making, and health care administrators often did not encourage or support nurse managers/leaders to participate in the financial side of health care. The inclusion of content related to health economics, finance, and business management into nursing curricula evolved slowly, which was a serious limitation as it prevented active nursing involvement in health care finance. This important content continues to require further development in graduate nursing programs. Gradually, nurse administrators developed an increased interest in budgeting; however, they have had to contend with hospital administrators who did not feel that nurse administrators needed to be involved in the budget.

In 1978, the National League for Nursing (NLN) published conference papers from a meeting of nurse executives, who represented acute care, long-term care, community health, and university settings (National League for Nursing, 1978). The conference focused on raising nurse executives' awareness of the need to be involved in budget preparation. An important impetus for this recognition was the development of prospective payment that was to be used by Medicare to control costs. Chief nursing officers and the management nursing level that includes nurse managers needed to have a better understanding of health care finances. One administrator stated, "The 1980s will find us even more concerned with belt tightening and intensifying voluntary efforts to contain health care costs. The future is in our hands" (National League for Nursing, 1978, p. 5). The belt tightening that was predicted for the 1980s occurred, and it continues today. Nurse administrators began to realize that they needed to play an active role in budget development in order to meet their goals for nursing services and to increase their understanding of health care reimbursement. Why is it important for nurses to understand reimbursement?

- Reimbursement affects patient care delivery: types of treatment, choice of provider, length of treatment.
- Reimbursement has an impact on provider performance and patient outcomes.
- Reimbursement affects financial resources that are available for health care organizations (for example, for staffing, equipment and supplies, renovation and expansion, and so on).

This early recognition of the need for involvement, however, focused only on the nursing management level: nurse executives and nurse managers. Staff nurses were, in most cases, still out of the loop; however, nursing can no longer afford to isolate staff nurses from financial issues. All nurses need a greater understanding of how financial decisions are made, by whom, why, and how these decisions make a difference in the care a patient receives; number of staff available to provide that care; access to services, supplies, and equipment; and so on.

## National Health Care Expenditures

The health care industry is an extremely large industry whose financing is influenced by many factors, particularly social expectation, economic trends, technological developments, and political factors, and in the last few years the U.S. economy has been the most critical factor. Financial issues affect all aspects of the provision of care, settings, and services, such as inpatient care, ambulatory care, home care, primary care, long-term care, public health, pharmaceutical, medical supplies, medical transportation, medical technology, medical research, and so on. Compared with other countries, the United States has the most expensive health care system with the highest living standard and economic status. Despite this, the United States has a large number of people without insurance coverage. The most recent statistics, 2007, identifies 45.7 million people without insurance, which represents a decline of more than one million people in 2006 (U.S. Census Bureau, 2010). Though a decrease is good news, it is still a large number of people. The largest portion of health care expenditures is found in the hospital industry, despite the fact that there is a decreasing length-of-stay rate and increasing use of nonhospital services. Health care expenditures are expected to continue to increase. An understanding of health care expenditures includes an appreciation of how the nation's health dollar is spent and also who pays for health care or the health care funding sources described in Figure 5-1. It is also important to recognize that health care expenditures change annually.

"As a result of more rapid growth in public spending, the public share of total health care spending is expected to rise from 47 percent in 2008, exceed 50 percent by 2012, and then reach nearly 52 percent by 2019" (Centers for Medicare and Medicaid Services, 2010). How does this description of projected health care spending impact current approaches to controlling health care costs and health care policy? Many experts believe that all of the "fat" has been removed from budgets, or rather the easier, more obvious methods to reduce costs have been used. To decrease costs further or even to just maintain the cost level so that it does not increase will now require more serious, difficult decision making. Health care reform legislation of 2010 will have an impact on these projections, hopefully decreasing costs, but its impact will really not be known for some time.

Decreasing hospitalization has been greatly influenced by the need to decrease costs; however, new advances in health care and new methods for providing health care have made it easier to lower hospitalization stays and costs. Factors that have helped to decrease hospitalization costs are early ambulation of patients so that they can be discharged sooner; prep time before admitted to hospital for surgery; greater use of ambulatory surgery with less use of inpatient surgery and stay; better use of medications such as antibiotics to prevent infections before the occur; greater use of home care and skilled nursing care; and more effective management of care within the hospital treatment period. Prescription costs have risen due to an increase in the cost of drugs, greater use of many new drugs that are effective but expensive, and broader health insurance coverage for prescriptions. Another aspect of the decreasing hospitalization is decreasing length-of-stay. Both of these changes have influenced patient acuity levels. Patients are admitted later and thus are sicker, and they leave quickly, which limits amount of time available to get patients and families ready for discharge. The patients then enter community services such as home care sicker, requiring more acute care than was true in the past. Home health care agencies now look for nurses who have had critical care experience to help with more complex care needs.

**FIGURE 5-1   The nation's health care dollar: Where it came from: 2004.**

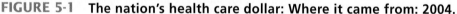

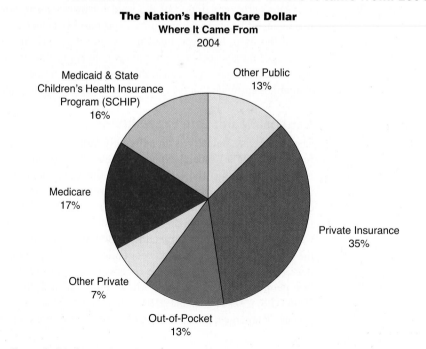

Source: Centers for Medicare and Medicaid Services (2006) Blue Cross Blue Shield Association, 2007 Medical Cost Reference Guide.

The largest portion of health care expenditures is found in the hospital industry, despite decreasing lengths-of-stay and increasing use of non-hospital services. Figure 5-2 provides another description of health care expenses: projected expenditures into 2030. These data indicate that health care expenditures are expected to increase, just about doubling from 2010 to 2020 and again from 2020 to 2030. These estimates are based on historical data and analysis.

Health care utilization and expenditures data are used to evaluate cost control outcomes. There is, however, another perspective of health care expenditures that is more complex than these data may indicate. Is spending more on medical care worth it in terms of its impact on the length and quality of life? Third-party payers must view health care expenditures from many perspectives using cost-benefit analysis. Nurses and nursing care do have an impact on these costs.

In 2008, with the worsening of the U.S. and global economy, health care was hit hard. In a survey of Americans conducted in February 2009, the news was not positive (Henry J. Kaiser Family Foundation, 2009a). More than half of Americans (slightly more than 53%) said that they limited their medical care due to cost in past year. The results indicated that there is grave concern about affordability and accessibility of health care when needed. Patients/consumers were relying more on over-the-counter drugs rather than visiting physicians (35%), and 34% were not keeping dental appointments. Twenty-one percent were not filling prescriptions, and 15% were cutting pills in half or skipping doses. Nineteen percent experienced major financial problems due to medical care that could not be put off. The survey also addressed the respondents' view of health care reform. The focus seemed to be more on getting help with costs of health care and getting coverage for those who did not have coverage rather than on improving the quality of care. Given that there is considerable concern about the quality of care as noted in recent Institute of Medicine (IOM) reports it is important to keep this part of the equation in mind. A dysfunctional health care system costs more money than a functional system that provides quality care and errors and prevents complications.

Experts agree that our health care system has many inefficiencies, excessive administrative expenses, inflated prices, poor management, and inappropriate care, waste, and fraud. All of these problems significantly increase the cost of medical care and health insurance for employers and workers and affect the security of families. With the growing economic crisis in 2008–2009 a greater number of families were affected. In 2008, health care spending in the United States reached $2.4 trillion, and was projected to reach $3.1 trillion in 2012, and $4.3 trillion by 2016 (Keehan, S. et al., 2008). The consumer's major concern in choosing a health plan today is personal cost. Employer and employee health insurance costs include the following (Henry J. Kaiser Family Foundation, 2009b):

- Premiums for employer-based health insurance rose by 5.0 percent in 2008. In 2007, small employers saw their premiums on average increase 5.5 percent. Firms with fewer than 24 workers experienced an increase of 6.8 percent.
- The annual premium that a health insurer charges an employer for a health plan covering a family of four averaged $12,700 in 2008. Workers contributed nearly $3,400 or 12% more

**FIGURE 5-2  Projected national health care expenditures, 2000–2030.**

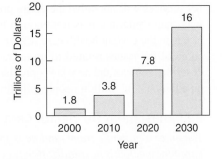

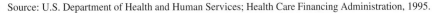

Source: U.S. Department of Health and Human Services; Health Care Financing Administration, 1995.

than they did in 2007. The annual premiums for family coverage significantly eclipsed the gross earnings for a full-time, minimum-wage worker ($10,712).

- Workers are paying $1,600 more in premiums annually for family coverage than they did in 1999.
- Since 1999, employment-based health insurance premiums have increased 120%, compared to cumulative inflation of 44% and cumulative wage growth of 29% during the same period.
- According to the Kaiser Family Foundation and the Health Research and Educational Trust, premiums for employer-sponsored health insurance in the United States have been rising four times faster on average than workers' earnings since 1999.
- The average employee contribution to company-provided health insurance has increased more than 120% since 2000. Average out-of-pocket costs for deductibles, co-payments for medications, and co-insurance for physician and hospital visits rose 115% during the same period.

The impact of rising health care costs has been dramatic as supported by the following descriptions and data.

- National surveys show that the primary reason people are uninsured is the high cost of health insurance coverage (Henry J. Kaiser Family Foundation, 2009b).
- A study by Harvard University researchers found that the average out-of-pocket medical debt for those who filed for bankruptcy was $12,000. The study noted that 68% of those who filed for bankruptcy had health insurance. In addition, the study found that 50% of all bankruptcy filings were partly the result of medical expenses (Himmelstein, Warren, Thorne, & Woolhander, 2005). Every 30 seconds in the United States someone files for bankruptcy in the aftermath of a serious health problem.
- About 1.5 million families lose their homes to foreclosure every year due to unaffordable medical costs (Robertson, Egelhof, & Hoke, 2008).
- Retiring elderly couples will need $250,000 in savings just to pay for the most basic medical coverage (Fidelity Investments, 2006). Many experts believe that this figure is conservative and that $300,000 may be a more realistic number.
- The United States spends six times more per capita on the administration of the health care system than its peer Western European nations (McKinsey Global Institute, 2007).

These examples illustrate how the economy is interrelated with health care, increasing the complexity when the economy worsens.

The concern about the uninsured has increased over the years. "The uninsured refers to persons with any form of public or private coverage for hospital and outpatient care, for any given length of time" (Institute of Medicine, 2004, p. 21). Along with this concern is the underinsured, an area that sometimes is ignored. The underinsured are "individuals or families whose health insurance policy or benefit plan offers less than adequate coverage" (Institute of Medicine, 2004, p. 21). When this happens, these individuals and families are left with debt because they cannot pay uncovered care, or they avoid getting care when they need it because their benefits do not cover required care. The U.S. safety net, which is represented by the health care organizations that disproportionately serve the needy and uninsured, has been stretched as the number of uninsured and underinsured increases (Institute of Medicine, 2004). However, increasing the safety net services will not solve the entire problem of the uninsured and underinsured. This approach may help some, but it is not enough to solve the problem. Both of these problems are major issues in the current health care reform debate. Health care reform legislation of 2010 addresses some of the issues related to uninsured, safety net, and increasing costs of care. Appendix B describes some of the new law's provisions. When full implementation of the law occurs in 2019 an additional 32 million people will have health care coverage.

## Reimbursement for Health Care Delivery Services

*You enter a patient's room, and he is speaking on the telephone. You overhear him say, "I don't care how much this hospitalization is costing. My insurance pays for it." You nod and agree. This example almost seems as if it came from another world, certainly not the real one, and both the patient and you, the nurse, need to enter the real one. Is it this simple?*

Health care reimbursement in the United States is a pluralistic payment system with multiple payers from both the public and private sectors. It is complex, with many players, motivations, and a long history of change. Insurance began in Boston in 1847. By the end of the 1860s, there were 60 health insurance companies. In 1911, Montgomery Ward and Company offered a plan that provided benefits to its employees who were unable to work due to illness or injury (Health Insurance Association of America, 1998). Employers began to offer health insurance coverage instead of increasing wages. Over time businesses offered employees insurance to get the tax benefit because employers' contributions for insurance benefits are exempt from federal and state taxes, which is a very important savings for employers.

From 1987 to 1997, the U.S. experienced the first major indication that health care costs would continue to have a critical impact on the economy when health insurance premiums increased 90%, which was an incredible increase for those earning low wages (Cooper & Schone, 1997), and since this time, costs have continued to increase. With the increase in premiums as well as the increase in other out-of-pocket expenses, people began to make choices about insurance. Some decided to not sign up for health insurance, and others limited their use of services to cut down on their personal costs. Employees who choose not to purchase coverage decide to take the risk and gamble that they will not need health care services.

Today, cost consciousness in the face of limited health care dollars has reached a level that crosses all care settings and patient populations to a much greater extent than in the past. Health care purchasers, typically employers and governments, are in a very influential position, because the purchaser makes the major decisions (e.g., approval of reimbursable services, provider choice, length-of-stay, length of treatment, quality). All nurses require a greater knowledge of reimbursement in order to understand how reimbursement affects care provided, denial of care, and numerous factors related to the nursing practice within all types of organizations. In the past, nurses did not discuss health care reimbursement with their patients. The business office typically is called to come and talk with a patient when questions arise. This is not an inappropriate intervention when a patient has billing questions; however, it has fostered a climate of separation. Nurses provide care, and "someone" pays. Patients, however, expect that nurses have some knowledge about reimbursement. The growth of managed care and other reimbursement changes has made this knowledge even more important. Nursing standards identify financial resource management as an important nursing responsibility.

KEY PLAYERS IN THE REIMBURSEMENT PROCESS    The key players in reimbursement strategies are the insurer (third-party payer), the customer, the consumer, and the provider. These players are identified in Figure 5-3.

1. **Third-party payer/managed care organization/insurer**    With the development of managed care the insurer, **third-party payer**, or MCO no longer carries all of the financial risk for health care. Reimbursement strategies used by insurers are primarily aimed at reducing insurer financial risk; however, these strategies are often difficult to separate from service strategies. The insurer may use any of the managed care models and may be a national or regional insurer. With the advent of managed care, the insurer gained more power to influence care, and third-party payers have been more successful in decreasing their financial risk by using reimbursement and service strategies.

**FIGURE 5-3    Key players in the health care environment.**

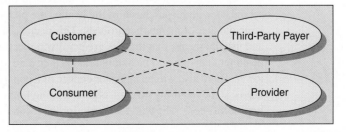

2. **Customer**    The **customer** is the person who contracts with the insurer. In most cases this is an employer or government through its insurance programs. The U.S. reimbursement system is employer-based. The employer looks for the most cost-effective plans to meet the needs of its employees.

3. **Consumer/patient/enrollee**    The patient or enrollee is a key player in the health care system. If patients did not exist, there would be no need for insurers or providers. When a person chooses a health insurance plan, the person is referred to as a plan member or enrollee.

4. **Provider**    Who is the provider? Provider is a generic term. Any of the following may be considered a provider: physician, advanced practice nurse or nurse practitioner, nurse-midwife, registered nurse, physician assistant, certified registered nurse anesthetist, pharmacist, dentist, optometrist, chiropractor, podiatrist, hospital, home health agency, hospice, long-term care facility, psychiatric hospital, skilled nursing home, infusion therapy agency, and so on. In short, a provider is any person or organization that provides health care.

WHAT IS HEALTH INSURANCE?    An insurer or third-party payer is the organization, private or public, that pays or underwrites coverage for health care for another entity, such as a business or individual. The third-party payer provides either group coverage or individual coverage. Most people who have insurance coverage receive it as an employee benefit or through membership in an organization, which is group coverage (e.g., a health care professional organization might offer health plans to its members). Most group insurers are commercial or for-profit insurers. Individual or personal insurance that is not part of employment is much more expensive for the purchaser or the enrollee. Sometimes individuals purchase personal insurance to cover gaps in their employment insurance. Others who are self-employed may have to purchase individual coverage plans. In the insurance schema, the patient is referred to as the first party, the provider as the second party, and the third party is the payer or insurance carrier, such as a commercial insurer, managed care organization, Blue Cross and Blue Shield, and the government programs (e.g., Medicare, Medicaid). The third-party payer actually pays the bills; however, the process is not simple. As insurance has grown, there has been an increase in insurer financial risk. The insurer could lose the money it invests, or it could miscalculate the amount of money it needs to cover all of its expenses, expected and unexpected. This could happen if too many of the health plan members require more health care than was estimated. If the insurer is a for-profit organization, it must also yield profits to pay its stockholders. Insurer administrative costs (e.g., staff, facilities, supplies, information systems, and other similar activities and functions) can also be very high.

How does the insurance process actually work to yield payment for health care services?

1. An individual experiences uncertainty about health care needs and treatment costs. Without this consumer uncertainty, there would be less need for insurance and less financial risk associated with health care. Given this uncertainty, there is a need to share the financial risk with other consumers to decrease individual risk.

2. When individuals decide to join an insurance plan, they put a specific amount of money into the pool or the insurance fund. The pool consists of the group of people that the insurer is covering for health care services.

3. The insurer takes on the role of managing or administering the pool of money. Plan members really do not want to do this for themselves.

For example, a large manufacturing company offers several health care coverage options to its employees. This company does not want to use its own resources to administer employee health care coverage, so it contracts with insurers to provide this service. The insurer will be better served, as will the purchaser of the health care plan (the employer) and the enrollees, if there are a large number of members/enrollees. This decreases the financial risk and the administrative costs and usually means that there is greater diversification in the health status of members, with some healthier than others. The amount that is then paid to obtain the coverage, the premiums, is usually lower. There also will be a greater chance of a pool of members who will have different health care needs: some requiring no care, others needing limited care, and some with major medical care and long-term needs. The worst scenario for the insurer is to have a group of unhealthy members.

PROSPECTIVE VERSUS RETROSPECTIVE PAYMENT    Typically, when a customer considers purchasing a product, such as a car, the price is known before the purchase. The seller sets the price, and then the purchaser decides to buy or not to buy the product, usually considering need, price, quality, and the like. This is **prospective payment**. The health care industry has had a different experience with setting prices. In the past, third-party purchasers of health care services devised a **retrospective payment** system. In this system, the provider spent money while providing the care, requested payment for these expenses, and then was paid. Providers liked this because they knew they would be paid for their services when they submitted their bills. This payment method was known as fee-for-service or billed charges for health care services. The provider establishes the fee-for-service, and the patient pays, usually through a third-party payer. For a long time was the major form of payment for health care. Fee-for-service payment typically did not put many limitations on the provider, and the insurer accepted the charges identified by the provider so the provider made most, if not all, of the treatment decisions with the patient. As a consequence, there was little incentive to be cost-effective when the provider knew that the requested charge would be paid in full. Box 5-1 describes indemnity insurance or the more traditional view of insurance coverage.

Third-party payers thought that retrospective payment or using a fee-for-service method was a good approach, but after a time, this became an expensive way to do business. Then, third-party payers began to put some limits on what they would reimburse, eliminating an automatic acceptance of all charges. The federal government, via its Medicare and Medicaid programs, was the first purchaser or third-party payer to develop a comprehensive **prospective payment system (PPS)**. The purpose of changing to this payment system was to decrease hospital costs. This system is not based on actual charges but rather on estimated, predetermined prices made by the payer, not the provider. The provider knows before the care is provided what the payer will pay for a particular service. Usually, additional resources such as specialty care that may be used are not figured into this amount. In changing to prospective payment, the health care industry moved to the approach used by most sellers of products—here is the price; you either buy it or do not buy it. Now, it is quite clear that health care is a much more complex product. Just consider: Do consumers (patients) usually have a choice when they need care? Getting sick is different from deciding to buy a book, chair, dress, or car.

COMPENSATION FOR HEALTH SERVICES    Since the product, health care services, is not as simple as other types of products, a number of different approaches are used to pay for these services. Compensation for health services has an impact on nurses and nursing care. It has a trickle down effect (for example, amount of available funds for hiring staff, buying supplies, paying for overtime, and so on). The typical types of reimbursement methods are discounted fee-for-service, per diem rates, diagnosis-related groups, capitation, and **resource-based relative value scale**. Home health care usually is reimbursed on a per-hour or per-visit basis.

*Discounted fee-for-service*    In the mid-1970s, early forms of managed care began to use discounts. **Discounted fee-for-service** is a payment method that offers to pay the provider a specific percentage of the provider's usual charge or a reduced rate. The percentage can be a straight one, in which only a certain percentage is taken off the charge, or it can be a sliding scale, with the percentage changing based on specified criteria. Discounted services are part of a contractual arrangement with a third-party payer. An insurer may contract with a health care facility or any other type of provider to receive a discount for services provided. For example, an

| **BOX 5-1** | **CHARACTERISTICS OF TRADITIONAL INDEMNITY INSURANCE** |
|---|---|

- Fee-for-service reimbursement for providers
- Insurer assumes all financial risk
- No restrictions on choice of provider
- Limited financial incentives to be cost-effective

- No organized interest in quality measurement
- No organized interest in appropriateness of services

insurer's enrollees who receive care at that facility receive a 20% discount, or rather are only charged 80% of the usual charge for the services. Clearly, this is an advantage for the insurer/MCO. Sliding scales, another type of discount, are reflective of the volume of services provided. If the insurer requires a specific level of service, the fee scale will be adjusted or decreased. Most health care facilities, such as hospitals, have many contracts with insurers that have different discounts. If not all care is reimbursed at 100% of the costs, this leaves the health care provider with expenses that are not covered. This can have serious ramifications for the provider over the long term if the provider cannot cover these unpaid expenses. Providers, such as hospitals, outpatient clinics, physician practices, and home care agencies, must be very careful about the amount of care that is discounted and consider how the unpaid portion will be covered. This insurer advantage can become a health care provider disaster. If a provider's expenses are not fully covered by reimbursement, then the provider (for example, a hospital) may have to decrease its operating costs (e.g., decrease staffing, postpone renovation or purchase of new equipment, decrease amount of educational programs provided to staff, and so on).

*Per diem rates*    A **per diem rate** is reimbursement that is fixed, based on each day in a health care facility (e.g., $600 per day). Services that may be covered, as well as expected length-of-stay and intensity of services, may be included in the agreed-upon per diem rate. This rate may also be discounted by the contract between the third-party payer and the provider. The per diem rate is an estimate of what the charges would be; however, this prospectively determined rate is all that is paid even if the actual expenses are greater. Usually, per diem rates vary for specialty areas; for example, daily rates for critical care, behavioral/psychiatric care, medical care, surgical care, or obstetrical care would not be the same (e.g., intensive care per diem would be higher than medical care per diem due to the staffing level, equipment, supplies, and so on). Per diem reimbursement is the negotiated rate per day times the number of days of care (e.g., $600 per day times the number of days in the hospital—3 days would equal $1,800 per diem reimbursement).

*Capitation*    The growth of managed care introduced one of the major changes in health care reimbursement—**capitation**. Capitation is a prepayment to a provider to deliver health care services to enrollees of a health plan. This is usually a monthly payment, but it can also be paid on an annual basis. The provider agrees to provide all care for the enrollee's health care needs that the provider is qualified to provide. If the enrollee requires no services in the allotted time period, the provider is still paid. If the enrollee's care incurs additional expenses, the provider receives no extra payment. The capitation method is dependent on a contract between the provider and a third-party payer. The focus is on covered lives or the number of persons who are enrolled in a health plan rather than individuals. For example, costs are typically described as inpatient days per 1,000, visits per 1,000, or cost per life. "Capitation changes the focus from how much a provider will be paid, as is the case with fee-for-service, to how much it costs to provide the care required" (Baldor, 1998). In doing this, the third-party payer no longer carries the full financial risk for the employer because much of it is shifted to the provider to keep costs down when decisions are made about care.

*Employee contributions to coverage*    The employee pays some parts of the insurance coverage with the employer paying another part. The amount an employee pays, the premium, varies depending on the amount paid by the employer, the insurer's contract, and the amount of health care services used and how they are used. **Premium rate setting** is one of the most important decisions that a third-party payer can make, and also an important decision for consumers. Rating is pricing. The third-party payer determines the premiums (price or rate) for its products or services. Premiums are usually calculated as an amount per member per month (PMPM). If the third-party payer miscalculates, it can mean that the insurer loses money and may become financially unstable because the third-party payer will then not have enough funds to pay for the health care services that its members require and to cover administrative expenses that are needed to manage the insurance plan.

Employee/member plan costs continue to increase. The employee contribution to medical coverage usually includes some form of a deductible, co-payment/coinsurance, and annual limits. Insurance plans are highly variable; these methods may not be included in all plans and can vary in how they are applied. Deductibles and co-payments/coinsurance represent the employee's out-of-pocket health care expenses and are used by the insurer to control its costs. When the insurer increases the out-of-pocket expenses, the insurer pays less and the enrollee or member pays more.

1. **Deductibles**   A **deductible** is the amount the employee must pay before the third-party payer will begin to pay for health care services. The deductible may be handled one of two ways. Some plans require that the employee pay a single deductible for the employee and also for family members, which is applied to all services in the plan. The deductible for family members often is higher. The second method is the use of separate deductibles for categories of services, such as hospitalization, ambulatory care, and so on. Usually, when employers and employees pay high premiums, the employee pays a lower deductible. Deductibles are usually not used by Health Maintenance Organizations (HMOs). Figure 5-4 describes the relationship of the deductible to other payments in the major medical model.

   Most major medical plans start with a deductible of $100, $250, or higher. This payment keeps the cost of the plan down because the enrollee is accepting responsibility for the initial, most frequent charges, those under the deductible limit. After the deductible is paid, the enrollee shares the expenses by paying the co-payment or coinsurance. Typically, this is shared with the insurer on an 80/20 basis. For example, each dollar above the deductible is paid in this manner—insurer 80 cents and enrollee 20 cents. If the medical bill is large, 20% can still be a sizable amount. A patient example illustrating how this is implemented is found in Box 5-2.

2. **Co-payments/coinsurance**   A **co-payment/coinsurance** is the fixed payment that the employee must pay per physician visit, procedure/treatment, or prescription. This is payment sharing between the insurer and the enrollee/patient. The payment typically is required at the time of the service and usually is an established amount, such as $5 or $10, or it can be a percentage. Co-payments may be found in all types of coverage. Box 5-3 describes an example of a patient's out-of-pocket expenses for an insurance plan.

*Annual limits*   **Annual limits** have been very important, particularly for employees and their families who experience major medical expenses in a year. All plans have has some type of limit on the amount that the employee is required to pay annually. However, health care reform legislation of 2010 prohibits the use of restrictive annual limits on coverage for care.

Employers are increasing their efforts to contain their own costs; to achieve this, out-of-pocket expenses for employees typically increase. Employees then carry more of the responsibility for paying for the costs of care. The new law of 2010 will result in major changes in

**FIGURE 5-4**  **Major medical model (deductible coinsurance, and high policy limits).**

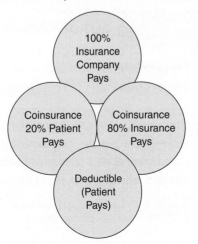

## BOX 5-2    DEDUCTIBLES AND CO-PAYMENTS: A PATIENT EXAMPLE

| | |
|---|---|
| **Hospital bill** | $20,000 |
| **Patient deductible** | –$    200 |
| | **$19,800** Medical charges after deductible paid |
| **Medical charges after deductible paid** | $19,800 |
| **Patient share/co-payment** | ×      .20 |
| | **$ 3,960** Amount of medical expenses to be paid by patient/co-payment |

Deductible must be paid before the insurer will pay its portion. Patient must pay deductible and co-payment.

| | |
|---|---|
| **Deductible** | $   200 |
| **Co-payment** | + $ 3,960 |
| | **$ 4,160** Total amount to be paid by patient |

**Despite insurance coverage, the patient must still pay $4,160, which is not a small amount.**

premiums or coverage for people who have been receiving their health coverage through large employers, improving the situation for patients/employees (Bernard, March 21, 2010).

When an employee joins a health plan or when an individual purchases insurance, the person becomes an enrollee/member/subscriber in the plan. The enrollee's family is not usually referred to as the enrollee. When they are included in the plan's coverage they are called dependents, if that is an option available to the enrollee. The contract or covered services plan describes the eligibility criteria, benefits, and payments. These criteria identify when the enrollee and dependents are eligible for the services as well as when they are not eligible. For instance, a dependent child typically is not covered after a specific age or when he or she is no longer considered a dependent; however, 2010 health care reform will change this as adult children may be covered until age 26 if this is the choice of the parents and the adult child.

Coverage renewability is particularly important with individual health insurance policies and long-term care contracts. The health care law passed in 2010 restricts insurers from refusing to sell or renew policies because of an individual's health nor can individuals be excluded for pre-existing conditions. This provision is effective 2014; however, another provision protects children, effective 2010. The law also provides temporary funding effective 2010 for people with pre-existing conditions who had been uninsured for at least six months.

## BOX 5-3    OUT-OF-POCKET EXPENSES: AN EXAMPLE

| | |
|---|---|
| Physician's bill for office visit: Bronchitis | $120 |
| Insurer's reasonable and customary charge for this visit | $100 |
| Patient's co-payment of 30% ($100 × .30) = | $ 30 |
| Uncovered part of bill to be paid by patient ($120 – $100) = | $ 20 |
| Patient's total out-of-pocket expenses | |
| Co-payment ($30) + uncovered portion ($20) = | $ 50 |

**The $50 represents 41.6% of the total charge, which was $120.**

Source: A. Finkelman. (2001). *Managed care. A nursing perspective.* Upper Saddle River, NJ: Prentice Hall, p. 32. Reprinted with permission.

The written **benefit plan** describes the benefits that are provided to the enrollee and the financial coverage for those benefits or the covered services. Before covered services can be described, it is important to understand the relationship between the enrollee and eligibility for the covered services. Federal law requires that all employees who are eligible for an employer plan be offered enrollment at the same price.

Benefits are a very important part of any health care plan. Important factors are the covered services, exclusions (services not covered), and limitations, which are impacted by health care reform. Great variability exists among plans in their benefit description and what is included or excluded. As an employee makes decisions about coverage, benefits can be a critical issue to consider, depending on the health and financial needs of the employee and the employee's family. In some cases, when there are major or chronic health problems, paying higher premiums to obtain maximum benefits may be the wisest choice. Health care reform of 2010 restricts insurers from discriminating for pre-existing conditions. Plan benefits are also important to the provider because medical decisions are often based on the benefits that will be covered, which may not necessarily be what the patient needs.

Covered services are the health care services that the plan will cover or reimburse; however, the care or services must be medically necessary. What are the criteria used to determine if care is medically necessary? These criteria include consistency among diagnosis, medical documentation, and the likelihood of acceptance by medical peers that the treatment is necessary for the patient (Casto & Layman, 2009). The insurer determines medical necessity with input from the provider. Clearly, this is an area that creates conflict because the insurer becomes the major decision maker, not the patient's health care provider. Typical benefits included in health care plans are the following:

- Hospital room and board
- Outpatient and inpatient surgery
- Office and inpatient physician visits
- Nursing services
- Diagnostic and radiological laboratory tests
- Ambulance services
- Medical equipment, such as might be used in the home

Some plans include more specialized care, such as home health care, extended care, hospice care, inpatient and outpatient mental health care, and alcohol and substance abuse treatment. When plans cover these services, specific descriptions are included in the covered services document or plan. Typically, home health care is used when skilled nursing care is required at home and usually covers required supplies and equipment. When hospice care is provided, it is usually covered for terminally ill patients who have 6 months or less to live though some insurers are more flexible. Extended care may be covered for patients who need less intensive care than hospital care and require skilled nursing care, rehabilitation, and/or convalescent services. Mental health services and alcohol and substance abuse treatment services usually have more stringent limitations. The insurer identifies not only the benefits that are offered but often who may provide these services, a requirement that must be met for the insurer to cover or pay for the health care service. Special health care needs are always a concern for the insurer because they increase costs. Dental and vision coverage are services that receive special attention. If an employer offers these services, it usually covers only one of them. Employers are beginning to pay a smaller portion of the premiums for these services. Some are only offering the option of dental HMOs. In addition, the use of medical technology has become an increased concern for insurers and for consumers. The development of new medical technologies is a positive step forward for health care delivery, but they cost money to develop and use. Insurers must evaluate new technologies carefully before agreeing to cover these new therapies.

Health promotion and disease prevention have become more important to insurers, particularly in the managed care environment though this has been a weak coverage area. In the past, traditional indemnity plans usually did not cover, or provided limited coverage for, these services. Examples of preventive care that might now be included are annual physical exams, childhood immunizations, and mammograms, usually within a specified age range. Health promotion examples are health education classes, wellness centers, and smoking cessation groups. Health care reform legislation of 2010 includes many provisions related to health promotion, prevention, and wellness. See Appendix B.

**Exclusions** are the services that will not be covered by a health care plan. Excluded conditions can vary from plan to plan. Some examples are cosmetic surgery, orthodontic treatment, experimental treatment, and artificial insemination.

## Government Health Benefit Programs

The federal government is the major player in the health care arena because it covers a large percentage of the population through is various insurance programs such as Medicare and Medicaid. The federal government benefit plans are Medicare, Medicaid, the Federal Employees' Health Benefit Program (FEHBP), TriCare, and the Civilian Health and Medical Program of the Uniform Services (CHAMPUS). Health care is the major item in the federal budget each year. Nurses are involved in the care of all of these groups of patients, civilian and military, and many of the changes made in government reimbursement eventually impact all reimbursement.

### An Overview of Medicare and Medicare

Medicare is the federal health care insurance program that was established in 1965 by Title XVIII, Health Insurance for the Aged, as an amendment to the Social Security Act of 1935. Medicare is funded by the Medicare Trust Fund, which includes payroll tax contributions, and it is the largest single payer in the United States. For many years, Medicare has played a major role in health care delivery despite the fact that it is a complex program that is difficult to understand. President Johnson signed the Medicare legislation in 1965, but earlier President Truman took the first steps toward this legislation. He envisioned this program as a critical step towards national health insurance (Daschle, 2008). Medicare has survived and changed over time. With the introduction of changes in Medicare reimbursement methods, such as DRGs, Medicare spending decreased. Interest in using managed care approaches to further decrease health care costs has increased over the years. As illustrated in Figure 5-5, Medicare spending, which is part of the federal budget, is expected to increase in the next 6 years, making the need for further cost reduction very important.

**FIGURE 5-5   Overall Medicare spending: 1980 actual through 2016 projected.**

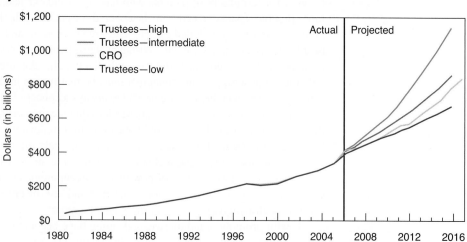

Note: CBO (Congressional Budget Office). All data are nominal, gross program outlays (mandatory plus administrative expenses) by calendar year.

Source: Medicare Trustees Report 2007. CBO March 2007 baseline.

The elderly are living longer, requiring longer periods of health care services, and medical prices are going up. These factors have a major impact on the size of the trust fund that will be available long-term for this federal program. There has been considerable concern about the growth of Medicare. The "baby boomers," people born between 1946 and 1964, are entering the Medicare beneficiary age range. This greatly increases the number of Medicare beneficiaries.

**LEGISLATIVE AND REGULATORY ISSUES RELATED TO MEDICARE**    The following discussion provides information about the legislation and regulations that have affected Medicare and its move toward managed care approaches to control costs.

- **Social Security Act of 1965 and Amendments**    The Social Security Act of 1965 with its subsequent amendments is the landmark legislation that established Medicare and also Medicaid and made the federal government the major player in health care. The creation of Medicare and Medicaid not only allowed many who could not afford care to receive care but also gave the federal government power to dictate standards, reimbursement methods, and influence other aspects of care. Few hospitals can avoid treating patients covered by these two programs, and when they do treat these patients, they must meet federal requirements and accept federal payment rates.
- **Tax Equity and Fiscal Responsibility Act of 1982**    The Tax Equity and Fiscal Responsibility Act of 1982 (TEFRA) established prospective reimbursement for Medicare acute care services using the diagnosis-related groups model (DRGs). The law also introduced Medicare to managed care by promoting the use of health maintenance organizations (HMOs) with Medicare contracts. Health Care Reform of 2010 revisited the issue of Medicare managed care plans, and by 2018 this type of plan will reduced.
- **Consolidated Omnibus Budget Reconciliation Act of 1985**    The Consolidated Omnibus Budget Reconciliation Act of 1985 (COBRA) affected most hospitals. It requires that all hospitals treating Medicare patients also treat all patients who request care in their emergency rooms to stabilize them, whether or not they are covered by Medicare or able to pay. This law has had a major effect on emergency services, their inappropriate use, and escalating costs. Once a hospital receives federal funding, such as Medicare this federal law applies to the hospital's emergency services.
- **Medicare Catastrophic Coverage Act of 1988**    The Medicare Catastrophic Coverage Act was signed into law in 1988. This law recognized the economic disparity that existed among the elderly. The decision was made that elderly with greater personal funds should pay more for Medicare; however, this law did not last long. Two years later, it was repealed. This is an example of the power of the consumer's voice, even a minority of the more affluent elderly, can have on legislation. This group of beneficiaries did not like paying higher premiums. In addition, the pharmaceutical companies were concerned about the drug benefit that was included, and they feared this would lead to greater price controls. They had a very strong, effective lobby in Congress.
- **Balanced Budget Act of 1997 (BBA)**    BBA expanded the ability of Medicare to offer managed care organizations (MCOs) to its beneficiaries. This included Medicare beneficiaries that had enrolled in HMOs since 1985. The law increased the options to not only include Medicare HMOs, but also Medicare **preferred provider organizations (PPOs)**, Medicare **point-of-service plans (POS)**, and several other MCO plans (Kongstvedt, 2009). Medicare contracts with nongovernmental insurers for these plans.
- **Medicare Prescription Drug Improvement and Modernization Act of 2003 (MMA)**    This legislation created Medicare Part D, the newest Medicare benefit part. The focus of Part D is prescription coverage, a long needed benefit for Medicare beneficiaries.
- **Patient Protection and Affordable Care Act of 2010 and Health Care and Education Reconciliation Act of 2010**    These two laws are the most significant health care legislation in decades. The Patient Protection and Affordable Care Act has many provisions, while the second law was used to reconcile differences between the Senate and House versions of this legislation. Additional information about the law is found in Chapter 2 and in Appendix B. Box 5-4 describes some of the reimbursement provisions including Medicare and Medicaid provisions found in the law.

| BOX 5-4 | EXAMPLES OF REIMBURSEMENT PROVISIONS IN HEALTH CARE AND EDUCATION RECONCILIATION ACT OF 2010 |
|---|---|

This legislation was signed into law on March 30, 2010, by President Obama. This information only represents some examples of the provisions, not all of the law's provisions.

### EFFECTIVE 2010

#### Provisions

Lifetime limits on benefits and restrictive annual limits will be prohibited.

Seniors will get a $250 rebate to help fill the "doughnut hole" in Medicare prescription drug coverage, which falls between the $2,700 initial limit and when catastrophic coverage kicks in at $6,154.

Insurers will be barred from imposing exclusions on children with pre-existing conditions. Pools will cover those with pre-existing health conditions until health care coverage exchanges are operational.

New plans must provide coverage for preventive services without co-pays. All plans must comply by 2018.

Young adults will be able stay on their parents' insurance until their 27th birthday.

Businesses with fewer than 50 employees will get tax credits covering 35 percent of their health care premiums, increasing to 50 percent by 2014.

Improve care coordination for dual eligible's (Medicare and Medicaid) to improve access and quality.

Medicaid to cover tobacco cessation programs for pregnant women.

Qualified health plans must cover a minimum coverage without cost-sharing for preventive services rated A or B by the U. S. Preventive Services Task Force, recommended immunizations, preventive care for infants, children, and adolescents, and additional preventive care and screenings for women. (See http://www.ahrq.gov/clinic/uspstfix.htm for information on the Task Force.)

Provide new options for home and community-based services through Medicaid.

Temporary funding (5 billion) for national high-risk insurance pool for coverage of individuals with pre-existing medical conditions who have been uninsured for at least six months.

Insurance plans may not place lifetime limits on benefits and restrictive annual limits.

Insurers may not rescind policies to avoid paying medical bills when a person becomes ill.

People receiving coverage from large employers are not expected to experience major changes in premium costs or coverage.

### EFFECTIVE 2011

#### Provisions

A 50% discount will be provided on brand-name drugs for Prescription Drug Plan or Medicare Advantage enrollees. Additional discounts on brand-name and generic drugs will be phased in to completely close the "doughnut hole" by 2020.

Cover only proven preventive services and eliminate cost-sharing for preventive services in Medicare and Medicaid.

The Medicare payroll tax will increase from 1.45% to 2.35% for individuals earning more than $200,000 and married filing jointly above $250,000.

States can offer home- and community-based services to the disabled through Medicaid rather than institutional care beginning October 1.

| BOX 5-4 | EXAMPLES OF REIMBURSEMENT PROVISIONS IN HEALTH CARE AND EDUCATION RECONCILIATION ACT OF 2010 (CONTINUED) |

Medicare will provide free annual wellness visits and personalized prevention plans. New plans will be required to cover preventive services with no co-pay.

Pharmaceutical companies will provide a 50% discount on brand name prescription drugs for seniors; additional discounts phased in over the next ten years.

A plan to provide a vehicle for small businesses to offer tax-free benefits will be created. This would ease the small employer's administrative burden of sponsoring a cafeteria plan.

Community Living Assistance Services and Supports (CLASS), a voluntary long-term care program, will be created. When employees contribute to the program for five years they would be entitle to a $50 per day cast benefit to pay for long-term care. CLASS does not cover all long-term care expenses. This is the first national government-run long-term care insurance program, primarily offered through employers.

Develop a Medicaid plan option for enrollees with at least two chronic illnesses, one condition and risk of developing another, or at least one serious and persistent mental health conditions to designate a provider as a health home.

Provide access to comprehensive health risk assessment and a personalized prevention plan for Medicare beneficiaries. Health risk assessment model to be developed with 18 months after law's effective date.

Provide incentives to Medicare and Medicaid beneficiaries to complete behavior modification programs (criteria need to be developed).

Community First Choice Option for Medicaid beneficiaries with disabilities to receive community-based attendant services and supports rather than institutional care.

Provides incentives to reduce Medicare readmissions due to infections or other preventable causes

## EFFECTIVE 2012

### Provisions

Create the Independence in Home demonstration program; providing primary care services in the home for high-need Medicare beneficiaries with goal of reducing preventable hospitalization, readmissions, improve health outcomes, improve efficiency of care, reduce costs, and achieve patient satisfaction.

Required mental health parity, which means deductibles, co-payments, and limits on the number of visits or days of coverage for mental health and substance abuse treatment, must be no more restrictive than for medical and surgical needs.

Establish more training for behavioral health professionals.

Develop nongovernmental research centers to investigate effective treatment for mental illness.

## EFFECTIVE 2013

### Provisions

Health plans must implement uniform standards for electronic exchange of health information to reduce paperwork and administrative costs.

Increase Medicaid payments for fee-for-service and managed care primary care services provided by primary care physicians (family medicine, general internal medicine, or pediatric medicine).

*(continued)*

| BOX 5-4 | EXAMPLES OF REIMBURSEMENT PROVISIONS IN HEALTH CARE AND EDUCATION RECONCILIATION ACT OF 2010 (CONTINUED) |
|---|---|

**EFFECTIVE 2014**

**Provisions**

Citizens will be required to have acceptable coverage or pay a penalty of $95 in 2014, $325 in 2015, $695 (or up to 2.5 percent of income) in 2016. Families will pay half the amount for children, up to a cap of $2,250 per family. After 2016, penalties are indexed to Consumer Price Index.

Companies with 50 or more employees must offer coverage to employees or pay a $2,000 penalty per employee after their first 30 if at least one of their employees receives a tax credit. Waiting periods before insurance takes effect is limited to 90 days. Employers who offer coverage but whose employees receive tax credits will pay $3,000 for each worker receiving a tax credit.

Insurers can no longer refuse to sell or renew policies because of an individual's health status. Health plans can no longer exclude coverage for pre-existing conditions. Insurers can't charge higher rates because of heath status, gender or other factors.

Health insurance exchanges will open in each state to individuals and small employers to comparison shop for standardized health packages.

Medicaid eligibility will increase to 133% of poverty for all nonelderly individuals to ensure that people obtain affordable health care in the most efficient and appropriate manner. States will receive increased federal funding to cover these new populations.

Sources: Health Care and Education Reconciliation Act of 2010 (P.L. 111-152); Health Reform http://www.healthreform.gov/; White House Health Reform http://www.whitehouse.gov/healthreform; The Henry Kaiser Family Foundation http://www.kff.org; Hossian, Farhana. (March 24, 2010). How people will be affected by the overhaul. *New York Times*, p. A18; Wolf, R. & Young, A. (March 23, 2010). Bill spreads the pain, benefits. *USA Today*, pp. 4A-3A; Span, P. (March 30, 2010). Options expand for affordable long-term care. *New York Times*, p. D5; Bernard, T. (March 21, 2010). For consumers, clarity on health care changes. *New York Times*. Retrieved from http://www.nytimes.com.

The Health Care Financing Administration (HCFA) is the agency within the U.S. Department of Health and Human Services (DHHS) that administers the Medicare program and the federal portion of Medicaid. It develops regulations to implement relevant federal laws. HCFA also grants all managed care contracts for Medicare beneficiaries and evaluates and reports on MCO performance. Medicare is financed from four sources. The most important source is the mandatory contributions made by employees and employers to the trust fund, which is used to provide hospital care. Employees contribute to the fund during their employment years, as do employers; however, the money that they contribute is actually used to reimburse care for people who are currently covered by Medicare. It is not saved to cover care for the contributing employees in the future. This means that current Medicare beneficiaries are actually covered by current employer and employee contributions. The other fund sources are general tax revenues, premiums paid by beneficiaries, and Medicare deductibles and copayments.

Some initiatives that are used to decrease Medicare costs include efforts to reduce hospital, home health, and provider payments. In some cases, these savings have exceeded expectations. There are, however, some results that are troubling, which have had a ripple effect throughout the health care system. Today, patients are sicker when they receive care, and thus need more intensive care at a time when nursing staff levels are reduced. Families are also greatly affected when they are left with the burden of caring for seriously ill family members at home with limited or no health care support such as home care. The 2010 health care reform law includes provisions to assist patients who want to receive care in their homes. (See Appendix B.)

**MS-DIAGNOSIS-RELATED GROUPS** **Diagnosis-related groups (DRGs)** is a statistical system that classifies care into groups. These groups, which include inpatient care, are then used to identify payment rates. This is a per-stay reimbursement that focus on a single episode of care related to a diagnosis and includes all predetermined services delivered for that episode. The DRG system is a prospective payment system that is used as the payment system for Medicare reimbursement. Some third-party payers also use it. Box 5-5 summarizes some information about DRGs.

The DRG system considers the types of patients a hospital treats or its case mix and the costs for treatment. Resources used and length of stay or bed days are important aspects of the incurred costs. Case-mix characteristics include severity of illness and intensity of service as described in Box 5-6.

This system focuses not on the number of patients, but rather on the types of patients and the resources they use. The major diagnostic categories (MDCs) are based on anatomical or pathophysiological groups and/or their clinical management. Within each MDC, there are a number of DRGs. The DRG rates are also affected by the following:

- Location of the hospital (rural or urban)
- Wage index, which affects hospital costs
- Teaching hospital status and house staff training
- Recognition of outliers

Outliers are patients with cost of care or length-of-stay that is outside the expected. If a patient's hospital stay is longer than expected or total costs are greater than expected for the patient's DRG, then the patient is considered to be an outlier. Hospitals are very concerned when they have outliers because they need to investigate the reasons to ensure that costs are controlled.

DRGs have had and continue to have an impact on care. Coordination of all aspects of care becomes critical in order to meet length-of-stay requirements for a specific DRG. Patients who stay longer incur more costs. Timely admissions and discharges are important components of cost-effective care. Decreasing the length-of-stay while maintaining quality care and meeting outcomes could lead to hospitals making a "profit" and not losing money. The nursing staff does most of the documentation, and it is this documentation that provides important information that is required to assign DRGs to actual patient services. The DRG is assigned after the patient is discharged, when it is too late to change the care or the documentation. The DRG system does consider outlier factors when determining payment. The hospital may need to consider changes in care and more effective coordination of care. The goal is to decrease the number of outliers,

---

**BOX 5-5     DIAGNOSIS-RELATED GROUPS**

### WHAT ARE DRGS?
Diagnosis-related groups (DRGs) are the basis of payment to hospitals under the Medicare prospective payment system (PPS). Each DRG represents a group of patients that are similar, both clinically and by use of resources. There is a specific payment rate for each DRG that is calculated by a formula. DRGs are the fixed payment amounts for each Medicare inpatient, regardless of length of stay. The location of the hospital, urban or rural, and wage levels are factored into this fixed price. Exceptions are those patients who are outliers or those with exceptional expenses.

### HOW ARE DRGS ASSIGNED?
The patient's physician documents the patient's principal diagnosis by using classifications and terminology found in the *International Classification of Diseases, 9th Revision, Clinical Modification* (ICD-9). In

addition to the principal diagnosis, the following are documented:

- Up to four secondary diagnoses
- Principal procedure and additional procedures
- Patient's age, sex, and discharge status

This information is reported to the hospital's Medicare fiscal intermediary. The information is used to classify the patient into one of 25 major diagnostic categories (MDCs). The principal diagnosis is the condition that caused the hospitalization. The patient is then assigned a DRG from within the MDC. Most MDCs are divided into surgical DRGs and medical DRGs. These DRGs may also be categorized by age, sex, and the presence or absence of complications or comorbidities.

### WHAT IS THE MAJOR COMPLAINT ABOUT DRGS?
Severity of illness is not adequately considered.

| BOX 5-6 | DRG CRITERIA: SEVERITY AND INTENSITY |
|---------|---------------------------------------|

**SEVERITY OF ILLNESS**

Clinical Findings

Chief Complaint Working Diagnosis

Vital Signs

Imaging

Diagnostic Radiology

Ultrasound

Nuclear Medicine Results

Hematology, Chemistry, and Microbiology
  Results

Other Clinical Parameters

**INTENSITY OF ILLNESS**

Physical Evaluation

Monitoring Clinical Elements

Treatment/Medications

Schedules Procedures

and thus decrease financial risk for the organization and risk of additional payment denials. There is no doubt that Medicare and DRGs have had a tremendous impact on health care. They have decreased lengths of stay in hospitals, but this has also increased the need for home health care, long-term care facilities, and ambulatory care. Costs have shifted to other settings, ones that were thought to be more cost-effective.

MEDICARE ELIGIBILITY    Eligibility requirements include the following (Center for Medicare and Medicaid Services, 2009). A person can receive Part A benefits at age 65 without having to pay premiums if the person

- Is eligible to get Social Security or Railroad benefits but has not yet filed for them,
- Or already receives retirement benefits from Social Security or the Railroad Retirement Board,
- Has a spouse with Medicare-covered government employment.

If the person is under 65, the person can receive Part A benefits without having to pay premiums if the person:

- Has received Social Security or Railroad Retirement Board disability benefits for 24 months.
- Has end-stage renal disease and meets certain requirements.

Employers are prohibited from forcing employees that are between the ages of 65 and 69 to use Medicare instead of their employer's health coverage, which would be a financial benefit for employers. If employers could do this, then they would not have to provide coverage for older employees in this age group, reducing health care insurance costs for employers. There continue to be new proposals to change benefits, eligibility, and funding for the Medicare program. Medicare has not been immune to managed care as the federal government does offer managed care options in the Medicare program.

MEDICARE BENEFITS    The Medicare program is composed of four parts: Parts A, B, C, and D (Center for Medicare and Medicaid Services, 2009).

- *Medicare Part A* is the hospital insurance plan, paying for inpatient treatment, skilled nursing facilities (not custodial or long-term care), home health care, and hospice care. Premiums are not paid if the beneficiary or spouse paid Medicare taxes while working. A person may purchase this coverage if the person does not meet past tax payment requirements but must meet citizenship or residency requirements and be 65 or older.
- *Medicare, Part B* is the supplementary medical insurance program, which includes coverage for physician services, outpatient treatment, laboratory testing, and some preventive services. This part is voluntary and requires that the enrollee or beneficiary meets the requirements to be entitled to Part A and is also willing to pay Part B premiums. The Medicare beneficiary must also pay deductibles and co-payments, which are not high. If

the person also qualifies for Medicaid by meeting the requirement of limited financial resources, Medicaid pays the Medicare deductibles and copayments.

Medicare Part B is very different from Part A. Part B resembles typical indemnity coverage and is supplemental medical insurance. Its benefits include physician services and outpatient hospital services, including emergency services, ambulatory surgery, diagnostic tests, laboratory services, durable equipment, and some preventive services. Though enrollment in Part B is voluntary, most beneficiaries enroll because it provides coverage at a reasonable cost. Part B benefits are funded by premiums paid by beneficiaries, annual deductibles, and copayments

- *Medicare, Part C* covers Medicare Parts A and B for all medically needed services, but it is covered by private insurance companies that are approved by Medicare—referred to as Medicare Advantage (MA). In many cases this is a cheaper plan than the original Medicare plan and also includes prescription drug coverage (Part D). Health care reform law of 2010 makes changes to this part, but they will be implemented over time. See Box 5-4.
- *Medicare, Part D* provides coverage for prescription drugs for Medicare beneficiaries. Coverage for prescriptions have improved since Part D was implemented, but there still are cost issues for beneficiaries, some of which are addressed in health care reform of 2010. (See Box 5-4.)

## Medicaid Legislative and Regulatory Issues

- **Social Security Act of 1965, Title XIX** The Social Security Act of 1965, Title XIX, established the jointly funded Medicaid program. Each state and the federal government share the costs associated with Medicaid. The federal government develops the federal guidelines for the program, with HCFA acting as the overall federal agency responsible for its implementation. This legislation was a major breakthrough in establishing a program to provide care for those who could not afford it. The regulations related to this program have grown more complex since 1965, and other laws have also affected the program.
- **Personal Responsibility and Work Opportunity Reconciliation Act of 1996** In 1996, there were several attempts to make major changes in Medicaid, and most were not passed. However, the Personal Responsibility and Work Opportunity Reconciliation Act of 1996 (also known as the Welfare Reform Act) was signed into law (Casto & Layman, 2009). While the law eliminated Aid to Families with Dependent Children (AFDC), families who were eligible for AFDC are usually eligible for TANF (Low-income families with children, including those who meet eligibility for Temporary Assistance for Needy Families (TANF). Prior to this law, Medicaid eligibility income thresholds were set by individual states, and thus there was great state variation in eligibility. Now, poorer states receive a greater percentage of federal matching funds to provide greater parity in state programs. The goal of this legislation is to move people off of welfare into jobs; however, many lose their health benefits when they take jobs that do not offer benefits. This law provides 6 to 12 months of Medicaid coverage during the transition to work. There has been improvement with more people employed; however, there are now more uninsured because of this change and other reasons such as the increased use of temporary staff who get no health coverage, increasing self-employment, and the economic crisis that increased unemployment in 2009–2010.
- **State Children's Health Insurance Program (SCHIP)** This law or Title XXI of the Social Security Act was signed into law in 1997. It is a "state/federal partnership that targets the growing number of children not covered by health insurance" (Casto & Layman, 2009, p. 73). It covers children from families whose incomes are too high to receive Medicaid but too low for private insurance. There is state variation in SCHIP. These children may then get their coverage through Medicaid or through a separate state program. SCHIP has been successful though it has had a rocky history. President Bush would not expand SCHIP; however, President Obama signed legislation expanding SCHIP as one of his first acts in 2009. SCHIP covers inpatient services, outpatient services, physicians' medical and surgical services, laboratory and radiological services, and well-baby and immunization services.

Examples of health care reform 2010 provisions related to Medicaid are described in Box 5-4.

Medicaid is not just a state program, but a program that is funded by the federal government and the states jointly. Each state has its own Medicaid program that provides funding for health care and long-term care or nursing home care. What is the role of the federal government? The federal matching funds are designed so that poorer states receive a larger percentage of the federal Medicaid funds to ensure more equity among the state programs. The state programs must meet federal guidelines established by HCFA. Each state, however, determines its own benefits, its eligibility requirements, and provider fee schedules based on federal guidelines. This is where problems and inequality occur. There is a difference in programs from state to state, particularly in eligibility requirements. All states by federal law, however, must include persons who qualify for AFDC, all needy children under the age of 21, persons who qualify for Old-Age Assistance, persons who qualify for Aid to the Blind, persons who are permanently and totally disabled, and the elderly over 65 years and on welfare. When states set eligibility standards below the federal poverty level, this can cause major problems for many people who need these health care services and cannot receive Medicaid reimbursement. Eligibility standards may have a major effect on providers who may provide care with no reimbursement to cover their costs.

The Medicaid program has also undergone many changes due to the need for cost containment and the increasing use of managed care models and strategies. Medicaid is a program that has been troubled with bureaucracy and inadequate funding. Because of these factors, many providers are not willing to care for Medicaid beneficiaries. Medicaid managed care, however, has made it easier for some providers to participate in the program. Medicaid is a complex program with many regulations. As cost-containment strategies increase, there is concern that coverage for some people will be eliminated or reduced to a point that many Medicaid beneficiaries may not have their health needs met. Advocacy for these patients is very important.

MEDICAID ELIGIBILITY    Welfare reform changed Medicaid eligibility. States may modify their AFDC eligibility criteria, which continue to be the criteria used for TANF to establish eligibility for Medicaid services (Casto & Layman, 2009). A state may lower its income standard but not any lower than what it was in May, 1998. This decreases the number of eligible persons. Second, a state may increase income or resource standards and expand eligibility. This increases the number of eligible persons. Welfare reform also established some specific provisions about eligibility. The most controversial provision is the refusal to work/transition. This gives states the option to discontinue Medicaid coverage for persons who refuse to work and lose TANF. Exceptions are children who are not heads of households and pregnant women. Legal immigrants are also included in these provisions.

Health care coverage for immigrants has long been a problem. "The passage of the Personal Responsibility and Work Opportunity Reconciliation Act (PRWORA) in 1996 changed the eligibility requirements for immigrants, making it more difficult for immigrants, especially those newly arrived in the U.S., to obtain Medicaid coverage. For the first time, the 1996 law tied legal immigrants' eligibility for Medicaid to their length of residency in the U.S. These restrictions also applied to SCHIP, which was established in 1997" (Henry J. Kaiser Family Foundation, April, 2006, p. 1). The following information summarizes Medicaid and SCHIP eligibility rules for immigrants today. Legal permanent residents (immigrants with green cards) are not allowed to apply for Medicaid or SCHIP for the first five years that they are in the U.S. Refugees do not fall under this rule. State Medicaid programs must cover the following groups (Casto & Layman, 2009, p. 71):

- Low-income families with children including those who meet eligibility for Temporary Assistance for Needy Families (TANF)
- People who receive federal Supplemental Security Income (SSI) based on state criteria
- Infants born to Medicaid-eligible pregnant women
- Children under the age of six whose families meet income criteria
- Recipients of adoption assistance and foster care
- Medicare recipients who are elderly and disabled and meet income criteria
- Special protected groups (short-term), for example, persons who lose SSI assistance because of increased wages or Social Security payments

Eligibility is usually influenced by poverty criteria, which are established annually by federal poverty guidelines. These guidelines are based on prospective estimates for a given year. Federal poverty threshold is retrospective data for a given year and used by the Census Bureau for their reports.

MEDICAID BENEFITS   Due to the great variation in the types of Medicaid beneficiaries, Medicaid must provide services across the health care continuum, from preventive care to long-term care and across the lifespan. Medicaid required benefits include the following (Centers for Medicare and Medicaid Services, 2009):

- Inpatient hospital care
- Outpatient hospital care
- Physician services
- Laboratory and radiological services
- Nursing facility services for beneficiaries 21 and older
- Home health care for individuals eligible for nursing facility services
- Medical and surgical dental services
- Family planning services and supplies
- Rural health clinic services
- Pediatric and family nurse practitioner services
- Federally qualified health center services
- Pregnancy-related services and service for other conditions that might complicate pregnancy
- Sixty days postpartum pregnancy-related services
- Nurse-midwifery services
- Early and periodic screening, diagnosis, and treatment services for individuals under 21

Optional benefits that states may offer are prescription medications, prosthetic devices, hearing aids, and care for people who are mentally retarded. The number of people without insurance and unemployed has overtaxed the Medicaid program. This problem is only increasing and is also addressed in health care reform initiatives of 2010. Patients who use Medicaid often have complex medical and socioeconomic issues and could benefit from case management. Every state Medicaid program provides pharmaceutical services, even though it is an optional service. It is provided in order to prevent the use of more costly services, such as surgery or extensive inpatient treatment. States try to control pharmaceutical use by requiring prior **authorization**, prescription caps, and prospective utilization review. Other services that may be provided are case management, transportation, hospice services, personal care services, inpatient psychiatric services, physical and occupational therapy for speech/language/hearing disorders, and respiratory services for children who are dependent on a ventilator. Home and community services may also be provided if the state receives a waiver to do so.

MEDICAID MANAGED CARE RISK   Medicaid, as has been true with other reimbursement methods, has turned to managed care strategies to decrease its costs (Kongvedst, 2009). There is, however, concern that some of the managed care strategies, such as capitation, may have led to underserving patients. In fact, some of these strategies, such as the use of co-payments and deductibles, are prohibited in traditional fee-for-service Medicaid. Proponents of managed care strategies emphasize that managed care focuses on better coordination, prevention, decreased hospitalization, and methods to predict and control costs. Traditional Medicaid pays only for services provided to Medicaid beneficiaries; however, in the managed care model, Medicaid must pay a capitated amount to providers even though services may not be provided. States must ensure that contracts with MCOs meet the following provisions: enrollment, marketing, emergency care, access to care, grievance procedures, and quality of care.

SPECIAL CONSIDERATIONS FOR PEOPLE WITH CHRONIC OR DISABLING ILLNESSES   Medicaid managed care must include care needs for people with chronic and disabling conditions even though these care needs are often not as important for other groups of Medicaid recipients. These needs are individualized care that usually is more complex than care required for other types of patients, comprehensive service systems, and care without cure. The latter is most important, as the need for treatment is typically long term. States have taken various approaches to meeting the needs of these patients in Medicaid managed care.

THE UNINSURED    The uninsured is a growing problem in the United States, as discussed in earlier chapters. There continues to be an increasing number of people without coverage. Children are at greater risk of having no insurance coverage. Sick people approaching 65 have the greater number of medical problems and higher costs. The people who are most likely to have insurance are those who are over 65, which is due to Medicare coverage. Adults who work for hourly wages often do not have insurance. Young adults also may decide not to pay for insurance, feeling that they have no need for it. People without insurance avoid preventive care and wait to receive medical treatment until it is an emergency, and thus frequently the care costs more. With the premiums rising, the problem of the uninsured will only increase.

One reason for this growth is the number of people who have lost Medicaid eligibility and thus health care coverage. Some people leave welfare for low-wage jobs though this is difficult in a time of high unemployment. Low-wage jobs typically do not offer health care coverage. Another group is people that are hired for temporary or contract positions. Many of these people had health insurance coverage in their full-time positions, which may have even been in high-level or professional positions. As more companies outsource, they hire people to fulfill only specific needs temporarily. These positions come without any benefits. In 2008, current numbers, the number of people without health insurance is 45 million, and this number continues to increase (Cover the Uninsured, 2009). The health care reform law of 2010 will have an impact on the uninsured by providing coverage for an additional 32 million people by 2019 and requiring most people to carry insurance or risk paying a fee.

FEDERAL EMPLOYEES HEALTH BENEFIT PROGRAM (FEHBP)    The FEHBP is a special insurance in that the employer is the federal government providing health care insurance to federal employees, retirees, and their dependents in the same way that any other employer might provide coverage. Because of this, it is not technically a government plan but rather an employer plan. This coverage is mandated by law and administered by the federal government's Office of Personnel Management. Members or enrollees of the FEHBP choose from a wide variety of health care plans, including managed care plans, during the government's annual enrollment period. Minimum benefits are required for plans to contract with the FEHBP. The federal government pays part of the premium. The enrollee must pay other costs. Managed care plans are an employee option through the FEHBP. In fact, it was the federal government's success, although limited, with managed care in the 1970s that encouraged the federal government to develop and enact the Health Maintenance Act of 1973. In 1990, the Omnibus Budget Reconciliation Act (OBRA-90) mandated the use of certain managed care strategies in the government's fee-for-service plans to reduce costs such using hospital precertification for nonemergency procedures and case management.

MILITARY HEALTH CARE    Health care coverage for military personnel and their dependents is another major health care expenditure for the government. The military health services system is not just an insurer but also a provider through its health care facilities globally. It provides health benefits to all active-duty military personnel and through its CHAMPUS program to retirees, dependents, and survivors. Many of these beneficiaries are over 65 years of age, and this proportion is expected to increase with the aging of the baby boomers. CHAMPUS was a fee-for-service insurance program for dependents; however, due to its increasing costs, the federal government also uses managed care approaches such as HMOs, point-of-service, and preferred provider plans. The Veterans Health Administration has also undergone changes (e.g., introducing primary care, regional centers and marketing, case management). This system provides ambulatory care, acute care, and in some cases long-term care, for military veterans.

STATE INSURANCE PROGRAMS    States also offer insurance to their state employees. Usually the state government is a state's largest employer and consequently largest insurer, and there is some degree of choice among plan options for state employees. The state or a contracted provider administrates these plans. State employees contribute to the payment of this coverage in the same way they would if they were employed in the private sector.

# Managed Care

Health care reimbursement is a complex process, which has been made even more complex by the use of managed care. Understanding how this process works and who the players are in the process helps health care providers advocate for their patients and intervene in the process to ensure that quality care is not compromised and that health care professional needs are considered. Today, reimbursement and managed care are inseparable. Nurses play active roles in the various models of managed care, and these models affect the practice of most health care professionals daily in many health care settings. Nurses are also employed by MCOs. They provide direct care, work with enrollees, determine allocation of benefits, and act as case managers. Some nurses hold management positions in MCOs. Over time managed care has become less important though managed care strategies have been integrated into many third-party payer health plans. Insurers have become more interested in consumer issues and recognize the need to attract consumers. This is partially due to managed care. There was a consumer backlash to the controlling aspects of managed care and this backlash emphasized the need to listen to consumers.

## Managed Care Models and Their Characteristics

The health maintenance organization (HMO) was the first managed care model; however, many others have been developed. Why did this happen? Consumers were not always happy with HMOs. The problem of increasing health care costs became a serious issue in the 1980s. Insurers, who were in competition with HMOs, began to develop new models for health care management, and employers were interested in these other options. Today, health care professionals and consumers experience a maze of different MCO models. Trying to compare and contrast their characteristics can be an overwhelming task; however, over time it has become more difficult to distinguish among the managed care models. In the earlier period of managed care development it was easier to see the major differences in the MCO models and other types of third-party payers. First, it is helpful to review a definition of managed health care, which has been described as "a regrettably nebulous term. At the very least, managed care can be described as a system of health care delivery that tries to manage the cost of health care, the quality of that health care, and the access to that care. Common denominators seen in MCOs include a panel of contracted providers, who are mostly physicians but may include other health care professionals such as advanced practice nurses, that is less than the entire universe of available providers, some type of limitations on benefits to subscribers who use non-contracted providers (unless authorized to do so), and some type of authorization system" (Kongstvedt, 2009, p. 230).

The most important difference in the managed care models is the relationship between the managed care organization and the participating providers, particularly physicians. The role of traditional indemnity insurance has been to process and pay medical bills. MCOs have a more comprehensive approach that has affected how MCOs are organized. MCOs continue to process and pay medical bills, but MCOs have become more involved in the management of their members' health care, focusing on appropriate care, when it is needed, and illness and disease prevention and even more health promotion.

## Provider Panels

The managed care **provider panel** is a key managed care concept. It is a group of providers that are contracted to provide service to enrollees in the MCO, the insurer. Examples of providers are physicians, advanced practice nurses, nurse midwives, hospitals, clinics, long-term care facilities, home health agencies, laboratories, durable equipment suppliers, pharmacies, and so on. Provider panels are selected and organized in a variety of ways. These differences are found in the descriptions of each MCO model. Providers are accepted or rejected based on the MCO's criteria. Clearly, this has serious consequences for providers, for example, physicians who may not be accepted for a provider panel, even causing providers to lose patients who have to select another provider when their insurer no longer includes their provider in its panel. If the person continues with the provider who is not in the panel then the person must pay out-of-pocket for the care.

Control is a major issue with MCOs. Physician providers may be selected as individual physicians or as groups of physicians. Medical groups contract with an MCO as a group, but the MCO still evaluates individual physicians within the group. A medical or practice group is typically two or more physicians that work together to provide medical services to patients. Nurse practitioners and nurse midwives may be part of a medical group and in some cases have formed their own groups. Usually, these provider groups share a single office or may have satellite offices to expand their geographic coverage. There is one medical record for each patient that is shared among all the providers in the medical group. This facilitates coordination of care for the practice and for the patient.

## Managed Care Models

HEALTH MAINTENANCE ORGANIZATIONS (HMOS)    The **Health maintenance organization (HMO)** was the first managed care model; however, many others have been developed. Health maintenance organizations have changed since the 1920s. The HMO pays the bills for its members' health services, but it also manages and provides care to its members. The HMO Act of 1973 describes an HMO as an organized entity that

- Ensures health care service delivery in a specific geographic area.
- Provides basic and optional benefits.
- Enrollees join voluntarily.

HMOs integrate the delivery of service with reimbursement for those services. The HMO is the original model or prototype of managed care. It develops incentives to encourage its providers to provide the lowest-cost care to the HMO members. An HMO contracts with providers for health care services required to meet the comprehensive health care needs of the HMO members and often are considered HMO employees. This is done on a prepaid basis. Employers pay the HMO to provide these services via premiums, and the HMO agrees to provide specific services. Typically, HMOs have focused on comprehensive care, illness and disease prevention, and health promotion. Patient volume and risk for illness and disease are important factors when an HMO seeks contracts with employers. There are several types of HMOs, and HMO control over its providers varies with each of these models. There are other types of MCO models whose major characteristics are summarized in Table 5-1.

## Managed Care Strategies to Control Cost and Quality

How do MCOs cut health care expenses and yet still ensure quality care? Service and reimbursement strategies are used to manage the health care services and to reduce costs. Today, many different types of third-party payers use many of these strategies. It is important for all health care providers, including nurses in all types of settings, to understand the strategies that are used and their purposes. Service strategies are methods used by MCOs and frequently are now used by other types of insurers that have adopted managed care strategies to manage delivery of care. The purpose of these strategies is to decrease cost and provide quality care. The MCO wants to find better, more cost-effective treatments; however, this is a strategy that has not been fully utilized. It is quite clear by now that as MCOs have been trying to decrease health care costs, provider roles, and responsibilities, provider–insurer/MCO relationships, patient needs, and at the same time societal health care needs have undergone major changes and will continue to do so. There is no doubt that health care delivery has been affected by managed care service strategies, but it is not always clear if costs have been better controlled with these strategies or if the quality of care has changed, positively or negatively.

Efficiency is a critical component of these strategies. The goal is to minimize costs and choose services with the maximum excess of benefits over costs. Just focusing cost-containment efforts on decreasing costs will not be enough in the long run. Achieving the desired outcome has become more important over the past few years, which definitely relates to achieving greater benefits over costs. Have MCOs been successful with strategies to increase efficiency? At this time, not much data are available to support linking costs with outcomes. The belief is, however, that managed care has more ability to do this than did traditional

| TABLE 5-1 | COMMON MANAGED CARE MODELS |
| --- | --- |

The following are several of the more common managed care models.

| Health Maintenance Organization (HMO) | Preferred Provider Organization (PPO) | Point-of-Service (POS) | Carve-Outs |
| --- | --- | --- | --- |
| The HMO is the original model or prototype of managed care, which integrates the delivery of service with reimbursement for those services. The HMO pays the bills for its members' health services, but it also manages and provides care to its members. An enrollee in an HMO such as Group Health goes to one site to receive care, both primary and usually specialty care. Most HMOs do require that the patient/enrollee pay a small co-payment. There may be limited provider choice. The HMO develops incentives to encourage its providers to provide the lowest-cost care to the HMO members. | A PPO is a delivery network of providers, physicians, advanced practice nurses, hospitals, and other providers. The PPO does not assume any financial risk or receive premiums, but it does charge for use of its provider network. The PPO itself is not directly involved in the delivery of health care services; rather, it acts as an intermediary to negotiate and manage the managed care contracts on behalf of the individual providers. Capitation is not common with a PPO, but rather reimbursement is usually based on the fee schedule identified by the PPO. Typically, members pay lower deductibles and coinsurance when they use providers in the PPO provider panel. PPOs do not focus on utilization management and quality assurance, which is not true of other MCO models. The PPO has become the most acceptable MCO model because consumers have the most choice in providers and do not have to get a referral from a primary care provider to see a specialist. | The POS model provides more choice for the enrollee/patient, but at a price to the enrollee. The enrollee may determine at the time that a health care service is needed whether to use a provider in the MCO panel or one outside the panel. If the enrollee chooses a provider outside the panel, then the enrollee pays higher co-payments and deductibles. When the enrollee goes outside the panel, the provider is paid on a fee-for-service basis. The MCO hopes that over time the enrollee will choose not to use the POS option. A POS option may be found in a number of different MCO models. | A carve-out is another method for organizing managed care services. These are health care services that are separated or carved out of a regular health care service contract and then are contracted separately in a separate plan. Services that are carved out are ones that are high volume or high cost. Psychiatric services, substance abuse treatment, prescriptions, radiology, laboratory, vision, and dental are typical services that are often carved out. The patient may need to pay an additional premium and meet different requirements for the use of these services, particularly related to referrals. Mental health treatment and substance abuse treatment are the two most common services offered in this manner. The enrollee usually does not even realize that a carve-out exists. |

indemnity insurance. Box 5-7 summarizes some of the service strategies, which may also be used by all types of insurers, not just MCOs.

PROVIDER PERFORMANCE    Provider performance has never been more important. Today, when MCOs contract with new providers to join their provider panels or renew contracts with providers, the MCOs base their provider selection on specific criteria. Why is this so important? The MCO wants providers who offer cost-effective, quality care that meets the MCO criteria. As managed care developed through the 1980s and 1990s, cost-effectiveness became more important than quality; today, quality issues are slowly becoming more important. The goal of performance-based reimbursement evaluation is to alter provider performance. How the MCO goes about reaching this goal can vary and can mean the difference in success or failure. Rewards work better than sanctions, but both may be used. The MCO may financially reward providers who meet the MCO's criteria for cost-effective care by offering bonuses or close the provider off from receiving new enrollees. The goal is to discourage the use of inappropriate and costly services. MCOs typically use continuing education, data and feedback, practice guidelines, and protocols to encourage providers to change their behavior. Examples of indicators that are used to evaluate provider performance are the following:

- Member satisfaction data
- Member complaint and grievance rates

## BOX 5-7    SERVICE STRATEGIES

### CHANGING PRACTICE PATTERNS

There is no doubt that managed care has affected how physicians, registered nurses, and all other types of providers deliver their care and services today. The greatest change in practice patterns has been the gradual move from the acute care setting to the home and community. Today, many providers focus on ambulatory care. There is also an increased emphasis on primary care. Providers are now more concerned with what treatment is really necessary and how to get the job done quickly. Hospitals have changed the way that they deliver care and are more interested in shortening length-of-stay, the utilization of resources, and the development of ambulatory services (e.g., clinics, wellness centers, ambulatory surgery, home care). Changing practice patterns has been positive for nursing and will continue to offer new opportunities for nursing. For example, physicians and health care organizations are recognizing the value of using advanced practice nurses and nurse-midwives to assist them in increasing their patient volume and reallocating their time. MCOs have gained more control over physician practice. With financial incentives driving many physician decisions, can the patient trust the physician to be completely honest about treatment options, even the expensive ones? This is one reason why it is important for all health care providers, such as nurses, to understand incentives and other service and reimbursement strategies used by MCOs. These strategies affect nursing care and the nursing profession; treatment patients receive or do not receive; length-of-stay and length-of-treatment; communication with providers; and trust in all health care providers. Consumers also need to be aware of these strategies, and they will turn to nurses for guidance and information.

### PRIMARY CARE

The **primary care provider (PCP)** plays a major role in the managed care environment. The major PCP responsibility is to coordinate comprehensive care and serve as a gatekeeper. Not all models of managed care require that every enrollee have a PCP. The managed care organization identifies the qualifications of the PCP, which may vary among MCOs. In addition, pressures from consumers and physicians have also changed how MCOs describe primary care providers. The traditional view was that the PCP should be a family practice physician. Other health care providers who may now be classified as PCPs are medical internists, pediatricians, obstetrician–gynecologists, and ophthalmologists, and some MCOs have contracted with advanced practice nurses to serve as PCPs. Another important characteristic of a PCP is the patient does not need a referral from a provider to see the PCP. The gatekeeping responsibility is used to control over-utilization of specialists and other medical costs. Patient choice is limited by this strategy. The PCP, in the role of the gatekeeper, does this for the patient. In addition, the PCP coordinates the patient's care, which should improve the outcomes. Concerns about cost and appropriate treatment utilization are not illegitimate; however, consumers have generally disliked the idea of having to go through a physician or another provider in order to see a specialist. The PCP may be paid using the capitation method to provide the contracted services identified by the MCO. This strategy provides additional cost control. In addition, MCO performance profiles provide descriptive data on the provider's utilization of services, such as laboratory testing, referrals to specialists, use of formulary, and the like, and are used to control costs.

### SPECIALTY CARE

In the managed care environment, the PCP and the authorization process have a major impact on specialty care. The rigid approach to specialty care used in the early 1990s, however, has been loosening up. This has occurred primarily because consumers dislike the lack of physician choice and have spoken out against this approach. Specialty physicians also found the rigid process associated with gatekeeping and authorization a major deterrent to practice survival. Open access, allowing for greater direct access to specialists, is provided in different ways by more MCOs today. The patient may have to pay an additional co-payment to have a choice of specialists, but some MCOs are not charging for the option of choice although still requiring authorization from the PCP. MCOs are providing more information to enrollees about the use of specialists and access to them. This information is often found on the Internet. There was concern about increased utilization and continuity of care; specialty referrals are not as tightly controlled. However, some MCOs have found that these concerns have not played out the way

## BOX 5-7 SERVICE STRATEGIES (CONTINUED)

they expected. Usually, these MCOs have developed systems to keep PCPs informed about their patient specialty usage.

### RESOURCE MANAGEMENT

Resource management is important to any MCO. The MCO's goal is to ensure that care is cost-effective, efficient, and of the appropriate quality. To do this, resources need to be used wisely. Resource management is interconnected with utilization and authorization. In the past the system of care was characterized by an independent array of disjointed providers and purchasers. Each provided many effective services for the consumers of health care, but they failed to overcome their independent interests to focus on the values of overall effectiveness. This led, in part, to oversupply of capacity, tremendous variability of outcomes, and duplication of resources. Managed care has influenced all types of insurers and all now recognize that resources must be managed better than in the past. Nursing needs to take a lead in defining how nursing resources should be managed in order to meet outcomes of cost and quality. It becomes more important to identify clear outcomes, use scientifically determined best practices to achieve outcomes, measure progress, and when required, to reinvent the processes through which care is delivered.

### UTILIZATION MANAGEMENT

Utilization management is the process of evaluating the necessity, appropriateness, and efficiency of health care services used by the enrollees/patients who receive care from a provider. Utilization data are used to assess care and by external organizations to assess the quality of the MCO's services. Authorization is the major method used in utilization management. This is the payer's approval for a health care provider to provide specific care. The MCO or payer identifies what services or benefits require authorization. To be truly effective in controlling costs, an insurer must be able to influence provider utilization behavior. For example, if an insurer or MCO cannot find a way to decrease a provider's number of hospital admissions or the number of referrals to specialists, costs will continue to be a problem. The purchaser of the plan, the employer, does not like the idea of health care costs increasing and may decide to drop the MCO and contract with another, more cost-effective MCO. Who can

authorize services is a critical decision. This decision is made in several ways. Probably, the most recognized method is to have authorization done by the primary care provider/ physician. If an enrollee wants to see the PCP, no authorization is required. Some MCOs require that plan staff authorize services. In this case, the physician or other type of provider calls a plan representative and describes the patient's problems and need for services. The staff representative compares this information with predetermined criteria. Often, this representative is a nurse. Nurses are finding many new roles in managed care, and this is one of them. The nurse discusses the patient's needs with the provider and determines whether authorization can be provided. If the provider does not agree with the decision, the provider is referred to a supervisor or the medical director. Some plans use a different system. They have the enrollee call the plan directly, using a nurse advice line. The enrollee does not have to go to the PCP to use a specialist but uses the advice line to gain authorization. The nurse uses predetermined criteria or protocols to assess the enrollee's needs for care and then tells the enrollee the type of provider that is required.

### HEALTH PROMOTION & DISEASE AND ILLNESS PREVENTION

Health promotion and disease and illness prevention are strategies that focus on encouraging the enrollee to become a partner in maintaining health. Education is a key method for accomplishing this partnership. Each time an MCO develops health promotion and disease and illness prevention services, it reassesses the costs and benefits of these services. MCOs vary in how much of this strategy is applied to its plan. The goals of health promotion are to help people modify their lifestyles and make choices to improve their health and quality of life. Health education is very important in helping enrollees/patients to accomplish this goal. After the MCO identifies the health promotion and disease and illness preventive services to offer, it must develop the services, ensure that providers provide the services, and then communicate their availability to the enrollees. MCOs use newsletters, personal letters, information provided at the worksite, and the Internet to share information with their enrollees. Models of managed care other than HMOs, such as PPOs, may cover

*(continued)*

## BOX 5-7     SERVICE STRATEGIES (CONTINUED)

the services or may set a dollar amount for preventive services. In the latter case, the enrollee has more choice as to how to use the money set aside for health promotion and prevention. Some plans may require co-payments and deductibles for these services.

### MANAGEMENT OF ANCILLARY SERVICES

Diagnostic and therapeutic services are ancillary services, and they greatly affect the costs of medical care. Typical diagnostic services are radiology, laboratory testing, electrocardiography, invasive imaging, and cardiac testing. Examples of ancillary therapeutic services are physical therapy, occupational therapy, speech therapy, and cardiac rehabilitation. Pharmacy service is also an ancillary service. These services are different from other services in that they require an order from a provider. Patients cannot just request a specific laboratory test or the like. These services have been identified as high-cost services with potential for overutilization. Their overuse or inappropriate use has often increased health care costs. How does the MCO control the utilization of these services? Collection of utilization data is very important. These data are collected so that individual providers can be evaluated. Standards of care and protocols are developed by the MCO to educate and guide the provider when decisions are made to use ancillary services. Another method used to control usage is the authorization process and limiting who can authorize services, which provides more rigid

control. Some MCOs also limit how many times the enrollee can receive the service before reauthorization is required. For example, how many physical therapy sessions can a stroke patient receive before reauthorization is required? The reauthorization typically requires reassessment of the patient's needs. This control of usage has been a problem for some patients and providers.

Service strategies have had an impact on changing health care and costs; however, reimbursement strategies probably receive the brunt of the criticisms directed at managed care. MCOs use a variety of strategies that focus on reimbursement to control medical costs, and these strategies require an understanding of the incentives that are important to managed care and buyers of health care (employers and government primarily). The incentive for MCOs is profit, which requires reduced costs. The incentive for the buyer, who is usually the employer, is reduced costs. The situation becomes complicated when one considers that the goal of the provider, especially the physician, advanced practice nurses, hospitals, and other health care professionals, is to provide quality care. Clearly, these may be conflicting goals, and this affects the outcomes. Even the choice of reimbursement strategies has caused conflict, more so than service strategies. The following provides a brief overview of some of these reimbursement strategies: provider performance, capitation, length-of-stay management, and formularies.

- Wait time for appointments
- Utilization rates
- Immunization rates
- Complication rates
- Overall medical costs or medical costs per member per month
- Hospital readmission rates
- Mammography rates
- Number and typed procedures
- Length-of-stay
- Number and type of prescriptions
- Capitation

LENGTH-OF-STAY (LOS) MANAGEMENT    Hospital occupancy rates and LOS for all types of patients have been decreasing, which has been supported by managed care. Managing LOS is an important method in controlling costs. This change to reduced LOS has increased the utilization of ambulatory care services, home care, subacute services, and other types of services that replace inpatient treatment. Nursing has been concerned about the decrease as it has affected patient care and patients' needs. There is increased nursing resource consumption as LOS is reduced. The first hospitalization days have higher requirements for nursing hours, particularly the first 2 days. Nurses are now encountering more acute patients on admission because patients are kept out of the hospital until it is absolutely necessary to admit them. This has increased care needs. There is also increased pressure to provide rapid patient and family education, with little time to provide it. Is money actually saved when LOS is shortened? At what point does the decreased LOS actually increase nursing costs? These are critical questions that require further research. It is important for nursing to continue to pursue further understanding of the impact of LOS on care needs and outcomes.

FORMULARIES   Advances in pharmaceuticals have helped patients to live normal lives and have decreased health care costs, but at the same time these advances have increased medical costs. This may seem contradictory; however, both have occurred. For example, new AIDS medications have decreased the number of hospitals days, but these drugs are also very expensive. Antibiotics prevent patients from becoming sick or sicker; however, some antibiotics are very expensive. Careful cost–benefit analysis is required. The federal government is more concerned about the increasing costs of drugs. To cope with these increasing pharmaceutical costs, the use of formularies is a critical reimbursement strategy that is used to control the ever-increasing costs of drugs. The **formulary** is the insurer's list of drugs or classes of drugs that the insurer prefers that providers use. There are three types of formularies: open, incentive, and closed. An *open formulary* means that the enrollee pays extra fees for using non-formulary drugs. With the *incentive formulary*, the insurer reimburses for drugs outside the formulary, but the enrollee is responsible for additional co-pay. This type of formulary is designed to encourage the enrollee not to use non-formulary medications. When a *closed formulary* is used, there is no reimbursement for drugs that are not in the formulary.

How does an insurer determine which drugs to include in its formulary? Most insurers use safety, effectiveness, cost, and cost-effectiveness as their criteria. No insurer formulary includes all of the drugs approved by the Food and Drug Administration (FDA). The formulary typically focuses on generic drugs because these tend to be less expensive than the brand-name products, though usually chemically equivalent. Many drugs are the same, but their therapeutic effect or their side effects may vary. For some patients, excluding drugs that they have found helpful may be a serious problem. This is particularly important for patients with chronic illnesses for whom a specific drug is more effective. When the insurer's formulary changes and the drug is not included or if the patient changes third-party payers and the new insurer formulary does not include the drug, the patient may suffer. Insurers must also consider the value of adding new drugs that are expensive, including biotechnology products. These drugs and products tend to be very expensive. Clearly, an insurer must weigh the costs and benefits of using these therapies. It needs data that demonstrate significant clinical advantages, but these advantages still may not be enough to support the decision to cover their use. Insurer protocols and authorization procedures are established for these highly expensive drugs. Another treatment issue is that most of the new biotech treatments are injectable, and typically insurers do not cover injectables under the category of pharmacy but rather as medical expenses. As these drugs become more common, this medical expense classification will require reconsideration. The pharmacy coverage may be different from other benefits, often more limited, and thus there may be some advantage in reclassifying biotech drugs as pharmacy expenses.

Many factors have an impact on the use of drugs today. Providers are inundated with drug information via the mail, Internet, and the ever-growing pharmaceutical sales force. Drug companies are also marketing directly to the consumer/patient, which has increased the number of patients going to providers requesting specific medications through all types of media. All of this increases drug costs and the pressure that providers feel to prescribe drugs and sometimes, specific drugs. The formulary presents other problems for the prescribing provider. Some providers have found that certain drugs work better than others or have fewer side effects, but the patient's insurer formulary does not reimburse for these drugs. This presents a conflict for the provider. In addition, most providers have contracts with many insurers. Each one has a formulary, and some are quite different from others. The provider, who is already inundated with paperwork and administration, is confronted with more information and differences. Many providers will choose the path of least resistance and use the least restrictive formularies, but these formularies may offer limited drug options. Authorization may also be required to receive reimbursement for non-formulary drugs.

Managed care is changing due to demands from providers and consumers. What will happen in the future with the managed care approach to reimbursement is still unknown. Some believe that the traditional approach or the managed care approach that is now used will not be successful in the long term. The ideal managed care delivery system will be an organized body of health services and financial mechanisms. It will operate in an integrated and systematic fashion to manage and provide the right wellness, medical, and related services at the right place and time. Health insurers in general have begun to use many of the MCO strategies that have been discussed so that they are no longer just MCO strategies at a time when managed care or MCOs are less important. They have, however, had a major impact on health reimbursement.

## Reimbursement Issues: Impact on Nurses and Nursing Care

Reimbursement has a major impact on nurses and on nursing care. What are some ways this impact has been felt? Nurses are not expected to be reimbursement experts, but understanding how care is paid for is important. It is particularly important if reimbursement affects which provider delivers care, to whom it is delivered, where and when it is delivered, what type of care can be provided, and when care might have to end. If one does not understand reimbursement and its role in health care delivery, one might think that these decisions have nothing to do with the payment of care and are only connected to the provider and the patient. This, however, is not true. Reimbursement is another layer to the complex health care delivery process and system that cannot be ignored. How have nursing and nurses been affected by reimbursement, and how can they affect reduction in costs? The following are some examples.

- Managing within fixed resources and decreasing costs by reducing waste and inefficiencies are more important to nursing today than they were in the past. Compared with other providers, nurses use the most resources, such as supplies and equipment, in the acute care setting, and through their usage they can make a difference in reducing waste and inefficiencies. The early history of nursing was one of "you don't need to know the budget or what things cost." This attitude is no longer acceptable if the organization expects to make a difference in reducing its costs.
- Nursing staff levels have also been affected by reimbursement as hospitals and other health care organizations have had to change staffing levels due to costs. This change requires that nurses assess how they deliver care and search for more efficient methods. In addition, nurses are speaking out more about staffing levels and their impact on patient care and quality and safety outcomes.
- Nursing has always been concerned with health promotion and prevention of illness and disease—important aspects of managed care. Nursing education emphasizes this content even more today. Nurses have even entered the primary care area with the increased usage of advanced practice nurses, who may serve as primary care providers.
- Quality and outcomes are not foreign to nursing, but nurses are not experts in these areas. Nurses, like other health care professionals, have yet to fully implement programs that access quality and outcomes. Much must be learned about these critical processes, and managed care seems to be driving the need for further development. Nurses could play an important role in this development. Health care professionals need to reexamine how they have assessed the quality of their care (see Chapters 16 and 17).
- Access to care has also been a concern of nursing, but again nursing has not been any more successful in this area than any other health care profession. Nurses have the opportunity to make major contributions when access to care is discussed in planning meetings in the acute care setting, and access issues are part of an important concern in community health. Nurses must participate actively in this planning, or they will be left out of the process.
- Nurses have been comfortable working in differentiated structures that are organized around specific diagnostic clusters (e.g., medicine, critical care, obstetrics, and support services such as nutritional or environmental services). More organizations are recognizing that this might not be the most effective way to structure the work. Greater emphasis is

now placed on coordination of work across parts of the organization. To survive the changes in the future and develop new roles, nurses need to be active participants in these new delivery systems. The following are some issues that are particularly affected by the macrolevel of health care financial issues.

1. Cost of care is more important than charges for care, which typically do not cover all the costs of care. This factor drives all decisions that are made, whether they are patient-related or not. Operating costs have to be covered.
2. Understanding health care reimbursement is critical, and not just by nurse leaders/managers, but also staff nurses.
3. The continuum of care has become more important and will continue to be so. What are its components? Are they easily accessible? What are the roles of nurses in helping the patient through the continuum and the roles of nurses within each component? Getting the appropriate care in the best setting from the most appropriate provider reduces costs.
4. There is an increased emphasis on patient education, promotion, and prevention, which are aimed at improving quality but also decreasing costs.
5. Caregivers (families, significant others) have taken on major roles in the health care delivery system supporting and caring for family members. Are they prepared for this? Are they available for this? How does their usage affect health care costs?
6. Provider performance evaluation is now the norm, even if it does cause stress. This includes performance data about hospitals, clinics, home care, long-term care, physicians, advanced practice nurses, and so on. Development of computer technology has helped move this along. These data are used to make reimbursement decisions.
7. The hospital discharge process has become more important. This affects the entire continuum of care and yet staff must care for sicker patients who are discharged, with less staff and less time.
8. Outcomes are constantly monitored. Paying for something that does reach expected outcomes is costly.
9. Quality improvement and costs are interconnected in all types of health care settings.

## Health Care Financial Issues: Microlevel

The microlevel focuses on an individual health care organization's financial issues. New nurses are typically not responsible for budgeting; however, a general understanding of the process as well as other related issues is important as they affect nurses and how they practice.

Prior to entering a more detailed discussion, it is helpful to review that some organizations are classified as for-profit and others as not-for-profit. It is not uncommon for staff to have only negative views of for-profit organizations. What do these two classifications really mean? In simplest terms, a for-profit organization must return some of its profits to its stockholders or owners. A not-for-profit organization does not have stockholders or owners who require returned profit; however, in this case the profit is reinvested in the organization. All organizations need to make a profit to stay in the "black" because, if this does not occur, debt will increase, the organization may be in the "red," and the organization over the long term will fail financially. This organization will be forced to reduce costs, which will impact care delivery and nurses. The key difference between these two types of organizations is how the profit is used. Even for-profit organizations need to use some of their profit on their organization; therefore, not all of it goes to stockholders or owners.

A second critical area in microlevel financing is the idea that budgeting is a very real description of the financial status of the organization. It is not something that is just described on paper. When the budget is prepared, it is just an educated guess. This process requires data that are as accurate as they can be. Change is a frequent theme in this text, and this is certainly true of budgets. Changes in many factors that affect health care delivery can mean the provider or organization must make budget adjustments. Examples of these factors are number of patients admitted, length-of-stay, decreasing amount of reimbursement, increased staffing costs or costs of staff benefits, change in the cost of supplies, need to renovate or expand space, expansion of computerized documentation, and need to purchase new medical equipment.

## APPLYING EVIDENCE-BASED PRACTICE

### Evidence for Effective Leadership and Management

**Citation:**  Pappas, S. (2008). The cost of nurse-sensitive adverse events. *JONA*, 38(5), 230–236.

**Overview:**  This non-experimental, descriptive research project examined a methodology to determine the cost of adverse events and effective levels of nurse staffing on two acute care hospitals including six units. Greater knowledge of quality and cost outcomes has led to changes to increase nurse staffing effectiveness. If we know the cost of complications and staffing and recognize staffing levels might reduce complications, then improving staffing could potentially make a difference in costs. The study does link patient-level clinical and financial outcome data, particularly in relation to adverse events to actual patient-level cost per case. This information can be used to support a need for higher levels of staffing to avoid increase costs for adverse events.

**Application:**  Nursing has struggled for a long time to take its place at the budget table—to make a case that what nurses do can reduce costs not just increase costs. This article provides a good example of a study that focuses on the need to be clearer about the impact of nursing care and that nurses can make important contributions to the budget process and financial management.

**Questions:**

1. *How do you think staffing impacts patient outcomes? Provide specific examples.*
2. *Discuss the relationship between adverse events, patient characteristics, and nurse staffing.*
3. *If you were a chief nurse executive for an acute care hospital, how might you use this study in your organization?*

The third critical issue is microlevel financial issues have a direct impact on the delivery of health care and on nursing. Much more will be discussed about this issue. These finances directly affect decisions about staffing, supplies and equipment, renovation of facilities, types of services provided, quality of services, accessibility of services, employee education and training, and much more. So even if staff nurses do not prepare the budget, it directly affects them.

This section of the chapter discusses an overall review of the financial component of hospital/other types of health care organizations, key financial management terminology, the budgeting process, productivity, and cost containment. Staff nurses typically do not become directly involved in these functions, although at times they may be asked for input on the budget at the unit level, and their work affects productivity and cost containment. Nurses who go into management positions need to become more involved in budgeting, and when this occurs, they need to devote more time to learning much more about financial health care issues at the microlevel.

### Financial Component of Hospitals and Other Types of Health Care Organizations

Each health care organization has its own financial system; however, there are some common elements of these systems that are helpful for nurses to understand. They affect nursing staff and nursing care. The governing body of the organization such as the board of directors is ultimately responsible for the financial activities and stability of the organization. The board oversees the organization's budgetary process and approves the final budget.

- The budget is prepared and submitted by the organization's chief executive officer (CEO).
- The CEO may delegate the day-to-day financial operations to other staff such as the chief operating officer (COO) and the chief financial officer (CFO) or comptroller.
- The chief nurse executive (CNE) is typically responsible for the nursing budget that is submitted to the COO along with assistance from the CFO and then to the CEO.

- The key high-level management staff should collaborate in the development of the overall organizational budget. Department heads, which should include directors of nursing for services and nurse managers, participate by developing budgets for their services and units, and then these budgets are passed up the line to become part of the overall budget.

This does not mean that all of these budgets are accepted as originally submitted. As the budgets go up the line, compromises need to be made—not everyone gets what they request. The final product or organization budget is a compilation of all of these budget requests.

This process takes time. Data from past budgets are used in developing subsequent budgets. Staff may participate at the unit or service level as managers request staff input about budgetary needs for the coming year. All through the budget process consideration should be given to the organization's vision, mission, and goals and marketing plan. For example, if an expansion of services is planned then this would need to be included in the budget planning with consideration given to additional staffing, equipment and supplies, physical plant changes, marketing expenses, staff training, the impact expansion will have on other services, and so on. This process is really the same in all types of health care organizations, but, of course, the smaller and less complex organizations may not have as many levels in the process.

## Key Financial Management Terminology

Financial management is highly complex and a specialty area in health care administration. The major goal is to obtain the funds necessary to meet the organization's goals. Nurses are not expected to be experts; however, they will hear some financial/budgetary terms and need to know what they are in order to participate as much as possible in this process. The organization needs accurate data to do the following: (a) guide operations of the organization, (b) make effective decisions about financial issues, and (c) monitor and control operations by using variance analysis.

The following are common budget terms.

- **Accounts receivable:** An amount owed to the health care organization (HCO) by a patient or customer for services. If these accounts are not paid in a timely manner, this does have an effect on the HCO's ability to pay its own bills.
- **Actual figures:** The exact amount of revenue and expenses the HCO experiences; these figures are not the amounts that were estimated or proposed for the budget, but rather the real numbers.
- **Asset:** An item owned by the HCO with value that can be identified objectively (for example, the value of equipment used in the operating room over a long period of time).
- **Bad debt:** An amount due to the HCO that will never be collected (for example, a patient who has no coverage for care and cannot pay the bill). Too much bad debt is a serious problem for an organization.
- **Balance sheet:** A financial statement identifying the HCO's assets and liabilities at a specific time. Assets are always found on the left of the balance sheet and liabilities on the right.
- **Budgeted figures:** The projected numbers the HCO expects in revenues and expenses that are identified in the budget.
- **Cost center:** The smallest functional unit that can be identified for cost control and accountability (for example, the cardiac care unit, the emergency department, pharmacy, etc.).
- **Cost per unit of service or unit cost:** The cost to produce a single unit of service (for example, provide a specific laboratory test, administer medications, prepare a meal, clean a room after discharge, or make a home visit).
- **Depreciation:** Allocation of cost of large capital assets by recognizing a portion of the cost for each year of its estimated life. If the HCO purchases equipment for the laboratory, it would estimate how long these machines typically last and then determine how much of the cost to allocate to the budget each year. For example, if the equipment costs $10,000, and the equipment is expected to last for 5 years, the organization would allocate a certain amount of the $10,000 for each year. At the end of the 5 years the equipment would not be an asset with value.

- **Direct costs:**   Costs that are incurred in giving direct care, which is not simple to allocate or determine as it depends on the type of service the cost is covering. For example, direct cost for a nurse working in a neonatal unit would be costs of the nurse's time to provide an infant care or the supplies required to provide that care. Allocating supply costs is much easier than allocating staff time.
- **Expenditure:**   A liability that is incurred from the acquisition of an asset (e.g., buying new equipment for the laboratory).
- **Expense:**   A decrease in the HCO's equity due to operations (e.g., funds to purchase medical supplies, staff hours). Important expenses include supplies, which is an area where nurses can assist in controlling costs.
- **Fiscal year:**   The identified time period for each budget cycle (July to July or January to January), which is then subdivided in a variety of ways—for example, biweekly, monthly, quarterly, semiannually.
- **Fixed costs:**   The costs that do not increase or decrease as a result of changes in volume or patient days (for example, specific salary levels, minimum staffing required, electricity, depreciation, telephone, or computer).
- **Income statement:**   A statement of revenues and expenses for a specific time period (see Box 5-8).
- **Indirect costs:**   Costs that are indirectly related to patient care; for example, supplies needed to provide care would be direct costs while the unit secretary's time to order supplies would be indirect. However, despite the distinction noted in this definition and the definition of direct costs, the salaries for all involved in the examples (nurses, supervisor, and unit secretary) would be listed under direct costs in the budget.
- **Indirect overhead:**   Costs that cannot be associated with a specific patient care provided or support services. These costs are usually allocated to a department (for example, time spent completing unit data logs or ordering supplies).
- **Liabilities:**   Money an organization owes to someone.
- **Overhead:**   Any cost of doing business that is not a direct cost of service and cannot easily be allocated to individual patients and even to individual units or services (e.g., utility costs).
- **PD:**   Patient day.
- **Per diem reimbursement:**   Payment for a day of care regardless of the specific services provided each day.
- **Prospective reimbursement:**   Payment schedules established prior to providing services.
- **Retrospective reimbursement:**   Payment for services after they are provided (e.g., DRGs).
- **Total costs:**   The combination of fixed and variable costs.
- **Unit of services:**   The specific unit of health care service that a department or unit provides to its consumers (e.g., patient day, specific treatment or procedures, meals served, patient visits to a clinic, number of home visits).
- **Variable costs:**   Costs that fluctuate with census or patient days, treatments, clinic visits, home visits, and so on. Costs that might be affected are number of meals, staffing levels, linen requirements, supplies, and so on.
- **Variance report:**   A report describing the difference between the budgeted and actual figures.
- **Wage index:**   The factor that is used to compare wages paid to specific categories of personnel in HCOs, such as hospitals, across the country (Finkler, Kovner, & Jones, 2007).

## The Budgeting Process: An Overview

The budgetary process is long and cyclic. As soon as it is complete for the year, it begins again. Effective and realistic budgets require reliable data. What is a **budget**? It is a statement, usually annual, that describes the expected revenues or money that will be made by the organization and expected expenses that will be required to provide the services. The budget should identify financial resources, who will use them, when, and the purpose of their use. Box 5-9 provides a sample departmental budget form.

| BOX 5-8 | SAMPLE INCOME STATEMENT FORM |
| --- | --- |

**Income Statement for Year Ended June 30, 2003**

| | | |
| --- | --- | --- |
| Patient Service Revenues | $_____ | |
| Less Allowances and Uncollectables | $_____ | |
| Net Patient Services Revenues | | $_____ |
| Other Operating Revenues | | $_____ |
| **Total Operating Revenues** | | $_____ |
| *Less Operating Expenses:* | $_____ | |
| Nursing Services | $_____ | |
| Other Professional Services | $_____ | |
| General Services | $_____ | |
| Administrative Services | $_____ | |
| Provision for Depreciation | $_____ | |
| **Total Operating Expenses** | | $_____ |
| **Loss/Gain from Operations** | | $_____ |
| *Nonoperating Revenues* | $_____ | |
| Unrestricted Gifts and Bequests | $_____ | |
| Unrestricted Income from Endowment Fund | $_____ | |
| Income and Gains from Board-Designated Assets | $_____ | |
| Total Nonoperating Revenues | | $_____ |
| **Income for the Year** | | $_____ |

Budgets must be live documents as they will need to be adjusted. Effective budgets are consistent with critical organizational qualifiers such as the vision, mission, goals, short-term and long-term strategic plans, and marketing plan. Budgets are composed of three parts:

1. **Salary and wage budget**, which is the largest part and includes salaries and wages, earned benefits (sick time, vacation time, health benefits, and so on), premium or overtime pay, and merit raises.
2. **Operational budget**, which includes the estimate of the volume and mix of activities and services, and the resources required to provide them.
3. **Capital budget**, which is the estimate of purchases of major capital items such as equipment, building, new furniture; it typically sets a cost amount to identify which items are to be included.

Management is responsible for three major budget functions.

- The first function is planning the budget, which is ongoing.
- The second function is management of ongoing activities and services in relationship to the budgeted items.
- The third function is control of spending, which requires careful identification of variances when the budget is not met and analysis of reasons for these variances. There has to be frequent review of the proposed budget and the actual budget. If there is a variance or difference between what was proposed in the budget and what was actually spent or money received, then this needs to be analyzed. For example, if the proposed annual budget allocated an

---

**BOX 5-9    DEPARTMENT BUDGET**

Department/Unit:_____Fiscal Year:_____

| Unit of Service/Patient Days | _____ | Revenue | _____ |
| Unit of Service/_____* | _____ | Revenue | _____ |
| Unit of Service/_____* | _____ | Revenue | _____ |
| | | Total Revenue | |

**Expenses**

| | |
|---|---|
| Productive Salaries | |
| Nonproductive Salaries | |
| TOTAL SALARIES | _____ |
| Employee Benefits | _____ |
| Medical Supplies | _____ |
| Dietary | _____ |
| Minor Equipment | _____ |
| Equipment Rental | _____ |
| Audiovisual Supplies | _____ |
| Recreational Supplies | _____ |
| Copying | _____ |
| Printing | _____ |
| Books/Literature Staff | _____ |
| Books/Literature Patients | _____ |
| Maintenance | _____ |
| Housekeeping | _____ |
| Linens | _____ |

**Total Expenses**

**Profit**

*Unit of service (UOS) may include more than patient days and should be identified in option categories such as UOS/procedure, group session, patient visit.

Comments:

Nurse Manager Signature:_____Date:_____

---

amount for staff recruitment and then the hospital finds that more staff have resigned than was expected, the hospital will need more funds for additional recruitment expenses. This may affect other aspects of the organization if there is a need to cut other expenses to cover these other important needs. Patterns are then analyzed. Critical variance questions are as follows:

1. What effect does the variance have?
2. Why did the variance occur?
3. What can be done to prevent its re-occurrence?
4. What needs to be done to make the best of the situation?

Data about variances are also used when the next year's budget is developed to better estimate needs. Box 5-10 provides an example of a variance analysis.

Why are budgets developed? Every organization has one, and it consumes staff time to develop the annual budget and then to implement it. The major reasons for developing the budget are to

**BOX 5-10    BUDGET VARIANCE ANALYSIS AND JUSTIFICATION FORM**

Budget Variance Analysis and Justification Form

Month_____Year_____Unit_____

**PART A:**

|  | Budgeted | Actual | Variance |  | Variance% |
|---|---|---|---|---|---|
| 1. Patient Days/Visits/Cases | _____ | _____ | _____ | Days/Visits/Cases | _____ |
| 2. Staff Vacancy (full-time equivalents [FTEs]) | _____ | _____ | _____ | FTEs | _____ |
| 3. Acuity | _____ | _____ | _____ | HPPD | _____ |
| Other: | _____ | _____ | _____ |  |  |
| 4. Orientation | _____ | _____ | _____ | hours | _____ |
| 5. Benefits | _____ | _____ | _____ | hours | _____ |
| 6. Charge Pay | _____ | _____ | _____ | hours | _____ |
| 7. Call Back | _____ | _____ | _____ | hours | _____ |
| 8. Minimum Staffing | _____ | _____ | _____ | hours | _____ |

**PART B:**

|  |  | Current Month | | | Year-to-date | | |
|---|---|---|---|---|---|---|---|
| Salaries | | Budgeted | Actual | Variance | Budgeted | Actual | Variance |
| **Staff** | _____ | _____ | _____ | _____ | _____ | _____ | _____ |
| **Agency** | _____ | _____ | _____ | _____ | _____ | _____ | _____ |
| **TOTAL** | _____ | _____ | _____ | _____ | _____ | _____ | _____ |

**PLAN OF ACTION/FOLLOW UP: JUSTIFICATION**

1. Patient Days/Visits/Cases Variance = $_____

2. FTE Variance Hours = $_____

 Agency ×_____Hour = $_____

 Other ×_____Hour = $_____

3. Acuity Variance* = $_____

4. Orientation Variance = $_____

5. Benefit Variance = $_____

6. Charge Pay = $_____

7. Call Back = $_____

8. Minimum Staffing = $_____

TOTAL JUSTIFIED VARIANCE = $_____

TOTAL UNJUSTIFIED VARIANCE = $_____

*In order to USE acuity in justification process, all acuity audits must be complete for the month and accuracy must be between 95 and 100%.

(continued)

| BOX 5-10 | BUDGET VARIANCE ANALYSIS AND JUSTIFICATION FORM (CONTINUED) |
|---|---|

| Items | Budgeted | Actual | $ Variance | $ Variance Year-to-Date | Justification | Follow-up | Plan of Action |
|---|---|---|---|---|---|---|---|
| Contract Service Fees | _____ | _____ | _____ | _____ | _____ | _____ | _____ |
| General Supplies | _____ | _____ | _____ | _____ | _____ | _____ | _____ |
| Food | _____ | _____ | _____ | _____ | _____ | _____ | _____ |
| Medical/Surgical Supplies | _____ | _____ | _____ | _____ | _____ | _____ | _____ |
| Drugs | _____ | _____ | _____ | _____ | _____ | _____ | _____ |
| Copies | _____ | _____ | _____ | _____ | _____ | _____ | _____ |
| Printing | _____ | _____ | _____ | _____ | _____ | _____ | _____ |
| Minor Equipment | _____ | _____ | _____ | _____ | _____ | _____ | _____ |
| Equipment Repairs | _____ | _____ | _____ | _____ | _____ | _____ | _____ |
| Equipment Rental | _____ | _____ | _____ | _____ | _____ | _____ | _____ |
| Books/Literature | _____ | _____ | _____ | _____ | _____ | _____ | _____ |
| Travel | _____ | _____ | _____ | _____ | _____ | _____ | _____ |
| Education | _____ | _____ | _____ | _____ | _____ | _____ | _____ |

*Items that require justification and plan of action/follow-up should be checked and the information attached to this report.*

| Total Expense | | Current Month | Year-to-Date |
|---|---|---|---|
| (includes salary plus agency) | | | |
| | Budgeted | $_____ | $_____ |
| | Actual | $_____ | $_____ |
| | Variance | $_____ | $_____ |
| | Justified | $_____ | $_____ |
| | Unjustified | $_____ | $_____ |

Source: Felteau, A., Budget variance analysis and justification. *Nursing Management, 23*(2), 1992 S-N Publications, Inc., Reprinted with permission.

1. Provide a financial and statistical expression of the plans for the organization.
2. Identify how resources (staff, equipment, space, finances) are to be allocated.
3. Provide a basis for measurement and evaluation of actual performance of the organization's plan.
4. Provide periodic reports that assist in management decision making.
5. Create cost awareness throughout the organization.
6. Assist management in determining rates or prices.

Budgets are more than just the initial financial data described; otherwise, these goals could not be met. As the budget is applied over the year performance data are monitored and analyzed. It is this performance that organizations use to guide budgetary decisions throughout the year. Is the organization making as much money (revenues) as it thought it would? If not, what impact does this have on expenses? If more money is made than was predicted in the budget, should the organization use that money or invest it? If expenses are higher than predicted in the budget, what steps need to be taken to insure cost containment and funds to pay expenses? All of these questions have an impact on nurses and nursing care.

There are several advantages to developing and implementing a budget. First, of course, budgets force the organization to plan. Just as a family that has a certain income should plan how money will be spent, saved, and invested, an organization has these responsibilities. It encourages many levels of staff to participate in overall and unit/service/department planning. Cost containment is another major advantage of budgeting—forcing staff to consider how they use resources (allocation of services) and to consider how money needs to be conserved. The budgetary process provides opportunity for self-analysis, motivating staff, and the organization to improve performance.

There are also disadvantages to budgeting. There can be disagreement among management staff about the budget, and consensus can be difficult to obtain. All levels of staff need to understand the process and its implications, which require education or training. Many organizations do not provide this to their staff. Budgeting does require flexibility as needs change, and sometimes making these changes is difficult. Another difficulty is some managers may focus too much on the budget without consideration of other organizational issues found in the vision, mission, goals, and strategic plans. Clearly, overbudgeting can lead to major problems, as can ignoring downturns and not adjusting the budget accordingly. The latter issues can lead to problems of survival for the organization as it might slip into "the red" and then not be able to meet its financial demands.

As budgets are developed, the two main components of the budget are revenues and expenses. Revenues are projected based on past experiences and plans for the probable future. Types of data that are important to consider are number of patient days, procedures, treatments, length-of-stay, number of clinic visits, number of home visits, types of patients, and so on. If the organization plans on adding new services, then data will have to be based on more speculation based on what might be. Data about other organizations might be used to project these revenues (for example, adding a new home care service and how this service might compete with other home care agencies). Strategic plans are also reviewed to identify possible revenues and expenses that might be affected by the plan. Probable expenses are carefully analyzed, again using past data. Examples of typical expense categories are as follows:

- Salary and wages
- Benefits
- Medical supplies and other supplies
- Depreciation
- Administration costs
- Housekeeping
- Dietary
- Professional fees and other fees the HCO may be required to pay
- Capital equipment
- Furniture and furnishings
- Maintenance
- Pharmacy
- Orientation and education
- Printing
- Information technology
- Utilities
- Landscaping
- Legal fees
- Parking and security

Some of the expenses are fixed as they do not change due to activity and service levels, and some are variable as they do change due to activity and service levels. For example, costs for orientation increase when the numbers of new staff increase; number of deliveries increases costs for the obstetrical department; and number of snowstorms increases the need for parking lot snow removal.

## *CASE STUDY*

### *Staff Role in Budget Development*

The nurse managers in a hospital have been asked to prepare budgets for their units. At the same time the managers are told that the hospital's budget has serious problems with being over budget last year. This is the first year that nurse managers have been asked to participate in the budget development. At the nurse manager meeting, several nurse managers were angry now that the hospital had serious problems they were turning to the nurse managers. Maybe if they had been asked to participate in the budget process before there were problems they might have been able to provide helpful strategies. Many nurse managers also felt they lacked the necessary skills to do the task. The nurse executive listened to their concerns at the meeting. After the meeting the nurse manager from a medical unit returned to his unit and met with team leaders to ask their advice about the budget and the deficit.

### Questions:

1. How might macrolevel financial issues affect micromanagement financial issues?
2. What might be the roles of staff nurses, team leaders, nurse managers, and nurse executives in budget development?
3. How might cost containment be used to address the deficit of the medical unit? Consider specific interventions or strategies that might be used.
4. How should the nurse executive respond to the nurse managers' concern about their lack of skills to cope with this request?
5. How might this be viewed as an opportunity for nursing administration?

### Productivity

Productivity must be considered during the budgetary process and also when changes occur in the health care arena. **Productivity** is the ratio of output (products and services) to input (resources consumed). The goal is to increase productivity, or at the minimum not to decrease it. To do this, factors that affect both input and output need to be evaluated.

Examples of factors affecting input are staff characteristics (mix, qualifications, experience, stability, length of shift, mandatory overtime), patients (number, ages, acuity, diagnoses, treatments), and organization (unit configuration, size, staffing, leadership and management, equipment, services, financial status).

Examples of factors affecting output are number of emergency visits, deliveries, admissions, clinic visits, meals served, radiological procedures, total number of patient days, surgical procedures, and acuity. What methods are used to assess productivity?

Some examples are application of a patient acuity or classification system, cost accounting, budget reports, position control, quality improvement monitoring, and **full-time equivalent (FTE)** analysis. An FTE is a full-time position that is equated to 40 hours of work per week, 80 hours per pay period, or 2,080 hours per year. It is not a person but a unit of time or time actually worked. Nonproductive time is included in the paid hours; productive time is actual time worked. The principal measure of input is worked hours, worked FTEs, or paid hours. However, it is also important to measure both "worked hours" productivity and paid hours productivity, which includes benefit allowances for sick time, vacation, and holidays.

Two critical issues in productivity are efficiency and effectiveness. Efficiency is doing things right while effectiveness is doing the right things. Both of these issues need to be assessed when productivity is analyzed. Cost containment and quality are related to productivity. Analyzing outcome variances is part of the process. Productivity is affected by staffing patterns, methods of organization, and the usage of nurse extender mechanisms such as other support staff to assist nurses (Eastnaugh, 2002). Productivity is described in Box 5-11.

| BOX 5-11 | PRODUCTIVITY |
| --- | --- |

**Productivity = output divided by input**

*Example:*

*Input:* 24 hours of nursing care (one patient day). Inputs are predetermined budgeted nursing care hours per patient day based on the patient's acuity and required patient care activities.

*Outputs:* the outcomes; achieved patient goals.

## Cost Containment

**Cost containment** must be part of the budgetary process, or the HCO may not survive. The problem with cost containment is it has a bad name. Seeing it only as a negative experience will limit the success of the effort. Quality and cost containment should be and are definitely connected. When decisions are made to control costs, there needs to be a balance. How does the cost of care affect quality? If costs are reduced, will quality of care be affected and in what way? These are critical questions that must be asked, and nurses who are involved in budgetary decisions should speak up and ask them. During this process ethical issues may be brought up when difficult decisions are made. The typical cost-containment methods are as follows:

- Decrease overtime expenses
- Decrease sick time expenses
- Adjusting staffing
- No filling empty positions
- Prevent costly expenses for repair of equipment
- Use supplies wisely
- Decrease the inventory of supplies that are infrequently used or not used at all
- Maintain productivity standards
- Prevent employee accidents
- Use methods to improve staffing decisions

There often is a fear in organizations that only financial staff make cost-containment decisions, and this is a legitimate concern. These decisions should be made jointly with other management staff that appreciates the clinical implications of these decisions. There is no doubt today that budget cuts do occur, and many are necessary. Staff needs to understand the reason for the cuts before the rumor mill about the cuts does major damage to morale. Nursing management should seek out facts to respond to budget cuts and to plan. If nursing management approaches all budget cuts with a negative attitude, assuming that all cuts are nonproductive, nursing management will not be able to work collaboratively with the HCO's other management staff. Cost-containment efforts require an honest appraisal of the needs and approaches to resolving them. Nurse leaders need to be team players and willing to step back and objectively assess a problem. This does not mean that they do not advocate for nursing and for patient care delivery, but rather they do this in a professional manner. They need to approach communication about the problems and the cuts openly with other staff, providing explanations and support as needed. Staff members too can be brought into the process as they may have some excellent ideas about how problems may be resolved. In the end, budget cuts need to be made carefully with consideration given to short-term and long-term effects. Nurse leaders must assume an active role in all phases of the process.

# APPLYING LEADERSHIP AND MANAGEMENT

## MY HOSPITAL UNIT

You have been told at the weekly nurse manager meeting that all units need to develop a cost containment plan. You need to develop two cost containment strategies for your unit. You begin by reviewing the content in this chapter. You might do some additional literature research on cost containment. After this you develop two strategies and describe them in a memo to the CNO. The memo should not be any longer than three double-spaced pages and should apply specifically to the unit you have been creating. You need to then develop an implementation plan considering how you will inform and involve the staff. How will you know that your strategies have been effective? Remember that other decisions you may have made about your unit may have an impact on this activity. Use the virtual unit site found on the textbook website to record the work that you do in the role of nurse manager for your unit.

## Critical Thinking Questions and Activities

1. Using the cost containment methods discussed in this chapter, describe how you would implement one of the methods in a specific type of health care organization.
2. Ask a nurse manager to see a unit budget. Review the budget and identify the items in the budget. Ask the nurse manager about the budgetary process and her role.
3. Visit the Centers for Medicare and Medicaid Services (CMS) website at http://www.cms .hhs.gov/. Review content on reimbursement and consider how it might apply to a Medicare or to a Medicaid patient.
4. Compare and contrast the macrolevel and microlevel perspectives of health care financing.
5. Why should staff nurses, nurse team leaders, nurse managers, and executive nurse leaders participate in the organization's financial planning? Describe ways in which each should participate.

## Media Links

- **URL: http://www.cms.hhs.gov/**

    Centers for Medicare and Medicaid Services (CMS)
- **URL: http://www.hhs.gov/about/opdivs/hcfa.html**

    Health Care Financing Administration (HCFA)
- **URL: http://www.statehealthfacts.org/**

    State Facts.Org (Health Care Financing State Facts)

### Pearson Nursing Student Resources

Find additional review materials at
**nursing.pearsonhighered.com**

Prepare for success with additional NCLEX®-style practice questions, interactive assignments and activities, Web links, animations and videos, and more!

# References

Baldor, R. (1998). *Managed care made simple* (2nd ed.). Malden, MA: Blackwell Science.

Bernard, T. (March 21, 2010). For consumers, clarity on health care changes. *New York Times*. Retrieved from http://www.nytimes.com

Casto, A. & Layman, E. (2009). *Principles of health care reimbursement*. Chicago: American Health Information Management Association.

Centers for Medicare and Medicaid Services. (CMS). (2009). Medicare and Medicaid Programs. Retrieved June 11, 2009, from http://www.cms.hhs.gov/MedicaidGenInfo/

Centers for Medicare and Medicaid Services. Retrieved June, 2009, from http://www.cms.gov

Centers for Medicare and Medicaid Services. (2010). National health expenditures projections, 2009–2019. Retrieved May 24, 2010, from http://www.cms.gov/NationalHealthExpendData/03_NationalHealthAccountsProjected.asp

Cooper, P., & Schone, B. (1997). More offers, fewer takers for employment-based health insurance: 1987–1996. *Health Affairs, 16*(6), 142–149.

Cover the Uninsured. (2009). Current Data. Retrieved July 8, 2009, from http://covertheuninsured.org/

Daschle, T. (2008). *Critical. What we can do about the health-care crisis*. New York: St. Martin's Press.

Eastnaugh, S. (2002). Hospital nurse productivity. *Journal of Health Care Finance, 29*(1), 14–18.

Finkler, S., Kovner, C, & Jones, C. (2007). *Financial management for nurse managers and executives.* (3rd ed.). Philadelphia: W. B. Saunders Company.

Health Insurance Association of America. (1998). *Managed care: Integrating the delivery and financing of health care, Part A*. Washington, DC: Author.

Henry J. Kaiser Family Foundation. (KFF). (April, 2006). *Kaiser Commission on Key Facts: Medicaid and the Uninsured.* Retrieved June 10, 2009, from http://www.kff.org/medicaid/upload/7492.pdf

Henry J. Kaiser Family Foundation. (2009a). News Release. Retrieved February 27, 2009, from http://www.kff.org/kaiserpolls/index2.cfm

Henry J. Kaiser Family Foundation. (2009b). Health Insurance. Retrieved June 27, 2009, from http://www.kff.org/

Himmelstein, D., Warren, D. Thorne, D., and Woolhander, S. (February 2005). Illness and injury as contributors to bankruptcy. *Health Affairs*. Web Exclusive W5-63: 02.

Institute of Medicine. (IOM). (2004). *Insuring America's health*. Washington, DC: Author.

Keehan, S. et al. (February 2008). Health spending projections through 2017. *Health Affairs*. Web Exclusive W146: 21.

Kongstvedt, P. (2009). *Managed care. What it is and how it works*. Boston: Jones and Bartlett Publishers.

McKinsey Global Institute. (2007, January). Accounting for the cost of health care in the United States. Retrieved July 6, 2009, from http://www.mckinsey.com/mgi/rp/healthcare/accounting_cost_healthcare.asp

National League for Nursing. (1978). *Financial management of department of nursing services*. New York: Author.

# 6

# Acute Care Organizations: An Example of a Health Care Organization

## CHAPTER OUTLINE

Before you begin, take a moment to familiarize yourself with the learning outcomes for this chapter.

- Critique the development of U.S. hospitals and the role they play in the health care delivery system.
- Differentiate the key methods for classifying hospitals.
- Compare the key departments found in most hospitals.
- Apply committee process to a policy and procedure committee as an example of committees.
- Analyze major changes that are occurring in hospitals and their impact on nursing.
- Examine the Magnet Recognition Program, its history, its process, and the impact it has had on nursing.
- Examine the forces of magnetism are important to new graduates as well as to any nurse considering a job change.

## KEY TERMS

- Accreditation
- Continuum of care
- Credentialing
- Differentiated practice
- Downsizing
- Faith-based hospital
- For-profit (investor-owned or proprietary)
- Government hospital
- Hospital

- Hospitalist
- Hospital system
- Intensivist
- Length-of-stay
- Network
- Not-for-profit organization
- Organizational characteristics
- Patient census
- Patient-focused health care organization

- Policy
- Privileging
- Procedure
- Standards
- Structural characteristics
- Teaching or non-teaching hospital
- Vertical integration

## WHAT'S AHEAD

This chapter explores acute care hospitals, an example of a health care delivery organization. There is greater emphasis on community-focused services today; however, since most new graduates begin their careers in hospitals, this is the appropriate place to begin to understand health care delivery settings. Hospital management is more complex than most businesses. As was discussed in Chapter 4, the hospital meets the criteria for an organization. It has a purpose and goals, people who work for it, and a systematic structure. Many hospitals continue to maintain a bureaucratic organization even if this is not the most effective type. Other hospitals, however, are undergoing restructuring and reengineering and thus changing into different types of organizations. Newhouse and Mills (2002) believe it is important for nurses to be informed about hospital organization factors and changes for the following reasons: (a) nurses coordinate the care of inpatients and play a major role in promoting continuity of care, (b) nursing is the largest labor source of health care services within the acute care organization, and (c) nursing is affected by each corporate decision to provide or discontinue selected services (p. ix).

This text also recognizes the critical need for nurses to understand some important elements related to hospital structure and functions to enable them to be more effective as care providers within this health care setting. The first part of the chapter focuses on the typical hospital organization, and the second part discusses important information about acute care nursing services by exploring the Magnet Nursing Services Organization.

# Development of U.S. Hospitals

The acute care hospital has long been the major focus in the U.S. health care delivery system. What is a **hospital**? This might sound like a strange question; however, the definition contains important descriptive criteria. It is an organization whose primary purpose is to deliver patient care both diagnostic and therapeutic for certain medical conditions. These medical conditions may be highly specialized, such as those found in psychiatric or rehabilitation hospitals, or in general, such as a hospital that provides a variety of services, the general acute care hospital. There is an organized medical staff, and continuous nursing services are provided under the supervision of registered nurses, which is a critical component of 24-hour care. All hospitals must follow certain laws and regulations: federal, state, and local. **Accreditation**, which is discussed in Chapter 17, is also a criteria used to describe a hospital. From this description several critical criteria can be identified.

- Organization with purpose
- Medical and nursing care and professionals who must meet their own professional requirements and standards
- Standards established by laws, regulations, and accreditation
- A complex organization
- The consumer must play a role (see Chapter 10)

The health care system's goals are to provide services that focus on (a) health promotion and illness prevention, (b) diagnosis and treatment, and (c) rehabilitation and health restoration and, if required, support during the dying process. To accomplish these goals the system is organized by the complexity of the services required to meet each of the goals: primary, secondary, and tertiary care. Some hospitals only focus on one of these goals (for example, a rehabilitative hospital or a hospice focusing on goal 3); however, others might meet all three goals. Hospital care is primarily secondary care, although other services related to primary care (such as clinic services and wellness programs) are also services hospitals might offer, as well as tertiary care, which may be found in a hospital organization (for example, when a hospital offers a hospital-based hospice program or a rehabilitation unit). The U.S. health care system is a multiprovider system, as is illustrated by the number of different providers identified in Box 6-1. These were discussed in Chapter 4.

Hospitals can be described in many different ways, and are constantly changing. Some terms that are helpful to understand when trying to define "hospital" are system, network, and organized delivery system, which describe organizational arrangements (Newhouse & Mills, 2002). A **hospital system** refers to a corporation that owns or manages health facilities, often using vertical integration as was described in Chapter 4. A **network** differs from a system in that it is a number of health care facilities that agree to deliver specific services, although each facility remains an independent organization. The organized delivery system can be found in some communities, and it "provides or arranges to provide a coordinated continuum of services to a defined population and is willing to be held clinically and fiscally accountable for the outcomes and the health status of the population service" (Newhouse & Mills, 2002, p. 3).

As hospital organizations have changed, more mergers are occurring. A merger occurs when two or more organizations come together to form one organization. This is a challenge for all of

**BOX 6-1     U.S. MULTIPROVIDER HEALTH CARE DELIVERY SYSTEM**

- Acute care hospitals
- Specialty hospitals
- Physician offices: Primary care and specialty
- Advanced Practice nurses and nurse midwives: Practices
- Clinics: Hospital and community
- Dental offices/clinics
- Urgent care centers
- Ambulatory care centers (e.g., one-day surgery centers, diagnostic centers)
- Industrial clinics as part of occupational health
- Extended care facilities, including skilled nursing (intermediate care) and extended care (long-term care)
- Retirement and assisted-living centers
- Rehabilitation centers
- Home health agencies
- Hospice services
- Psychiatric services and community mental health centers
- Substance abuse treatment centers (inpatient and outpatient)
- School health clinics
- Public health includes government agencies, federal, state, and local, funded primarily by taxes and administered by elected or appointed officials.

the organizations and their staff. Organizations have cultures, and when a merger is created the various organizational cultures merge to form one organization. Otherwise, the organizations and their staff will continue to view themselves as separate organizations rather than one organization. (See Chapter 8 on organization culture.) The community will also need to change its view of the health care organizations, recognizing that individual organizations no longer exist and the merged organization is one organization. None of this is easy to accomplish, and some attempts at mergers have not been successful. Barriers to success are poor planning, lack of collaboration, territoriality, ineffective communication systems, lack of organization-wide leadership, and loss of control. All of this has a major impact on the organizations' nurses. Much work needs to be done to develop one organization. How this is accomplished and how much independence each organization in the merger may have is highly variable.

## Acute Care Organization and Governance

As acute care hospitals are described, three elements are important to consider: the system, the patient, and the outcome (Newhouse & Mills, 2002).

- System characteristics include organizational, structural, and patient-focused characteristics. Each of these characteristics affect outcomes (Wolper, 2004). Examples of **organizational characteristics** are governance (for-profit or not-for-profit), number of beds, teaching status, urban-rural location, technology level, **patient census** (both number admitted and length-of-stay), and operating expenses. **Structural characteristics** are teaching status, urban density, profit status, percentage of board-certified physicians, RN hours per patient day, volume of cases, technological availability, and operating expenses. With the increased emphasis on patient-centered care this element is critical today. Hospitals are trying to figure out how to better ensure patient-centered care (Institute of Medicine, 2002; 2003).
- In addition to these characteristics, some of which overlap, it is important to remember that each patient comes with individual characteristics such as age, gender, race, severity, illness, and health history, and experiences with the health care system, probably some of which are positive and some of which are negative.
- All of these characteristics can affect outcomes, which "is the result of the affect of the system, patient characteristics, and intervention" (Newhouse & Mills, 2002, p. 13).

Levels of management in acute care include top management, middle management, and first-line management. Every hospital has a board of trustees or board of directors, which acts as the governing body. This board is responsible for developing the organization's mission and goals, as well as setting the overall hospital policies. The board ensures that the hospital provides the services that have been designated by the board. Typically, these boards are made up of community and business leaders. Top management includes the chief executive officer (CEO) of the hospital, who reports to the board and is hired by the board, and other key management staff. The chief nurse executive (CNE), who in some hospitals also reports to the board but more typically to the CEO, is also part of top management. The board has great influence over the functions and management of the hospital, and thus has a great impact on nurses and nursing care. It is important for the CNE to understand the board and develop strong communication mechanisms to get information to the board in order to ensure that patient care is of the highest quality and that nursing staff are supported. The chief financial officer (CFO), another member of top management, is responsible for the organization's financial management. Other high-level/top level administrative staff may also be considered top management, but this can vary from hospital to hospital. If a hospital has a CNE, the hospital may also have a director of nursing who may be included in middle or in top management. In this case the CNE may be responsible for more than just nursing. For example, the CNE may also be responsible for medical records, social services, laboratory, and so on. The inclusion of other services or departments can vary from hospital to hospital. Supervisory staff is middle management, while nurse managers are examples of first-line managers. Coordinating the work of the three levels is key to an effective organization. Many organizations are flattening their administrative or management staff levels by eliminating layers. When this occurs, there may be fewer than the three layers or levels described here.

The medical staff organization has great power in any hospital. This is a formal organization of the medical staff that provides services in the hospital, and it is part of the total hospital organization. These physicians may be on staff (paid by the hospital) or may have admitting privileges (which allows them to admit their patients and provide care within the hospital, although they are not paid directly by the hospital). In order to become a member of the medical staff, physicians have to complete a formal appointment process, which is described in the medical staff organization bylaws. References and credentials are checked as well as information about involvement in malpractice suits. "Credentialing and privileging are the most direct means for an organization to ensure that patients receive quality care from skilled practitioners" (Payne, 1999, p. 8). What is the difference between these two processes? **Credentialing** focuses on ensuring that practitioners meet certain qualifications. This is done by obtaining, verifying, and assessing qualifications such as licensure and certification to ensure that the person is qualified based on required position criteria. **Privileging** occurs when a health care organization "authorizes a specific scope and content of patient-care services for a licensed independent practitioner based on evaluation of the individual's credentials and performance" (Payne, 1999, p. 8). There would be a clear statement of what the physician is allowed to do within the hospital. For example, a physician who was not a qualified surgeon would not be allowed to perform surgery. The Joint Commission requires that independent licensed practitioners go through these two processes. Advanced nurse practitioners (NPs) and nurse midwives who want to admit and practice in a hospital must also go through this process. If the hospital is a university medical center, the medical school faculty also serves on the medical staff. House staff, interns, residents, and fellows can be found in all types of hospitals, not just university medical centers, but they provide care as "students," not as official members of the medical staff. They are paid by the hospital.

The medical staff is typically organized by committees such as medical records, credentials, utilization review, infection control, and quality improvement committees. The committees focus on these areas to ensure that the patient care goals are met. A medical director or, in some hospitals, the chief of staff, is usually elected by the medical staff to serve as their leader. In some hospitals, however, the medical director may be selected by the board of directors. Larger hospitals may also have service leaders or department heads for departments such as surgery, medicine, pediatrics, obstetrics/gynecology, psychiatry, emergency, pathology, and radiology. It is critical that the CNE develop a strong, positive relationship with the medical staff organization and its leaders. Collaborating together will allow for greater, positive outcomes for patients and nursing staff.

Although the formal organization is very important in a hospital, so is the informal organization. Recognizing the informal organization and using it to the fullest to reach desired outcomes is a sign of an effective leader. Nurses at all levels can benefit from a greater understanding of "what makes the organization run" other than the formal structure. There are many times when it is the informal organization that actually gets the job done, as sometimes the formal organization interferes or puts up barriers to effective functioning. Chapters 1 and 4 discussed leadership and organization in more detail, and this content is certainly applicable to this chapter's content.

## Classification of Hospitals

Hospitals are classified according to the following characteristics: public access, ownership, number of beds, length-of-stay, accreditation, licensure, teaching, vertical integration, and multihospital system organizations (Wolper, 2004).

PUBLIC ACCESS    Public access characteristics describe hospitals as community or non-community hospitals, determined by the amount of access that the public has to the hospital. Community hospitals are nonfederal, short-term, or other special hospitals, which the public may use. Non-community hospitals are characterized as federal, long-term, hospital units of institutions (prison hospitals, college infirmaries, psychiatric hospitals), hospitals for chronic diseases, (for mentally retarded, alcoholism, and other chemical dependency problems), or psychiatric/mental health. Public access hospitals serve as a critical safety net resource for patients who either have no health insurance, limited insurance, or on Medicaid coverage. This part of the health system experiences great stress. There are an increased number of patients requiring services from these hospitals, and these hospitals frequently have fewer resources. They form the safety net for patients who have nowhere else to go.

OWNERSHIP    Identifying the owner of a hospital provides critical information about the organization—particularly who makes decisions and what is done with the profits. All hospitals need to make a profit to maintain financial stability and to maintain their physical plant and equipment. The following are different perspectives of ownership.

1. The **not-for-profit** hospital is funded by reimbursement, just as all hospitals are, and also with donations and endowments. It is important to remember that this type of hospital must also make a profit. The key difference with investor-owned (for-profit) hospitals is that the not-for-profit hospital invests its profits back into the hospital, and none of the profit is given to others outside the organization.
2. The **investor-owned or proprietary** organization is owned and administered by corporations who are shareholders or stockholders and own stock in the corporation. The hospital is responsible to the shareholders, and the shareholders expect that the organization will make a profit so that they can make money on their investment. As is true of hospitals in general, this type of organization will also have a board of directors or trustees that reports to the shareholders. This is the fastest growing type of ownership. Typically, the corporation is a large, national corporation. Examples are Hospital Corporation of America (HCA) and Tenet. These health care corporations own hospitals and other types of health care provider settings throughout the country. Each of the components of the corporation is required to meet the corporate standards and to provide profit for the corporation.
3. **Faith-based hospitals** are owned and administered by a faith-based group such as Catholic hospitals, Jewish hospitals, and so on. They maintain not-for-profit status.
4. **Government hospitals** are owned by the government. Examples of these hospitals are military hospitals; state psychiatric hospitals; hospitals owned and operated by states, counties, or cities; Veteran's Administration hospitals; National Institutes of Health Clinical Center; and hospitals on Indian Reservations, which are administered by the U.S. Public Health Service. Government hospitals maintain not-for-profit status.

NUMBER OF BEDS    The number of beds is another hospital characteristic that is considered. Typical bed number ranges that are used to classify hospitals are 6 to 24, 25 to 49, 50 to 99, 100 to 199, 200 to 299, 300 to 499, 400 to 499, and 500 or more (Wolper, 2004).

LENGTH-OF-STAY    **Length-of-stay (LOS)** is also used to classify hospitals. A hospital's average length-of-stay is used to determine if a hospital has a short-term (average LOS of less than 30 days) or long-term stay (average LOS of over 30 days). Length-of-stay has been decreasing for acute care hospitals and specialty hospitals such as psychiatric hospitals. This has been affected by pressure from managed care organizations/insurers, technological advances, scientific advancement, and more effective drugs and treatment, leading to more care provided in the community.

ACCREDITATION    Accreditation is another hospital characteristic, as hospitals are classified as accredited or non-accredited. The Joint Commission, which is discussed in more detail in Chapter 17, is the voluntary accreditation organization that accredits hospitals and other health care organizations. Hospital accreditation has been in existence for 60 years. A health care organization uses its accreditation status in marketing and communicating to consumers that it provides quality care, though accreditation does not guarantee quality. Insurers want their plan members to receive care in accredited hospitals. For a school of nursing or medicine to use a hospital as a clinical site for students, it must be accredited.

LICENSURE    In addition to accreditation, licensure and certification are also important. Licensure of hospitals is done by states when the hospital meets certain state standards and requirements. Hospitals must be licensed through the state to provide services though Joint Commission accreditation is optional. However, hospitals that are not accredited may encounter reimbursement difficulties and will not be able to have students such as nursing and medical students in their organization for training. For a hospital to receive Medicare and Medicaid reimbursement, it must be certified or given authority to provide this care by the Centers for

Medicare and Medicaid Services (CMS), and it must be accredited. Accreditation, licensure, and certification all involve meeting specified standards and some type of routine inspection. This can consume much staff time and is costly, but it is important.

TEACHING    Hospitals are also classified as teaching or non-teaching. **Teaching hospitals** offer residency programs for physicians. These residency programs vary in size. Hospitals may be university-affiliated (with a major connection to a university) or freestanding (not connected to a university but still maintains a residency program). The latter might be a community hospital that has medical residents on their staff.

VERTICAL INTEGRATION    **Vertical integration** is another hospital characteristic that considers whether or not a hospital focuses on primary, secondary, or tertiary care services. To be classified as a primary care hospital the hospital provides services on "an as needed basis to the public" (Wolper, 2004). These services are part of a comprehensive health care system, providing outpatient or ambulatory care services. Secondary care facilities require greater sophistication in terms of equipment and skills. Examples are acute care hospitals and specialized outpatient services such as ambulatory surgical centers. Tertiary level hospitals require even greater skills and equipment, and are much more specialized in need. Examples of this level are university medical centers and specialty hospitals such as pediatric hospitals and burn centers.

MULTIHOSPITAL SYSTEM    A multihospital system is a newer characteristic that is used to classify hospitals. When large health systems or national health corporations first began, the emphasis was on horizontal integration or bringing together hospitals of like characteristics— similar size and purpose. After a time, these organizations have expanded, and diversification has occurred more and more. Now, these multihospital systems actually include more than just hospitals; they often also include other types of provider organizations. For example, a corporation might include acute care hospitals, home health agencies, long-term care facilities, hospice care, and various ambulatory care provider organizations.

## Typical Departments Found in an Acute Care Hospital

Hospitals are complex organizations with many departments and services. Some departments provide direct care services to patients, and others provide support services to facilitate the provision of care. The following are examples of typical departments and services.

- **Administration.** Administration may not be an official department but rather a description of administrative staff that supports the work of the organization—it provides direction. Typically, administrative staff includes the CEO, CNE, CFO, and other high-level management staff. Titles can vary from hospital to hospital.
- **Admissions.** The admissions department ensures that patients are admitted in a timely and efficient manner, and reimbursement issues are resolved related to covered medical services during the admissions process. This department is involved in a great deal of paper work and assigns patients to rooms and services. The department may be part of billing (financial) services or may work closely with these financial services.
- **Ambulatory care/outpatient services.** This department or service provides services to persons who generally do not need the level of care associated with the more structured environment of an inpatient or a residential program. Typically, these services are organized by specialty (for example, medical, pediatrics, and orthopedics clinics). Usually these services are provided Monday through Friday during daytime hours, although there is now a greater recognition that consumers/patients need access to these services in more nontraditional hours due to work, child care, and other scheduling issues.
- **Clinical laboratory.** This department or service is equipped to examine material derived from the human body to provide information for use in the diagnosis, prevention, or treatment of disease; it is also called a medical laboratory. Some hospitals may contract out for these services to a company that would run the tests and then provide the hospital with the results. This may be more cost-effective for the hospital, although it can lead to communication problems if there are no clear policies and procedures for this service and it is less in

the control of the hospital. The hospital is still responsible for the quality of the services, but some or all of the staff that delivers the services are not hospital employees. More hospitals are considering it to be more cost-effective to contract out for some services.

■ **Clinical respiratory services.** This department or service provides goal-directed, purposeful activity to patients with disorders of the cardiopulmonary system. Such services include diagnostic testing, therapeutics, monitoring education, and rehabilitation. Nurses are part of the staff.

■ **Diagnostic procedures.** This department or service provides laboratory and other invasive, diagnostic, and imaging procedures. Nurses are part of the staff (e.g., endoscopy services).

■ **Dietetic services.** This department or service delivers optimal nutrition and quality food services to individuals. This is a service that may be contracted out. Nurses need to work closely with this staff to ensure that patients' needs are met.

■ **Finance and budget.** This department ensures a financial plan (budget), financial analysis, and the financial solvency of the organization.

■ **Housekeeping/environmental service.** This department or service ensures the environment is clean. This is a service that may be contracted out or outsourced.

■ **Infection control program.** This department or service ensures there is an organization-wide program or process, including policies and procedures for the surveillance, prevention, and control of infection. Nursing is very involved in this area.

■ **Infusion therapy services.** This department or service provides therapeutic agents or nutritional products to individuals by intravenous infusion for the purpose of improving or sustaining an individual's health condition. Nursing is very involved in this area.

■ **Information management.** This department or service is responsible for ensuring that information can be collected, linked, is accurate and reliable, monitors use of data, and ensures that legal regulations are met and ethical issues are addressed such as confidentiality and providing secure systems. Computer equipment is a major concern. It needs to be appropriate to the needs of the organization, as well as efficient and effective. This department must work closely with nursing and medical services as well as other clinical departments who require access to information. It also must input data into the system.

■ **Material/resource management.** This department or service ensures the hospital has the needed supplies by selecting, purchasing, storing, distributing, and obtaining reimbursement for their use when appropriate. This is another service that may be outsourced.

■ **Medical equipment management.** Hospitals need to assess and control the clinical and physical risks of fixed and portable equipment used for the diagnosis, treatment, monitoring, and care of individuals. Medical equipment management provides this service. Nurses use equipment daily and need to be involved in monitoring safety issues and their application to the needs of patients.

■ **Medical records.** This department or service ensures that the documentation process is maintained, develops relevant policies and procedures, and provides availability of data as required. This is a department that works closely with clinical departments and medical records as well as quality improvement. Nurses are the staff members who are responsible for most of the documentation, and they need to be very active in all aspects of medical records functions.

■ **Nursing service/patient care.** Nursing service is the key service in any acute care hospital as patients are admitted primarily for more intensive nursing care. This is not to say that patients do not receive other services that are important, but nursing care is critical to reaching patient coordination and reaching patient outcomes.

■ **Occupational therapy services.** The department or service that provides goal-directed, purposeful activity to evaluate, assess, or treat persons whose function is impaired by physical illness or injury, emotional disorder, congenital or developmental disability, or the aging process. Nurses assist in referring patients for these services.

■ **Pharmacy/pharmaceutical care and services.** The department or service that is responsible for procuring, preparing, dispensing, and distributing pharmaceutical products and the ongoing monitoring of the individual to identify, prevent, and resolve drug-related problems. Nurses administer most of the medications and thus need to work closely with this department.

- **Physical therapy services.** This department or service provides treatment with physical agents and methods such as massage, manipulation, therapeutic exercises, cold, heat, hydrotherapy, electric stimulation, and light to assist in rehabilitating individuals and in restoring normal function after an illness or injury. Nurses assist in referring patients for these services.
- **Radiology.** This department or service provides diagnostic services such as x-ray, magnetic resonance imaging (MRI), and computed tomography (CT) scans. Nurses prepare patients, and may provide care, during radiological procedures.
- **Respiratory care services.** This department or service delivers care to provide ventilatory support and associated services for individuals. Nurses monitor these services and assist.
- **Social work services.** This department or service assists individuals and their families in addressing social, emotional, and economic stresses associated with illness or injury. Nurses need to communicate, coordinate, and collaborate with social workers.
- **Staff development/education.** This department or service provides organized education designed to enhance skills of staff members or teach new skills relevant to their responsibilities and disciplines. This department is critical for maintaining nurses' competencies.
- **Quality improvement performance.** This department ensures that the hospital meets standards (local, state, federal, and accrediting bodies) to ensure quality and safety of care. Risk management (RM) is typically part of this department. RM addresses prevention, monitoring, and control of areas of potential liability exposure and safety for patients, staff, and visitors. Chapters 16 and 17 focus on these critical topics. Nurses must be active participants in all phases of quality improvement (Joint Commission, 2004, pp. 311–344).

This description of hospital departments and services is not complete; however, the descriptions identify some of the key departments found in many hospitals.

## Organizations and Committees

Committees are used by organizations for planning, obtaining staff input, and getting some of the organization's work completed. Including staff from various levels and areas of the organization in committee membership offers greater opportunity for staff participation and buy in to changes. Committees can also be very problematic—they can take time, can be unproductive and disorganized, and can lead to ineffective management. These problems need to be addressed so that committees can be productive. Nurses do not like working on committees that are unproductive, as they do not have the time. To prevent some of these problems the organization needs to consider the following.

- Establishment of clear purpose and goals
- Appropriate committee membership
- Effectiveness of communication
- Support from management/administration
- Collaboration and sharing committee results
- Recognition that some problems are not appropriate for committee decision making
- Ensuring that appropriate data is used
- Scheduling of committee meetings

Later in this chapter the work that the policy and procedure committee does will be described as an example of a committee and its process. This is an example of a committee that is very important to nursing care.

DESCRIPTION OF TYPICAL COMMITTEES    Acute care hospitals typically have many committees. These committees may be within a department or service, professional group such as physicians or nurses, or hospital wide. Committees are usually classified as standing or ad hoc.

A standing committee is one that meets regularly for a particular purpose and submits reports to designated management staff. Examples of standing committees might be policy and procedures, quality improvement, medical records, and infection control. Hospitals may have different titles for committees, but the titles given here represent typical titles or focus areas.

Ad hoc committees are established for a specific purpose with a specific time frame in mind. Some organizations may call these task forces. How long this type of committee exists can be highly variable and depends upon the need and focus. Examples of this type of committee might be a committee that is formed to address a major change in the information management system.

Another characteristic of committees is they can be composed of members from one profession or be interprofessional. The latter type is best for any issue that crosses disciplines, which describes the majority of issues today. Committees have designated meeting times, keep minutes, make decisions, and develop reports. Members need to prepare for meetings and attend regularly. There are two very common errors made with committees. The first error is having too many committees and too many meetings. When this occurs, staff members get tired of committee work and feel that they are just attending meetings. The second error is meetings that are not effective. Both of these errors lead to problems—staff apathy, lack of effective results, loss of work time, lack of staff interest to participate, and so on.

NURSING ROLES ON COMMITTEES   Nurses need to be very active in the committee work in an acute care hospital and in any health care setting in which they work. Depending upon how the hospital and its committee structure are set up, nurses may be selected or may volunteer for committee membership. Becoming involved in a committee provides a different perspective of the hospital and its needs. Nurses have much to add when planning is done and decisions are made that affect patient care. The CNE needs to take on the leadership of ensuring a nursing presence on hospital committees.

# Framework for Effective Care

Chapters 16 and 17 discuss quality improvement in more detail. Quality improvement relies on standards as well as policies and procedures; however, the following provides information on these two topics as they relate to acute care hospitals and their operation and services.

## Standards

Standards are used by hospitals to provide guidelines for care provided and professional responsibilities. They can have an impact on the quality of care, patient outcomes, and the workforce environment. The American Nurses Association (ANA) and specialty nursing organizations have developed many standards. These standards may be used within a hospital and other health care settings such as a home health agency, city health department, behavioral health hospital, or a hospital that may use the standards to provide guidance that is specifically developed by the hospital. Many hospitals use a combination of both approaches to develop their internal standards. There typically are overall nursing standards and then standards for specialty areas. These standards, however, should be consistent with the professional standards. Other sources of information about standards are local, state, and federal laws and regulations and accreditation organizations. Evidence-based practice (EBP) also emphasizes the use of standards and the development of standards based on what research demonstrates as effective care. Chapter 15 discusses the evidence-based approach as a tool that is used in health care.

There can be confusion about the different types of standards. A **standard** is an "authoritative statement defined and promoted by the profession by which the quality of practice, services, or education can be evaluated" (American Nurses Association, 2004, p. 49). Clinical nursing standards include standards that focus on care, nursing practice, and professional performance (American Nurses Association, 2004, p. 116).

**Standards of Care:**   Authoritative statements that describe a competent level of clinical nursing practice demonstrated through assessment, diagnosis, outcome identification, planning, implementation, and evaluation.

**Standards of Nursing Practice:**   Authoritative statements that describe a level of care or performance common to the profession of nursing by which the quality of nursing practice can be judged. Standards of clinical nursing practice include both standards of care and standards of professional performance.

**Standards of Professional Performance:**    Authoritative statements that describe a competent level of professional behavior of the nurse in the areas of quality of care, performance appraisal, education, collegiality, ethics, collaboration, research, and resource utilization appropriate.

## Policies and Procedures

**Policies** and **procedures** are found in every hospital and other types of health care organizations. They are the "formal, approved description of how a governance, management, or clinical care process is defined, organized, and carried out" (Joint Commission, 2004, p. 335). Policies and procedures provide guidelines for staff when decisions are made or procedures are done. This section describes the policy and procedure development process in some detail and is an example of how a health care organization develops its processes and how a committee might work.

In addition to the general overriding concerns of quality care, risk management, and cost containment, each hospital department within a general hospital and nursing department needs to consider eight factors that have an impact on policy and procedure development. When a hospital or department decides to develop or revise its policies and procedures, these factors should not be ignored, and they are also important for most major changes that nursing might consider in a health care organization. If a nursing department attempts to operate in isolation from other departments in the hospital, from the hospital organization itself, or from the external environment, this leads to communication problems and work performance barriers. Because change is inherent, each of these factors requires frequent review to maintain relevant policies and procedures.

1. **Joint Commission.** The Joint Commission provides accreditation surveys for health care facilities and details the requirements for accreditation in its manuals and on its website. It is the first resource for any nursing department to use in policy and procedure development; however, the detailed content of policies and procedures needs to be individualized. The Joint Commission manual and its standards are not written to be used as an individual hospital's or a nursing department's policy and procedure manual. It does not include specific policies and procedures for hospitals, but rather it provides guidelines for content and direction. (See Chapter 17 for additional information about the Joint Commission and accreditation.)

2. **Professional standards.** Professional standards reflect a specific professional group's views on what is acceptable professional performance. The professional nursing standards, along with the Joint Commission standards, identify many additional issues to consider in policies and procedures. For example, nursing standards describe the nurse's role in assessment. A hospital would use this guideline in the development of a policy and procedure related to the admission assessment.

3. **State and federal legislation.** State legislatures determine regulations that need to be monitored carefully, such as state nurse practice acts and rules and regulations, reimbursement requirements, safety requirements, facility requirements, and staffing level regulations. In the federal arena, the most important issue is reimbursement. It is particularly critical for hospitals reimbursed by Medicare and/or Medicaid to understand current reimbursement legislation and regulations. Emergency department issues are affected by laws, and these would have to be incorporated in policies and procedures about emergency admissions and transfers.

4. **Court decisions.** Court decisions have affected many areas of patient care, particularly when related to patient's rights, length-of-stay, commitment, discharge planning, patient and staff protection, and informed consent. The hospital's legal counsel often provides guidance in this area.

5. **Reimbursement.** Reimbursement governs or is a strong factor in many decisions made in hospitals, including decisions related to length-of-care and type of treatment as well as discharge plans. In addition, staffing cuts and increased stress to patients and families caused

by concern about the cost of care and the duration of care that is covered by their personal health endurance directly affect the health care environment. Hospitals have policies and procedures about checking health coverage, what is covered, and other aspects related to reimbursement.

6. **Patients' rights.** Patients' rights are part of both the Joint Commission standards and the ANA standards and greatly impacted by HIPAA. These rights are identified in writing and shared with patients, families, and staff. In addition, the rights need to be incorporated into policies and procedures. For example, in a procedure that describes preoperative care, patients' rights would be included by identifying how informed consent should be obtained, by whom, when, and how it is to be documented.

7. **The Community.** The community in which the hospital is located must not be ignored. The hospital develops both a relationship with, and an image in, the community. Two areas of consideration are of particular importance. The type of support available to the patient and family in the community has a major effect on the hospital's ability to discharge patients and prevent complications and readmission. Examples of issues that need to be considered are availability of home health care, medical supplies and equipment, general support such as Meals-on-Wheels, social services, case management, and so on, and ambulatory care clinics. With the increasing movement to care in the community, hospitals need to develop more strategies for connecting their services with the community.

8. **Evidence-Based Practice (EBP).** The nursing department that is interested in maintaining an up-to-date department and providing quality nursing care will utilize research results and professional literature to develop and revise its policies and procedures, ensuring that they are evidence-based. EBP needs to be integrated throughout the hospital and is a critical health care profession competency (Institute of Medicine, 2003; 2008). It is hoped that this external influence will also encourage the nursing department to support its own research and the development of literature for publication, and thereby share its experiences with other nurses. The continuing progress of nursing care depends on nursing research conducted in the clinical setting. For these reasons, policies and procedures related to nursing research should be included. Evidence-based practice, as discussed in Chapter 15, supports the need to collect and analyze data to support decisions. This includes management decisions such as the development of policies and procedures. Figure 6-1 describes the key issues related to policy and procedure development.

**FIGURE 6-1   Key issues related to the development of policies and procedures.**

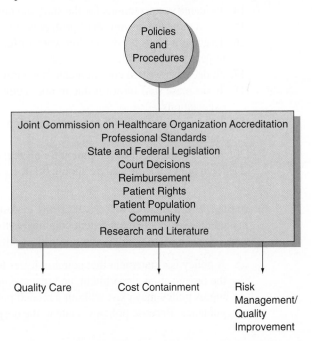

After considering the major influences on policies and procedures, the policy development process has begun. Policy and procedure development is a complex process that ultimately affects both management of the nursing department and all of the care provided. The entire process takes place in the context of the critical concerns and influences previously described. It needs to involve all of the nursing staff. It is a process that flows from the chief nurse executive to the nursing management staff, and then to staff at all levels in the department. Policy and procedure development is typically the responsibility of a committee designated for this purpose. The following discussion describes the objectives, definitions, and format of policies and procedures as well as the development and implementation processes. This also provides an example of how committees function in organizations. As each nursing department is different, this information serves only as guidelines. It should be noted that typically a hospital has an organization-wide committee on policies and procedures; however, in some hospitals the nursing department also has its own policy and procedure committee that interrelates to the hospital-wide committee. Regardless of the type of structure, the process that is described applies to both types of committees.

The first step in developing policies and procedures for the nursing department is for nursing administration to identify the objectives for the members' development and their implementation. If this is not the first step, policy and procedure development will be neither organized nor helpful to the nursing staff. Each hospital and its nursing service are different, and objectives can therefore vary. The following is a list of possible objectives that can serve as guidelines for individual nursing departments.

1. To promote quality care and EBP
2. To implement the hospital's and the nursing department's vision/mission and objectives
3. To support effective implementation of the nursing care model
4. To incorporate changes in health care into the hospital
5. To increase the quality and quantity of work through consistent decision making and action
6. To maintain cost containment through efficient use of staff, time, and supplies
7. To meet accrediting agencies' requirements
8. To maintain professional nursing standards
9. To increase the quality of communication at all levels in the organization
10. To promote a risk management program by preventing negligence and maintaining safety of patients, visitors, and staff
11. To delineate lines of authority
12. To increase interprofessional collaboration
13. To assist in developing sound judgment
14. To identify expectations for the staff and promote job security
15. To promote the resolution of problems closer to the problem situation
16. To act as a focus for discussion when differences occur and thus decrease the opportunity to personalize conflicts
17. To decrease written communication regarding daily problems
18. To decrease staff turnover due to poor communication and inadequate identification of expectations
19. To assist with orientation for new, transferred, promoted, or temporary staff and for nursing faculty and students
20. To assist with staff development for all nursing staff
21. Each policy and procedure should relate to at least one of the objectives

**DEFINITIONS OF POLICY AND PROCEDURE**    Many definitions for policy and procedure are found in the literature, but one consistent comment is that the terms are different from and yet related to each other. How are policies and procedures different or similar?

- A policy is a statement that communicates to staff the expectations and vision/mission of the organization, department, and management. It provides a guideline for decision making. A policy may exist without a related procedure if staff requires no further specific guidance. Because policies relate to the hospital's and the department's objectives and do not change very often, policies are revised less often than procedures. Review of a nursing department's policy manual should provide a total picture of the particular department's beliefs concerning its management and the nursing care it provides. Identifying a policy does not negate the need for individual judgment, nor does it negate the professional nurse's accountability for decision making.

- A procedure is a definite statement describing the step-by-step actions required for a specific outcome. It provides a recipe for reaching a specific goal and that goal is often a completed treatment that is safe for the patient and efficient in the use of staff, time, supplies, and equipment. A procedure is more detailed than a policy, and changes in routine or treatment directly affect procedures, which then require revision. Written procedures support quality care and prevent errors that might be detrimental to the patient and to the department or hospital. Procedures and policies both help to maintain consistency and continuity; however, to do so, they need to be written in concise, easy-to-understand language and contain appropriate and up-to-date information. If policies and procedures are just words on paper, they will not be utilized by the staff, and all the effort, time, and money spent to develop them will therefore be wasted.

POLICY AND PROCEDURE FORMATS    Formats for policies and procedures also vary greatly from hospital to hospital; however, certain elements always need to be included. These elements are the title, effective date, review date, purpose, and identification of the responsibility for final review. Boxes 6-2 and 6-3 describe examples of policy and procedure formats.

| BOX 6-2 | **EXAMPLE OF A POLICY FORMAT** |
|---------|-------------------------------|

DEPARTMENT OF NURSING POLICY MANUAL
POLICY NUMBER

TITLE:
POLICY AREA:
EFFECTIVE DATE:
REVIEW SCHEDULE:
FINAL APPROVAL RESPONSIBILITY:
PRIMARY RESPONSIBILITY:


PURPOSE:


POLICY:


SUPPORTING EVIDENCE:


Approved by:


Date: _____                    Review Dates: _____

| BOX 6-3 | EXAMPLE OF A PROCEDURE FORMAT |
|---------|-------------------------------|

DEPARTMENT OF NURSING PROCEDURAL MANUAL
PROCEDURE NUMBER

TITLE:

PROCEDURE AREA:

EFFECTIVE DATE:

REVIEW SCHEDULE:

FINAL APPROVAL RESPONSIBILITY:

WHO MAY PERFORM:

PURPOSE:


EQUIPMENT AND SUPPLIES:


ACTION:


SUPPORTING EVIDENCE:

More and more organizations are putting their policies and procedures online, moving away from hard copies or manuals. This makes the information more accessible as long as staff can access a computer and get into the hospital intranet. It is also easier to update the policies and procedures, and changes can be quickly communicated to staff. As changes are made, it is easier to find related material that needs to be changed (for example, other policies and procedures) by searching for content.

POLICY AND PROCEDURE COMMITTEE   The policy and procedure committee is a very active committee and requires members who are willing to do work that at times may be tedious. As an advisory committee, the committee does not have the ultimate authority for the approval of a policy or a procedure. The final approval process and responsibility must be clearly defined. The best size for this committee is six to eight members with a chairperson. If the committee is too small, the members may feel burdened with work, and if it is too large, getting the members together efficiently becomes difficult. With at least a 2-year term of membership, the members will have time to be productive on the committee. Since it is also important to get new ideas, committee membership should include both new and old members; therefore, it should have rotating changes in membership. This will ensure that there will be some experienced members on the committee at all times. The purpose of this committee is to develop the policies and procedures for the nursing service/department and to maintain a system for periodic review and revision of policies and procedures. This committee's work is never completed, and it thus requires active participation and an interest in this work from all members. With the increasing emphasis on EBP it is important for all hospitals to ensure that current policies and procedures are evidence-based. This requires time and work.

ROLE OF NURSING ADMINISTRATION/MANAGEMENT   The CNE typically does not serve on the committee but has many responsibilities related to this committee. Examples of these responsibilities include the following.

1. To clarify with hospital administration the nursing committee's relationship to the hospital policy and procedure committee and to provide written communication on this issue to the nursing committee

2. To appoint a chairperson (unless the chairperson is to be elected)
3. To identify needs for policies and procedures
4. To communicate specific policy and procedure issues to the committee
5. To review and approve all new and revised policies and procedures
6. To communicate to all nursing management staff and all nursing staff the importance of policies and procedures and encourage their input in the development process
7. To ensure that policies and procedures are implemented and evaluated
8. To review and respond to the committee's annual report
9. To provide secretarial assistance for the preparation of the policies and procedures

Through the fulfillment of these responsibilities, the CNE communicates the importance of policies and procedures and coordinates the committee's work both within the department and with other departments, acting as a facilitator.

ROLE OF THE COMMITTEE CHAIRPERSON   The chairperson should be a nursing staff member who can organize well and work effectively with others. The committee is very busy, and consequently, the chairperson should not have many responsibilities on other committees. The chairperson has the following responsibilities:

1. Select committee members using the designated approval process.
2. Establish a meeting schedule and attendance requirements.
3. Establish a process for electing a committee secretary who will keep the minutes.
4. Maintain contact with secretarial assistance provided by nursing administration/ management.
5. Ensure that all records are up-to-date (attendance, minutes, location of all manuals, annual reports, individual files on each policy and procedure, records of review dates for each policy and procedure).
6. Ensure that the committee selects appropriate methods for identifying need and content of policies and procedures.
7. Ensure that the committee develops the content for the policies and procedures and that the approval process is maintained.
8. Establish a system for review of each policy and procedure.
9. Select reviewers for policies and procedures and maintain a list of the reviewers, the policies and procedures reviewed, and deadlines.
10. Participate in staff development related to policies and procedures.
11. Prepare an annual report.

ROLE OF THE COMMITTEE MEMBERS   The policy and procedure committee's work will be more efficient and more responsive to actual needs if there is broad nursing representation on the committee. This representation allows for greater input and participation by nursing staff. Coming to the meeting prepared helps the committee do its work more efficiently and effectively. Committee members' responsibilities include the following:

1. Attend meetings regularly.
2. Complete designated work by deadlines.
3. Assist in selecting appropriate methods for identifying need and content of policies and procedures.
4. Collect data for policies and procedures.
5. Review policies and procedures for committee approval before moving the policy or procedure through the committee approval process.
6. Participate in staff development related to policies and procedures.

THE PROCESS OF POLICY AND PROCEDURE DEVELOPMENT   It is important to remember that policies and procedures do not make robots out of the nursing staff. No two situations are exactly alike, and as a consequence, policies and procedures will be interpreted differently at different times. Professional nursing staff members are taught and encouraged to think through their decisions using the policies and procedures as guidelines. They are developed to help the staff, not to freeze creativity. This flexibility does not negate the importance of implementing policies and procedures, but supports the idea that effective decision making requires more than just following a set of written rules.

1. **Identification of need.** After the committee structure is organized, the next step is to determine the policy and procedure needs of the nursing department. The best way to begin is to review existing policies and procedures. Some may require no changes; some may require changes; some may need to be eliminated; and some may need to be added. In addition, the major influences on policies discussed earlier in this section should be considered. A thoughtful evaluation of policies and procedures with input from nursing staff that uses them is very helpful in making these decisions.

   Many of the decisions in nursing departments are made in crisis situations. Health care is not static, and consequently, changes frequently occur suddenly and require immediate decisions. Decisions to develop a policy and procedure often are made during crises. However, responding to a crisis by saying, "We need a policy on this" is not always the best approach and can result in many infrequently used policies or procedures. Too many policies and procedures can be just as harmful as too few. Staff may begin to see all policies and procedures as paper with little substance. If nursing administration and the committee are aware of changes occurring in the department, the hospital, the community, and health care, then policies and procedures will more likely be developed in non-crisis periods with a less harried approach. The critical word in policy and procedure development is change, a recurrent theme in this text. Changes may or may not affect policies and procedures, but it must always be considered. Changes in any of the following areas should be an indication for the committee to evaluate the policies and procedures:

   - Hospital's policies and procedures
   - Evidence; research and other types of evidence
   - Departmental organization
   - Vision/mission and objectives for the department and the hospital
   - Factors related to other departments that affect nursing
   - Patient population and needs
   - Medical procedures and treatment modalities
   - Nursing routines
   - Documentation
   - Equipment changes
   - Staffing
   - Position descriptions
   - Incidents and consultations with attorney and insurance carrier
   - Reports from reviewing agencies and their criteria
   - Reimbursement
   - State and federal laws
   - Current, relevant professional literature

   There are many ways to obtain data that are useful in identifying policy and procedure needs. It is best to employ multiple methods and to evaluate these methods periodically to determine whether they provide relevant, timely data. Staff interviews and questionnaires are two methods; however, they both require time to develop, collect, and analyze. A poorly conducted interview or poorly written questionnaire will not result in helpful information, and consequently, the committee's time and effort will be wasted. Nursing staff members will also feel their time has been wasted. Surveys of other institutions may also be helpful, but again, surveys need to be well written and short. The response to a survey may not be great, so committees should not depend on this method for a major portion of the data.

   Some data collection methods do not require as much preparation as interviews and questionnaires but do require thoughtful analysis after data collection. One of these methods is observation. One important reason for rounds by nursing management staff is to have the opportunity to observe, and committee members can also use this method. Not all that is observed is relevant to a policy or a procedure, so careful analysis of observations is important. Talking with nursing staff and physicians informally rather than using a structured interview can often reveal concerns and needs, but decisions cannot be made on what just a few people say. After informal discussion, further investigation will be necessary. Material that is already available, such as audits, incident reports, annual reports from nursing and other departments, requests for staff development on particular topics, and minutes from staff meetings, may reveal many needs for new policies and procedures or needs for change in existing ones. Another method that may provide data is interviewing new staff members after their orientation to find out what information was difficult for them to obtain and what problems they encountered. Still another source is one that is often not considered: patients and their families, who frequently have concerns that relate to policies and procedures.

Need identification is a process. It does not happen once, and it is never complete. Communicating the nature of need identification to the nursing staff helps to emphasize that their input into the process is always useful. Staff members should never put off communicating questions or concerns that they may have about policies and procedures. A committee or nursing management that does not listen to the nursing staff will soon encounter problems and will not have effective policies and procedures.

2. **Development of content.** Before developing the content for a particular policy or procedure, the committee identifies the policy or procedure's purpose. The committee asks, "What is the decision to be made?" and "Why make the decision?" At the same time, the committee identifies who will make the decision or perform the procedure. Policy and procedure content must support the vision, mission, and objectives of the department and the hospital, and the state nurse practice act and nursing standards. Content should be evidence-based. The committee also needs to be alert to conflicts between policies and procedures. It is important to compare new or altered policies and procedures with other policies and procedures and determine if there is conflict or overlap, or if the policy or procedure will cause problems with other departments.

   In developing policies and procedures, there are several factors to keep in mind. First, terminology needs to be clear and concise. As lengthy, cumbersome statements do not communicate information quickly, short sentences are preferable. Abbreviations and acronyms may be used; however, when initially used, they need to be defined and not conflict with the hospitals approved abbreviation/acronym list. Their meanings should be included for reference. Second, so that staff can make decisions efficiently, the information in a policy or procedure should be organized in logical steps. Committee members provide multiple checks of logical steps by asking questions such as the following: "Does this make sense? Can it be followed easily? Is it complete? Could it be stated more simply?"

3. **Approval.** After the content is developed, the approval phase begins. The approval process needs to be clearly designated. No policy or procedure should be implemented without written approval. This rule must be strictly enforced, particularly since there are probably copies of the draft that could be interpreted as official policy or procedure. All nursing staff should be told to check for the approval signature and date before applying a policy or procedure.

4. **Implementation and communication.** Implementation of a policy or a procedure requires planning and participation from the committee and nursing management. The goal of implementation is to make all nursing staff aware of the new or changed policy or procedure and to get them to apply it in appropriate situations. Implementation requires that staff knows about the policy and procedure, understands it, and knows when to apply it. All of these factors influence the implementation process. It is not always easy to get the nursing staff to use a policy or procedure. Management staff members become important in this effort, but they need a thorough understanding of the purpose and the content of the policy or procedure. All of this makes communication a very important part of the implementation process to assure that nursing staff knows about the policy or procedure content; when it is in effect; who may make the decision or perform the procedure; and what the process is for providing feedback about a policy or procedure.

A critical question about implementation that often arises is, "What keeps staff from using policies and procedures?" There are many answers to this question, and consideration of these answers will help to combat underutilization of policies and procedures. Some of the most frequent reasons for not using policies and procedures are that staff members

- Cannot find the policy and procedure manual.
- Do not know what is in the manual.
- Do not know how to use the manual.
- Do not know how to access the computer; unable to access a computer when need; unable to find information on the computer.
- Do not understand how policies and procedures reflect the philosophy of the department and the hospital.
- Do not feel the policies and procedures are practical or helpful.
- Do not like someone telling them what to do and how to do it.
- Do not understand how the policies and procedures protect the patient and staff and support quality care.
- Feel that poor communication in the department results in a poor relationship between the staff and administration.
- Feel policies and procedures represent more paperwork.

Staff may, however, have an appropriate reason for ignoring the policies and procedures. Each complaint needs to be discussed, and if necessary, resolved. It is, therefore, important to plan all steps of the development and implementation processes. Anticipation of some of the possible problems before they occur may provide a better chance of successfully implementing a policy or procedure.

Staff development or education plays an important role in the implementation of policies and procedures. Staff development personnel frequently are directly involved in preparing staff for a new policy or procedure by providing programs about content related to a policy and procedure (for example, what happens during a code). As a consequence, staff development personnel need to be kept fully informed of changes. In fact, it might be helpful to have a staff education representative on the policy and procedure committee. Staff development nurses frequently are the first to recognize that a policy or procedure requires a change or that a new one is needed. When all of this information is filtered through appropriate channels, the result is a more comprehensive, useful policy and procedure manual that is utilized on a daily basis by the staff.

Through staff development, nursing staff develop an understanding of why a policy or procedure exists and what the content means to their practice. It is clear that because the staff nurse cannot know everything, the nurse needs to know where to find information quickly. How can nurses be made to look in the manual or on the computer for the policies and procedures? Reminding them whenever situations occur that require implementation of a policy or a procedure is one way; however, more structured methods are also necessary such as written communications, inclusion of information in staff meetings, posters reminding staff of new policies and procedures, and staff development programs on these topics.

5. **Evaluation and revision.** In most departments evaluation and revision is probably the weakest part of policy and procedure development. It is, however, critical to the success of implementation. An outdated policy or procedure can be just as detrimental to care and to the organization as no policy or procedure. Changes never come easily and usually involve some risk, but a system designed to ensure that every policy and procedure is evaluated regularly and that records are kept on this evaluation can ease change. Box 6-4 provides an example of an evaluation form that can be used to get feedback from staff that is using the policies and procedures.

Why has so much content been presented about policies and procedures and the development process? They provide guidelines or expectations to assist staff members as they make decisions and provide care. In addition, understanding one example that describes how an organization develops and provides direction to staff, such as through policies and procedures, helps in understanding project development—there is a problem and then the organization goes about solving it.

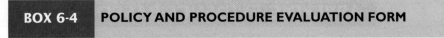

| BOX 6-4 | POLICY AND PROCEDURE EVALUATION FORM |
|---|---|

**POLICY OR PROCEDURE NUMBER**
**TITLE:**



What is the problem(s) you encountered with this policy or procedure?



What recommendations do you have for changes?



**SIGNATURE:**
**UNIT:**
**DATE:**

# Changes That Affect Acute Health Care Delivery

The acute care delivery system has experienced many major changes over the last decade, for example the change toward more community and primary care; emphasis on health care delivery and financial issues; such as growth of managed care and other reimbursement issue; and changes in organizations such as mergers or closing of hospitals. These changes have led to problems for many communities (such as rural areas) when their hospitals close. Community members then have to travel longer distances to get health services. The key factors that have affected health care delivery and the acute care hospital system are as follows:

- Problems with access (eligibility for government benefits such as Medicaid, transportation, hours of operation, number and type of providers, child care, cost of care)
- Reimbursement and managed care
- Increased number of the uninsured and underinsured
- Demographic changes (increasing age of population, single-parent families, immigrant growth, limited access to extended family members, diversity)
- Aging population with chronic illness and greater acuity and complications when hospitalized
- Improvement in technology that extends lifespan and increases costs
- Uneven distribution of health care services (for example, more services in urban areas as compared to rural areas)
- Increase in homeless population with limited health care access
- Increase in new drug therapies that are costly
- Increase in specialty usage leading to fragmentation of care and increased cost

Newhouse and Mills (2002) note that "Ackerman's (1992) description of the health care environment still rings true. Health care organizations are still engulfed in efforts to control spiraling costs, provide care for an aging population with increasing health demands, and obtain human resources to provide care. Technology has provided a means to affect the health of patients and reduce their length of stay, but has also increased the cost of care" (p. 6). The Institute of Medicine (IOM) reports on quality identify that the system is dysfunctional (2001). The following is a discussion of some of the important changes affecting hospitals.

## APPLYING EVIDENCE-BASED PRACTICE

### Evidence for Effective Leadership and Management

**Citation:**   Storey, S., Linden, E., & Fisher, M. (2008). Showcasing leadership exemplars to propel professional practice model implementation. *JONA, 38*(3), 138–142.

**Overview:**   This qualitative study examined the question: What are the aspects of successful leadership in implementing a professional practice model (PPM)? "As leadership begins to role model the components of the PPM, staff nurses are given autonomy and are empowered to influence patient outcomes through change. But what is the nature of leadership's best practices that reflect the PPM?" (p. 139). This question was explored through in-depth interviews of four directors identified by their peers as exemplar leaders at one acute care hospital. The interviews were recorded, and three independent reviewers analyzed the verbatim interviews for themes. Results indicate that these leaders demonstrated leadership and themes (reflective practice, aspirational thinking, interdisciplinary approach, risk taking, attitude, and passion) that were directly related to the model (core values, professional development, professional practice and behaviors, community connections, and outcomes).

**Application:**   Best leadership practices have an impact on implementation of a PPM such as the Synergy Model and others. This study, though it includes a small sample, indicates that understanding how this process works and the implication of leadership to move professional practice model implementation forward is critical.

**Questions:**

1. *Discuss the implication of best leadership practice on a change to a professional practice model.*
2. *Why is it important to move nursing to a higher level of responsibility?*
3. *What does "modeling behaviors" mean, and why is it important?*

### Emergency Services

Emergency services (ED) are not only provided in emergency departments that are part of hospitals, and also by urgent care centers, which may be freestanding, separate from hospitals, or part of a hospital organization. In hospitals with trauma centers the emergency services play a critical role in trauma services. The Institute of Medicine has recently published several reports on emergency services. These services are described as "overburdened, underfunded, and highly fragmented" (2007a, p. 1). Frequently patients have to be sent to other hospitals due to overburdened ED units. Emergency care for children is also a problem (Institute of Medicine, 2007b). These patients have unique needs, and this service is also not performing at required levels. Emergency medical services are described as "the initial stages of the emergency care continuum. It includes emergency calls to 9-1-1; dispatch of emergency personnel to the scene of an illness or trauma; and triage, treatment, and transport of patients by ambulance and air medical service. The speed and quality of emergency medical services are critical factors in a patient's ultimate outcome" (Institute of Medicine, 2006, p. 1). The 2006 report describes the system as having insufficient coordination, disparities in response time, uncertain quality of care, lack of readiness for disasters, divided professional identity, and limited evidence base. The 2010 health care reform legislation recognizes the national emergency service problem and includes providing trauma care, establishing a new trauma care center program to strengthen emergency department and trauma capacity, and developing new models for emergency care.

**Downsizing** has also had a major impact on the emergency care services/department (ED). This service is one of the areas of care that has received much media attention, primarily focused on reimbursement denial when insurers consider the care non-emergent. Health plan benefits usually state that emergency care requires preauthorization. Laypeople may consider many conditions an emergency, particularly when they are not sure what is happening to them. They go to the emergency room to have a health care professional diagnose their problem and need for treatment. Health plans, however, set their own standards for what constitutes an emergency; some plans do this more than others. There has been concern for a long time that an increasing number of patients are using emergency services as their primary care provider. This is especially true for the uninsured. This is not the best treatment for continuity or for most medical problems. It also increases the patient load in the emergency department and provides less staff to treat true emergencies. Emergency staff also becomes frustrated with these patients who should receive care elsewhere, and the frustration spills over onto the patients and their families.

Not only are emergency services experiencing an increase in the number of patients who do not need emergency services, but in many hospitals the emergency room is often used to hold patients who are admitted and should be transferred to appropriate inpatient units. With decreased staff working on the inpatient units and some beds closed, patients cannot be transferred out of the ED quickly. Staff find this to be very frustrating, and these patients require staff time that should be used for patients who do need emergency services. Emergency room nurses need to be involved in recommending strategies for coping with these problems. This requires collaboration and an ability to assess these problems objectively. With the expertise that ED nurses have they should participate in the development of solutions. A place to begin is to consider some of the following questions: Do local community providers need to extend their hours? Do patients know what care is available to them and how to access it? Could advanced practice nurses be used to assist with triaging patients or running urgent care clinics? Should the hospital develop urgent care center, or is it best for the hospital to collaborate with existing urgent care providers? There are many other possibilities, and with staff input hospitals can resolve these critical problems. The health care reform legislation of 2010 includes provisions about emergency and trauma services, recognizing the need for changes. A new trauma center program is to be established to increase emergency service capacity, fund research on emergency care, and develop demonstration programs to design, implement, and evaluate innovative care models in the emergency and trauma setting.

When decisions are made about emergency services' policies and procedures, their content must meet the requirements of the federal law, Emergency Medical Treatment and Active Labor Act of 1986 (EMTALA), or the hospital can be fined. In addition to the extension of coverage, EMATAL established a federal requirement that all hospitals with emergency services that participate in Medicare—and this is most hospitals—must treat all patients requiring emergency treatment or who are in labor. Inability to pay cannot be used as a reason to deny emergency treatment. This offers a major protection for the patient; however, the critical issue is the definition of an emergency and who defines it. Some patients use the local emergency department as their personal physician office. Insurers are concerned about this use, but the patients for whom this law is addressed often have no insurance. How does this affect emergency service expenses? What is the hospital's moral obligation? Neither of these questions can be ignored, nor are they simple to answer. The following are aspects of this problem, which affect the ED, the entire hospital, and the entire health care delivery system in a community.

TRIAGE   Triage is the process of determining which patients need immediate treatment, a process to prioritize patient needs. There are several issues pertinent to triage. The first is to perform a medical screening examination and to stabilize the patient. What constitutes a screening is not described by federal regulation. It could be as limited as taking vital signs and identifying a chief complaint to a complete workup or referral to a specialist. Clearly, the patient's condition should determine the type of screening that is required. Patients may refuse care at any point, and to protect the emergency room and its staff, this refusal should be obtained in writing. This prevents questions about the staff refusing treatment to the patient. The troubling issue arises when the insurer refuses to authorize the emergency care. The critical factor for emergency staff is the patient's condition, and care should be provided if the patient accepts it. Patients may at times become upset with their insurer's response. Staff needs to listen but avoid being judgmental, which is not easy to do. Emergency staff receives different directions about who is responsible for calling the patient's insurer to obtain authorization of emergency treatment. Hospitals need to have well-defined steps for this procedure because it can make a major difference as to whether or not reimbursement is covered. Many patients today are very aware of the need to contact their insurer and will bring it up themselves. Reaching the insurer with the information may vary depending on time of day and the staffing level for authorization calls. These efforts to call should be documented by ED staff. Because this really is a financial issue, the patient is the best person to speak with the plan representative, but in many cases the patient is unable to do this due to his or her condition, and because family members may not be available.

MEDICAL EVALUATION AND THERAPY    There are times when the insurance plan representative insists that the patient be sent elsewhere for treatment or testing. This can cause a conflict for ED staff. The first priority is to stabilize the patient and ensure that the best care is provided. The physician may need to speak with the plan representative. Insurers want their patients seen and treated by contracted providers (e.g., physicians/hospitals who have been approved by the plan to treat the plan's members), something that is not always possible. When permission is given to use a non-contract provider, emergency staff must document this with details, such as authorization number, insurance representative spoken to, time, date, and so on. Another treatment issue that occurs is the problem of reimbursement for specific medications. It is often easier to change the prescription to one that is covered than to argue about one that is not covered, unless there is no other appropriate medication available. Providers should never alter a diagnosis in order to ensure reimbursement. Any injury that occurred while the patient was working must be reported as an employment injury because this affects workers' compensation. If this is not done, it may be viewed as defrauding the patient's insurer.

MEDICAL DISPOSITION AND DISCHARGE    If patients are stable with little likelihood of deteriorating, they can be transferred. The patient must agree to the transfer; however, the patient must be legally competent to agree. Patients in this situation must realize that they can receive emergency treatment regardless of their ability to pay. As is always true, transferring patients from one unit to another (or in this case to another facility) requires that the nurse and/or physician give a report to staff in the receiving facility or unit, and that the receiving facility or unit must have the resources to provide the care that the patient needs. The receiving admission office or the ED staff must be notified of the transfer and time of arrival of the new patient. Discharge against medical advice (DAMA or AMA) occurs when a patient decides to leave treatment when the physician or health care provider feels that treatment should continue.

Emergency care is a specialty area that has been affected by legislation and will likely be important in health care legislation in the future. Questions related to denial of emergency services and the need for these services, the patient's view of emergency services, and emergency care provided outside the plan's geographic area need to be addressed and clearly described to consumers. Hospital staff frequently encounters problems such as the ones described with ED patients that then affect inpatient units and patient care.

## Patient Access to Services

Patients have to get into and out of hospitals, and this process is one that can lead to problems for patients, their families, and the staff. As this content is discussed, consider how patients are admitted and discharged in local hospitals. What are the problems that occur? What can be done to improve the process for all concerned? It is not uncommon for staff that is responsible for the "paperwork" part of admission and discharge to be disconnected from the direct care providers, particularly nurses. This gap is where problems occur, and frustration increases. This is when nursing staff is heard saying, "Don't they realize we don't have a clean room yet?", "How many more admissions can we handle this shift?", "This patient should have been sent to another unit because he does not meet our admission criteria.", "Why is it taking so long to get those discharge papers?", and "Where is the transport staff to take the patient down to her car?" The comments can go on and on. In the meantime, admissions staff members are also frustrated. They are saying, "Why can't they get those rooms cleaned up faster so that we can move these patients out?", "We don't have the doctor's order for discharge.", "This admission information is incomplete.", "Where is the patient going after discharge?", and "The nursing home will not accept his insurance." As was mentioned earlier in the content about committees, it is important to have interdisciplinary input for effective patient access services—admission and discharge. Transfers also cause problems, whether they are internal from unit to unit or external to other health care facilities. Transfers or handoffs are also times of increase in errors, which can lead to complications for the patient. Handoff errors are discussed further in Chapter 17. All of this can lead to less cost-effective care. Admission and discharge problems take time, and this means additional costs to the organization. There is always the need to make sure that the admission is appropriate to ensure that reimbursement for care is approved. However, patients who stay too long may find that there is no or limited reimbursement for their care. These are major problems for hospitals.

## Patient Education

For many years acute care settings have been required to provide patient education to meet accreditation requirements. Nursing education and the profession also have a long history of emphasizing the role of nurses in providing patient education. Despite this emphasis on patient education, health care still has not been very successful in providing it. Insurers have begun to recognize the importance of patient education, believing that it will reduce costs and increase patient satisfaction. Patient education methods and evaluation of outcomes are still not fully understood. Providing patient education in acute care has become even more difficult with the decreasing length-of-stay. Patients are sicker when admitted because efforts are first made to keep the patient out of the hospital, and then they stay only a short time. Patients are then often too sick to absorb patient education content, and when they begin to improve, they have less time to absorb the information because they are quickly discharged. Family members also have similar experiences—they are unable to focus on education when their family member is acutely ill, and then when they can, it is time for discharge. Nurses are tired, stressed, and have problems including patient education with the rapid turnover of patients. Hospitals are turning more toward standardized patient education material, which they purchase. Nurses, however, need to assess these materials carefully and should participate in the development of these materials and their adaptation to meet individual patient needs. Standardized educational materials can be excellent resources if they meet the needs of the hospital and patients/families. These resources can also reduce staff preparation time and increase content consistency, which are both important factors in today's busy acute care hospitals. Rapid discharge also means that hospital nurses must develop effective communication and collaborative relationships with agencies and other providers who will care for patients after discharge. Patient education needs to continue, and hospital nurses must share what educational content has been provided and the response of the patient/family to ensure that additional patient education meets the needs of the patient/family.

## Expansion into New Areas and Approaches

There are many changes in acute care services occurring almost daily, and due to the increasing use of outpatient surgery, surgical services have experienced major changes. Hospitals are increasing the size of their outpatient or ambulatory surgery departments and adjusting to the need of moving patients into and out of the surgical service in one day or even a few hours. This has affected many departments, particularly preadmission testing, admissions, nursing, clinical laboratories, pathology, radiology, pharmacy, anesthesiology, post-anesthesia recovery, and patient transportation. In some hospitals nurses call surgical patients at home prior to surgery to begin the nursing assessment and to give the patients brief preoperative education. Patients are coming in several days prior to surgery for their preadmission testing on an outpatient basis and then arriving at the hospital a few hours before their surgery for admission, which for some may be in the very early morning hours. Nursing staff may call patients a few days after surgery to assess their status. Surgical inpatient units are finding that their census has dropped because patients do not stay in the hospital after their surgery. Nurses have had to make adjustments in patient education that is typically provided after surgery because patients are now going home nauseated, barely recovered from anesthesia, and in pain. In these cases, family members receive the patient education.

USE OF HOSPITALISTS/INTENSIVISTS  Some hospitals have been using **hospitalists** or intensivists, as was discussed in Chapter 4. These are physicians who focus on inpatient care and are employees of the hospital. In some hospitals nurse practitioners are also in these positions. They serve as liaisons between the primary care provider in the office and specialists in the hospital. Primary care physicians trade off reduced income for fewer hospital visits to gain increased income for more billable time spent with patients in the office. "Hospitalists, therefore, attend to patients during hospital stays, rather than the primary care physicians who no longer visit their patients in the hospital. Hospitalists link specialists and coordinate care so that all physicians for one patient know the diagnoses, what has been ordered, and the patient's progress" (Milstead, 2002, p. 19). The goal in using hospitalists is to increase coordination and continuity of care. The **intensivist** works primarily in the intensive care unit in a similar role as a hospitalist. The expectation is the hospitalists and intensivists will be more up-to-date in hospital treatment than physicians in private practice since they provide hospital care daily.

## CASE STUDY

### Health Care Delivery Systems: Changing

You have been chosen to be on a committee that will plan the implementation of critical new changes within a hospital. Administration and medical staff have decided to open up some new positions: two intensivists and four clinical nurse specialists. You are serving on the newly formed interprofessional planning committee. The plan is due in 3 months and should include critical implementation issues. This is the first time the hospital has had an interprofessional team work on descriptions of new staff roles function within the hospital. You are not sure why you are on the committee, although you have worked on a number of units over the last 7 years. You still lack confidence in this type of setting (a committee, especially one that is interprofessional). The first meeting is used to discuss purpose and plan the work of the committee.

### Questions:

1. Why would the new roles of intensivist or clinical nurse specialist be helpful to the hospital and its staff?

2. What might be some reactions from medical and nursing staff about these new roles?

3. What needs to be done to prepare staff for the change?

4. Describe the critical elements that need to be clarified before staff is hired into these positions.

### Advanced Practice Nurses, Clinical Nurse Specialists, Clinical Nurse Leaders, and Nurse-Midwives

The roles of nurse practitioners, clinical nurse specialists, and nurse-midwives have been expanding in many hospitals just as advanced practice nurses in primary care are increasing. Nurse practitioners who work in acute care are acute care nurse practitioners (ACNPs), but some of these nurse practitioners have completed educational programs that focused on hospitalized patients. "Nurse practitioners are licenses independent practitioners who provide primary and/or specialty nursing and medical in ambulatory, acute, and long-term settings. They are registered nurses with specialized advanced education and clinical competency to provide health and medical care for diverse populations in a variety of primary care, acute care, and long-term care settings. Master's, post-master's, or doctoral preparation is required for entry into practice" (American Academy of Nurse Practitioners, 2006). Hospitals are also returning to using clinical nurse specialists (CNSs) in areas such as neonatal units, cardiology, critical care, trauma, internal medicine, and behavioral health/psychiatry. They work closely with families. Some hospitals are using ACNPs and CNSs in the same way they use house staff or as hospitalists. The new role of the clinical nurse leader (CNL) is also expanding. The Veteran's Administration (VA) has found that use of CNLs, who is seen as the "pivotal clinician; an 'attending' staff nurse at the point of care responsible for patient-driven, evidence-based, outcome-oriented nursing practice" (Ott, et al., 2009, p. 363). Many of the decisions to expand the usage of these nurses are driven by costs and the pressure of managed care for hospitals to reduce costs. Health care reform legislation will increase the need for more advanced practice nurses, with the increasing number of insured over the next 4 years; physician shortage; increase need for primary care; and the recommendation from the IOM to increase primary care services provided by nurse practitioners (Institute of Medicine, 2011).

## Alternative/Complementary Therapies

Alternative/complementary therapies are now found in almost all types of health care settings. Acute care hospitals are no exception to this growth. Insurers are beginning to cover some of these services. Acute care hospitals might offer massage therapy, acupuncture, and other methods within the hospital setting, in their ambulatory care services, and in their wellness centers. It is not yet clear the direction this will all take so it bears watching. Nurses may find that they are more involved in these services.

## Continuum of Care and Acute Care

Understanding and participating in the changing health care environment requires an appreciation of the importance of the continuum of care and its relationship to acute care. **Continuum of care** is "matching an individual's ongoing needs with the appropriate level and type of medical, psychological, health, or social care or service within an organization or across multiple organizations" (Joint Commission, 2004, p. 317). The goal is to avoid fragmented care, which only increases cost (Newhouse & Mills, 2002). The Institute of Medicine emphasizes the need for greater care coordination across the continuum by identifying care coordination as a major priority area (2003). The continuum includes health promotion, disease and illness prevention, ambulatory care, acute care, tertiary care, home health care, long-term care, and hospice care as it takes place within health care organizations and across organizations. Today, patients move into and out of the acute care setting quickly due to shorter lengths-of-stay. Acute care nurses are caring for sicker patients in shorter periods of time while they are overworked, short-staffed, and stressed. Nurses must become facilitators, actively using coordination skills to ensure that patients receive the care they need despite the shortened length-of-stay. Many nurses feel that they do not accomplish much with patients who often leave the hospital ill and in need of more care.

Using standardized operating procedures supports work processes to better ensure continuity (Newhouse & Mills, 2002). Case management has become common in many hospitals, and it is considered to be an important insurer strategy to reduce costs and ensure quality as the patient moves through the continuum of care (Finkelman, 2010). Hospitals have also found that case management is useful in assisting with care coordination and rapid discharge, which are both critical to cost reduction. The case manager is also used to ensure that quality care is provided throughout the stay. Nurses are frequently chosen to be case managers in hospitals. "Care coordination must include the following elements: a comprehensive plan of care; a multidisciplinary team approach for patients with complex needs; use of specialists as primary care providers (PCPs) as appropriate; collaboration with providers across the continuum of care; communication of postdischarge home and community arrangements; and medical record integration" (Newhouse & Mills, 2002, p. 87).

## Primary Care Providers

Primary care has grown in the last decade, and it has affected acute care. This care is provided by a particular level of provider (for example, family medicine, general internal medicine, general pediatrics, obstetrical/gynecology, and advanced practice nurses). Managed care has pushed the use of primary care providers to reduce costs. The primary care provider should serve as the gatekeeper to the health care system, providing care at the primary care level, and referring the patient to others for specialty care. The primary care provider should be aware of the patient's entire treatment plan and monitor the patient's progress. Does this always happen? Not always, but the goal is to improve in this area. However, most recently there have been fewer physicians going into primary care, mostly due to low reimbursement rates. Health care reform legislation should alter this picture and a return to increasing use of primary care providers.

## Nurses and Acute Care Hospital Changes

Nurses in hospitals are members of the system, and they need to learn to be more assertive in order to ensure that nursing care is recognized as critical to successful acute care. Nurses have much to offer in acute care settings, although they do not always get recognized. They also need to use their leadership skills to improve their position and role in hospital decision making.

Unwillingness to change and inability to explore new ideas that might be more cost-effective and yet provide quality care have a negative impact on improvement. Nurses with this attitude will eventually find that they are not part of the team, feel left out of the health care system, and may be out of jobs. This victim mentality acts as a barrier to the roles that nurses could assume within health care organizations, acute care, and others.

## Staffing Issues

It is difficult to discuss acute care without discussing the major nursing shortage. Chapter 9 discusses this topic in more detail; however, it is important to recognize the problem in this chapter on acute care. Acute care hospitals are not only adjusting staffing levels but also the staffing mix to reduce costs. Registered nurses (RNs) are finding themselves supervising unlicensed assistant personnel (UAP) more and more. Many nurses have not been adequately prepared for the supervisory role and delegation (see Chapter 14). RNs all carry the same license but may have completed diploma, associate's degree, or baccalaureate degrees for entry into nursing practice. Later chapters discuss differences in patient outcomes based on nursing education background. In some cases, patients are seeing fewer RNs and more UAP. This has increased staff stress and concern for errors and potential legal consequences. Consistent UAP training and educational background is also a concern in some areas of the country; however, other areas require certification for UAP. Due to the RN shortage the trend of using UAP will probably not change, and nurses must provide leadership and direction to ensure that quality, safe care is provided. UAP are not only used in acute care but also in home care, skilled nursing facilities, rehabilitation, behavioral health/psychiatry, and long-term care.

Outcomes and staffing levels continue to be critical issues in acute care. Chapter 9 discusses some of the recent studies on this topic. If patients do not reach expected outcomes and then experience complications, this increases the cost of health care. Hospitals and managed care organizations do not want their patients/enrollees to experience complications that then require longer hospital stays, additional treatment, and extended care after hospitalization. Complications usually mean more medications are prescribed, and this is of particular concern since the cost of drugs is increasing. Nurses need data to demonstrate that decreasing nursing staff in hospitals will increase patient complications and affect outcomes negatively. Nurses need to gather more data about the positive effects that nursing care has on patient outcomes in the acute care setting.

Nurses who work in acute care settings have found that their work has changed. Skills that are more important now are advocacy, negotiation with a variety of internal and external staff, collaboration, coordination, delegation, and an understanding of the need to provide culturally appropriate care that considers language, religion, nutrition, and culture and family relationships. All of these are leadership competences and are discussed in this text.

# Magnet Nursing Services Recognition Program

It is important that nurses take active roles in determining the quality of care and the nurse's role in the process. Nurses run the risk of blame for some of the problems that are found in acute care today. "Politics in health care may not end at the bedside, but it certainly begins there. It would be a tragedy if patients and family members blamed nurses for system failures. But the more nurses detach from their patients, the easier it becomes for the rest of us (consumers) to lose sympathy" (Kaplan, 2000, p. 25). The Magnet program is one way to address this issue and many others. What is the Magnet Nursing Services Recognition Program, its impact, and why is it important to new graduates? The following discussion explores some of the critical issues related to Magnet hospitals as an important consideration in any discussion about acute care hospitals today.

## Research: The Pathway to the Magnet Nursing Services Recognition Program

The Magnet program was developed unexpectedly as a result of a study in 1981 conducted by the American Academy of Nursing entitled *Magnet Hospitals: Attraction and Retention of Professional Nurses* (McClure, Poulin, Sovie, & Wandelt, 1983). This study explored variables that helped some hospitals create a magnet or force that assisted in the recruitment and retention of nurses. The study considered hospital nursing practice and combination of variables that helped to create staff personal and professional satisfaction. The Magnet Nursing Services Recognition Program began in the 1980s to recognize hospitals that provided quality nursing care or excellence in nursing care. Throughout the country, 165 hospitals were nominated for consideration in the study, with 155 responding by submitting applications and information. From this group of hospitals, task force members reviewed the information and selected 46 hospitals. As five of the hospitals were unable to participate, 41 hospitals were actually included in the sample, all predominately private, nonprofit institutions and all affiliated with some educational program in nursing (McClure, Poulin, Sovie, & Wandelt, 1983). Interviews were conducted to gather the data, creating one of the limitations of the study—self-reported data. In addition, interviews were conducted by different task force members, and staff nurses who participated were selected by their directors of nursing.

Results from this first study indicated that there were great similarities between how staff nurses and directors of nursing identified the variables that helped create the "magnet" so that the hospital environment was able to retain nurses or attract nurses to their hospital. These early results established the foundation for the Magnet Recognition Program. When administration was described in these hospitals, the most common management style identified was participant management in which managers listened to staff and used two-way communication. Leadership was important, and leaders were able to describe the philosophy of care so that it meant something to the staff. These nurse leaders also supported nurses so that they received the resources and services they needed to do their job. This relates to content presented in earlier chapters about the most effective leadership styles and organization structure particularly transformational leadership. Nurse managers were also critical to the success of these hospitals. Directors of nursing were of high quality and had high levels of education. When organization structure was discussed, decentralization was common, which led to more staff control. Nurses were also very active in hospital committees. Staffing, the ever present concern, was considered to be adequate, and they had a higher number of nurses who had baccalaureate degrees. Personnel policies are always important, and this study explored some of these policy issues. Work schedules often were innovative, and consideration was given to staff needs. Promotion opportunities not only included management tracks but also clinical tracks. Professional practice was very important, and these hospitals were found to have higher levels of quality of care, autonomy, primary nursing, mentoring, professional recognition, respect, and the ability to practice nursing as it should be (McClure, Poulin, Sovie, & Wandelt, 1983). These hospitals also recognized the importance of professional development—orientation, inservice and continuing education, formal education, and career development. There were some differences between staff and manager viewpoints; however, there were "no instances of 'we versus they' dichotomy of employee-management relations" (McClure, Poulin, Sovie, & Wandelt, 1983, p. 20).

The original study led to six other studies that indicated hospitals that receive the Magnet recognition have better outcomes such as lower burnout rates, higher levels of job satisfaction, and higher quality of care than non-Magnet hospitals (Laschinger, Shamian, & Thomson, 2001). A critical study completed in 2001, *Staff Nurses Identify Essentials of Magnetism* (Kramer & Schmalenberg, 2002), included 14 Magnet hospitals and 279 staff nurses who worked in them. The study objectives were as follows:

1. To update the variables staff nurses in Magnet hospitals today consider most important for nursing effectiveness in giving high-quality care
2. To define what staff nurses mean by good nurse-physician relationships, control over nursing practice, and autonomy
3. To quantify the preceding two variables empirically
4. To ascertain the degree of relationship between these variables and nurse job satisfaction, effectiveness, and competence of co-workers
5. To identify degree of value congruence among staff nurses, nurse managers, and chief nurse executives (Kramer & Schmalenberg, 2002, p. 27)

The results from this study identified eight variables that are important in providing quality care. Future research will undoubtedly further explore these variables. The following are the critical variables:

1. Working with other nurses who are clinically competent
2. Good nurse–physician relationships
3. Nurse autonomy and accountability
4. Supportive nurse manager-supervisor
5. Control over nursing practice and practice environment
6. Support for education
7. Adequacy of nurse staffing
8. Concern for patient is paramount (Kramer & Schmalenberg, 2002, pp. 53–55)

When these variables are reviewed it is easy to see how they connect to the results from the first study. These are the variables that create magnetism—the process of attracting nurses and keeping them.

## Magnet Hospital Framework

As the research about Magnet hospitals has developed, there is greater indication of the positive impact that the Magnet program has on patient care. "Nurses in hospitals, because of their employment status, are agents of the bureaucracy but hold professional values and seek peer relationships with other professionals and professional modes of organizing their work. Nurses are accountable to both the bureaucratic structure as headed by management and the professional structure as exemplified and headed by physicians" (Aiken, 2002, p. 62). This puts nurses in potential conflict situations. This conceptual framework considers the patient surveillance system that assists in identifying medical errors and adverse events. Nurses are the key players in the surveillance system, which is strongly emphasized in an Institute of Medicine report on nursing (2004). Other key factors are staffing, skill mix, and management decisions. Staffing looks at the total numbers of all types of nursing staff, and skill mix is the proportion of registered nurses compared to other nursing staff. The nurse work environment, which is a critical factor for any nurse in any type of health care setting, includes resource adequacy, administrative support, and nurse–physician relations. All of these variables come together in the implementation of the process of care that results in nurse and patient outcomes. Research results indicate that Magnet hospitals tend to provide quality care that leads to positive outcomes for patients and better work environments for nurses (Aiken, 2002).

There are other interesting results from recent research on Magnet hospitals. Cost is always a critical concern in health care, and so it is with Magnet hospitals. Since Magnet hospitals tend to have higher staff–patient ratios and staffing is the most expensive budget item, they do have higher nursing staff costs. Some research, however, does indicate that some patients in these hospitals have lower length-of-stay rates, which decreases health care costs (Aiken, 2002). This might balance out the costs of increasing the number of nurses or nurses with higher degrees. As would be expected, these hospitals have better nurse outcomes or job satisfaction. There were also fewer needlestick injuries in the hospitals that were in the study. If nurses are more satisfied with their work, less frustrated, and work with the same staff over a longer period of time, then nurse workplace safety may improve. There is no doubt that further research about cost-benefit issues and Magnet hospital characteristics are needed and will be conducted. There also needs to be further exploration of nurse and patient outcomes (McClure & Hinshaw, 2002).

## Building Magnetism

Forces of magnetism or organizational elements of excellence in nursing care are the critical elements that make a difference in whether or not a hospital receives Magnet status, and these forces or magnets seem to affect how a hospital attracts and retains nurses. How does a hospital get to the stage that it can demonstrate these elements? Hinshaw (2002) has described some of the strategies that might be used; however, a key point is to have competent nursing staff. Nurses want to know that they can count on their colleagues to know their job and what needs to be done to care for patients. This competency directly affects autonomy and control over nursing practice, which are part of the forces of magnetism. Hospitals need to ensure staff competence and provide educational opportunities—to maintain skills and enhance skills through staff education and to develop further (for example, by obtaining additional degrees or certification). These hospitals are willing to invest in staff by providing education within the hospital, assisting staff in identifying the need to pursue formal education, providing flexibility with scheduling, and assisting with reimbursement of educational costs.

Staffing is, of course, critical, and this has been demonstrated in Magnet hospitals, which appear to have adequate staffing. Staffing includes not only numbers of staff but also their education, expertise, competence, and skill-mix. The goal is high-quality care, and this is supported with recent research indicating positive patient outcomes (Aiken, Havens, & Sloane, 2000; Havens, 2001; Sovie & Jawad, 2001). Magnet hospitals have used a number of strategies to improve their staffing such as establishing recommended levels of patient–staff ratios, limiting use of substitution (Sovie & Jawad, 2001), using teams of competent nurses that include agency or float nurses, and developing float teams that are used for particular types of patients (Kramer & Schmalenberg, 2002). Some states, led by legislation passed first in California, are establishing required nurse–patient ratios. Magnet hospitals have higher RN–patient ratios, and more of the RNs have baccalaureate and master's degrees.

Autonomy is an important characteristic found in Magnet hospitals and in the forces of magnetism. Autonomy is "the freedom to act on what you know" (Kramer & Schmalenberg, 2002, p. 36). Responsibility and accountability are important components of autonomy. How is autonomy supported? Nursing leadership that is strong and visible is important, as is decentralization. Empowering staff members to feel that they can make decisions and that they are competent is a strategy that helps to develop autonomy. It is difficult to separate autonomy from control over practice—to understand and participate in what needs to be done to ensure that nursing care meets nursing standards. Again leadership, empowerment, and decentralization are important, and hospitals have found that shared governance does make a difference. Communication at all levels is critical in providing care and for nurses to control their practice.

Finally, nurse–physician relationships are also important; typically, this can be problematic. The goal is to have positive relationships that are collaborative so that both work together to meet the needs of patients and reach positive outcomes for the patients. The requirement for interprofessional care is the norm today and emphasized by the IOM quality reports though teamwork is not always effective. Health care reform legislation, 2010, even comments on teams in the requirement to create an Independence at Home demonstration program. This requires communication and coordination to ensure that ongoing needs are met, plans are implemented, and that there is no unnecessary duplication of services. Information needs to be shared, clear, and reported in a timely manner. This also means that nurses and physicians need to respect one another and recognize the expertise of each other. Strategies that have been shown to be effective in improving nurse–physician relationships in Magnet hospitals are clearly defined communication procedures and structures, interprofessional committees, and the development of teams of nurses and physicians so that they can develop working relationships. Newhouse and Mills (2002) have identified some key points related to nurse–physician relationships and forming interprofessional teams.

- All teams are not created equal, but careful development of working relationships and clear goals can make all the difference.
- Successful teams are composed of competent team members with the necessary skills, abilities, and personalities to achieve the desired objectives.
- Teams composed of many professional disciplines are able to expand the number and quality of actions to improve health care systems.
- Interprofessional teams work collaboratively to set and achieve goals directed toward innovative and effective care and efficient organizational systems.
- The nurse team member represents the voice of nursing as a discipline responsible for the holistic care of patients.
- Positive relationships with physicians benefit the patient and enhance the work environment for nurses.
- Nurses must develop the skills to work collaboratively as a professional member of the interprofessional team (pp. 64–69).

Chapters 11 and 12 discuss teams in more detail.

There is no doubt that management is important. The content of this textbook is a testament to that as is the requirement of leadership and management content in nursing curricula. Magnet hospitals have demonstrated that nursing leadership needs to be strong and supportive of nursing staff—to be the advocate for the nursing staff and the care that they provide. Leadership provides the vision and ensures that it is implemented, ensures that staff has the resources needed to provide quality care, ensures that staff is competent, develops communication procedures and structures that work, provides information technology that supports the work that needs to be done, and ensures that nursing leaders play an important role in the organization of the hospital—thus representing the nursing staff.

In a study done by Havens (2001) that compared nursing infrastructure and outcomes in Magnet and non-Magnet hospitals, the results noted that there were some structural differences in the hospitals in addition to the characteristics that have been identified as part of Magnet hospitals such as autonomy, control of practice, quality care, and other critical elements. More of the Magnet hospitals had discrete departments of nursing. This might be more supportive of an organization that supports and respects nursing. Nursing was seen as visible—a distinct profession within the organization. The chief nursing executive also had more control of nursing practice and the nursing practice environment. These hospitals also had more doctorally prepared nurse researchers who supported staff participation in nursing research, affecting the quality of care. A critical difference was the Magnet hospitals had not responded to reengineering and restructuring in the same way as non-Magnet hospitals (Havens, 2001).

Whereas the non-Magnet hospitals had made major changes by eliminating the department of nursing, reconfiguring skill-mix, and reducing the number of RNs, the Magnet hospitals had taken different approaches. The result was actually an expansion of the chief nurse executive role to include non-nursing departments or services. The results of the study also re-confirmed the importance of applying the *ANA Scope and Standards for Nurse Administrators* (2009). "Based on research and grounded in professional standards (American Nurses Association, 1996), the Magnet Recognition Program may present a prescriptive model for administrative 'best practice' by recognizing excellence in four areas: (a) management philosophy and practices, (b) adherence to standards for improving the quality of care, (c) leadership of the CNE in supporting professional practice and continued nursing competence, and (d) attention to the cultural and ethnic diversity of patients, their significant others, and providers. The findings from this research further suggest that the ANCC Magnet Program may also offer an evidence-based approach to solve two crucial problems confronting hospitals: recapturing public confidence and recruiting and retaining high-quality employees" (Havens, 2001, p. 266). These specialty standards correlate with general nursing standards, *Nursing Scope and Standards of Practice* (American Nurses Association, 2004).

Other studies have examined the impact of Magnet recognition. Improving professional practice in the work environment and clinical competence does have an positive impact on retention of staff (Stone, Larson, Mooney-Kane, Smolowitz, Lin, & Dick, 2006). Aiken, Clark, and Sloane (2008) study determined that "nurses reported more positive job experience and fewer concerns with care quality, and patients had significantly lower risks of death and failure to rescue in hospitals with better care environments" (p.223). Armstrong, Laschinger, and Wong (2009) demonstrated "an important link between the quality and nature of hospital nurses' work environments and the level of patient safety climate in those same environments" (p. 61). More research is needed to examine the impact of Magnet recognition. One issue that is of concern is what happens after a hospital gets Magnet recognition. It is easy to get complacent. Ulrich, Buerhaus, Donelan, Norman, and Dittus (2007) state an important point: "It is clearly not sufficient to obtain Magnet status, declare victory, and move on. Although obtaining Magnet status is a defining moment for an organization, it is much like completing a college degree with honors—the true outcomes and worth of the effort are only evident in future years by what you do with it" (p. 220).

## Description of The Magnet Recognition Program

The Magnet Nursing Services Recognition Program for Excellence, established in 1993, is administered by the American Nurses Credentialing Center (ANCC), the Commission on the Magnet Recognition Program. This program not only recognizes excellence in hospital nursing, but as of 1998, it also offers this recognition for long-term care facilities. The objectives of the program are to do the following (American Credentialing Center, 2009a):

- Promote quality in a setting that supports professional practice.
- Identify excellence in the delivery of nursing services to patients/residents.
- Disseminate "best practices" in nursing services.

The recognition program is available to any size hospital that meets the standards. Its focus is on quality patient care and the nurses within the institution. How does a hospital receive Magnet Recognition? First, it is important to understand the difference between accreditation, certification, and recognition. The ANCC has defined "Accreditation as a voluntary process used to validate that an organization and an approval body meets established continuing education standards. Certification focuses on the individual and is a process used to validate that an individual registered nurse possesses the requisite knowledge, skills, and abilities to practice in a defined practice specialty. Recognition is a third credentialing process operationalized in ANCC to evaluate an organization's adherence to excellence-focused standards" (Urden & Monarch, 2002, pp. 102–103). The Magnet Program is a recognition program. The evaluation process uses the *Scope and Standards for Nurse Administrators* (American Nurses Association, 2009) and the forces of magnetism identified in Box 6-5 to determine excellence in nursing care (American Nurses Credentialing Center, 2009b).

---

**BOX 6-5** | **FORCES OF MAGNETISM: ORGANIZATIONAL ELEMENTS OF EXCELLENCE IN NURSING CARE**

### FORCE 1: QUALITY OF NURSING LEADERSHIP

Knowledgeable, strong, risk-taking nurse leaders follow a well-articulated, strategic, and visionary philosophy in the day-to-day operations of the nursing services. Nursing leaders, at all levels of the organization, convey a strong sense of advocacy and support for the staff and for the patient. *(The results of quality leadership are evident in nursing practice at the patient's side.)*

### FORCE 2: ORGANIZATIONAL STRUCTURE

Organizational structures are generally flat, rather than tall, and decentralized decision-making prevails. The organizational structure is dynamic and responsive to change. Strong nursing representation is evident in the organizational committee structure. Executive-level nursing leaders serve at the executive level of the organization. The Chief Nursing Officer typically reports directly to the Chief Executive Officer. The organization has a functioning and productive system of shared decision making.

### FORCE 3: MANAGEMENT STYLE

Health care organization and nursing leaders create an environment supporting participation. Feedback is encouraged and valued and is incorporated from the staff at all levels of the organization. Nurses serving in leadership positions are visible, accessible, and committed to communicating effectively with staff.

### FORCE 4: PERSONNEL POLICIES AND PROGRAMS

Salaries and benefits are competitive. Creative and flexible staffing models that support a safe and healthy work environment are used. Personnel policies are created with direct care nurse involvement. Significant opportunities for professional growth exist in administrative and clinical tracks. Personnel policies and programs support professional nursing practice, work/life balance, and the delivery of quality care.

### FORCE 5: PROFESSIONAL MODELS OF CARE

There are models of care that give nurses the responsibility and authority for the provision of direct patient care. Nurses are accountable for their own practice as well as the coordination of care. The models of care (i.e., primary nursing, case management, family-centered, district, and holistic) provide for the continuity of care across the continuum. The models take into consideration patients' unique needs and provide skilled nurses and adequate resources to accomplish desired outcomes.

### FORCE 6: QUALITY OF CARE

Quality is the systematic driving force for nursing and the organization. Nurses serving in leadership positions are responsible for providing an environment that positively influences patient outcomes. There is a pervasive perception among nurses that they provide high-quality care to patients.

*(continued)*

| BOX 6-5 | FORCES OF MAGNETISM: ORGANIZATIONAL ELEMENTS OF EXCELLENCE IN NURSING CARE (CONTINUED) |
|---|---|

### FORCE 7: QUALITY IMPROVEMENT

The organization has structures and processes for the measurement of quality and programs for improving the quality of care and services within the organization.

### FORCE 8: CONSULTATION AND RESOURCES

The health care organization provides adequate resources, support, and opportunities for the utilization of experts, particularly advanced practice nurses. In addition, the organization promotes involvement of nurses in professional organizations and among peers in the community.

### FORCE 9: AUTONOMY

Autonomous nursing care is the ability of a nurse to assess and provide nursing actions as appropriate for patient care based on competence, professional expertise, and knowledge. The nurse is expected to practice autonomously, consistent with professional standards. Independent judgment is expected to be exercised within the context of interdisciplinary and multidisciplinary approaches to patient/resident/client care.

### FORCE 10: COMMUNITY AND THE HEALTH CARE ORGANIZATION

Relationships are established within and among all types of health care organizations and other community organizations to develop strong partnerships that support improved client outcomes and the health of the communities they serve.

### FORCE 11: NURSES AS TEACHERS

Professional nurses are involved in educational activities within the organization and community. Students from a variety of academic programs are welcomed and supported in the organization; contractual arrangements are mutually beneficial. There is a development and mentoring program for staff preceptors for all levels of students (including students, new graduates, experienced nurses, etc.). Staff members in all positions serve as faculty and preceptors for students from a variety of academic programs. There is a patient education program that meets the diverse needs of patients in all of the care settings of the organization.

### FORCE 12: IMAGE OF NURSING

The services provided by nurses are characterized as essential by other members of the health care team. Nurses are viewed as integral to the health care organization's ability to provide patient care. Nursing effectively influences system-wide processes.

### FORCE 13: INTERDISCIPLINARY RELATIONSHIPS

Collaborative working relationships within and among the disciplines are valued. Mutual respect is based on the premise that all members of the health care team make essential and meaningful contributions in the achievement of clinical outcomes. Conflict management strategies are in place and are used effectively, when indicated.

### FORCE 14: PROFESSIONAL DEVELOPMENT

The health care organization values and supports the personal and professional growth and development of staff. In addition to quality orientation and in-service education addressed earlier in Force 11, Nurses as Teachers, emphasis is placed on career development services. Programs that promote formal education, professional certification, and career development are evident. Competency-based clinical and leadership/management development is promoted and adequate human and fiscal resources for all professional development programs are provided.

Source: American Nurses Credentialing Center. (2009). Retrieved from http://www.nursecredentialing .org/Magnet/ProgramOverview/ForcesofMagnetism .aspx. Reprinted with permission.

When a hospital is interested in pursuing magnet recognition, it must first conduct an environmental assessment and begin the Pathway to Excellence. From the results of this self-assessment, the organization can determine if there are gaps between what exists and what is expected for Magnet status recognition. At this point, the hospital may decide that the gap is too large and more work needs to be done to improve before seeking recognition. If the hospital decides to seek recognition, the hospital must organize for the process, identify leaders for the process, make plans, and set timelines. Following this, there are four major phases (Urden & Monarch, 2002). Staff nurses need to be included in all phases.

1. The first phase is the application and designation process.
2. The second phase is documentation review when the hospital sends required documentation to ANCC for review. This material is reviewed and scored, which takes several months.
3. The third phase is the site visit. Several appraisers visit the hospital to meet with staff, administration, patients, families, and other critical people.
4. The final phase is review and decision. When Magnet status is awarded, the hospital maintains this status for 4 years. Then the hospital can apply for recognition again, but it must continue to meet the required standards.

What must a hospital do to maintain its Magnet recognition? The following is expected.

1. Submit annual monitoring reports.
2. Participate in the ANA's quality indicator study coordinated by the National Center for Nursing Quality.
3. Notify the Magnet Recognition Program office if any of the following occurs:

   - significant increase in staff turnover
   - significant increase in the nurse vacancy rates
   - significant decrease in nurse decision-making positions/activities
   - significant negative change in the organization's nurse–patient ratio
   - significant negative change in the licensed/unlicensed ratio of the nursing staff
   - significant increase in the organization's nurse absentee rate
   - significant amount of mandatory overtime worked by nurses reporting to the Department of Nursing
   - Nursing-Sensitivity Quality Indicator data fall significantly below the threshold established by the Magnet organization
   - Nursing-Sensitive Quality Indicator data fall significantly below the national average as determined by the National Database of Nursing Quality Indicators (*The American Nurse,* 2002, p. 17)

This list of what a hospital must report provides a good example of the key acute care issues that should concern new graduates as they search for jobs.

## Benefits of the Program

Typically, hospitals that are recognized as Magnet hospitals publicize this in their marketing. Clearly, this recognition can affect patients' interest in receiving care in the hospital if they understand its significance. The information can also be used in the recruitment and retention of nursing staff. Hospitals that receive this recognition become models of excellence for other hospitals. Consumers want more and more information about the quality of their health care. The usual benchmark for hospitals has been receiving a high rating on Joint Commission accreditation; however, the Magnet Recognition Program offers another method to determine quality—one that has been largely ignored and focuses primarily on nursing (Aiken, Havens, & Sloane, 2000). "The slow rate of ANCC Magnet hospital recognition is problematic. This potentially useful quality indicator must be propelled into the public domain" (Aiken, Havens, & Sloane, 2000, p. 33). More needs to be done to educate the public about the recognition, and hospitals that are designated as Magnet hospitals of nursing excellence need to publicize this status and explain what it means.

Why is this information about Magnet hospitals important to new graduates? The research over the last decade or more indicates that some hospitals are more successful than others in attracting and retaining staff. These hospitals also demonstrate critical positive outcomes for patients and for staff. As new graduates consider their first nursing positions, understanding Magnet hospitals, the related research results, and the forces of magnetism can help new graduates assess potential employers and decide if a particular hospital is the place for them. The description of a Magnet hospital via the forces of magnetism can provide a checklist when assessing hospitals and their nursing services.

## A Conclusion and the Future

In 2009 The Institute of Medicine in collaboration with the Robert Wood Johnson Foundation (RWJF) held three forums in three different areas of the country to begin the IOM Initiative on the Future of Nursing. The focus of these forums was acute care nursing with the goal of gathering more information. The summary recognizes the complex issues of acute care practice, stress nurses experiences, and the need for new practice models. The summary (see link to summary in Media Links at the end of the chapter) identifies concepts for imagining the future of nursing (Institute of Medicine, 2010):

Core Concept 1: Leverage the power of the electronic health record.

Core Concept 2: Achieve a balance among technologies, disruptive business models, and human needs.

Core Concepts 3 and 4: Implement rapid translational teams and interdisciplinary teams of designers.

Core Concept 5: Create an infrastructure for rapid network exchange of successful system design innovations.

In the fall of 2010 the IOM released a major report on nursing that resulted from these earlier forums. This report emphasizes that nurses must become partners and leaders in improving health care and specifies some critical recommendations to accomplish this. The report is based on the IOM Quality Series reports and supports the need for a greater role for nursing (Institute of Medicine, 2011).

Key recommendations are as follows:

1. Remove scope of practice barriers.
2. Expand opportunities for nurses to lead and diffuse collaborative improvement efforts.
3. Implement nurse residency programs.
4. Increase the proportion of nurses with a baccalaureate degree to 80 percent by 2020.
5. Double the number of nurses with a doctorate by 2010.
6. Ensure that nurses engage in lifelong learning.
7. Prepare and enable nurses to lead change to advance health.
8. Build and infrastructure for the collection and analysis of interprofessional health care workforce data.

# APPLYING LEADERSHIP AND MANAGEMENT

## MY HOSPITAL UNIT

Now it is time to return to the unit you created when you started this textbook to apply some of this chapter's content to your own unit. The hospital is getting its application ready for the Magnet Recognition Program®. Describe the approach you would take on your unit. What would be in your preparation plan? How would you communicate the importance of the recognition program to the staff? How would you include the staff? What would you share with the medical staff on your unit? You may want to visit the Magnet Recognition website to get current information at http://www.nursecredentialing.org/Magnet.aspx. Use the virtual unit site found on the textbook website to record the work that you do in the role of nurse manager for your unit.

## Critical Thinking Questions and Activities

1. What do you know about the health care organizations in your community? Select a hospital and learn more about its organization and services. You may find the some of the information on the hospital's website, in hospital documents, through interviews with managers, and discussion with staff. Share your information with your classmates. You may want to do this activity in small teams. Then compare the different hospitals that different teams examined. There is no right answer. This response requires you to search for information and apply chapter content. Describe the levels of management. Have any mergers occurred in the last 5–10 years? Is so, describe them. Is the hospital accredited and by whom? What the accreditation status? When is the next scheduled accreditation? Is this a teaching or non-teaching hospital? What difference does this make? Does the hospital have Medicare certification? What is this and why is it important? How is the hospital organized (review and organizational chart)? Is it a Magnet hospital or on the Pathway to Excellence?

2. Many health care professionals and different departments in an acute care hospital are required to provide care. Explore more about the hospital you examined in #1. Select one non-nursing department described in this chapter. What can you find out about the service or department? Consider its purpose, type of staff, and how this department relates to other departments. What are two problems that the department staff feels need to be improved? How does the department staff relate to nursing?

3. Committees can be found in most organizations—student organizations, employer-related, professional, and other organizations. What has you been your experience with committees? Describe an experience you have had on a committee. Consider whether you understood the purpose of the committee, leadership of the committee, your role or reason for participating, and whether or not this was a valuable experience for you.

4. What can you learn about specific health care policies and procedures? Ask to see a policy or procedure manual in one of your clinical sites. Some hospitals now have them computerized. You do not have to choose a hospital. You could do this in any clinical site where you are for practicum. Get an idea about the types of policies and procedures that are available. What have you learned about policy and procedure development? Consider the following: focus, primary responsibility, content, evidence-based, reaction of staff to the policy or procedure, problems that have been encountered with the policy or procedure, and usefulness of the policy or procedure.

5. Debate the benefits of the Magnet Recognition Program. Be specific about the benefits and apply to a hospital in which you have had clinical experiences.

6. Review the Institute of Medicine *The Future of Nursing: Leading Change, Advancing Health.* Divide into teams with each team selecting one of the four areas that require transformation. Discuss each area and then share the discussion with the entire class. Access at http://iom.edu/Reports/2010/The-Future-of-Nursing-Leading-Change-Advancing-Health.aspx.

## Media Links

- **URL: http://www.jointcommission.org/**
  Joint Commission
  Information about the Joint Commission; access to some of their accreditation documents
- **URL: http://www.nursecredentialing.org/Magnet.aspx**
  ANCC Magnet Recognition Program®
- **URL: http://www.nursingworld.org/mainmenucategories/anamarketplace/anaperiodicals/ojin.aspx**
  *Online Journal of Issues in Nursing*
- **URL: http://www.nacns.org/**
  National Association of Clinical Nurse Specialists
  National Organization of Nurse Practitioner Faculties (NONPF)
- **URL: http://www.nonpf.com/displaycommon.cfm?an=1&subarticlenbr=14**
  Competencies for Acute Care Nurse Practitioners
- **URL: http://www.aha.org/**
  American Hospital Association
- **URL: http://www.nursecredentialing.org/default.aspx**
  American Nurses Credentialing Center
- **URL: http://www.aacn.nche.edu/cnc/index.htm**
  Clinical Nurse Leader Certification
- **URL: http://www.midwife.org/**
  American College of Nurse-Midwives
- **URL: http://www.aana.com/aboutaana.aspx?id=46**
  American Association of Nurse Anesthetists
- **URL: http://books.nap.edu/openbook.php?record_id=12855&page=8**
  Institute of Medicine *Summary of October 2009 forum on the future of nursing: Acute care* (2010)

**Pearson Nursing Student Resources**

Find additional review materials at
**nursing.pearsonhighered.com**

Prepare for success with additional NCLEX®-style practice questions, interactive assignments and activities, Web links, animations and videos, and more!

## References

Ackerman, F. (1992). The movement toward vertically integrated regional health systems. *Health Care Management Review, 2,* 81–88.

Aiken, L., Clarke, S., Sloane, D., Lake, E., & Cheney, T. (2008). Effects of hospital care environment on patient mortality and nurse outcomes. *JONA, 38*(5), 223–229.

Aiken, L. (2002). Superior outcomes for magnet hospitals. In M. McClure & A. Hinshaw (Eds.), *Magnet hospitals revisited* (pp. 61–82). Washington, DC: American Nurses Publishing.

Aiken, L., Havens, D., & Sloane, D. (2000). The magnet nursing services recognition program: A comparison of successful applicants with reputational magnet hospitals. *American Journal of Nursing, 100*(3), 26–35.

*American Nurse.* (2002, September–October). New law, JCAHO report recognizes success of Magnet concept, 16–17.

American Nurses Association. (2009). *Scope and standards for nurse administrators.* Silver Springs: MD: Author.

American Nurses Association. (2004). *Scope and standards of practice.* Silver Springs: MD: Author.

American Nurses Credentialing Center. (2009a). Goals of Magnet Program. Retrieved December 30, 2009, from http://www.nursecredentialing.org/ Magnet/ProgramOverview/ GoalsoftheMagnetProgram.aspx

American Nurses Credentialing Center. (2009b). Forces of Magnetism. Retrieved December 30, 2009, from http://www.nursecredentialing.org/ Magnet/ProgramOverview/ ForcesofMagnetism.aspx

Armstrong, K., Laschinger, H., & Wong, C. (2009). Workplace empowerment and magnet hospital characteristics as predictors of patient safety climate. *Journal of Nursing Care Quality, 24*(1), 55–62.

Finkelman, A. (2011). *Case management for nurses.* Upper Saddle River, NJ: Pearson Education.

Havens, D. (2001). Comparing nursing infrastructure and outcomes: ANCC magnet and nonmagnet CNEs report. *Nursing Economics, 19*(6), 258–266.

Hinshaw, A. (2002). Building magnetism into health organizations. In M. McClure & A. Hinshaw (Eds.), *Magnet hospitals revisited* (pp. 83–102). Washington, DC: American Nurses Publishing.

Institute of Medicine. (2001). *Crossing the quality chasm.* Washington, DC: Author.

Institute of Medicine. (2003a). *Health care professions education.* Washington, DC: Author.

Institute of Medicine. (2011). *The future of nursing: Leading change, advancing health.* Washington, DC: The National Academies Press.

Institute of Medicine. (2003b). *Priority areas for national action.* Washington, DC: Author.

Institute of Medicine. (2004). *Keeping patients safe. Transforming the work environment for nurses.* Washington, DC: Author.

Institute of Medicine. (2008). *Knowing what works in health care.* Washington, DC: Author.

Joint Commission. (2009). *Hospital accreditation standards.* Oakbrook Terrace, IL: Author.

Kaplan, M. (2000). Hospital caregivers are in a bad mood. *American Journal of Nursing, 100*(3), 25.

Institute of Medicine. (2010). *A summary of the October 2009 forum on the future of nursing: Acute care.* Washington, DC: Author.

Kramer, M., & Schmalenberg, C. (2002). Staff nurses identify essentials of magnetism. In M. McClure & A. Hinshaw (Eds.), *Magnet hospitals revisited* (pp. 25–59). Washington, DC: American Nurses Publishing.

Laschinger, H., Shamian, J., & Thomson, D. (2001). Impact of Magnet hospital characteristics on nurses' perceptions of trust, burnout, quality of care, and work satisfaction. *Nursing Economics, 19*(5), 209–219.

McClure, M., Poulin, M., Sovie, M., & Wandelt, M. (1983). *Magnet hospitals: Attraction and retention of professional nurses.* American Academy of Nursing Task Force on Nursing Practice in Hospitals. Kansas City, MO: American Nurses Association.

McClure, M., & Hinshaw, A. (2002). The future of magnet hospitals. In M. McClure & A. Hinshaw (Eds.), *Magnet hospitals revisited* (pp. 117–128). Washington, DC: American Nurses Publishing.

Milstead, J. (2002). Leapfrog group: A prince in disguise or just another frog? *Nursing Administration Quarterly, 26*(4), 16–25.

Newhouse, R., & Mills, M. (2002). *Nursing leadership in the organized delivery system for the acute care setting.* Washington, DC: American Nurses Publishing.

Ott, K., et al. (2009), The clinical nurse leader: Impact on practice outcomes in the Veterans Health Administration. *Nursing Economics, 27*(6), 363–370.

Payne, D. (1999). Credentialing and privileging ensure skilled care. *Nursing Management, 30*(8), 8.

Sovie, M., & Jawad, A. (2001). Hospital restructuring and its impact on outcomes. *The Journal of Nursing Administration, 31*(12), 588–600.

Stone, P., Larson, E., Mooney-Kane, C., Smolowitz, J., Lin, S. & Dick, A. (2006). Organizational climate and intensive care unit nurses' intention to leave. *Critical Care Medicine, 34*(7), 1907–1912.

Ulrich, B., Buerhaus, P., Donelan, K., Norman, L., & Dittus, R. (2007). Magnet status and registered nurse views of the work environment and nursing as a career. *JONA, 37*(5), 212–220.

Urden, L., & Monarch, K. (2002). The ANCC Magnet Recognition Program: Converting research findings into action. In M. McClure & A. Hinshaw (Eds.), *Magnet hospitals revisited* (pp. 103–116). Washington, DC: American Nurses Publishing.

Wolper, L. (2004). *Health care administration.* (4th ed.). Boston: Jones and Bartlett Publishers.

# CORE COMPETENCIES

This section focuses on the Institute of Medicine health care profession core competencies. The competencies are as follows:

- Provide patient-centered care
- Work in interprofessional teams
- Employ evidence-based practice
- Apply quality improvement
- Utilize informatics

The eleven chapters in this section emphasize these core competencies and include content related to managing patient-centered care, diversity and disparities, recruitment and retention to meet staffing requirements, consumers, building interprofessional teams, improving teamwork through collaboration, coordination, conflict resolution, and effective communication. Two chapters focus on health care quality and policy issues and the second on implementation of quality improvement. The last chapter addresses the fifth competency: informatics. These core competencies relate to practice in all settings but also to effective leadership and management.

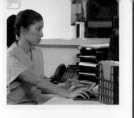

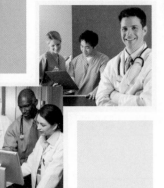

# 7

# Managing Patient-Centered Care

## CHAPTER OUTLINE

## LEARNING OUTCOMES

Before you begin, take a moment to familiarize yourself with the learning outcomes for this chapter.

- Explain how patient-centered care impacts the health care delivery system and nursing care.
- Analyze the implications of care planning, clinical reasoning and judgment, and patient/family education to patient-centered care.
- Examine the relationship between self-management and patient-centered care.
- Apply health promotion and disease and illness prevention to nursing management.
- Apply the chronic illness model to a specific chronic illness and relate to patient-centered care.

- Compare and contrast clinical pathways and practice guidelines.
- Compare and contrast tools used to manage care such as a clinical pathway or practice guideline so that care is more patient-centered.

## KEY TERMS

- Clinical judgment
- Clinical pathway
- Clinical reasoning
- Collaboration

- Disease management
- Health promotion
- Patient-centered care
- Practice guideline

- Primary prevention
- Secondary prevention
- Self-management
- Tertiary prevention

## WHAT'S AHEAD

**Collaboration** is important within clinical settings and between organizations and is an important part of each patient's care. Because health care is complex, working together to reach goals is more successful and usually more efficient. Collaboration is "the recognition of the expertise others within and outside the profession, and referral to those other providers when appropriate. Collaboration involves some shared functions and a common focus on the same overall mission" (American Nurses Association, 2003, p. 8). Collaboration is critical and integral to effective patient-centered care (Finkelman & Kenner, 2010). This chapter examines the Institute of Medicine (IOM) patient-centered care core competency. The content includes a discussion about patient-centered care and factors that impact it such as care planning, clinical reasoning and judgment, patient/family education, self-management, and health promotion. The IOM emphasizes the need for patient-centered care for all patients and highlights the increasing number of patients with chronic illnesses. Chronic illness and disease management are examined. Two examples of tools used by different health care settings and providers to assist in managing care for individuals, families, and communities are described: clinical pathways and practice guidelines.

## The Core Competency: Patient-Centered Care

The Institute of Medicine (2003) identifies five core competencies for health care professions, all of which are emphasized in this text. Provide patient-centered care is the key competency around which the other four competencies (work in interprofessional teams, employ evidence-based practice, apply quality improvement, utilize informatics) function. The core competency of **patient-centered care** is described by the IOM (2003): "identify, respect, and care about patients' differences, values, preferences, and expressed needs; relieve pain and suffering; coordinate continuous care; listen to, clearly inform, communicate with, and educate patients; share decision-making and management; and continuously advocate disease prevention, wellness, and promotion of healthy lifestyles, including a focus on population health" (p. 4). With the IOM (2001) describing the health care system as "in need of fundamental change" (p. 1), providing patient-centered care is a critical need. Health care delivery systems need to be "carefully and consciously designed to provide care that is safe, effective, patient-centered, timely, efficient, and equitable. Such systems must be designed to serve the needs of patients, and to ensure that they are fully informed, retain control and participate in care delivery whenever possible, and receive care that is respectful of their values and preferences" (Institute of Medicine, 2001, p. 7). The main issue is to move away from a focus on disease or medical problems to focus on the individual. Patients who are involved in their own care have better outcomes (Institute of Medicine, 2003). Over the last fifteen years researchers and experts have examined the skills required by health care professionals to provide effective patient-centered care. The following are identified as important (Institute of Medicine, 2003, pp. 52–53):

- Share power and responsibility with patients and caregivers.
- Communicate with patients in a shared and fully open manner.

- Take into account patients' individuality, emotional needs, values, and life issues.
- Implement strategies to reach those who do not present for care on their own, including care strategies that support the broader community.
- Enhance prevention and health promotion.

The concept of patient-centered care is not a universal concept across different health care professions, and there needs to be more done to improve this and arrive at a common language and terms (Lewin, Skea, Entwistle, Zwarenstein, & Dick, 2001).

Effective patient-centered care requires that staff collaborate and coordinate care. The patient, and when appropriate the patient's family, needs to be engaged in the care delivery process. Diversity issues need to be considered to better ensure that the patient's values and preferences are integrated in the care process. As will be discussed in a later chapter, consumerism is more important today in health care. Patient-centered care is directly related to consumerism and the need for patient advocacy—advocacy in which the patient is supported and makes decisions not the health care provider making the decisions for the patient. Informatics is also an area that supports patient-centered care. Patients can get more current information and access experts when they need it, and staff can get information easily in order to plan care with the patient. Chapter 18 discusses the core competency of employing informatics.

## The Role of Management and Patient-Centered Care

A nurse manager or a team leader must recognize the need for patient-centered care and keep this need in the forefront when making decisions. How does management actually relate to providing patient-centered care? The following are some examples:

- The structure of a unit is designed to meet individual patient needs through an interprofessional team.
- Care planning is interprofessional and includes the patient.
- Patient care rounds include the patient and when possible the patient's family.
- Shift report focuses on the individual patient, recognizing the patient's values, preferences, diversity, rights, and needs.
- Patient–staff relationships and communication focus on the patient, e.g., listen to the patient, take time to focus on the patient, avoid acting hurried, use open communication, and so on.
- Nursing management should routinely visit patients to assess status, talk with patient and family, and determine issues that need addressing.
- The unit processes put the patient first for example how meals are served, communication system with the patient, and so on.
- The organizational culture considers the patient to be the center of the culture influencing systems, communication, and the environment so that the patient feels comfortable, providing a healing environment.
- Errors are disclosed in an effective manner to patients, and patients are considered a part of quality improvement—engaged in identifying possible risks.
- Quality improvement evolves around patient outcomes.
- Delegation is guided by patient needs.
- Assignment is guided by patient needs.
- Staffing includes patient needs and acuity, consideration of required staff, and competencies of staff to ensure effective patient outcomes.
- Staff education is designed so that patient needs and the patient is the center of content and learning experiences—to ensure that care is effectively and efficiently provided.
- Self-management is incorporated into care so that patients will be better able to care for self long-term; family is included as appropriate.
- The admission process focuses on the patient with a complete assessment and identification of needs and problems; engaging the patient in the process when appropriate the family. Patient is oriented to the unit and care processes.
- The discharge process prepares the patient for discharge and care needs after discharge; engaging the patient in the process and when appropriate the family.

- Performance appraisal focuses on the ability of the employee to provide patient-centered care and achieve effective patient outcomes.
- Support services recognize that the patient is the center of concern.
- Patient privacy and confidentiality (Health Insurance Portability and Accountability Act of 1996, HIPAA) is maintained, for example sharing of patient name and other information is controlled.

Just as transformational leadership engages staff and focuses on inclusion in the decision-making process transformational leadership should keep the patient at the center of the process. Davis, Schoenbaun, and Audet (2005) identify seven attributes of patient-centered care.

1. *Superb access to care.*   Patients can easily make appointments and select the day and time. Waiting times are short. E-mail and telephone consultations are offered. Off-hours service is available.
2. *Patient engagement in care.*   Patients have the option of being informed and engaged partners in their care. Practices provide information on treatment plans, preventive and follow-up care reminders, access to medical records, assistance with self-care, and counseling.
3. *Clinical information systems that support high-quality care, practice-based learning, and quality improvement.*   Practices maintain patient registries; monitor adherence to treatment; have easy access to lab and test results; and receive reminders, decision support, and information on recommended treatments.
4. *Care coordination.*   Specialist care is coordinated, and systems are in place to prevent errors that occur when multiple physicians are involved. Posthospital follow-up and support is provided.
5. *Integrated and comprehensive team care.*   There is a free flow of communication among physicians, nurses, and other health professionals. Duplication of tests and procedures is avoided.
6. *Routine patient feedback to doctors.*   Practices take advantage of low-cost, Internet-based patient surveys to learn from patients and inform treatment plans.
7. *Publicly available information.*   Patients have accurate, standardized information on physicians to help them choose a practice that will meet their needs.

### Implications of Care Planning, Clinical Reasoning, and Clinical Judgment to Patient-Centered Care

Patients need to be as active in the care planning process as possible given their medical status. Planning that is done separate from the patient and then delivered as a final decision acts as a barrier to patient-centered care. Patients will tolerate this type of care approach less today then they did in the past. They expect to be the decision maker. Communication with the patient needs to be clear and open. Health literacy has been a concern in health care as discussed in Chapter 8. Health literacy is "the ability to read, understand, and act on health care information" (Institute of Medicine, 2004, p. 52). Health literacy can be a major barrier to patient-centered care. Care plans that are developed by an interprofessional team with an emphasis on collaboration, coordination, and continuity of care are more patient-centered focused. The plan guides the care for individual patients but also informs teams and unit management about patient needs and interventions that need to be considered in the management of services such as staff number, mix, and competencies. Throughout the care process nurses need to actively use clinical reasoning and clinical judgment. **Clinical reasoning** is the "practitioner's ability to assess patient problems or needs and analyze data to accurately identify and frame problems within the context of the individual patient's environment" (Murphy, 2004, p. 227). This is the ability to reason as a clinical situation unfolds (Benner, Sutphen, Leonard, & Day, 2010). **Clinical judgment** requires that a nurse apply, analyze, and synthesize knowledge considering the patient context. It is the "ways in which nurses come to understand the problems, issues, or concerns of clients/patients, to attend to salient information, and to respond in concerned and involved ways" (Benner, Tanner, & Chesla, 1996, p. 2). This is deliberate, conscious decision making. If done effectively it should allow the nurse to reflect on the patient, communicate effectively, respond to uncertainty, and avoid snap judgments. The 2010 national report on nursing education expresses strong concern that nursing education is not preparing students to use clinical reasoning and clinical judgment and that this has an impact on care (Benner, Sutphen, Leonard, & Day, 2010).

### Implications of Patient/Family Education to Patient-Centered Care

Patient and family education has long been a nursing responsibility. It has become more difficult to provide effective education, particularly in the acute care setting due to the acuity of patients and shorter lengths-of-stay. Different methods are being used to deliver patient education such as videos, downloads onto computers or smart phones, and the typical brochures and handouts. Health literacy needs to be carefully monitored as the nurse determines if the patient understands the information and can apply it. Follow-up with home health care may be required. Families should be involved whenever possible as they typically are the primary caregivers when patients return to their homes. All patient education needs to focus on the individual patient and not just provide broad information. Understanding the patient's medical history, assessment data, needs, and home situation is important in developing patient-centered patient education. This also requires patient engagement—asking what the patient identifies as needs, problems, and so on and getting active feedback from the patient and listening to the patient (and/or family).

### Self-Management

Self-management support is the "systematic provision of education and supportive interventions to increase patients' skills and confidence in managing their health problems, including regular assessment of progress and problems, goal setting, and problem-solving support" (Institute of Medicine, 2003b, p. 52). "The existing health care system also does not support the practice of patient self-management. The current system adheres to the traditional model of patients following "doctor's orders" and does not encourage a patient to perform such activated behavior as seeking information, defining problems, setting priorities, establishing goals, creating treatment plans, and solving problems along the way. Patients currently do not have a central role in determining their care, one that fosters a sense of responsibility for their own health" (Institute of Health Improvement, 2010). A patient-centered focus requires that patients play a greater role in their care and in some instances providers play less of a role. The IOM identifies four areas that need improvement and lead to effective programs (Glasgow, Funnell, Bonomi, Davis, Beckham, & Wagner, 2002 as cited in 2003b, p. 52).

1. Providers communicate and reinforce patients' active and central role in managing their illness.
2. Practice teams make regular use of standardized patient assessments.
3. Evidence-based programs are used to provide ongoing support.
4. Collaborative care planning and patient-centered problem solving result in an individualized care plan for each patient and support from the team when problems are encountered.

### Health Promotion and Disease and Illness Prevention

Health promotion and disease and illness prevention are strategies that focus on encouraging people to become partners in maintaining their own health. The IOM includes health promotion, prevention, and wellness in its perspective of patient-centered care. These are also critical strategies used by insurers, primary care, and community/public health. Medicare is also providing more reimbursement for these strategies. Health promotion and prevention are found in the health reform legislation of 2010. (See Appendix B.) Education is a key method for accomplishing this partnership. Each time an insurer develops health promotion and disease and illness prevention services, it reassesses the costs and benefits of these services. The Health Maintenance Organization (HMO) is the managed care model that is most likely to cover preventive services. How much reimbursement coverage is provided for these services varies and still is minimal coverage for most; however, there is greater emphasis on covering this service in the health care reform legislation of 2010. The three major health promotion and prevention methods used by health care organizations, community health, and insurers are as follows.

1. **Screening.** This method includes periodic physical examinations and laboratory tests based on the patient's medical history and risk assessment, such as family history and smoking and exercise habits.

2. **Counseling.** The primary care doctor or other medical professional explains the relationship between risk factors and health. Through counseling, the health plan assists patients in obtaining knowledge and skills, and developing the motivation to adopt and maintain healthy behavior.

3. **Immunization and chemoprophylaxis** (Korczyk & Witte, 1998, p. 128). The goals of **health promotion** are to help people modify their lifestyles and make choices to improve their health and quality of life. Health education is very important in helping enrollees/patients to accomplish this goal.

There are three types of disease and illness prevention strategies: primary, secondary, and tertiary.

1. **Primary prevention** focuses on wellness behaviors and prevention of illness or prevention of the natural course of an illness. Examples of interventions are prenatal clinics, stress management courses, AIDS prevention education, nutrition education, safety for children, smoking clinics, alcohol usage, and seat belt safety.

2. **Secondary prevention** focuses on early diagnosis of symptoms and treatment after the onset of disease or illness and recognizes that early treatment may decrease complications. Examples of interventions are mammograms, parent education, and screening for diabetes or glaucoma.

3. **Tertiary prevention** focuses on rehabilitative strategies to decrease disability from a disease or illness. Examples of interventions are chemotherapy education for a cancer patient and bladder training for a stroke patient.

How do insurers determine which health promotion services or interventions to offer? The Agency for Healthcare Research and Quality (AHRQ) publishes up-to-date prevention guidelines on a variety of topics through is website (http://www.ahrq.gov/whatsnew.htm). This resource provides information about preventive services categorized by age and sex.

Examples of some of the topics covered are the following:

- Skin cancer
- Colorectal diseases
- Prostate cancer
- Promoting breastfeeding
- Sexually transmitted diseases
- Behavioral health

The U.S. Preventive Services Task Force publishes a preventive guide that can be accessed through its website at http://www.ahrq.gov/CLINIC/uspstfix.htm, and this guide is even mentioned in the health reform legislation of 2010. (See Appendix B.) Preventive services are frequently inadequately provided. Some of the reasons for this have been inadequate reimbursement, fragmentation of health care delivery, and insufficient time with patients. Even when these factors have been removed, the services are often not provided. This is partially due to lack of knowledge about what to provide and questions about their effectiveness. Patients may also be unaware of their own needs for preventive services, and thus, do not request them. Some preventive services are best provided on a community basis rather than with an individual focus in a clinical setting. This approach may become more common in the future. In addition, insurers may develop their own clinical guidelines for preventive services, which increases the variability of these services.

After an insurer identifies the health promotion and disease and illness preventive services to offer, it must develop the services, ensure that providers provide the services, and then communicate availability of preventive services to the enrollees. To share information with their enrollees insurers use newsletters, personal letters, information provided at the worksite, and the Internet. The National Committee for Quality Assurance (NCQA) includes some preventive services in its quality indicators, for example, vaccination rates, cervical cancer screening, mammography, and retinal exams for diabetics. The inclusion of preventive services by the major quality assessment organization for insurers is an indication of the increasing importance of these services to insurers. As insurers determine which preventive services to offer, cost-effectiveness is an important consideration. "Cost-effectiveness analysis is a method for assessing and summarizing the value of a medical technology, practice, or policy. Underlying the methodology is the assumption that the resources available to spend on health care are constrained, whether from the societal, organizational, practitioner, or patient point of view. Cost-effectiveness information is intended to inform decisions about health care investments within this finite budget. The cost-effectiveness ratio summarizes information on cost and effect, allowing interventions to be compared on the basis of their worth and priority to the patient, society in general, or some other constituency. Although the cost-effectiveness ratio takes the form of a price—that is, a dollar cost per unit of effect—it is generally interpreted in the inverse manner, as a measure of the benefit achievable for a given level of resources" (U.S. Preventive Services Task Force, 2001).

The central purpose of cost-effectiveness analysis (CEA) is to compare the costs and the values of different health care interventions in creating better health and longer life (Agency for Healthcare Research and Quality, 2009). Many new medical devices, procedures, diagnostic tests, and prescription drugs are expensive. Cost-effectiveness analysis can help to evaluate whether the improvement in health care outcomes justifies the expenditures relative to other choices. This understanding of the costs and outcomes of comparative interventions is essential for public- and private-sector decision makers to make informed decisions about using health care resources efficiently.

## CASE STUDY

### Is the Patient First?

A rehabilitation hospital wants to implement a patient-centered approach. The chief executive officer has requested this change after reviewing the Institute of Medicine reports on quality and health care professions. The senior management team has just concluded a meeting discussing this topic. The hospital has many patients with chronic illnesses and disabilities. These patients are often referred to the rehab hospital after acute care and stay long periods of time for physical therapy, occupational therapy, and nursing care. The hospital looks like a typical hospital with little personal features. Visiting hours tend to be regulated with staff members saying that they want patients to focus on their treatment. Considering the content in this chapter and earlier chapters on change and organizations, what would you recommend as chief nursing executive to respond to this directive?

### Questions:

1. What does patient-centered care mean?
2. Identify strategies that this organization could take to implement a patient-centered approach.
3. How might patient-centered care impact nursing care in this hospital? How might patient-centered care impact other services?
4. How might the hospital use its consumers (patients and families) in this change process?
5. You recommend that the hospital use clinical pathways. Why would this recommendation be connected with patient-centered care?

# Chronic Illness: A Key Health Care Concern

More people are living longer and often with multiple chronic illnesses, mostly because of advances in medical-science and technology. It is not uncommon for these patients to have co-morbid conditions, increasing the complexity of their problems and requiring more collaboration and coordination. Many people are in relatively good health though chronic illness is a problem. Patients over 75 average three chronic conditions and may take four or more medications (Institute of Medicine, 2008). Given the growing number of people with chronic illnesses, which in 2004 accounted for more than two-thirds of the U.S. $1.6 trillion medical bill and the increasing need to respond to the growing number of persons with chronic illness, the need for effective services for this population is critical. From 2003 to 2004, employer-sponsored health plans that included a disease management service increased from 41 percent to 58 percent (Landro, 2004). The health reform legislation of 2010 has numerous provisions about chronic illness from reimbursement to delivery provisions. (See Appendix B.) Typical disease management goals are to improve quality of life, decrease disease progression, and reduce hospitalizations. Chronic illnesses that are typically monitored are diabetes, heart disease/hypertension, asthma, cancer, depression, renal disease, low back pain, and obesity.

### Chronic Illness Care Model

Wagner (1998) developed a chronic care model, which is described in Figure 7-1. This model is also described on the website Improving Chronic Illness Care sponsored by the Robert Wood Johnson Foundation (http://www.improvingchroniccare.org). The model focuses on an informed, activated patient who is supported by a prepared proactive practice team. The elements of the model are the health system, delivery system design, decision support, clinical information systems, self-management support, and the community. In 2003 five new themes were added:

- Patient safety (in Health System)
- Cultural competency (in Delivery System Design)
- Care coordination (in Health System and Clinical Information Systems)
- Community policies (in Community Resources and Policies)
- Case management (in Delivery System Design)

It is easy to see the influence of the Institute of Medicine reports and recommendations on the additions to the model and the impact of patient-centered care. Nursing needs to consider the impact of increasing chronic illness on its practice and nursing delivery processes.

**FIGURE 7-1    Chronic Care Model.**

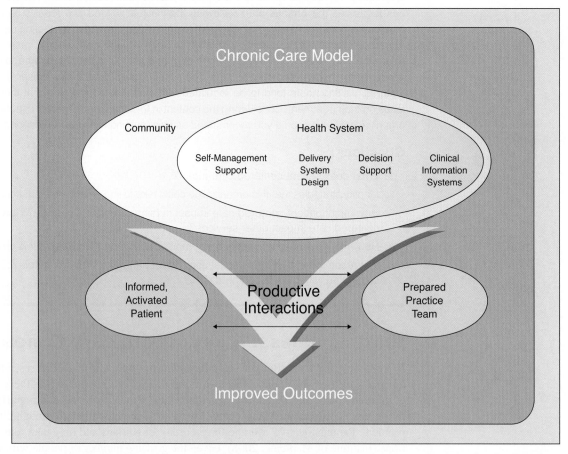

Source: Reprinted with permission from the Institute of Healthcare Improvement. Retrieved May 26, 2008, from http://www.ihi.org/IHI/Topics/ChronicConditions/AllConditions/Changes/

There are six fundamental areas identified by the Chronic Care Model making up a system that encourages high-quality chronic disease management. Organizations must focus on these six areas, as well as develop productive interactions between patients who take an active part in their care and providers backed up by resources and expertise.

## Disease Management

Disease management can be an effective tool to use to assist patients with chronic illness to better ensure patient-centered care.

DEFINITION AND PURPOSE    Disease management is another service strategy or method used by third-party payers to control costs and improve care. Disease management focuses on the whole patient who has a specific disease or illness, typically a chronic, long-term illness. Examples of illnesses that are often targeted for disease management are asthma, arthritis, cancer, diabetes, hypertension, osteoporosis, high-risk pregnancy, congestive heart failure, depression, high cholesterol, and human immunodeficiency virus/acquired immune deficiency syndrome (HIV/AIDS). **Disease management** is "a system of coordinated health care interventions and communications for populations with conditions in which patient self-care efforts are significant" (DMAA, 2009). Why would an insurer develop a disease management program that takes time to develop and is expensive to develop and offer? The following are some disease management program goals that help to understand the advantage of using this strategy (Kongstvedt, 2009):

- Improve patient outcomes.
- Encourage self-management and patient-centered care.
- Reduce costs.
- Support preventive care.
- Increase patient adherence to recommended medical care.

Disease management programs are similar to continuous quality improvement (CQI) programs that have been used by organizations to improve their functioning. CQI programs focus on identification, intervention, and measurement, just as do disease management programs. Disease management programs can vary from one insurer to another, but they usually include all or some of these elements:

- Prevention
- Early detection/diagnosis
- Treatment
- Management

Some programs just monitor medication treatment. Other programs offer only patient education or behavior modification. The more complex disease management programs use case management for their patients in order to provide coordinated care over a long period of time and to ensure that there is collaboration within interprofessional teams. HMOs offer more control over the physician and can more easily encourage physicians to use disease management programs. Usually, the role of the physician is to continue to provide appropriate interventions for the patient; however, other health care professionals, often nurses or case managers, provide education that focuses on prevention and health maintenance based on the disease and individual needs of the patient. The major goal is to prepare the patient to understand the disease and increase the patient's self-management of the disease.

The purpose of disease management programs is to provide patients with education and preventive care that improves the quality of their lives and prevents complications that may increase health care costs. Examples provided in the previous paragraph are problems that are of higher risk.

How does a disease management program really work? The insurer groups its enrollees into disease-specific populations and, based on the numbers within a specific disease category, it then focuses its disease management program on this population, and it usually is one whose care incurs higher costs. Disease management programs focus on prevention and health maintenance for the selected disease-specific groups. Patients chosen for disease management services typically have high cost, long-term problems and at risk for complications, increased hospitalizations, and longer lengths-of-stay. Patients with chronic illness are the most common type of patient for whom disease management can be effective. Usually, the physician's role is to continue to provide appropriate interventions for the patient; however, other health care professionals—often nurses—provide education that focuses on prevention and health maintenance based on the disease and individual needs of the patient. Case managers may be involved to help coordinate care. Case managers may be nurses and in some cases are social workers. The major goal is to prepare the patient to understand the disease and increase the patient's self-management of the disease. Disease management programs typically focus on chronic illnesses such as the examples found in Box 7-1.

Developing disease management programs takes time and is costly. Many insurers are turning to other groups or organizations that have developed these programs or contract with experts to design a customized program. Health care organizations, insurers, and health care businesses, such as consulting businesses, have developed disease management programs that are then sold as a package or contracted to providers and insurers. Disease management also provides an opportunity for partnerships between insurers and other organizations to create innovative programs. Some of these programs offer nurse call lines and nurse-led education programs and support, consider readiness to learn and behavior modification, encourage partnerships that are formed between the patient and the primary care provider, and track critical data such as hospital admissions and use of emergency services and prescriptions. These programs offer great opportunities for nurses.

## Provider Response to Disease Management Programs

Provider concerns about disease management programs are similar to those with practice guidelines and clinical pathways. Is this "cookbook" health care with little regard for the individual? Program supporters and developers insist that these programs offer individual assessment of needs and an opportunity to incorporate individual treatment needs. Some providers do not understand the concept, and thus they have problems accepting disease management programs. Others are concerned that this is an effort to take over their treatment. Supporters of disease management emphasize that the programs augment the provider's treatment and help patients better accept treatment and encourage compliance. Co-morbidities continue to be a problem, particularly with older patients. To increase physician support, physicians need education about the program and its purposes. They need to be recognized as coordinators of patient care and understand that disease management programs offer support to their treatment.

In addition to physicians benefiting from disease management programs, advanced practice nurses can benefit by using these programs, but they must also understand disease management and its application to their practice. Including the nurses and physicians, as well as other health care providers, in the development or adaptation of these programs is critical for their success. Insurers collect data on the outcomes, and then use these data to demonstrate results to physicians and other providers. Nurses can play major roles in the development and implementation of these programs because they are highly suited to teaching patients and monitoring progress.

Pharmacists have also taken an active role in disease management programs. Pharmacy costs are a major insurer concern. Disease management programs can focus on the use of medications and medication education for specific diagnoses in order to decrease costs. Pharmaceutical companies are also developing disease management programs that they sell or

---

**BOX 7-1    DISEASE MANAGEMENT: EXAMPLES OF COMMON DISEASES**

- Arthritis
- Diabetes
- Asthma
- Cardiac diseases

- Chronic obstructive pulmonary disease
- Mental illness
- Stroke

contract to insurers. The danger with these programs is the potential of pushing specific drugs on the insurer and its providers. This could result in ethical dilemmas. The companies are, however, providing a variety of services that could be very helpful such as development of patient information resources.

# Examples of Tools to Manage Care

Several tools or methods can be used to help providers manage care. In addition to disease management two other examples are described: clinical pathways and practice guidelines. Even though these tools are developed from a general patient standpoint, any time they are used the nurse, physician, or other provider must ensure that the pathway or the guideline is individualized to meet the patient's needs and to ensure that all care is patient-centered.

## Clinical Pathways

DEFINITION AND PURPOSE OF CLINICAL PATHWAY   Health care organizations are dependent on providing effective, efficient care, which requires a clear framework of practice for the interprofessional team. Collaborative care and interprofessional care are intertwined, as the development of clinical pathways and their implementation requires interprofessional collaboration. This section describes definitions, historical background of clinical pathway development, purpose, the clinical pathway development process, implementation, the effect of pathways on outcomes, and providers' responses to clinical pathways.

There is no universally accepted definition of **clinical pathways**. Reviewing a variety of definitions is helpful in appreciating their differences and similarities. The following are some examples of clinical pathway definitions.

- An optimal sequencing and timing of interventions by physicians, nurses, and other staff for a particular diagnosis or procedure, designed to minimize delays and resource utilization and to maximize the quality of care (Coffey et al., 1992)
- A visualization of the patient care process (Coffey et al., 1992)
- A timeline that identifies expected patient outcomes and associated interventions for a specific diagnosis or class of cases, often defined by a diagnosis-related group (DRG) (Griffin & Griffin, 1994)
- A tangible method for linking the patient, family, and the achievement of definable outcomes to the direct caregivers, interprofessional team, and continuous quality improvement (Zander, 1992)
- Tools to define practice and guides for patient care activities; delineate the best/ideal practice (Cesta, Tahan, & Fink, 2002)
- Tools for managed care that provide the interprofessional team with desired outcomes and identified time frames in which they should be accomplished; predict the critical targets a patient will achieve within specific time intervals, coupled with efficient use of resources (Flarey & Blancett, 1996)
- A proactive set of daily prescriptions that has been prepared following a particular timeline to facilitate the care of a specific patient population from preadmission to postdischarge (Cesta, Tahan, & Fink, 2002)
- Important tools to link patients, clinicians, and managed care organizations and other payers to achieve both high-quality and cost-effective care; effective tools to improve the planning, coordination, communication, and evaluation of care foster collaborative goal setting among multiple care providers for specific case types (Coffey et al., 1996)

One can conclude from these definitions that there are some common characteristics, including the following:

- Provide guidelines for practice
- Define outcomes
- Focus on timelines

- Use resources efficiently
- Emphasize the need for coordination, communication, and collaboration
- Include the patient and family
- Provide interdisciplinary effort
- Collaborate

Pathways provide direction in the coordination of care and ensure that outcomes are met within a designated time frame. The emphasis is on efficient use of resources and controlling costs (Ireson, 1997). Pathways have an interprofessional focus, and thus include all aspects of the patient's care that are critical to meeting outcomes. They can be used to demonstrate compliance with standards of care, accreditation, and regulatory requirements. These tools assist staff during orientation and in teaching nursing and medical students and others. Some institutions have developed patient versions of pathways that are given to the patient/family on admission or when treatment begins. They can be used to help the patient and family understand the patient's care and what to expect (Cesta, Tahan, & Fink, 2002).What are the advantages and disadvantages of using clinical pathways? Because they have been used for some time, there is considerable information about their use and difficulties in using them. Figure 7-2 identifies some of the advantages of using clinical pathways. These advantages relate to all of the major aspects of patient care delivery and help to explain why clinical pathways have become so common.

Critics of pathways question pathways as rigid requirements and with limited individuation. This could be a major disadvantage; however, health care organizations have considered this potential problem. They usually require that pathway content is assessed each time it is used with a patient to ensure that individual patient needs are met. Pathways should not be used without thought and consideration of the individual circumstances because this can lead to errors and care that is not appropriate for the patient. Patient-centered care requires that patient values and preferences along with needs are integrated into the decision making that must include the

**FIGURE 7-2   Advantages of clinical pathways.**

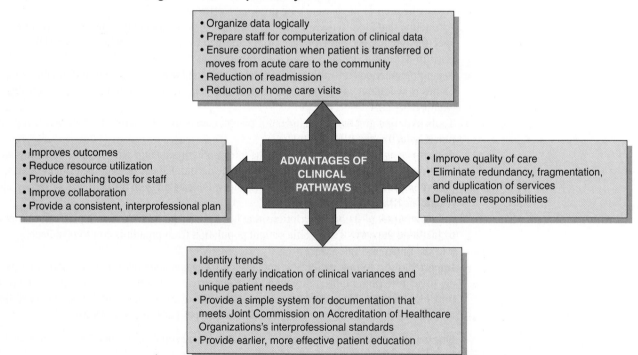

Source: Author, content summarized from Griffin, M., & Griffin, R. (1994). Critical pathways produce tangible results. *Health Care Strategic Management, 12*(7), 1, 17–23; Critical paths concept evolves into more comprehensive system. (1992). *Hospital Peer Review, 17*(2), 27–30; Hague, D. (1996, May). Clinical pathways: The careplans of the 90s. *Ohio Nurses Review*, 15–19; and Cesta, T., Tahan, H., & Fink, L. (1998). The case manager's survival guide: Winning strategies for clinical practice. St. Louis, MO: Mosby-Year Book, Inc.

patient. The physician, nurses, and other providers need to document changes or adaptations. Another disadvantage is the cost and time required to develop and implement pathways. For any health care organization, the development of its first pathway is the most expensive part of the project. It takes time to develop the process, policies and procedures, and forms, and then conduct the research that is required to get started as well as time to educate the project committee, interprofessional teams, and all of the staff. This process is described later in the chapter.

Selection of the illnesses or conditions that require pathways should be done carefully. If there are few patients in a category (illness or condition), it may not be cost effective to spend time on developing pathways that may make little difference in care, outcomes, and expenses. For example, if a hospital does not do transplants of any kind, developing a pathway for transplant care is not useful. A negative staff attitude toward pathways can also be a major disadvantage. If staff views the development of pathways as just another project with excessive paperwork, redundant documentation, and a new gimmick to endure, then the process of implementing pathways will be an arduous one. Staff will be waiting for it to pass and will not feel committed to the project. This is particularly problematic in organizations that have instituted many "new projects" only to have them fall by the wayside due to a lack of commitment, a lack of knowledge about their use and implications to practice, or a lack of funding to complete the project. If care and systems do not change as a result of pathway outcomes, staff will wonder about all the effort that is expended on the project. If staff is fearful that pathways may be used to identify individual staff performance problems rather than assessment of process and systems to improve care, the staff will be reluctant to participate. Health care organizations that spend time considering these disadvantages and staff concerns, resolving them, and increasing staff commitment and participation will be much more successful.

EVOLUTION OF PATHWAYS    Why have health care organizations developed clinical pathways? Oil and chemical refineries were the first industries to use pathways as a method for defining their work processes, and then pathways were adopted by engineering, construction, and computer industries, as they discovered that it was a good tool for managing projects. Karen Zander, a nurse, then borrowed the idea in the mid-1980s and adapted it to the acute care setting. These early clinical pathways focused on nursing interventions and use of technology to provide care. Zander was interested in decreasing the cost of care without decreasing quality. The process to develop clinical pathways was very similar to the nursing process and the nursing care plan. As is true of all new ideas, they grow and change, and hopefully improve.

The initial efforts to use pathways were restrained by limitations. Because of the generic nature of these plans, they did little to control the use of resources, types of medications, route of administration, or other factors related to cost and quality. Although the pathways did suggest the appropriate number of hospital days to allocate to a diagnostic-related group (DRG), they did little beyond this to control the kinds of product resources applied to the particular broad groupings of patients (Cesta, Tahan, & Fink, 2002). Pathways, however, have changed and improved as they no longer focus only on nursing interventions. Instead, they focus much more on interprofessional treatment and the effect of interventions on cost and quality.

An unresolved issue with the evolution of pathways is their name. Initially, they were called critical pathways. Now, pathways may be called care paths, CareMaps®, case management plans, anticipatory recovery plans, care guides, collaborative plans, coordinated plans, integrated plans, plans of action, and, probably the most common name, clinical pathways. This does cause confusion, as some health care professionals think that each of these represents a unique tool, and yet they are all basically the same. There are other tools that add to this confusion (for example, algorithms, practice guidelines, practice parameters, and the newest, disease management programs).

Practice guidelines focus on general treatment for a specific illness or condition, whereas pathways are more specific and unique to the health care agency or managed care organization in which they are used. Pathways are also individualized for patients and meet the practice concerns of the providers. These characteristics make it more difficult to use pathways developed by other institutions and organizations. Pathways need to be adapted to meet the individual needs of the institution, its providers, and its patient population.

A common misperception is that clinical pathways and case management are the same. How did this come about? The case management plan used by case managers confuses the issue, as it focuses on case manager responsibilities, while the clinical pathway focuses on shared accountability of the interprofessional team. More case managers are using pathways as they coordinate care with the interprofessional team.

## Pathway Development and Implementation Process

The pathway development process must be considered carefully as this is not a simple project. Typically, a project committee develops the framework that will be used for all pathways and oversees the project. This committee should have a broad-based representation. Some of the departments or services in an organization or agency that might be included are nurses, physicians, and representatives from social service, case management, admissions, finance, administration, medical records, utilization review, quality improvement, risk management, and materials management. Laboratory, radiology, claims processing, and other specialized areas, such as respiratory therapy and physical therapy, may also be on the interprofessional teams that develop the content for specific pathways.

Before any specific plans are made for this project, the organization's environment for change needs to be assessed. As is true of all change efforts, the commitment of key staff is the critical element for the success of pathway development. Change has become an all too common experience in health care today, and it is unlikely to go away. There are steps that can be taken, however, to make it easier on the staff and to maintain an environment that is supportive of change. If pathways are to be used, the organization's leaders must support the effort, communicate this support to all staff, and ensure that the project is completed. Too frequently, projects are begun but never seem to be completed. A lack of commitment to complete projects affects future projects in the organization. Staff is then not enthusiastic or supportive, knowing the organization's history of failure with new projects. Open and consistent communication assists staff members as they adjust to new requirements.

Because instituting the use of pathways or any of the other tools or strategies highlighted in this chapter is a major undertaking, beginning other major projects at the same time needs to be considered carefully. Too much stress at one time may affect the success of all new projects. There must also be a clear definition of the goals and identification of those staff members who will have leadership responsibilities in instituting clinical pathways. Because this is not a quick fix, a reasonable timeline is required, with identified key points for reassessment of progress. With these decisions made, the project committee can begin work on specific pathways. The first phase of the project is the development of the pathways, and the second is implementation. Evaluation is incorporated throughout the project.

Pathway development requires an interprofessional team/committee that is (a) willing to openly discuss issues and research information, (b) receptive to change, and (c) committed to the project. It is, however, helpful to have some staff members who are skeptical as they provide the "other viewpoint" that is critical in the development of realistic pathways. Hopefully, these team members will not be so negative that they are destructive to the process, but rather they will identify issues and concerns that staff will undoubtedly experience. The committee works its way through the phases highlighted in Box 7-2.

The project committee and interprofessional teams need education about project development, change, and clinical pathways. It is helpful to provide this education prior to beginning the project or in the initial stages. Content should include the following:

- Project development and organizational change
- Definition and purposes of a pathway
- Advantages and disadvantages of pathways
- Implementation of pathways
- Research resources
- Variances and variance analysis
- Project evaluation

## BOX 7-2 PATHWAY DEVELOPMENT PROCESS

### PROJECT COMMITTEE SELECTED

- Assess environment for change
- Identify target populations
- Design pathway format
- Select medical record and documentation issues
- Develop variance tracking and analysis requirements
- Develop policies and procedures
- Select interprofessional teams for specific pathways
- Provide education about pathways to the teams
- Develop and implement general staff education

### INTERPROFESSIONAL TEAMS

- Research to prepare content for specific pathway
- Retrospective chart review
- Current practice patterns
- Benchmarking
- Standards of practice
- Literature review

- Review pathway samples from other institutions and literature
- Review financial data
- Review utilization data
- Review outcome studies
- Request expert opinions
- Identify outcomes, length of stay, and timeline
- Define required content
- Pilot test
- Make changes based on pilot test data
- Repeat pilot as necessary

### FINAL APPROVAL OF PATHWAY BY PROJECT COMMITTEE AND ADMINISTRATION

### IMPLEMENTATION OF PATHWAY

### VARIANCE TRACKING AND ANALYSIS

### CONTINUE OVERALL PROJECT EVALUATION

Source: Author created; summarized from A. Finkelman. (2001). *Managed care.* Upper Saddle River, NJ: Prentice Hall, p. 154.

Providing committee members and teams with resources such as current articles on pathways, books, and even sample pathways from similar organizations is a good way to begin. The project committee and the teams that develop the content for specific pathways need access to data such as length-of-stay (LOS), common admission diagnoses, laboratory tests, and quality improvement data. Some staff may not know what data are available within the organization, so including information management system (IMS) staff that can assist the committee and the teams is very helpful.

It is best if there is a standard pathway format that will be used throughout the organization. Reviewing formats used by other organizations is a good way to understand what can be done, and many examples are found in the literature. The committee may also want to contact similar organizations and ask about their pathway formats as well as their experiences with using clinical pathways. The format that is chosen needs to be easy to use, clear, and should not seem so overwhelming that staff will immediately complain that it will only add more work. Staff appreciates brevity, relevance, and conciseness.

What is included in the clinical pathway format? The scope of clinical pathways can vary; for example, a pathway might focus on inpatient care, a complete episode of care, specialized applications, or life and health management. Box 7-3 describes the scope in more detail.

Specific pathway content may also vary among organizations; the most common categories of information that are included in pathways are identified in Box 7-4; however, a pathway does not have to include all of these categories. The committee selects the categories of information that are important to include for specific patient population and its providers.

Key indicators are a very important part of the pathway. These indicators are the interventions that must be implemented in order to attain specified outcomes. During the development phase of pathways, it is important to understand the key indicators; however, overemphasis on indicators can be a problem. This usually happens when staff is concerned about missing something important. Nurses and other health care providers need to continuously remind themselves

**INPATIENT CARE**

Focus is on admission to the inpatient setting to discharge. This is the most common.

**COMPLETE EPISODE OF CARE**

Focus is on the time that care is requested at the physician's office to termination of post-hospitalization treatment.

**SPECIALIZED APPLICATIONS**

Focus is on the patient's special needs (e.g., renal dialysis, ambulatory surgery, management of outpatient treatment of a problem).

Source: Author created; summarized from A. Finkelman. (2001). *Managed care.* Upper Saddle River, NJ: Prentice Hall, p. 158.

to focus on the most important care needs. This is not easy to do in today's stressful health care environment with its complex patients.

The development team needs to document its work so that there is a record of the planning and development process. The organization must make a decision about whether or not the pathways will be a permanent part of the medical record. If it is optional, confusion and inconsistency often occur. Accrediting agencies may question records that are not consistent. Pathways that are not part of the medical record may be viewed as less important by the staff. In the past nurses experienced this with nursing care plans when some hospitals included them in their medical records and others did not. If staff members are concerned that using the pathways does not really cover documentation needs, they may over-document. As the interprofessional teams develop specific pathway content, it is essential to review the present documentation system and how it relates to the specific content and use of pathways. How will documentation need to change in the medical record and on the clinical pathway? Organizations or providers that use computerized information management systems need to incorporate their pathways into these systems. These are critical questions that need to be repeated for each new pathway that is developed. In addition, the following questions are helpful to consider as documentation needs are reviewed.

- Is the pathway replacing existing forms?
- Will the pathway meet the documentation needs of the organization, accreditation bodies, and third-party payers?
- Will documentation result in duplication, thereby possibly contributing to a decrease in compliance?
- Who will be documenting on the pathway?
- Do policies and procedures need to be revised to reflect the changes in the documentation process (Mateo, Newton, & Kanatas, 1996, p. 81)?

- Assessment and monitoring
- Psychosocial assessment
- Actual and potential problems
- Treatment interventions: prevention and therapeutic
- Tests and procedures
- Expected outcomes
- Consults
- Required observations
- Predetermined length-of-stay
- Timeline with trigger points
- Key indicators

- Medications
- Patient activity
- Nutrition
- Intravenous therapy
- Patient/family education
- Variance tracking
- Delineate responsibilities of interdisciplinary team

Source: Author created; summarized from A. Finkelman. (2001). *Managed care.* Upper Saddle River, NJ: Prentice Hall, p. 158.

Including medical records staff on the project committee is critical. Their participation and input will prevent many future documentation problems.

Identification of the target population is a critical decision for the project committee, as time should not be wasted on the wrong population. It is costly and will only aggravate staff. A typical way to approach classifying diagnoses for pathway development is to use the International Classification of Diseases, Version 10 Conversion Manual (ICD-10-CM) (Centers for Disease Control and Prevention, 2010). This is the primary resource for medical diagnoses and third-party payer reimbursement coding. Diagnoses with the highest cost are the best ones to select. In addition, the committee considers the following as it reviews the typical illnesses or conditions in its patient population (e.g., patients in the hospital or home care agency, insurer enrollee, etc.):

- High volume
- High risk
- Complex care requirements
- High cost
- Variations in length-of-stay compared with the "norm" or benchmarks
- Variations in practice patterns
- Payer request or interest in the illness or condition
- Opportunity for improved care

With increasing emphasis on interprofessional issues, interprofessional staff teams that are selected to develop specific pathway content need to be qualified in the particular clinical area or some aspects of the delivery of care. For example, a pathway for a surgical condition should include surgeons, registered nurses from surgical units, operating room, and recovery room, and might include representatives from anesthesia, transportation, pharmacy, laboratory, medical records, admission, finance, utilization review, quality improvement, risk management, and information management system (IMS). The team begins by brainstorming but must focus on the routine, not the exceptions. Developing a flowchart often provides a helpful picture of the steps required from the routine care for the identified illness or condition. The team considers all aspects of care, a timeline that corresponds to the LOS goal, outcomes, and the key indicators for reaching the outcomes. As the team prepares to develop content, they review medical records of cases with the same diagnosis or condition, literature, outcome data, current practice, and local practice patterns (both internal and external), and seek expert opinions. Identification of outcomes is a critical aspect of the process. Outcomes need to be specific, objective, and quantitative, and they should be reviewed periodically to ensure that they are current with new research, technology, medications, and clinical practice. There is now a greater emphasis on evidence-based practice, and pathways need to be evidence-based.

It is important, and yet often difficult, for staff members to question current practices within their own organization as they often feel that they are criticizing their colleagues or themselves. Serious questions, however, need to be asked.

- What criteria are really necessary for the patient to meet for discharge?
- What care can be provided at home or on an outpatient basis?
- What intermediate patient care objectives or outcomes are really necessary to accomplish the desired long-term outcomes?
- What activities contribute to meeting outcomes?
- What activities are unnecessary or not directly related to the key discharge criteria?
- Do different practices really result in different outcomes (Coffey & LeRoy, 2001)?

These questions certainly apply to nursing and all types of care that is provided in any setting. With the increasing emphasis on care in the community, acute care hospitals need to consider what is the best setting in which to deliver the care and how to better collaborate with community providers and resources. The development of pathways is a good time to discuss these questions.

Another approach to the development of pathways is to use pathways that have been developed by other health care or professional organizations or are found in the literature. It is critical that all selected pathways are then adapted to the specific provider organization. Questions that the team considers as they review external pathways to use in their own organization include the following:

- Does the provider base its pathways on national standards and large national studies?
- Does the pathway define a population that fits our patients?
- Does the pathway consider long-term outcomes?
- Does the pathway contain information about long-term services that may be required?
- Does the author (organization) have a reputation of honesty and integrity ("Algorithms and paths," 1995, pp. 146–147)?

The reviewers must also consider how current the references are that were used to develop the pathway's content. Outdated references can be a problem in reflecting the currency of the pathway content. "One of the most significant criticisms of critical pathways is that they are rarely evidence-based" (Renholm, Leino-Kilpi, & Suominen, 2002, p. 201). With the increasing emphasis on evidence-based practice it is important that practice guides such as pathways are based on best practice. (See Chapter 15.)

Many drafts of the pathways are required as the team works through the content, discusses it with other staff, and reviews the literature. The project committee identifies the final review process that should be followed for all pathways that are developed. This process includes key persons in the organization and the project committee. Consensus is critical for successful implementation, but it is not always easy to reach. Negotiation and collaboration often are needed to reach consensus.

Clinical pathways need to be pilot tested prior to their final approval. The project committee determines the pilot testing process, including its length, number of times the pathway is implemented with patients, and data collection procedures. Issues that are important to consider during pilot testing are pathway quality, feasibility of use, appropriateness of timeline and LOS, delays or variations in care practice patterns, and compliance (Cesta, Tahan, & Fink, 2002). Undoubtedly, changes need to be made, and some of these may be major. If so, another pilot may be required. Obtaining staff members' feedback as they use the pathway in the pilot is critical for obtaining helpful information. If this feedback is ignored, staff feels left out and less inclined to support the pathways when they are implemented. Once pathways are approved, implementation begins; however, there are two issues that are important throughout the development and implementation phases: collaboration with other health care organizations that might require the use of clinical pathways (MCOs and other third-party payers) or receiving patient referrals for additional services and the liability and ethical issues related to the use of pathways.

Implementation of clinical pathways requires time and patience. Staff members will be uncomfortable and have concerns about how their use will affect their practice. Pathways should not be seen as a method for improving all of an organization's problems. For example, using clinical pathways probably will not improve overall communication in an organization that has a long-standing problem of poor communication. During the implementation of pathways, problems are often encountered that need to be resolved to prevent project failure. The following are examples of potential problems that may interfere with pathway implementation.

There is concern that pathways represent cookbook medicine in that they standardize care without regard to individual patient needs or individual provider practice. Pathways ignore practice pattern differences that occur when physicians and nurses care for the patients with the same diagnosis. Staff education is required to ensure that clinical staff understands the purpose of pathways and that appreciates the need for individualizing pathways to meet individual patient needs.

Pathways can become just one more record to keep or follow, particularly if the documentation system is not evaluated at the time of pathway development. Duplication is a frequent complaint and serves only to frustrate staff and increase documentation errors. Consolidating the progress notes often helps. In addition, there is a tendency to include too many indicators or too much detail in the pathways. This makes them cumbersome to use. If a pathway is long, staff may assume that using it is a complex process that will only increase the workload.

If pathway outcomes are based only on data from within the institution and do not consider relevant external information and outcomes, the pathways may represent only the internal current standards rather than the optimal. In this case, patient care may not improve.

Turf battles may become very serious, particularly if they were present prior to implementing pathways. Who is in charge of the pathways? Utilization review? Nursing staff? Case managers? Job boundaries need to be reviewed prior to implementation. When project leadership is defined, staff needs to be included in discussions. Gaining consensus is an important part of the implementation process for all levels of staff. As was discussed in Chapter 3, effective change requires understanding and buy in from staff. Clearly defining purpose and responsibility will help to prevent many future problems.

A common problem in pathway development is to overestimate or underestimate the expected LOS. This can lead to increased staff stress. Using pathways is the best way to assess the LOS, and their use helps to determine the best expected LOS.

Co-morbidities are also problematic. Pathways usually are developed for one illness or condition; however, patients often have more than one. How should staff use the pathways for these patients? This needs to be clarified before implementation. One way to resolve this problem is to develop co-paths. This prevents confusion and problems with increased documentation. The co-path is usually used across departments, as typically these are problems that are experienced with different types of patients. Physicians usually are concerned about pathways, as they need to be reassured that pathways do not replace physician orders. They are also concerned about losing their autonomy. To decrease this fear, physician input is absolutely necessary during pathway development, implementation, and evaluation. Some institutions have even gone so far as to require a physician's order for the use of a pathway; however, there is usually a method for physicians to alter or choose not to use a pathway. This is important to ensure patient-centered care. Of course, these approaches could defeat the purpose of the pathways, and the health care organization would need to monitor the use of these alternatives to ensure that pathway implementation is not sidetracked. Data obtained from the pathways about patient outcomes may also be affected by these physician options.

Staff resistance to the use of pathways must be dealt with directly. Often, recognizing that it might be a problem and taking steps to alleviate staff concerns can prevent it. Cesta, Tahan, and Fink (2002) have discussed examples of such measures and advantages to emphasize.

- Increase staff involvement in all phases of development and implementation
- Share critical literature with staff
- Identify pathway benefits to specific health care professionals
- Ensure that pathways are recommendations, not rigid requirements
- Emphasize that pathways affect the quality of care: coordination, collaboration, patient/family education, outcomes, and data assessment
- Decrease costs, achieve expected LOS, increase consistency and improved care, and decrease risk management issues
- Increase compliance with accreditation and regulatory requirements
- Increase marketing ability to attract more plans and MCO contracts
- Provide data for research
- Serve as staff education tools

LIABILITY AND ETHICAL ISSUES   Clinical pathways can be introduced as evidence in court to demonstrate a standard of care or to illustrate expected patient outcomes or timelines. There are two areas of concern. The first is liability for staff that develops pathways, and the second is provider liability for those who use the pathways. Pathway developers have been named in liability cases. It is important that pathways are based on best practice (evidence-based practice). What can be done to prevent this experience? The committee should be an interprofessional team, with representatives who have expertise in the pathway focus area. Their résumés should be kept on file in case questions about expertise arise later. Written policies and procedures about the pathway development process and implementation, including a clear description of how pathways are individualized and how this is to be documented, should also be kept on file. It is important that all of this material is dated. A file should be kept for each pathway that includes the pathway tool, all of its major drafts, reference material, pilot testing data, and evaluations. All relevant organizational policies and procedures need to be evaluated to ensure that there is no conflict with new pathways. It is best that risk management staff and legal counsel review final pathways, policies, procedures, types of records that should be kept, and the like. Staff that develops and use the pathways need to have appropriate education about them, and attendance needs to be documented. The evaluation process should be clearly defined, and compliance with the process documented.

What is the liability for the provider? There are four provider responses to pathways that may lead to liability problems.

1. The provider follows the clinical pathway but delivers negligent care.
2. The provider follows the clinical pathway, but the clinical pathway outlines substandard care to be delivered to the patient.
3. The provider does not follow the clinical pathway and fails to document the variance and the reason for noncompliance.
4. The provider misinterprets the clinical pathway or applies it incorrectly (Sheehan & Sullivan, 1998, p. 118).

An important point to make is that the provider is at risk if a pathway is blindly followed. If a pathway contains errors or represents substandard care, the provider is still responsible for the care provided. Nothing relieves the professional, such as a nurse, of the responsibility for using professional judgment. If pathways are used, every health care professional who uses them must be responsible for learning how to use them correctly in the best interest of individual patients or take the risk of making an error. Variances are tracked and used to assess achievement of outcomes. Comments about general variance data should never be documented in individual medical records. Disclaimers may be used with pathways. General disclaimers should state that the pathway provides guidance for the plan of care, but staff recognizes that each patient requires individualized care. The disclaimer should convey that the practitioner makes treatment decisions after an assessment of the patient's condition. The patient's version of the pathway should contain a statement that the guidelines are provided to inform the patient and that, because every patient is different, treatment and outcomes differ (Sheehan & Sullivan, 1998).

**PATHWAY EVALUATION**     Pathway evaluation should not be made into a complicated process. The areas of most concern are whether costs are changing per patient diagnosis and for itemized costs, such as laboratory tests, pharmacy, physical therapy, and radiology, and whether the quality of care is compromised. Are outcomes met? Evaluation also focuses on the LOS or the length of treatment. Particularly important in evaluation process is variance analysis.

Variances are deviations from the expected or that which is defined in the clinical pathway. They may be positive or negative. Negative variances indicate that the patient has not achieved expected outcomes or that activities have not been completed. A positive variance indicates that the patient achieved an outcome or activity prior to the expected deadline. If the trend is toward more positive variances, it may mean that the deadlines need to be reviewed and could be shortened. Negative variances might relate to organization, provider, or patient issues. With today's complex health care organizations and concern about quality it is important to analyze the causes for negative variances. System or operational variances focus on hindrances in the system or the organization that prevent the achievement of patient outcomes. Examples are delay in laboratory results, lack of bed space, hours of service, delayed transfers to a long-term care facility, lack of supplies, and so on. Provider variances focus on the variances that may be caused by the provider. Examples include the following:

- The physician does not respond to a telephone call from a nurse about a patient's condition.
- A mislabeled medication is given to a patient.
- A staff member is unable to do a procedure due to lack of experience or knowledge.
- Orders are misread, and a patient is sent for the wrong procedure.
- Inadequate nursing staff decreases the time a nurse has to review a patient's history.

- A patient variance identifies factors related to the patient that prevent the achievement of patient outcomes; for example, a patient refuses medication; a patient experiences complications (e.g., elevated temperature that interferes with proceeding with treatment); a patient experiences inadequate pain relief; or a patient arrives late for his admission for ambulatory care surgery.

It is important to avoid blame when assessing variances but rather to look at reasons and resolution; this is a key recommendation from many of the Institute of Medicine reports about quality and patient safety. Staff needs to consider all aspects of an issue (for example, a patient's medication problem). Why is the patient refusing medication? Is the patient afraid of the medication and its side effects? Does the patient lack understanding of the purpose of taking the medication? Does the patient not have the money to pay for the medication? Does the patient lack transportation to pick up the medication or feel that the medication will not help? Jumping to conclusions is not helpful and limits true understanding as to the reason for the variance. Variance data are most critical in understanding outcome achievement or lack of achievement and also provide direction for change. Data should be shared with the pathway development team and relevant staff. Involving them in resolution development is also important.

Variance analysis assists in identifying patterns of concern or problems that are seen in a number of patients. These problems may require more intensive action for every patient who experiences these problems. It might, however, be due to a repetitive problem in the system. Algorithms are created to resolve these variances and prevent future variances. Generally, algorithms are not developed until variance data indicate a need. Algorithms are developed in the same way as pathways. Typically, they are formatted as decision-making trees. For example, if a patient experiences an elevated temperature, then specific treatment is begun.

Documenting these variances can be problematic due to liability risk. Staff needs to avoid blaming a staff member in the medical record; for example, to state in the medical record that because a physician did not respond to a call from the nurse about the patient's condition the patient developed a complication. Documenting variances must be done with care. Reasons for the variance, if known, need to be identified but should be based on factual data. When treatment that is not in the pathway is added or deleted, this must be documented. Nurses document most of the variances because they have the most contact with patients, particularly in acute care, home care, and long-term care. Variance documentation requires accurate and complete documentation. The health care organization develops documentation policies and procedures and prepares staff in their use.

Patient and staff satisfaction are also critical evaluation issues. Patient satisfaction is a very important factor in the evaluation of the use of pathways and should consider three key questions:

1. Does the patient/family feel involved in the care?
2. Were the patient's goals met?
3. Did staff discuss the patient's progress with the patient?

Patients need to first understand what a clinical pathway is and how it is used. Individual nurses best provide this explanation because they interact more with patients and families. Several studies have indicated that the use of pathways seems to increase patient satisfaction (Goode, 1995; Leibman et al., 1998; Renholm, Leino-Kilpi, & Suominen, 2002). Other issues that have been discussed as factors that might be affected by the use of pathways are patient education, continuity of information, continuity or care, quality of care, length-of-stay, and reduction of costs. All these appear to be affected positively by the use of pathways, although additional research is clearly necessary (Renholm, Leino-Kilpi, & Suominen, 2002).

Staff satisfaction should also not be overlooked in pathway evaluation. Important questions to consider include the following:

- Do you understand the reasons for using pathways?
- Did you feel prepared to use the pathways?
- If you participated in the development of the pathways, do you feel that your input was respected?
- How has the use of pathways affected your daily practice/work?

- How has the use of pathways affected your relationship with your patients/families?
- Do you think that pathways support interprofessional collaboration? If so, how?
- How has the use of pathways affected your documentation?
- What would you like to see changed with pathways and their implementation?
- Is staff using the pathways and using them correctly?

These questions are particularly important for health care organizations that use temporary nurses, part-time staff, and travel nurses, which may make it difficult to ensure that all staff is knowledgeable about the pathways and are committed to using them. Full-time staff may carry the burden of ensuring that pathways are used correctly. This can lead to increased staff stress and affect patient care delivery.

There are many questions that can be asked in the evaluation process. Health care organizations need to develop questions relevant to their environment, patients, and staff. Gathering data can be overdone, so question selection and related data should be carefully considered. When evaluation is complete, a summary of the results and any pathway revisions must be shared with the staff. In many organizations, staff finds out about changes when changes affect them, but this is too late. Staff members should not pick up a copy of a pathway when they need to use it and find out it has been changed. This does not allow time for staff to understand the changes and how they affect patient care delivery. Studies have indicated that pathways can make a positive difference in care (Renholm, Leino-Kilpi, & Suominen, 2002; Panella, Marchisio, & Stanislao, 2003; Dy, et al., 2005).

## Practice Guidelines

Managed care organizations' interest in practice guidelines has made a difference in their acceptance by other types of insurers and the federal government insurance programs. Health care professional organizations have also recognized the value in using guidelines. This interest in tools to manage care stems from the need to decrease costs and yet provide quality care. Guidelines have been used in conjunction with clinical pathways. The goal is to narrow the gap between an organization's current care and optimal care. Practice guidelines are used to assist with treatment decision making and to evaluate care. The Joint Commission does not require the use of practice guidelines but does require that hospitals consider their use and application to the hospital's services and processes. Several questions about practice guidelines that could also be applied to disease management programs include the following:

- Are clinical practice guidelines (or disease management programs) a means for improving the quality of health care?
- Are clinical practice guidelines (or disease management programs) a means for saving money in the health care system?
- Are clinical practice guidelines (or disease management programs) a means for solving the malpractice problem?
- Are clinical practice guidelines (or disease management programs) a means for making the health care system work better for all?
- Or are they a recipe for disaster (Lohr, 1995, p. 51)?

The last question is of concern, but for now, there is no answer to this question. As with all new changes, such as these and clinical pathways, experience data will help to answer these questions. Early studies on the use of clinical pathways indicate that this patient care management tool has had some positive impacts on cost containment and quality (Lohr, 1995). There has been less research on practice guidelines and disease management programs, so less is known about their effect.

DEFINITION AND PURPOSE    **Practice guidelines** are "systematically developed statements that assist practitioners in making decisions about appropriate health care for specific clinical conditions" (General Accounting Office, 1996). As with clinical pathways, practice guidelines are called by many names. Some of the more common ones are appropriateness indicators, practice parameters, medical review criteria, and standards. Their purpose is to pull together research information from the literature, evaluate these results, and access expert opinion about the clinical condition. They should be evidence-based. This information is then prepared in a usable form. Practice guidelines are different from standards of care in that guidelines do not define treatment but rather provide information and options. See Media Link for examples of evidence-based practice guidelines.

**INSURER INTEREST PRACTICE GUIDELINES** Insurers often support the use of practice guidelines. The common reasons for this support are to do the following:

- Reduce health care costs.
- Improve the quality of care.
- Ensure consistency of care.
- Provide performance data for comparison with other MCOs, as well as comparison of individual provider performance levels.
- Comply with accreditation and regulatory requirements.

In 1996, the General Accounting Office reported to the House Subcommittee on Health on the use of practice guidelines within the managed care environment (General Accounting Office, 1996). Interviews were conducted with medical directors from 19 managed care plans representing multiple states, with a combined enrollment of 7 million people. In addition, professional literature was reviewed, and interviews were conducted with representatives from health care organizations, condition-specific organizations, and the Agency for Healthcare Research and Quality (AHRQ). What did this report tell the health care community about the use of practice guidelines? The first important fact is that by March 1996, 2000 practice guidelines had been developed, and this number is even higher today. This indicates potential problems because many of these guidelines are on the same topics. Some of these guidelines may also offer conflicting guidance. As providers and insurers consider the many different practice guidelines, conflicts do arise. The report's conclusions identified the following:

1. Clinical practice guidelines promote greater uniformity within physician networks, encourage improved efficiency and clinical decision-making, and eliminate unnecessary care.
2. Several health care plans have adopted clinical practice guidelines to control costs, improve performance on standardized measures, receive accreditation, and comply with regulatory requirements.
3. Due to time and fiscal constraints, many health care plans customize published clinical guidelines rather than generate original guidelines.
4. Physicians are more likely to use a clinical practice guideline if local health providers develop it.
5. Managed care plans customize existing clinical practice guidelines to suit alternative treatments, available resources, population needs, and format and currency concerns.
6. While health care plans modify existing clinical practice guidelines to varying degrees, extensive changes could jeopardize the guidelines' effectiveness.
7. Some health plans would prefer that the federal government publish and update evidence on medical conditions and services, develop useful practice guideline tools, and perform outcomes research and medical technology assessments that would help them to develop, modify, and update their guidelines. Since the time of this report the federal government has developed many more practical guidelines.

Typically, insurers select practice guideline content based on services or conditions that have high cost, high liability risk, and a high incidence in their particular enrollee population, which are the same key criteria used to select pathway focus. If an insurer has few enrollees with renal problems, it does not make sense for it to expend efforts to institute the use of practice guidelines for renal problems. The insurer must reduce its costs but also must consider the expenses that are incurred to make changes that might reduce costs.

Most insurers do not develop their own practice guidelines. They review guidelines that have been developed by professional organizations, the AHRQ, or other resources. Guidelines are then selected and adapted to meet the needs of the insurer. This is less costly, expedites the development process, and, more importantly, the final product meets the individual needs of the insurer, its providers, and its enrollees. For example, lengthy guidelines—and there are many that are quite long—have not been found to be as helpful to the provider. Many providers do not even take the time to read them. Some guidelines may make recommendations that the insurer considers too costly. The insurer must recognize that once it adapts a practice guideline, it is no longer the same guideline and thus loses the integrity of a published guideline as agreed upon by the publishing organization or authors. The insurer must then take the responsibility of periodic evaluations to ensure that the content is current and accurate.

DEVELOPMENT AND IMPLEMENTATION OF PRACTICE GUIDELINES    Public and private sector organizations develop practice guidelines, including professional organizations, health care organizations, and researchers. Condition-specific organizations (e.g., American Heart Association, Arthritis Foundation) have also developed guidelines. As members of these various organizations, nurses have been active in the development of guidelines. Governmental agencies that have been involved in the development are the AHRQ through the National Guideline Clearinghouse, the National Institutes of Health, the Centers for Disease Control and Prevention, the U.S. Preventive Services Task Force, Centers of Medicare and Medicaid Services, and the Department of Health and Human Services. Active participation from many types of organizations indicates the level of interest in practice guidelines. The AHRQ guidelines are well-known sets of statements that may be used to assist practitioners and/or patients in making health care decisions for specific clinical problems. Interprofessional panels of experts develop these guidelines. The guidelines include the following:

- Supporting materials, such as methodology, scientific evidence, and comprehensive bibliography
- A desktop reference, the *Clinical Practice Guideline*, for the practitioner that includes recommendations, algorithms, flowcharts, tables, figures, and references
- A quick reference guide for practitioners that is an abbreviated version of the *Clinical Practice Guideline*
- *The Patient's Guide*, which provides information for the patient about the clinical problem and treatments

Physicians are using practice guidelines, but the level of use is variable. How might physicians and other providers such as advanced practice nurses use these guidelines? Examples of their purposes that are important for practitioners are to establish immunization schedules for patients and to provide evidence-based practice for example by following a treatment guideline for adult asthma.

What are the problems or factors that are keeping providers, such as physicians and nurse practitioners, from using practice guidelines? One major problem is the accessibility of the information while the provider (such as a physician, nurse, or nurse practitioner) is with the patient. If the provider has access to a computer in the examining room, then this information could be discussed with the patient in the examining room. This would save time and be more relevant to the patient. This is, however, an expense. With so many guidelines in existence, making decisions about which ones to use is problematic. Information overload is a major complication today, and it can actually increase stress rather than decrease it or control it. A common approach made by providers is to amalgamate the guidelines by considering providers' personal experiences and approaches with the specific condition.

Non-adherence to guidelines can often be traced to limited provider input in guideline development, after which the provider does not accept the guidelines. Change that is instituted from outside is rarely successful. In addition, change that brings limited rewards often fails. Some insurers encourage guideline use by paying incentives to providers who use them and by tracking their use when they evaluate provider performance. A final concern with practice guidelines is coverage of co-morbidities, which is also true with clinical pathways. For example, what does the provider do when a patient has a cardiac condition and diabetes? There are guidelines for the cardiac condition and also guidelines for diabetes. The guidelines may not consider the impact of one illness on the other and may actually offer conflicting treatment options. Often, the provider chooses not to use any practice guideline rather than deal with conflicting and confusing recommendations.

Nurse practitioners also encounter the same problems with practice guidelines as they use them in their practice. As more nurse practitioners enter private practice and clinics, they will need to review these guidelines and determine their relevance to advance practice nursing. Nurses who work in the community can make use of the guidelines to help plan community health education and services that focus on specific problems.

Informatics can be used to support implementation of guidelines as well as assist with evaluation of their use and outcomes. As noted in Chapter 18, informatics has become more important in all areas of health care. Informatics can provide quick access to the guidelines. Within the information system staff should be able to get to the guidelines when they are needed, review them, and then apply them to planning and patient education. The information system can also be set up to remind staff to use guidelines and integrate these guidelines into the documentation system. Information systems also allow for easy updates of guidelines, but for this to be successful it must be built into the system to ensure that it gets done.

Evaluation of the implementation of practice guidelines is important, and the key questions are as follows:

- How does the guideline improve practice?
- Is the guideline still scientifically based?
- Does the guideline continue to meet the needs of the patient population?
- Are clinicians implementing the guidelines as designed (Poniatowski, 2000, p. 13)?

## APPLYING EVIDENCE-BASED PRACTICE

### Evidence for Effective Leadership and Management

**Citation:** Needleman, J. et al. (2009). Overall effect of TCAB on initial participating hospitals. *AJN, 109*(11), Supplement TCAB: 59–65.

**Overview:** Transforming Care at the Bedside (TCAB), a Robert Wood Johnson Foundation partnership initiative with the Institute for Health care Improvement (IHI), focuses on improving inpatient care and work environment. The goal is to have front-line staff recognize need for change, identify innovations to improve, test these changes, and then decide whether or not to adopt changes permanently. Teamwork and nurse retention are a critical part of TCAB. This study is an evaluation of TCAB participating hospitals' experiences. Surveys, interviews, and hospital data are used in the evaluation of 10 participating hospitals and 533 tests of change. The results indicate that staff is more likely to participate in further change projects as a result of participating in TCAB. There is a positive impact on falls, codes, and readmission rates. The study highlights selected innovations that focus on safe and reliable care, patient-centered care, value-added processes, and vitality and teamwork.

**Application:** Acute care hospitals are struggling with many factors that work against them such as financial losses, increasing demands to improve care but with limited resources to do so, staff shortages, retention problems, staff morale, and need for more effective leadership. As the title of this article implies, TCAB moves the focus to the bedside—to more patient-centered care.

TCAB is an initiative that makes change possible, change that comes from the bottom up. Change was discussed in Chapter 3, but it is a critical force in any acute care hospital. Change will happen, but will it be controlled and effective or chaotic and nonconstructive? This evaluation of TCAB supports an approach to improving the functioning of acute care hospitals.

**Questions:**

1. *Why do you think TCAB is particularly important to nursing? To nursing management?*
2. *What is your opinion of the examples identified for each of the selected innovation categories?*
3. *If you were involved in a TCAB project for an acute care unit, what would you focus on?*

# APPLYING LEADERSHIP AND MANAGEMENT

## MY HOSPITAL UNIT

You have to decide on your priority strategic goal for your unit for the coming year. You and your staff decide that it will be to improve patient-centered care. A meeting is scheduled with the staff to discuss how this might be achieved. You do not want the plan to be broad and want clear direction of strategies. What might you and your staff develop to describe the strategies you will use to meet this goal and how you will measure goal achievement and apply to your specific unit? The strategies need to be clear and specific; measurable. Use the virtual unit site found on the textbook website to record the work that you do in the role of nurse manager for your unit.

## Critical Thinking Questions and Activities

1. Discuss examples from a clinical setting to illustrate that the health care organization is patient-centered. Identify examples that are not patient-centered and assess why they are not patient-centered and how you would improve them.
2. Find an example of a clinical pathway from a clinical site, nursing literature, or Internet. Review the example. Apply what you have learned in this chapter. Describe the critical elements of the pathway and, if possible, how it was developed. You should consider the following: purpose of the pathway, the process used to develop it (including who did it, how it was reviewed, what type of data was used to develop it), the target population and why it would be selected, type and quality of content, identification of any possible legal and ethical issues, use of the clinical pathway (Is it easy to use? What does staff think about using it? Could you follow it for a patient?), and what is the evaluation process for the pathway (frequency of review, by whom, and who can provide feedback about its use).
3. Find an example of the application of health promotion or illness prevention in one of your clinical sites. What is the example? How is it used? Is it effective, and what do you base this on? What is the role of the patient or consumer of health care?
4. Visit the National Institute of Health website on patient-centered research at http://outcomes.cancer.gov/areas/pcc/. What can you learn about current research? How might it be relevant to nurses?
5. Visit the Institute of Health Improvement site at http://www.ihi.org/IHI/Topics/PatientCenteredCare/PatientCenteredCareGeneral/Tools/StrategiesforLeadership PatientandFamilyCenteredCareToolkit.htm and explore the toolkit of strategies for hospital leaders to improve patient-centered care. Explore the tools offered. Discuss in small teams.

## Media Links

- **URL: http://www.ahrq.gov/clinic/cpgsix.htm**
  Agency for Healthcare Research and Quality: Clinical Practice Guidelines
- **URL: http://www.ahrq.gov/browse/hpdp.htm**
  Agency for Healthcare Research and Quality: Health Promotion
- **URL: http://www.uspreventiveservicestaskforce.org/about.htm**
  Agency for Healthcare Research and Quality: U.S. Preventive Services Task Force
- **URL: http://www.ihi.org/IHI/Topics/PatientCenteredCare/PatientCenteredCareGeneral/**
  Institute of Health Improvement: Patient-centered Care
- **URL: http://www.improvingchroniccare.org/**
  Improving Chronic Illness Care
- **URL: http://www.guideline.gov**
  National Guideline Clearinghouse

# References

Agency for Healthcare Research and Quality. (AHRQ). (2009). Focus on cost-effectiveness analysis at AHRQ. Retrieved June 15, 2009, from http://www.ahrq.gov/research/costeff.htm

Algorithms and paths: Use them to monitor, improve quality care. (1995). *Case Management Advisor, 6*(11), 145–146.

American Nurses Association. (2003). *Nursing's social policy statement.* (2nd ed.). Silver Spring, MD: Author.

Benner, P., Tanner, C., & Chesla, C. (1996). *Expertise in nursing practice: Caring, clinical judgment, and ethics.* New York: Springer.

Benner, P., Sutphen, M., Leonard, V., & Day, L. (2010). *Educating nurses.* San Francisco: Jossey-Bass Publishers.

Centers for Disease Control and Prevention. (2010). International Classification of Diseases, Version 10 Conversion Manual (ICD-10-CM). Retrieved February 8, 2010, from http://www.cdc.gov/nchs/icd/icd10cm.htm

Cesta, T., Tahan, H., & Fink, L. (2002). *The case manager's survival guide: Winning strategies for clinical practice.* St. Louis, MO: Mosby-Year Book, Inc.

Coffey, R., et al. (1992). An introduction to critical paths. *Quality Management in Health Care, 1*(1), 45–54.

Coffey, R. & LeRoy, S. (2001). Critical paths: Linking outcomes for patients, clinicians, and payers. In P. Kongstvedt (Ed.), *The managed health care handbook* (pp. 521–538). Gaithersburg, MD: Aspen Publishers, Inc.

DMAA. (2009). Disease Management. Retrieved July 6, 2009, from http://www.carecontinuum.org/

Davis, K., Schoenbaum, A., & Audet, A. (2005). A 2020 vision of patient-centered primary care. *Journal of General Internal Medicine, 20*(10), 953–957.

Dy, S., et al. (2005). Critical pathway effectiveness: assessing the impact of patient, hospital care, and pathway characteristics using qualitative comparative analysis. *Health Services Research, 40*(2), 499–516.

Finkelman, A. & Kenner, C. (2010). *Professional nursing concepts. Competencies for quality leadership.* Boston: Jones and Bartlett Publishers.

Flarey, D., & Blancett, S. (Eds.). (1996). *Handbook of nursing case management: Health care delivery in a world of managed care.* Gaithersburg, MD: Aspen Publishers, Inc.

General Accounting Office. (1996). Practice guidelines: Managed care plans customize guidelines to meet local interest. (GAO/HEHS-96-95). Washington, DC: Author.

Gerteis, M., Edgman-Levitan, J., Daley, J, & Delbanco, T. (Eds). (2003). *Through the patient's eyes.* San Francisco: Jossey-Bass.

Glassgow, R., Funnell, M., Bonomi, A., Davis, C., Bechham, V., & Wagner, E. (2002). Self-management aspects of the improving chronic illness breakthrough series: Implementation with diabetes and heart failure teams. *Annals of Behavioral Medicine, 24*(2), 80–87.

Goode, C. (1995). Impact of a care map and case management on patient satisfaction and staff satisfaction, collaboration, and autonomy. *Nursing Economics, 13*(6), 337–349.

Griffin, M., & Griffin, R. (1994). Critical pathways produce tangible results. *Health Care Strategic Management, 12*(7), 18–23.

Institute of Health Improvement. (2010). My shared plan. Retrieved February 8, 2010, from http://www.ihi.org/IHI/Topics/HIVAIDS/HIVDiseaseGeneral/Tools/My+Shared+Care+Plan.htm

Institute of Medicine. (2001). *Crossing the quality chasm.* Washington, DC: National Academies Press.

Institute of Medicine. (2003a). *Health professions education.* Washington, DC: National Academies Press.

Institute of Medicine. (2003b). *Priority areas for quality improvement.* Washington, DC: National Academies Press.

Institute of Medicine. (2004). *Health literacy.* Washington, DC: National Academies Press.

Institute of Medicine. (2008). *Retooling for an aging America: Building the health care workforce.* Washington, DC: National Academies Press.

Ireson, C. (1997). Critical pathways: Effectiveness in achieving patient outcomes. *Journal of Nursing Administration, 27*(6), 16–23.

Kongstvedt, P. (2009). *Managed care. What it is and how it works.* Boston: Jones and Bartlett Publishers.

Korczyk, S., & Witte, H. (1998). *The complete idiot's guide to managed care.* New York: Alpha Books.

Landro, L. (October 20, 2004). Disease management: Pro and con. *Wall Street Journal,* D4.

Lewin, S., Skea, V., Entwistle, V., Zwarenstein, M., & Dick, J. (2001). Interventions for providers to promote a patient-centered approach in clinical consultations (Cochrane Review). *Cochrane Database System Review* 4: CD003267.

Lohr, K. (1995). Guidelines for clinical practice: What they are and why they count. *Journal of Law, Medicine & Ethics, 23*, 49–56.

Mateo, M., Newton, C., & Kanatas, K. (1996). Developing and implementing critical paths in case management. In D. Flarey & S. Blancett (Eds.), *Handbook of nursing case management: Health care delivery in a world of managed care* (pp. 80–99). Gaithersburg, MD: Aspen Publishers, Inc.

Murphy, J. (2004). Using focused reflection and articulation to promote clinical reasoning. *Nursing Education Perspectives, 24*, 226–231.

Panella, M., Marchisio, S., Di Stanislao, F. (2003). Reducing clinical variations with clinical pathways: do pathways work? *International Journal Quality Health Care, 15*(6), 509–21.

Poniatowski, L. (2000, February). Clinical practice guidelines: Consider, adopt, or do your own. *Nursing Management, 31*(2), 13.

Rehnholm, M., Leino-Kilpi, H., & Suominen, T. (2002). Critical pathways: A systematic review. *Journal of Nursing Administration, 32*(4), 196–202.

Sheehan, J., & Sullivan, G. (1998). Psychiatric clinical pathways, documentation, and liability. In P. Dykes (Ed.), *Psychiatric clinical pathways: An interdisciplinary approach* (pp. 115–124). Gaithersburg, MD: Aspen Publishers, Inc.

U.S. Preventive Services Task Force. (2009). Cost effectiveness. Retrieved August 19, 2009, from http://www.ahrq.gov/CLINIC/uspstfix.htm

Zander, K. (1992). Quantifying, managing, and improving quality. Part II: The collaborative management of quality care. *The New Definition, 7*(3), 1–2.

# 8

# Diversity and Disparities in Health Care

## CHAPTER OUTLINE

## LEARNING OUTCOMES

Before you begin, take a moment to familiarize yourself with the learning outcomes for this chapter.

- Analyze the status of patient diversity in health care.
- Discuss the problem of health disparities.
- Apply strategies to improve health literacy and the role of the nurse manager.
- Examine the implications of a multicultural patient population for the staff and organization.
- Explain how a dissonance culture can affect an organization and patient care.
- Compare and contrast staff culture and patient culture.
- Apply the concept of organizational culture to a health care organization.
- Describe a healing organization.
- Apply strategies that may be used to improve an organization's culture.

## KEY TERMS

- Baby boomers
- Culture
- Cultural competency
- Consonant culture

- Dissonant culture
- Generation X
- Generation Y (Nexters)
- Health disparity

- Health literacy
- Organizational culture
- Values
- Workforce diversity

## WHAT'S AHEAD

The U.S. health care system has seen an increase in diverse patients representing many cultural backgrounds. The Institute of Medicine (IOM) examined the health care system, and now there is recognition of a serious problem with health disparities in the U.S. understanding culture and diversity as part of the strategies to improving the disparity problem as well as other strategies. Organizational culture plays a role in how consumers view health care organizations (HCO) and influences staff that works in the organizations. The following discussion focuses on patient culture and diversity, health disparities, health literacy, health care organizational culture, and workforce diversity.

# Health Care Diversity and Disparities

The Institute of Medicine's core competencies for health care professions ensure patient-centered care includes cultural issues: *identify, respect, and care about patients' differences, values, preferences, and expressed needs* (2003). The IOM states that "a culturally diverse population poses challenges that go beyond simple language competency and include the need to understand the effects of lifestyle and cultural differences on health status and health-related behaviors; the need to adapt treatment plans and modes of delivery to different lifestyles and familial patterns; the implications of a diverse genetic endowment among the population; the prominence of nontraditional providers, as well as family caregivers" (2003, p. 40). Nurses play a major role in health care 24/7, and they have a major impact on improving care for all patients and ensuring equitable care.

What is cultural competency? It is an issue that is in the forefront of health care delivery and health care education. "The process of developing cultural competence is a means of responding effectively to the huge ethnic and racial demographic shifts and changes confronting our country's health care system. Cultural competence is defined as a set of policies, behaviors, attitudes, and practices that enable individuals and organizations to work effectively in cross-cultural situations. **Cultural competency** is the ability of systems to provide care to patients with diverse values, beliefs, and behaviors, including the tailoring of delivery to meet patients' social, cultural, and linguistic needs" (Salisbury, 2006, p. 90). The American Association of Colleges of Nursing (AACN) emphasizes the five IOM core competencies in its 2009 publication *Essentials of Baccalaureate Education for Professional Nursing Practice*, including cultural competency, and has also developed an online toolkit to assist in developing cultural competency. (The link for the toolkit is found in the Media Links at the end of the chapter.) Nursing education has been making improvements in including content and learning experiences to improve cultural competency, though current reports on disparities indicate that more improvement is required. Health care diversity is also mentioned in the 2010 health care reform legislation. The new law requires that beginning in 2010 there needs to be improved collection and reporting of data on race, ethnicity, sex, primary language, disability status, and for underserved and frontier populations. Access to treatment for persons with disabilities must also be monitored. Data must be analyzed to monitor trends in disparities.

## A Diverse Patient Population

The Institute for the Future (2000) forecasted more diversity for the United States. While the population is still primarily white non-Hispanic, the number of African American, Hispanic, Asian, and Native Americans is increasing because of birth rates and immigration. It is predicted that by 2010 the country's population will be 32% minority ethnic. Absolute numbers will still be small until after 2050 (The Institute for the Future, 2000). The important issue with the diverse population is its regional impact. The regions with higher concentrations of diverse populations, in order of size, are the South, the West, Northeast, and Midwest. This prediction was accurate as growth and change continues across the country.

There is no doubt that nurses are caring for patients who come from a variety of cultural backgrounds. It is also important for nurses to consider how their own cultural backgrounds affect the care they provide and their leadership. What is done with this information? How does it impact the health care delivery system? Why should a nurse leader be concerned? "One of the newest requirements of a nurse leader is to function as a bridge person between people of different cultures" (De Ruiter & Saphiere, 2001, p. 62). This means that nursing leaders must understand the implications of staff members' personal cultural background, and how this relates to patient cultural background, the cultures in the local community, and of course, the culture of the health care organization. The American Organization of Nursing Executives (AONE) has identified nursing leadership diversity principles, which are found in Box 8-1.

---

**BOX 8-1    AONE GUIDING PRINCIPLES FOR DIVERSITY IN HEALTH CARE ORGANIZATIONS**

The following principles are intended to guide the nurse leader in achieving a diverse workforce by becoming an advocate for resources to implement and support a diversity program, encouraging a commitment to education, and leading diversity research initiatives that are based on performance improvement outcomes.

**Health care organizations will strive to develop internal and external resources to meet the needs of the diverse patient and workforce populations served.**

1. Designate fiscal resources to develop programs and policies to meet the needs of diverse patient populations served.
2. Establish system processes to ensure the needs of all patient populations are met. Include members from the local community with diverse backgrounds in organizational planning processes.
3. Educate the community on the importance of collecting data, including patient and workforce race, ethnicity and primary language spoken, for use in improving patient safety and quality.
4. Develop processes and policies to ensure that non-English speaking and limited English proficiency patients will be assured of access to interpretive services and written translated patient education materials and documents.
5. Implement processes to promote both the consistency of quality of care across various patient populations and a balance in demographics between the patient and the workforce populations.

6. Execute employment recruitment plans and strategies to attract a workforce that is reflective of the populations served.
7. Train staff members in the importance of understanding the diversity of the patient population served and provision of culturally competent care.
8. Support staff members in obtaining training and education in health care interpretation.

**Health care organizations will aim to establish a healthful practice/work environment that is reflective of diversity through a commitment to inclusivity, tolerance, and governance structures.**

1. Encourage the employment of diverse groups of health care professionals. Actively involve all people in a shared decision-making process, when appropriate.
2. Aim to establish a diverse healthful practice/work environment at all levels, including leadership and governance teams.
3. Celebrate the diversity of talent as a source of strength, pride, and team spirit throughout the organization.
4. Emphasize the promotion, recognition, and acceptance of diversity by all staff members in a nonbiased and sensitive manner.
5. Facilitate the creation of a work environment that is conducive to open communication, flexibility, and acceptance of differences.
6. Lead staff members without stereotypes or assumptions and with sensitivity to their gender, race/ethnicity, knowledge, skills, cultural backgrounds, values, and beliefs.
7. Establish metrics to monitor targeted diversity benchmarks.

| BOX 8-1 | AONE GUIDING PRINCIPLES FOR DIVERSITY IN HEALTH CARE ORGANIZATIONS (CONTINUED) |
| --- | --- |

**Health care organizations will partner with universities, schools of nursing, and other organizations that train health care workers to support development and implementation of policies, procedures, programs, and learning environments that foster recruitment and retention of a student population that reflects the diversity of the United States.**

1. Encourage use of admission criteria that focus on both qualitative and quantitative data.
2. Recognize and appreciate the social and cultural barriers to college attendance that may exist for students from diverse population groups.
3. Enter into collaborative agreements between education and practice that offer nursing staff from diverse groups the opportunity to serve as student mentors, guest lecturers, participants in school-based health centers, and/or clinical faculty.
4. Encourage and support graduate education for nurses from diverse populations in order to build a more diverse pool of nurse leaders including nursing faculty.
5. Develop and implement career plans for potential candidates for nursing careers from current employees with an emphasis on those from nonmajority groups.
6. Create and support community outreach programs such as "shadow a nurse day," health care career fairs, and high school tutoring programs for targeted cultural groups in collaboration with members of the local community.
7. Create a clinical rotation environment that supports a diverse nursing student body and learning styles.

**Health care organizations will collect and disseminate diversity related resources and information.**

1. Utilize technology to heighten awareness and share information and resources related to diversity.

2. Collect data (including, but not limited to, race and primary language spoken) as a part of routine patient registration processes and human resources management programs in order to better document and reflect the components of the patient and workforce populations.
3. Establish formal policies and procedures to reflect these data collections.
4. Support health care information technology (IT) systems that enhance the collection of diverse patient and workforce demographic data.
5. Provide education to all staff regarding the relevance and value of collecting patient and workforce data including race, ethnicity, and primary language spoken.
6. Train staff on effective strategies and appropriate mechanisms for obtaining these data elements.
7. Inform communities why it is necessary for health care organizations to collect patient and workforce race, ethnicity, and primary language data.
8. Routinely review quality and utilization data by race, ethnicity, and primary language of patients to eliminate potential inconsistency in quality of care across various patient populations and to balance patient population demographics and the workforce population.
9. Utilize data to develop action plans toward improving the state of diversity in the workplace.
10. Conduct research to measure the effectiveness of improvement plans.
11. Review evidence-based practice related to diversity and incorporate "best practices" into the organizations' own settings.

Source: The American Organization of Nurse Executives (2007). Reprinted with Permission.

How do these demographic facts affect the health care delivery system? There will be new demands to provide more culturally appropriate health care. This means more than language competency, which is highly problematic in many areas and for individual health care organizations that must provide interpreters when needed. Where to find this resource and the cost factors are major problems. There are, however, other considerations. These are as follows:

- The effects of lifestyle and cultural differences on health status
- The implications of the diverse genetic endowment of the population

- The impact of patterns of assimilation on health status
- Underdiagnosis and treatment differences among minority groups (The Institute for the Future, 2000, p. 20)

The last issue of differences in health care quality for minority Americans was addressed in a report, *Diverse Communities, Common Concerns: Assessing Health Care Quality for Minority Americans* (Collins et al., 2002). It identifies "three factors in ensuring that minority populations receive optimal medical care: effective patient–physician communication, overcoming cultural and linguistic barriers, and access to affordable health insurance" (p. 6). Minority groups are the primary groups that have been affected by uninsurance, underinsurance, and limited access to providers in many communities. Migrant health care is also a critical issue in many areas—and a complex one. The State Children's Health Insurance (SCHIP) program established by President Clinton to increase the number of children with health insurance coverage has made an important impact on these disparity problems, but there have been problems with it, too. The money is there for the coverage; however, many states struggled with getting families to register for it. One barrier is families who are concerned about sharing information required for registration, such as illegal aliens. Additionally, in some states the process is complex. Language and culture also affect willingness to share information. Fear of government intervention(s) is a concern with some groups. Many states have been successful in addressing some of these critical barriers, and others have been less successful. President Obama signed a law renewing and expanding SCHIP. Programs that assist multicultural populations need to consider these concerns as they can act as barriers to success.

Another aspect of a diverse health care system is staff education about other cultures. How should this be done to ensure that staff have the needed information and apply it? More of this content is included in nursing education today. This, however, does not get to staff that has practiced for a time and yet still need updates. The Mayo Clinic developed a transcultural patient care website to assist its staff, which is an effective method to provide easy, quick access to staff members for information when they need it (De Ruiter & Larsen, 2002). This site is available to staff 24/7, whenever the information is needed, and includes information related to the following categories.

- Information about countries, ethnic groups, religious groups, and special populations
- Communicating with the non-English-speaking patient/family
- Cultural assessment guide
- Nutritional assessment tool/resources
- Patient education database
- Departmental information
- Classes on a variety of diversity issues
- Internet transcultural websites

This type of resource would be helpful for any health care organization that has a diverse patient and/or staff population. Obviously, the Mayo Clinic site is for its staff; however, that does not exclude other organizations from developing their own sites that can serve as useful resources for staff with easy, quick access when information is required.

## Health Care Disparities

The Institute of Medicine report, *Unequal Treatment* (2002b), opened up an area of major concern for health care delivery by identifying that there are problems in the health care system with bias, prejudice, and stereotyping issues. The report recommended that the U.S. needed to monitor the problem routinely. Health care disparities occur consistently, which is a difficult fact for health care professionals to accept. "Discourse on provider bias has been silent in health care literature. Medicine and nursing as predominantly white professions have failed to acknowledge the White domination inherent in and perpetuated by its research, clinical, and educational practices" (Baldwin, 2003, p. 8). Health care organizations must deal with this issue daily. The Sullivan Commission report (2004) also supports this concern by commenting on the disparity in the health care workforce as a major contributor to the health care delivery disparity problem. The report recommends an increase in minority representation in health care professions. Additional comments about workforce issues are found later in this chapter.

What are health care disparities? The American Association of Colleges of Nursing summarizes some key definitions: "**Health disparities** are differences in the incidence, prevalence, mortality, and burden of disease and other adverse health conditions that exist among specific population groups in the United States (NIH, 2002–2006). The definition of health disparities assumes not only a difference in health but a difference in which disadvantaged social groups—who have persistently experienced social disadvantage or discrimination—systematically experience worse health or greater health risks than more advantaged social groups (Braveman, 2006). Consideration of who is considered to be within a health-disparity population has policy and resource implications. The IOM defines health care disparity as a difference in treatment provided to members of different racial (or ethnic) groups that is not justified by the underlying health conditions or treatment preferences of patients (1OM, 2002b). These differences are often attributed to conscious or unconscious bias, provider bias, and institutional discriminatory policies toward patients of diverse socioeconomic status, race, ethnicity, and/or gender orientation (Finkelman & Kenner, 2009). The reasons for disparities are varied and can be a "function of the overall performance of the health system where one lives or of the quality of providers that care for many minorities" (Mead, Cartwirght-Smith, Jones, Ramos, & Woods, 2008, p. 1).

Health care disparities also have an impact on emergency care. The most common response to the problem of overburdened Emergency Departments is the uninsured abuse the emergency system; however, this is not necessarily the case. Minority patients typically do not come to ED for minor illnesses. This is done more by the insured using the ED for minor illnesses (Carmicahel, 2008). The disparity issues that are found are barriers to effective communication such as the lack of interpreters. Safety net hospitals struggle the most as they often do not have the economic resources to provide quality care and many of their patient populations are diverse with complex medical, sociological, economic, and psychological needs (Werner, Goldman, & Dudley, 2008). These hospitals care for the majority of the Medicaid patients and the uninsured.

The annual National Health Care Disparities Report (NHDR) provides extensive data on the status of health care disparities (see link to report in chapter Media Links). The IOM recommendations include the following (IOM, 2002, p. 7):

- Analyze racial and ethnic disparities, considering socioeconomic status.
- Conduct research to determine how to best measure socioeconomic status as it relates to health care access, service utilization, and quality.
- Recognize that access is a critical element of health care quality.
- Measure high and low utilization of certain health care services; include data state by state.
- Work with public and private organizations that provide data to increase standardization.
- Provide Agency for Healthcare Research and Quality (AHRQ) with resources to compile an annual survey of disparity in health care.

The health care disparities monitoring matrix developed by the IOM for the National Healthcare Disparities Report (NHDR) is used as the guide for data collection and analysis. *Equality* is the absence of disparities. *Disparity* is less evidence-based care for racial and ethnic minorities that provided for the majorities. *Hyperdisparity* is care that is disproportionately provided to racial and ethnic minorities from lack of care to poor prior care. This annual national report includes data about racial, ethnic, socioeconomic, and geographic disparities in health care. Quality of health care includes effectiveness, patient safety, timeliness, and patient centeredness. Access to care covers facilitators and barriers and health care utilization. The report also focuses on priority populations: racial and ethnic minorities, low-income groups, women, children, older adults, residents of rural areas, and individuals with disabilities and special health care needs. The most current report (2008) identified three key themes:

- Disparities persist in health care quality and access.
- Magnitude and pattern of disparities are different within subpopulations.
- Some disparities exist across multiple priority populations.

Health care organizations can use the data in the annual NHDR to identify current national disparities problems and then compare with their own disparity issues. The NHDR is correlated to the National Healthcare Quality Report recommended by the IOM. (See Chapter 16.) The web link to access the most current NHDR is found in the end of chapter Medial Links. Figure 8-1 describes the matrix.

**FIGURE 8-1   Matrix for the Annual National Healthcare Disparities Report.**

| Consumer Perspectives on Healthcare Needs | Continuum of Disparities | | |
|---|---|---|---|
| | Healthcare Equalities | Healthcare Disparities | Healthcare Hyperdisparities |
| Staying Health | | | |
| Getting Better | | | |
| Living with Illness or Disability | | | |
| Coping with the End-of-Life | | | |

Source: Institute of Medicine. (IOM). (2002). *Guidance for the National Healthcare Disparities Report.* Washington, DC: National Academies Press, p. 86. Reprinted with permission.

As a follow-up to the IOM work on health disparities, the National Quality Forum (NQF) announced in 2009 that it was endorsing guidelines to reduce health disparities and make care patient-centered and culturally appropriate. NQF emphasizes that we cannot use "one size fits all" approach to this problem.

## APPLYING EVIDENCE-BASED PRACTICE

### Evidence for Effective Leadership and Management

**Citation:**   Chin, M., Walters, A., Cook, S. & Huang, E. (2007). Review of interventions to reduce racial and ethnic disparities in health care. *Medical Care Research and Review, 64,* October, 29S–100S.

**Overview:**   This systematic review of more than 200 published articles addresses the question: What actually works for reducing racial and ethnic disparities in health care? The review focused on care for patients with cardiovascular disease, diabetes, depression, and breast cancer and disparities. The conclusions indicate that the following strategies are often part of successful interventions: multifaceted programs that include providers, patients, and the community; a focus on cultural relevancy or culturally tailored interventions to ensure that the patient's culture is included; and nurse-led programs.

**Application:**   As has been discussed in this chapter and by the Institute of Medicine reports on diversity, there is a major problem with health disparities. Much more needs to be known about the impact of culture on care and what interventions can be more effective. What needs to be considered to redesign interventions so that they include cultural issues? Cultural leverage is identified by this study as very relevant to care delivery. This is "a focused strategy for improving the health of racial and ethnic communities by using their cultural practices, products, philosophies, or environments as vehicles that facilitate behavior change of patients and practitioners. Building upon prior strategies, cultural leverage proactively identifies the areas in which a cultural intervention can improve behaviors and then actively implements the solution" (Fisher et al., 2007: 245S).

Source: Fisher, T., Burnet, D., Huang, E., Chin, M., & Cagney, K. (2007). Cultural leverage: interventions using culture to narrow racial disparities in health care. *Medical Care Research and Review, 64* (5 Suppl.), 243S–282S.

Questions:

1. *What is your opinion of "cultural leverage"?*
2. *What has been your experience with the impact of culture on patient care?*
3. *Why do you think nurse-led programs are considered successful strategies?*

## Health Literacy

**Health literacy** is "the ability to read, understand, and act on health care information" (Institute of Medicine, 2004, p. 52). This impacts patient–provider communication, both verbal and written communication. Health care organizations (HCOs) need to carefully review forms and information given to patients to ensure that the content is understandable and to check with patients and families to confirm that they understand the information. Vulnerable populations are more at risk for health care literacy problems; however, staff needs to be alert to this potential problem with all patients. The major barriers to quality health care associated with health literacy are inabilities to access care, manage illness, and process information (DeWalt & Pignone, 2008).

1. *Accessing care:*   Critical issues are obtaining health insurance, finding health care providers, and knowing when to seek health care (for example, making an appointment, finding the number, and keeping a record of the appointment may all be difficult for someone who cannot read).
2. *Illness management:*   Managing illness today, both acute and chronic illness, can be complex with complicated prescription recommendations, testing schedules, and appointments at different providers; patients need to know the right questions to ask as information is often not freely shared. Health care transitions are very common; patients move from provider to provider even within the same health care organization, increasing the risk of errors but also requiring that the patient adapt to changes and new providers.
3. *General information processing:*   Patients are presented with informed consents and other documents, often written in a manner that they cannot understand, especially under stressful situations. Family members can be very helpful with this type of information. Medical bills can easily overwhelm even someone who reads English well, and for those who do not, this inability to read bills can lead to major problems and stress.

What impact does health literacy have on care? A review of 44 studies examining the relationship between health literacy and adherence to clinical outcomes indicated the following (DeWalt, Berkman, Sheridan, Lohr, & Pignone, 2004):

- People who have low literacy are 1.5 to 3 times more likely to have adverse outcomes than those with higher literacy.
- Medicare enrollees with lower literacy have a greater chance of never having a Pap smear, not having a mammogram within the past two years, and not receiving influenza and pneumococcal immunization than those with higher health literacy.
- Lower literacy is associated with increase risk for hospitalization.

These outcomes are important and indicate the negative impact of health literacy on health care. The Joint Commission identifies the following as strategies to decrease problems with health care literacy, all of which are related to nursing practice (Joint Commission, 2007, p. 5).

- Create patient-centered environments where the patient is involved in decision-making and safety processes.
- Increase awareness and understanding of health literacy.
- Ensure that interpreters are available when needed.
- Develop cultural competence.
- Understand how communication affects quality care.
- Teach consumers how to better access the care that they need.
- Review and improve informed consent materials and processes.
- Utilize a disease management approach to better individualize care and reduce errors.
- Standardize handouts.
- Give patients clear information.

Recognizing the importance of culture to each patient and family is the first step. Then it is important to incorporate cultural competency into health care education and practice to decrease health disparities and improve care for all. Connected to all of this is the health care organization. The organization has its own culture that then interacts with the diversity in its patients and also its workforce diversity.

# Culture and Climate: Building Organizational Cultural Competency

What is it that makes an organization feel like a comfortable place to work or receive services? How is an organization described? How do individual staff members affect an organization's culture? Understanding this part of an organization is not easy. It is even harder to change an organization's culture. For an organization to build its cultural competency, it must first understand what **organizational culture** is and then assess its present culture. Is it a **consonant** (functional, effective) culture or a **dissonant** (dysfunctional or ineffective) culture? The goal is to be an effective culture. As this process occurs, there are legal issues that also need to be considered related to the organization's culture. Staff, of course, plays a key role in the organization's culture. This section of the chapter discusses these critical issues.

What competencies are needed to develop a culturally competent organization? Four primary skills are needed for the culture competencies:

- Human resource diversity planning: translates diversity requirements from strategic and business planning into specific human resource recruitment and retention practices.
- Development of diverse work teams focuses on job design, work structures and processes, and how the organization enables, integrates, and supports diversity so that high performance can be achieved.
- Diversity education, training, and development address how the organization develops employees regarding diversity awareness, biases, and skills building. The approach to reinforcing, evaluating, and improving employees; performance related to diversity is also examined.
- Development of a respectful work environment focuses on how the organization creates, maintains, and improves the work environment and work climate that is conducive to the well-being and development of all employees (Frusti, Niesen, & Campion, 2003, p. 33).

This approach views diversity development from four key perspectives. It is not simple to address diversity issues in a health care organization when the organization as a whole and all its component parts need to be considered: staff, patients, and families. The community in which the organization exists is also an important factor that impacts organization culture.

## Definition of Organizational Culture and Climate

In the late 1920s and early 1930s, a study conducted at an electric company focused on employee performance, productivity, and motivation (Milgram, Spector, & Treger, 1999). Why would this study be important to the topic of organizational culture today? The results of this study identified a phenomenon, which became known as the Hawthorne Effect. During the study environmental factors such as light and noise were altered, and productivity was monitored. Changes in the environment affected productivity. The study also noted that when employees participated in decisions their job satisfaction increased. In the long term these particular experiments have been questioned; however, they did begin the process of increased interest in productivity, work environment, and job satisfaction factors, which are related to an organization's culture.

This interest in the culture of organizations has grown in all types of businesses including health care. Curtin (2001), a nursing leader, has written about this very important issue. "There is in each institution an implicit, invisible, intrinsic, informal, and yet instantly recognizable *welenschaung* [sic] that is best described as 'corporate culture.' Like most important things, it is difficult to define or even describe. It is not 'corporate climate,' 'organizational climate,' or 'corporate identity.' The corporate culture embodies the organizational values that implicitly and explicitly specify norms, shape attitudes, and guide the behaviors of the members of the organization" (Curtin, 2001, p. 219). Health care organizational culture is more complex than culture found in other businesses as it also includes professional culture due to the presence of health care professionals. Professional culture focuses on highly skilled individuals who are members of a profession and their performance of skilled tasks, whereas bureaucratic culture focuses more on defining "discrete roles carefully and specific role rights and obligations clearly" (Curtin, 2001, p. 220). Health care organizations have struggled to develop their own cultures, blending the typical organizational culture factors with the professional culture factors. The result is often "a dysfunctional production-oriented overlay to their traditional bureaucratic-professional culture" (Curtin, 2001, p. 220). This culture is discussed in this chapter and has been reflected on throughout this text. The Institute of Medicine also describes the health care delivery system as dysfunctional (Institute of Medicine, 2001). Schein (2004) defines the **culture** of a group as "a pattern of shared basic assumptions that was learned by a group as it solved its problems of external adaptation and internal integration, that has worked well enough to be considered valid and, therefore, to be taught to new members as the correct way to perceive, think, and feel in relation to those problems" (p. 17). The organization's culture is passed on to new members through the process of socialization. Schein identifies three levels of organizational culture. The *artifacts* are the visible structures and processes. The *espoused beliefs and values* are found in the vision, mission, goals, and strategic plans. The *underlying assumptions* are the taken-for-granted beliefs and perceptions.

## Consonant and Dissonant Organizational Cultures

If an organization ignores its culture, this can lead to major problems for the organization. To prevent this, leaders within the organization must recognize the importance of culture to the organization and work toward developing a consonant or an effective organizational culture. This culture includes shared **values**, which are the important concerns and goals shared by most of the people in the organization, and group behavior norms, which are the most common ways of acting within the group in the organization (Jones & Redman, 2000). New people come into the organization and learn about the culture by making a connection between behaviors and their consequences. An adaptive organizational culture is able to meet the challenge of change to become more effective and meet their outcomes. Rigid organizational cultures are not able to do this and become a dissonant or ineffective organizational culture.

Values have a major effect on organizations and provide direction for organizations, which can be demonstrated in staff loyalty and commitment to the organization. "Values encompass the abstract of what is right, worthwhile, or desirable" (McNeese-Smith & Crook, 2003, p. 261). They influence when decisions and judgments are made. Do values always mesh? No, they do not, and when they do not, problems often arise. "Lack of congruency between a nurse's personal values and those of the organization decrease satisfaction and effectiveness and may lead to burnout and turnover" (McNeese-Smith & Crook, 2003, p. 260). There is no doubt that there are major problems with burnout and turnover in health care delivery systems today. As these health care organizations struggle to understand these issues and resolve them, gaining a better understanding of the status of the culture—whether it is dissonant or consonant—may help. It is initially important to identify what is a dysfunctional or dissonant culture. Sovie (1993) identified characteristics of dysfunctional or dissonant hospital cultures. These included the following:

- Organized to serve the providers and not the patients
- Unclear about individual and department expectations
- Do not regularly measure quality of service
- Lack of patient involvement in decision-making
- Limited concern about employee satisfaction
- Limited educational/training programs for employees
- Frequent turf battles
- Do not recognize staff accomplishments (as cited in Jones & Redman, 2000, p. 605)

Characteristics such as these can be used to assess the status of an organization's culture. These characteristics have been discussed in earlier information about leadership and management styles; these styles are directly related to organizational culture.

Today, some health care organizations are experiencing an evolving culture of oppression, which affects organizational culture. One reason this has happened is the limited input that staff nurses have in decisions about nursing practice. Certainly retention and recruitment problems have made this problem worse. Along with these problems, the loss of trust in people and systems has become a critical problem (Aiken et al., 2001). Nurse leaders are needed to resolve this loss of trust. "Trust involves a risk of one person approaching another in the hope of a response. Trust is a central aspect of human existence and within a trusting relationship we care for the lives of others" (Ray, Turkel, & Marino, 2002, p. 1). Making ethical choices is also related to trust. Without trust, there can be no security, no cooperation, no communication, no community, and ultimately no business (Cuilla, 2000). The health care workplace appears to be out of sync—something is missing (Parker & Gadbois, 2000). This missing piece may be the need for more community in the workplace—a place where the staff is valued and trust is present. There is also a need to decrease mechanized practice and make practice more human and caring. This is difficult to accomplish when the environment is struggling with staff shortages, stress, rapid change, and organizations that frequently have dissonant cultures.

## An Effective, Creative, and Productive Workplace

The organization's culture identifies the acceptable attitudes and values within the organization. Formal and informal frameworks define the culture (Milgram, Spector, & Treger, 1999). The formal framework includes the organization's structure, chain of command, and rules and regulations. The informal framework includes use of open-door policies, accessibility of management, dress codes, special events and rituals, and standard manners of speech and behavior. Both frameworks are important and interrelated.

Some health care organizations are more driven by financial issues, and in other organizations staff interpret that this is the case when it may not actually be true. Both perspectives affect the organization's culture. Why is this the case? Many health care professionals feel a real conflict in their work environment. They want to advocate for the patient and yet they feel extreme stress at work, which makes it difficult to provide the required care. While blaming administration for real and unreal problems, perceptions can become part of an organization's culture, making it an ineffective culture. Organizational caring has been studied within the hospital organizational culture. The bureaucratic caring theory focuses on the complex nature of the meaning of caring and how health care staff members implement caring in their practice (Ray, Turkel, & Marino, 2002). Developing an environment of caring must come from leadership so that it is part of the entire organizational environment. "Caring, financial and managerial knowledge, and ethics are integrated by leaders who will create a work environment that encourages autonomy and creativity and where organizational caring is supported by structures and systems devised in the organization" (Ray, Turkel, & Marino, 2002, p. 5). Transformational leadership supports this type of environment.

Ray, Turkel, and Marino (2002) also investigated the loss of trust, as well as decreased loyalty to employers (hospitals) and the disillusionment of nurses. The study included 46 hospitals, one military hospital, and three civilian not-for-profit health care systems, involving 32 registered nurses and 14 top-level administrators. Semi-structured, 30- to 60-minute participant interviews were used to collect data. The results indicated that the nurses felt administration's decision making centered only on financial issues, which is a common theme heard when nurses discuss organizational culture. Some nurses were concerned about the loss of supplies or running out of supplies, which interfered with their practice. Others noted that administrators made comments about nurses not making the hospital money, but the nurses acknowledged that without nurses there would be no hospital care. The nurses were also concerned about hospitals not covering the cost for people who did not have insurance. They were disillusioned with nursing practice as well as with the impact of the work environment on the nurse–patient relationship. They commented that they were not able to connect with their patients in the best ways possible. Nurses wanted to feel respected and valued as professionals in the organization, but they did not. They felt that improved communication at all levels in the organization was a key strategy for rebuilding trust. Nurses needed to know what was going on when decisions were made. Other nurses complained about the lack of visibility of administrators, which decreased trust. Administrators agreed that visibility was important, but they were too busy with work, which kept them from the clinical areas. Nurses wanted to be seen as equal partners without fear that they would lose their position or be labeled as troublemakers if they made complaints or voiced their opinions about decisions. Participative decision making is critical to autonomy, which allows the nurses to make more decisions about what they can do and cannot do. This was another important way for administration to demonstrate trust in staff. Nurses wanted to feel empowered, but instead they felt that they had little voice in decision making. What is really described in the results of this study is the organization's culture. Culture involves key factors that affect how people work together, pleasure or dissatisfaction in work, and understanding how these factors interact within an organization is important.

The Competing Values Framework is a method that can be used to define an organization's culture. This framework includes four orientations (Cameron & Quinn, 1994; Jones & Redman, 2000).

1. **Group/clan orientation** in which the organization focuses on concern for people and sensitivity to customers. This type of organization has a friendly work environment that emphasizes loyalty, high cohesion, and tradition. The leader(s) emphasizes teamwork and consensus building.
2. **Developmental/"adhocracy orientation"** is a type of organization in which the focus is on innovation and individual initiative and freedom. This is a dynamic and creative environment with many entrepreneurs. Risk-taking is highly valued.
3. **Irrational/market orientation** focuses on getting the job done with positive results. In this organization the staff is competitive and goal-oriented.
4. **Hierarchy orientation** is a formalized structure organization. The focus here is on procedures and not on people. Efficiency is most important with staff following the rules.

Jones and Redman (2000) have applied these four cultural orientations to two dimensions: (a) flexibility versus control and (b) internal versus external. Considering these two dimensions, how do the four orientations apply? Clan and adhocracy cultural orientations would be placed in the flexibility dimension while market and hierarchy orientations would be placed in the control dimension. Clan and hierarchy orientations also focus on internal processes while adhocracy and market orientations focus on external challenges. Box 8-2 provides a summary of this view of organizational culture.

Strategies have been developed to assist organizations to change their orientation and culture. In today's health care environment, most health care organizations recognize the need to be more flexible and to respond more to both external and internal factors, not just one. These organizations then need to change their orientations to accomplish this effectively. They should promote adhocracy and clan values and decrease hierarchy and market values. The study discussed earlier conducted by Ray, Turkel, and Marino (2002) highlighted nurses' concerns about organizations that focus on financial factors over and above other critical issues. This overemphasis on market values suggests the organization would need to change its focus to other goals and emphasize quality. Examples of strategies that might be used to promote group/clan values would be to survey staff members about their needs and ideas, improve team-building skills, and improve employee recognition programs.

■ To promote developmental/adhocracy values, the organization might encourage and reward innovative ideas and develop an effective continuous quality improvement program.
■ To reduce hierarchy values, the organization would need to eliminate ineffective policies and procedures and decrease micromanagement.

Many HCOs have incorporated a shared governance model to improve organizational culture, as discussed in Chapter 4. An organization's culture can be changed, but it takes leadership and a planned effort to accomplish this change. The first step should be to assess the culture.

| BOX 8-2 | COMPELLING VALUES FRAMEWORK: ONE APPROACH TO ORGANIZATIONAL CULTURE |
| --- | --- |

| Flexibility | vs. | Control Dimension | Internal | vs. | External Dimension |
| --- | --- | --- | --- | --- | --- |
| Team/Clan Orientation | | Market Orientation | Team/Clan Orientation | | Adhocracy Orientation |
| Adhocracy Orientation | | Hierarchy Orientation | Hierarchy Orientation | | Market Orientation |

## Assessment of Organizational Culture

A place to begin the assessment is to consider the many factors within the organization that have an impact on the organizational culture. These factors include the following:

- Structure and process
- Communication, both formal and informal (e.g., use of memos, e-mail, effect of gossip, accessibility of information, secrecy, how soon does staff know about changes, how effective is its communication, information overload, grapevine, and so on)
- Acceptance of new members/staff
- Willingness to allow new members to offer suggestions or new ideas
- Management's willingness to include staff in change process
- Management and staff morale
- Staff turnover rate
- Staff vacancy rate
- Feedback (staff, patients, families)
- Reputation in the community

The organization's vision, mission statement, goals, and strategic plans reveal important information about the organization and how the organization views itself and its staff; however, these documents may be just more paper to put into binders. The key is to decide if what is written in these documents is actually demonstrated in behavior and communication. Organizations with a consonant culture emphasize the sum of their parts rather than their many separate parts. An organization that is tied up in focusing on its parts and has problems with viewing itself as a whole would have a dissonant culture. It will feel out of sync. From a systems perspective, the organization will not be as effective as it could be. Some aspects of an organization are helpful in describing and understanding the organizational culture. These are the cultural artifacts, which are "the obvious signs and symbols of corporate culture, such as written rules, office layouts, organizational structure, and dress codes" (Dessler, 2002, p. 54). Patterns of behavior can be used to identify traditions, written and verbal comments, and staff behaviors. The values and beliefs are a critical part of the culture. "Stories illustrating important company values are also widely used to reinforce the firm's culture" (Dessler, 2002, p. 55). Managers, team leaders, and preceptors play an important role in clarifying expectations about organization values to the staff and to the students, but to do this effectively they need to understand the culture.

Curtin (2001) comments on some key terms often mentioned when discussing organization culture. Staff members, of course, have personal values, and as they interact and function in their positions within organizations, *role-related values* are developed when personal values are shared with others within the culture. *Attitudes* are also important, but what does this mean? Attitudes are formed when staff applies values to real situations. *Institutional values* are critical in understanding organizational structure, and these are developed "over time and reflect shared beliefs about desirable rules of conduct and desirable states of existence" (Curtin, 2001, p. 219). The greater the consistency between the staff values and values of the organization and its managers, the better the organization will function.

## CASE STUDY

### What Is It with This Place?

Tom has been working in the local acute care hospital for about 10 years. The hospital has grown from a 150-bed facility to a 200-bed facility in that time, but recently there have been comments made about cutting some beds due to a lower census. He works on a cardiac unit as one of the team leaders. Sue graduated from nursing school 2 years ago and has recently joined the staff. This is her second position since graduation. After working on the unit for 3 months, Sue comes to Tom and says, "What is it with this place?" He is confused and asks what she means. Her response is spoken with much emotion, "People here don't seem to care about one another. I don't trust anyone I work with, do you?" He responded, "Sure I do. Seems like a comfortable place to me. Just go with the flow, and you will be fine." Sue ponders this but still struggles. Another new nurse begins to work on the unit. This nurse has 5 years experience and recently moved from out-of-state. A few weeks after her arrival she and Sue have lunch together. The new nurse tells Sue that she is discouraged. She has always liked working and now dreads coming in. "I just don't feel that staff is connected here. No one really talks to one another. I don't even think that staff members have any pride in their work." Sue connects with these comments and discusses how she has felt. It is great to have someone who understands, but she wishes that staff that has been working on the unit longer would be more helpful and connect to these concerns.

### Questions:

1. Why do you think Tom responded in the way he did?
2. How would you describe the culture of this organization?
3. Do you think that the culture that is described applies to the specific unit or the entire organization? What would you base your answer on?
4. Is this a consonant or dissonant culture, and what is your rationale?
5. What possible effects can an organization's culture have on patient care delivery?
6. If you were either of the new nurses, what would you do?

# Workforce Diversity

The people within an organization—its staff, patients, and families that receive the health care services—affect an organization's culture and how the staff responds to the diverse patient population that exists in the health care system today. "**Workforce diversity** refers to the mix of people from varied backgrounds in the labor pool" (Shea-Lewis, 2002, p. 6). The critical federal regulations and state labor laws that affect workforce diversity are Title VII of the Civil Rights Act of 1964 and Executive Order 11246, which prohibits employer discrimination on the basis of race, color, religion, sex or national origin, and the American Disability Act of 1990. It should be noted that since most health care organizations receive reimbursement from Medicare, which is a federal payment system, and Medicaid, which is a joint federal and state reimbursement system, most health care organizations must meet the requirements of these laws and regulations. This means that staff must be prepared with education and training for work in a culturally diverse environment. As noted in earlier comments about the Sullivan Commission report, diversity within the workforce must also be improved within health care organizations. It is necessary to evaluate the effectiveness of diversity education programs to improve a culturally diverse work setting. "Workforce diversity in health services organizations is of extreme importance. Diversity provides a more comprehensive range of knowledge and abilities. Diversity allows for better decision making based on different life experiences and perspectives. A diverse workforce can better provide health services to diverse populations" (Shea-Lewis, 2002, p. 6). There is an ongoing problem with diversity within the profession of nursing. Efforts have been made to improve this. Workforce data from 2008 indicates a positive change in RN diversity: "White, non-Hispanics (65.6 percent of U.S. population) comprise 83.2 percent of licensed RNs, a decrease since 2004, when 87.5 percent of RNs were white. Asian, Native Hawaiian and Pacific Islanders (non-Hispanic) are the next largest group at 5.8 percent (4.5 percent of U.S. population). African Americans (non-Hispanic) are 5.4 percent of RNs (12.2 percent of U.S. population) and Hispanics/Latinos of any race are 3.6 percent of RNs (15.4 percent of U.S. population). Women outnumber men by more than 15 to 1 in the overall number of RNs, but among only those who became RNs after 1990, there is one male RN for every 10 women" (Health Resources and Services Administration, 2010).

Cultural barriers for staff and patients within the organization must be assessed and resolved. Language barriers are particularly important as noted by the IOM and its comments about health literacy. This, of course, includes availability of interpreters when they are needed to assist staff. Family members are not the best choice for interpreters; they are too personally involved, and their culture may affect how and what they translate. For example, in some cultures the husband is the decision maker and the wife simply agrees. In this situation, if the husband interprets for his wife (the patient), the husband's attitude would probably limit the wife's participation. Another issue with language is the health care provider needs to be in control of the conversation, and this is difficult to accomplish when staff does not know the language (Griffin, 2002). Patients from different cultures need time to understand what is said and what it means, and they will also process the communication through their own cultural filter. Cultural filters are the way that individuals perceive the world and their experiences. These filters are created and adopted by members of a culture. For example, how a person communicates, verbally, nonverbally, and behaviorally, goes through this filter. If staff members are not sensitive and aware of culture and do not have knowledge of other cultures, they may misinterpret words and behaviors. This filter also affects how people define health and illness, whether or not they seek care, from whom they seek care, and their attitudes about the quality of their lives.

Organizational culture includes how staff responds to persons with disabilities as employees. Laws dictate some of this response. The American Disability Act (ADA) of 1990, which became effective in 1992, has had a major impact on health care workforce issues (Sullivan & Decker, 2001). This law makes it illegal for employers to discriminate against persons with disabilities in employment, and provides for enforcement of equal access to jobs and accommodations. Employers of 15 or more are affected by this law, which certainly includes most health care organizations. How is a disability defined in the law? A disability is (a) a physical or mental impairment that substantially limits one or more of the major life activities of such individuals, (b) a record of such impairment, and (c) being regarded as having such impairment. Examples of disabilities that would apply to the health care workforce include the following: emotional or mental illness, alcoholism/drug abuse (person would need to be participating in a supervised rehabilitation program), multiple sclerosis, HIV infection/AIDS, cancer, diabetes, heart disease, orthopedic impairments, hearing/vision/speech impairments, communication disorders, and learning disabilities (Sullivan & Decker, 2001). The law does more than prohibit discrimination. It also requires reasonable accommodation, which means that efforts must be made to provide leaves of absence with or without pay, job reassignment, or job restructuring. In addition, this law affects the hiring process. A qualified person is a person who can perform the essential job functions, with or without reasonable accommodation. During the process questions about general medical conditions, state of health, specific diseases, or nature/severity of disability cannot be asked. The focus must be on whether or not the person meets essential job functions. It is thus critical that employers clearly define essential job functions, which should be based on the employer's judgment, the job description, and the amount of time spent performing the given function (Guido, 2001). The presence or lack of an atmosphere of acceptance is an important factor in an organization's culture.

## The Staff and Its Culture

Health care staff affects an organization's culture and is also affected by the culture. The staff brings its own personal culture into the organization; in addition, the staff represents several generations, which has a major impact on the organizational culture. Staff members and their personal cultures represent a critical component of building cultural competency in an organization. Many organizations now have required staff education about culture. Despite these efforts there continue to be health care disparities. The Media Link section, at the end of the chapter, provides some links to this type of information and related staff training.

## Management and a Culturally Diverse Staff

Managers need to understand the impact of cultures on the organization, the daily work, and the staff, and know how to use cross-cultural management. This requires an open mind and understanding. Acceptance of others who may be different is critical, as is encouragement of staff members to share their feelings and reactions appropriately. Staff members need to be appreciated for their individual strengths. The focus is on differences, not on right and wrong.

There has been an increase in nurses from other countries who have come to work in the United States due to the nursing shortage, and there is also a more diverse physician pool today. The common reasons for this migration are differences in income, job satisfaction, organizational environment, governance, protection and risk, and social security and benefits (International Council of Nurses, 2010). In 2008 the U.S. implemented the Voluntary Code of Conduct for the Ethical Recruitment of Foreign-Educated Nurses to the U.S. through the Alliance for Ethical International Recruitment Practices with the goal of increasing transparency and accountability. Those who participate must agree to monitoring through surveys, including surveying of nurses coming to the U.S., to identify issues and problems (International Council of Nurses, 2010).

Diversity, however, is not just found in staff that comes from other countries for short periods of employment. There are many staff members from other cultural backgrounds who have lived in the U.S. for some time or were born in the United States though they are members of minority cultures. The multicultural work environment means that nurse leaders must consider its impact on productivity, recruitment, and retention. This requires an awareness of cross-cultural issues. Staff members may respond to other staff and patients from cultures different from their own in ways that may be ineffective. This must be addressed in order to build cultural competency.

Seago (2000) investigated "thinking and behavioral styles that are used to measure the concept of organizational culture among registered nurses and unlicensed assistive personnel in acute care hospitals" (p. 278). This study surveyed staff members who worked at least 20 hours per week in selected hospitals. The results indicate that there were differences in how staff members think and behave in these organizations. Why is this so important? Managers whose staff that includes people of color need to implement management strategies that promote behaviors to improve patient care. Understanding cultural diversity from the perspectives of thinking and behavior may help managers and other staff understand differences in how staff approaches problems and how staff responds. Though this study was done some time ago it is an example of an application of Cooke and Lafferty's (1987) *Organizational Culture Inventory*. This inventory is based on a definition of organizational culture: "the shared norms and expectations that guide the thinking and behavior by the group members" (Cooke & Rousseau, 1988, p. 246). This is a typical definition of organizational culture. The inventory includes 12 thinking and behavioral styles. These self-reported thinking and behavioral styles are used to measure the ways that group members are expected to think and behave within the organization's culture. This particular inventory is mentioned here as it provides one viewpoint of organizational culture, highlights some important factors and styles, and has had an impact on current surveys or assessments. The Internet has examples of other types of surveys. In this inventory or survey there are three thinking/behavioral factors, and each has specific styles of thinking and behavior.

1. *Constructive factor:* This factor is satisfaction-oriented and includes the following styles. The humanistic or helpful style assumes that people are basically good and that the staff members enjoy assisting and teaching others. The affiliative style is described as warm, accepting, and cooperative. Staff members prefer friendly work relationships. The achievement style focuses on the need to do well, planning, ambitiousness, and enthusiasm. The fourth style is self-actualization, which is the need to meet individual goals, seek growth, and enjoy self-respect.
2. *Passive-defensive factor:* This factor is people-security-oriented and includes the following styles. The approval style focuses on the need to be accepted and trying to please. The second style is conventional, which means staff follows rules and meet expectations. The dependence style also includes following the rules, with an emphasis on the good follower. The avoidance style focuses on self-blame and guilt, and the staff member avoids conflict.
3. *Aggressive-defensive factor:* This factor is task-security-oriented and includes the following styles. The oppositional style focuses on staff resistance to authority. The second style is power, in which staff needs to use influence, power, and control. The competitive style includes staff that needs to win, and everything is a challenge. The fourth style is competence/perfectionist, when staff needs to appear independent and competent and will try harder to reach higher goals to seek perfection (Seago, 2000, p. 279).

Box 8-3 highlights the thinking/behavioral factors and their related thinking and behavioral styles. Of these three factors, the constructive factor allows for the most positive organizational culture.

| BOX 8-3 | THINKING AND BEHAVIORAL FACTORS RELATED TO THINKING AND BEHAVIORAL STYLES |
|---|---|

| Thinking and Behavioral Factors | Thinking and Behavioral Styles |
|---|---|
| Constructive Factor | • Humanistic or Helpful Style<br>• Affiliative or Cooperative/Warm Style<br>• Achievement or Enthusiastic/Ambitious Style<br>• Self-Actualization Style |
| Passive-Defensive Factor | • Approval or Need to Please Style<br>• Conventional or Need to Follow the Rules Style<br>• Avoidance of Conflict or Guilt Style |
| Aggressive-Defensive Factor | • Oppositional Style<br>• Power Style<br>• Competitive Style<br>• Competence/Perfectionist Style |

Seago (2000) applied these thinking and behavioral factors to health care organization redesign. The findings indicate that many organizations are hiring and using more unlicensed assistive personnel (UAP) resulting in a greater staff skill mix, typically with more UAP than RNs. Therefore, it is important that managers understand how this change in skill mix might change staff culture and behavior. Since in this study UAP scored much higher on dependence and opposition than RNs, it is important to understand what this might mean to a nurse manager. UAP may feel that they need to use these thinking and behavior styles (dependence and opposition) to be successful and a "good follower." Typically, this is interpreted as not being threatening or challenging; however, is this really what organizations need in today's health care environment? There is no doubt that teams need good followers to be effective, as is discussed in other chapters in this text; however, health care organizations today also need staff, RNs and other staff, who challenge themselves and the organization to do better. The nurse manager and staff nurses need to provide more positive recognition of the UAP and their work. They need to listen to them more and try to facilitate more decision making within this group, but still provide appropriate recognition of UAP job position limitations as to what they can do. This all needs to become part of the culture of the unit, service/department, and organization. The results of the study also indicate the following.

- Both groups of staff, RNs and UAP, want positive interpersonal relationships, are generally accepting and cooperative, need to do well, and enjoy helping and assisting others.
- Staff members of color, regardless of position, scored higher on the thinking and behavioral styles of approval, avoidance, and competitiveness, whereas UAP, regardless of race or ethnicity, scored higher on the thinking and behavioral styles of dependence and opposition.
- Participants in this study who were people of color, regardless of the position, gender, or education, scored higher than Caucasians on approval, avoidance, and competitiveness. They tended to want to please more, required more acceptance, and avoided conflict. They also tended to try harder and set high goals for themselves (Seago, 2000, pp. 278, 285).

This study provides information about how changing the skill mix of a unit or workgroup (team) will change the culture of that team. If the goal is to change the culture so that staff members work better as a team and feel that they can participate in decision making, the three factors (constructive, passive-defensive, and aggressive-defensive), and their respective styles can make a difference in the success of this effort.

## Generational Issues and Their Effects on Organizational Culture

Some authors have discussed the importance of understanding the generation that staff members represent and how this influences their different responses to the work environment (Zemke, Raines, & Filipczak, 2000; Ulrich, 2001; Gerke, 2001; Wieck, Prydum, & Walsh, 2002).

"Managing diversity here is defined as creating and maintaining an environment in which each person is respected because of his or her differences" (Davis, 2001, p. 161). Nursing now has the unique experience of including four generations working in the same place (Gerke, 2001). This situation can lead to a rich diversity of viewpoints and practice; however, it can also lead to conflict and problems within the organizational culture. Key questions to consider are (a) What are the four generations? (b) What are their characteristics? (c) What can be done to gain the most for this matrix of generations? The focus of this discussion will be on the last two generations; however, to appreciate these two generations it is necessary to briefly describe the first two generations. Box 8-4 highlights the four generations.

**The traditional, silent, or mature generation, born from 1930 to 1940.** This generation is less apparent due to its age, but it had a major impact on nursing. Many from this generation were nurses in World War II. They can be characterized as hard-working, loyal, valuers of duty, and family focused. They accepted hierarchy as an important characteristic of the organizations in which they worked.

**Baby boomers, born from 1943 to 1960.** This generation fills most of the nursing positions, both in practice and nursing education. Typically, this group had a choice of only two careers, nursing or teaching (Bertholf & Loveless, 2001). This group is beginning to retire, leading to a greater nursing shortage in both practice and education. This generation works independently, accepts authority, causes few problems, feels that loyalty is an important work value, is less able to cope with new technology, and has been described as workaholics (Bertholf & Loveless, 2001). Gerke (2001) describes this group as preferring consensus leadership, competitive, and more focused on material gain. It is important to recognize that there is variation within the generational group (for example, many in this generation have been the leaders and pushers for greater use of technology in health care). This can be supported by the increased use of computer technology in nursing education and in practice documentation. This would have never happened if some members of the generation had not pushed for it.

**Generation X**, who were born from 1960 to 1980, and **Generation Y**, who were born from 1980 to 2000, will be discussed in more detail in this chapter. Why is it important to understand the differences in the last two generations of staff? At this time, they are the major age groups that are increasing in nursing and will take on the leadership of the profession as the baby boomers retire. It is believed that characteristics of the age groups affect how they work, why they work, and leadership that is required within organizations (American Hospital Association, 2002). Generation X is different from the baby boomer generation (Santos & Cox, 2002). Generation X nurses are described as the "original 'latch key kids' and have grown up mastering information technology and creative thinking" (Bertholf & Loveless, 2001, p. 169). They have grown up during a time of extreme change. Generation X nurses want to be led, not managed. They need to develop self-confidence and empowerment. They want effective, intelligent leaders who mentor staff, and they want to be trusted and respected by their leaders. Nurturing is a key leadership characteristic that is important to Generation X, and it forms the base for their other important characteristics: motivational, receptive, positive, good communicator, team player, good people skills, approachable, and supportive (Wieck, Prydun, & Walsh, 2002). This generation is not made up of joiners, and this is a problem for professional organizations. They do not value job longevity, which has an impact on loyalty to employers. They also feel strongly about maintaining a balance between work and personal life.

| BOX 8-4 | THE FOUR KEY GENERATIONS IN NURSING |
|---------|-------------------------------------|

| | |
|---|---|
| 1. Traditional Generation | Born 1930–1940 |
| 2. Baby Boomers | Born 1943–1960 |
| 3. Generation X | Born 1960–1980 |
| 4. Generation Y | Born 1980–2000 |

The core values of Generation X staff are diversity, thinking globally, balance, technoliteracy, fun, informality, self-reliance, and pragmatism. The job assets of this generation are adaptable, technoliterate, independent, intimidated by authority, and creative. How might their values affect their assets? Generation X staff is motivated by organizational messages such as

- "Do it your way."
- "We've got the newest hardware and software."
- "There aren't a lot of rules here."
- "We're not very corporate."

"Generation Xers are pessimistic and rightfully so given the world they grew up in. They are loyal to themselves and the people with whom they have familial-like relationships. They like to feel that they are part of something bigger. They expect and respond well to things that contribute to their own professional knowledge and competency. Xers are flexible and very comfortable with change. . . . They are technoliterate. . . . Because Generation X often views a job as a stepping stone to the next job, benefits and rewards geared to the present rather than the future are the most valuable in recruitment and retention" (Ulrich, 2001, p. 152). This description of Generation X explains some of the conflict or tension that can be seen between these nurses and baby boomer nurses, who are just ahead of them. Baby boomer nurses are more willing, although not happy about it, to work overtime and are often shocked when younger nurses say they are leaving. This is driven by the fact that more baby boomer nurses have a long-term commitment to employers (Santos & Cox, 2002). These are not characteristics found in the generation that is replacing the baby boomers.

Generation Y (**Nexters**; Millennials, Generation Next, MyPod generation, GenY, and other titles) (Kogan, 2001), the newest generation entering nursing, demonstrates the core values of optimism, civic duty, confidence, achievement, social ability, morality, street smarts, and diversity. Their important on-the-job assets are collective action, optimism, tenacity, heroic spirit, multitasking capabilities, and technology savvy. They are interested in technology and feel competent around it. Compared to Generation X, they have more trust in centralized authority (Gerke, 2001). Change is part of their lives, and thus they tolerate it better. Related to this, they are seen as being greater risk-takers and want to be challenged and excited about their work.

The first step is to recognize the importance of distinguishing between generations, and the second is to develop strategies that improve collaboration and culture. It is clear that these generational groups need to communicate with one another to increase understanding of where each group is coming from and recognize the values that are important to each group. Some strategies that have been recommended to accomplish this include the following:

- Develop coaching behaviors in preceptors/educators to enable learning by doing and supporting the newer employee in asking "why" questions.
- Design care delivery models to support collaborative practice.
- Utilize participatory management strategies to develop relationships.
- Recognize and accept that all employment is temporary.
- Lighten up.
- Be specific.
- Realize that you have more in common than different.
- Assess the organization for its ability for inclusion.
- Discuss openly how you see your team working with new members (Bertholf & Loveless, 2001, pp. 170–171).

# Facilitating Cultural Diversity Within Health Care Organizations

If an organization has a dysfunctional or dissonant culture, what should be done? Many authorities recommend that this be approached carefully as the problems may not be major ones (Curtin, 2001). "Three key steps related to an assessment and analysis of the culture are (a) identify and develop an appropriate list of organizational values, (b) measure the degree to which employees and managers share those values, and (c) measure the degree to which they perceive the institution as demonstrating those values" (Curtin, 2001, p. 222).

As organizations assess their cultures and then realize that changes are needed, they will find that increasing participation from all levels of the organization will go a long way in improving the organization and increasing trust among staff and between staff and the organization. Lack of trust can be a major barrier to improving the organization's culture, as was noted earlier in this chapter. How do organizations get a better match between employee values and those of the organization? ". . . we should hire to values, seek diversity, and train to skills. Shared values help create a culture that sends the consistent message and focus. Through shared values and beliefs organizational cultures emerge. Diversity of the team, not simply ethnic diversity but also diversity in thinking, creates a true opportunity for organizational learning to occur. Through this diversity we are able to challenge our own thinking or think out of the box. Through diversity of thinking conflict can emerge and true dialogue can occur. Through this new level of dialogue more creative approaches can emerge and better decisions can be made" (Tornabeni, 2001, p. 7). Tornabeni identifies a key issue. Typically, one thinks of diversity as different cultures; however, it can and should be more than this. Diversity in thinking is also important. McNeese-Smith and Crook (2003) recommend that managers annually discuss and examine employee values in relationship to the organization's values. A good time to do this is at the time of performance evaluations. The goal should be to help staff members and support their values as this may help to prevent burnout and loss of staff. This goes along with comments made earlier in this text about the need for leaders to help staff grow and develop, to encourage self-assessment and development of goals, and to recognize the need that to keep staff members they must feel a part of the system and the culture.

If an organization concludes after an extensive assessment of its culture that improvement is needed, what should the organization do? Leaders who want to change an organization's culture need to follow these key principles as they develop and implement strategies to improve the organization's culture.

- Involve people in the problems and programs that affect them.
- Do not place blame.
- Clarify battles, objectives, purposes, and tasks.
- Focus on short-term and long-term results.
- Work from a sound information base.
- Use multilevel change strategies.
- Integrate concern for people and achievement of organizational goals. Emphasize sustained culture change (Allen & Kraft, 1982; as cited in Jones & Redman, 2000, p. 605).

A key aspect of the organization's culture is how staff and managers view diversity and their level of cultural competency. The basic components of cultural competency in nursing care that continue to be important in effective cultural competency are as follows:

1. An awareness, sensitivity, and tolerance to differences in culture and language
2. An ability to refrain from making assumptions (or judgments) about the beliefs, behaviors, needs, and expectations of patients or colleagues of a different cultural background from oneself
3. An understanding of the role culture plays in forming the health/illness prevention, beliefs, and practices of patience
4. The ability to recognize the role that one's own culture and background plays in determining one's attitudes and beliefs about such factors as what constitutes acceptable behavior, cleanliness, a happy lifestyle, the roles of family and friends, and so forth
5. Enough knowledge about the cultures that one serves to avoid breaching the patient's taboos, health care beliefs, or rules of interaction
6. Enough knowledge about the cultures that one serves to anticipate possible barriers to access or compliance with care

7. The skill to deliver culturally and linguistically appropriate patient advice and education
8. The skill to utilize interpreters effectively so that language barriers do not impact the extent or quality of care
9. The knowledge and flexibility to modify both one's mode of interaction and one's manner of delivering care so that it is culturally and linguistically appropriate to the patient while it meets the hospital's or clinic's standards of quality patient care
10. Confidence in one's ability to offer quality care to patients of other cultures (Salimbene, 1999, p. 31)

These are helpful guidelines for developing staff/manager competencies. Do they have these competencies? If not, training and education need to be addressed to increase the level of cultural competency. Culture is a sensitive subject so it is important that education programs consider the best learning methods and relevancy of content to the staff and organization. It is important to avoid a paternalistic approach, stereotyping, and biases when this content is presented.

The recent Institute of Medicine report *Crossing the Quality Chasm* (2001) addresses some key issues related to organizational culture in health care delivery systems. The process of developing this report included the participation from experts in medicine, nursing, safety, pharmacy, and health administration, which resulted in a broad base of viewpoints.

**Care based on *continuous healing relationships:*** Patients need a health care system that is responsive to their needs when they need care. The type of services or entry into services should consider all possible methods, including innovative ones when necessary, such as Internet, telephone, and so on.

***Customization* based on patient needs and values:** Health care delivery must consider the needs that are frequently found in the population; however, it must be flexible enough to address those unexpected needs and consider individual patient choices and preferences.

**The *patient as the source of control:*** To be in control patients need information, and health care providers need to be able to accommodate differences.

***Shared knowledge* and the free flow of information:** Patients need access to their health information in an easily accessible manner. The focus should be on sharing information.

***Evidence-based* decision making:** The best possible scientific information needs to be used in providing care.

***Safety* as a system property:** All health care provider settings and providers need to offer a safe environment in which to receive safe and appropriate care.

**The need for *transparency:*** Information needs to be shared with patients, which includes information about the provider's performance on safety, evidence-based practice, and patient satisfaction.

***Anticipation* of needs:** Health care providers need to be proactive in relationship to patient needs.

***Continuous* decrease in waste:** Resources should not be wasted, and this includes patients' time.

***Cooperation* among clinicians:** Individual providers and provider organizations need to collaborate to ensure appropriate, timely care and exchange of information (Institute of Medicine, 2001; as cited in Curtin, 2001, p. 218).

Each one of these descriptors is directly related to nursing care, although some have been addressed more effectively than others.

The most effective organizational cultures will be those that have a credible culture. These cultures build and maintain trust, and feature leaders who are role models and set the culture's tone. Communication is recognized as important and is viewed as being effective. Staff and management are clear about expectations. How do an organization and its leadership go about building a credible culture?

- Reward people who communicate openly and build trust in the workplace; punish those who don't.
- Talk about the values of your organization from the top down and encourage conversation about issues.

- Build your own credibility bank by practicing open communication; if you make a mistake, you will get the benefit of the doubt.
- Encourage questions. Trust thrives on open lines of communication. The people who work for you need to know it's OK to question a decision or priority.
- Do not assume people know what is expected; be clear about the kind of behavior and communication you expect and find acceptable (Bates, 2003, p. 38).

The Magnet Recognition Program, discussed in earlier chapters, has had an impact on HCO organizational culture. Magnet hospitals demonstrate more effective and innovative work environments, more shared governance, empowerment of nurses, and better quality care (Armstrong, Laschinger, & Wong, 2008; Aiken, Clarke, Sloan, Lake, & Cheney, 2008; Drenkard, 2009). Positive workplace environments do impact positively on patient outcomes.

# Cultural Perceptions of Health and Illness: Need for a Caring, Healing Environment

As organizations and their cultures are considered, it is important to recognize that health care delivery organizations are more than just organizations in which people work. This is one part of the culture but not the only part. Whether or not the organizational culture supports an environment in which patients can be cared for is another critical issue. This section discusses factors related to a caring, healing environment.

## What Is a Healing Environment?

Curtin (2001) has indicated that "today's hospitals do not have to change their cultures; they have to heal themselves" (p. 219). This is a different perspective of organizational culture. She concludes that the growing emphasis on market-based culture in health care with all of its concern for financial issues and getting a bigger piece of the market has had a serious detrimental effect on the health of health care organizations. She concludes that this value approach needs to be addressed to help hospitals heal. This certainly relates to comments made earlier in this chapter about nurses' concerns about the overemphasis on financial issues. Related to this problem are intrinsic and extrinsic values, which are values that are affected by age, life cycle, and professional status (McNeese-Smith & Crook, 2003). At the same time, some organizations are describing themselves as healing environments. Can this really happen? Can organizations that need to heal themselves be healing environments?

Defining healing environments is not easy. There are a variety of components that are associated with healing environments such as privacy, air quality, noise levels, views, and visual characteristics. As needs among people vary, there is no doubt that the perfect environment for healing cannot be developed, but there has been recognition that efforts should be taken to develop healing environments. "Throughout history health care providers, architects, and psychologists have noted a strong link between the environment and human behavior" (McCullough & Wille, 2001, p. 111). Florence Nightingale commented on the need for healing environments that she associated with fresh air, warmth, cleanliness, quiet, diet, and light (McCullough & Wille, 2001). "Traditionally, physicians and nurses have been the center of action in health care, and patients were expected to adapt to the routines of the facility. Today, patients and families are the central focus of health care, and health care facilities are being designed to address their needs. Regulations, market pressures, and a desire to improve the health care experience foster patient-centered movements" (McCullough & Wille, 2001, p. 110). When health care organizations began to change their focus, they had to confront their weaknesses and try to make difficult changes. Some have been more successful than others.

If one reflects on personal experiences in acute care facilities as well as other types of health care settings, the environment often is not all that conducive to healing—noise interferes with rest and relaxation, lack of cleanliness, difficulty finding one's way around, the lack of warmth as far as color and furnishings, confusion over staff identities, and unresponsive staff.

Some organizations, of course, have made successful efforts to improve their environments. One particular example is the California Pacific Medical Center, the Planetree Unit, begun in 1995. This unit was actually created by a health care consumer (McCullough & Wille, 2001). The approach was based on a concept that became known as the Planetree concept: "The model of care is a patient-centered, holistic approach to health care, promoting mental, emotional, spiritual, social, and physical healing. It empowers patients and families through the exchange of information and encourages healing partnerships with caregivers. It seeks to maximize positive health care outcomes by integrating optimal medical therapies and incorporating art and nature into the healing environment" (Planetree, 2010). In this type of environment the focus of care is on the whole patient—body, mind, and spirit—with active consumer involvement. The following beliefs are part of the Planetree concept (Planetree, 2010):

- We are human beings, caring for other human beings.
- We are all caregivers.
- Care giving is best achieved through kindness and compassion.
- Safe, accessible, high quality care is fundamental to patient-centered care.
- Use a holistic approach to meet people's needs of body, mind, and spirit.
- Families, friends, and loved ones are vital to the healing process.
- Access to understandable health information can empower individuals to participate in their health care.
- The opportunity for individuals to make personal choices related to their care is essential.
- Physical environments can enhance healing, health, and well-being.
- Illness can be a transformational experience for patients, families, and caregivers.

The Planetree concept and organization was developed prior to the IOM reports. The concept emphasizes the need for a patient-centered approach to care. This concept recognized a need and responded to it. Due to the IOM reports there is greater movement to embrace and operationalize patient-centered care.

Some hospitals have been applying the Planetree concept to make necessary changes to improve their healing environments. In reviewing the key strategies that support the Planetree concept, they are clearly strategies that are integral to quality nursing care. They are also highly supportive of a positive culture that not only moves the patient into an important role but also provides a more positive work culture.

The Picker Institute and the Center for Health Care Design conducted research on the patient's perspective of the health care environment, which included over 350,000 interviews. From these interviews, eight dimensions of care valued by patients have been identified:

- Respect for patients' values, preferences, and expressed needs
- Coordination and integration of care
- Information communication and education
- Physical comfort
- Emotional support and alleviation of fear and anxiety
- Involvement of family and friends
- Continuity and transition (Picker Institute, 2010)

## The Physical Environment as Part of a Healing Environment

Making health care organizations more appealing spaces is also important to developing healing environments. In the last 15 to 20 years, more efforts have been made by hospitals to make their environments more comfortable and soothing (Leighty, 2003). The Center for Health Design identified consumer environmental rights in health care facilities. Environments should do the following:

- Be easy to navigate.
- Offer restricted access to nature through views, gardens, landscaped patios, terraces, courtyards, atria, and natural elements.

- Have an easy-to-control personal environment including lighting, noise and sound reduction, odor elimination, thermal comfort, and privacy.
- Offer the capability to select positive distractions including television, games, videotapes, computers, art, telephone, music, social opportunities, access to nature, and reading material.
- Have activities in spaces conducive to their purpose.
- Make it easy for staff to bring food, medicine, and other supplies related to the care.
- Have access to furniture and equipment that is comfortable and user-friendly.
- Allow maximum opportunities for regular lifestyle activities.
- Have access to a continuous sequence of environments that support one's dignity and the dignity of others.
- Be clean, neat, and orderly.
- Be free from hazards.
- Provide for personal safety and security for personal possessions. Inspire trust and confidence.
- Symbolize values appropriate to patients and others.
- Provide for local cultural backgrounds and diversity in the community.
- Be appropriate for the various ages, genders, and physical and cognitive abilities of the people who use it.
- Support interaction with others including care-partners.
- Decrease unnecessary stress for all patients or residents, visitors, and staff.
- Be aesthetically appealing (The Center for Health Design, 2000).

This effort can also be seen in other types of health care settings, too (for example, clinics, M.D. offices, and long-term care facilities).

Some evidence exists that these strategies actually have an important impact on patient outcomes and staff. The study described in this chapter's evidence example emphasizes unit design factors and their impact on patient outcomes. A nurse-friendly environment is one in which the work environment is conducive to safe practice. Examples of these strategies are reducing travel time between work areas, better lighting, connecting areas that relate, and providing space for staff to take breaks. These efforts decrease staff stress, fatigue, and physical burden and thus improve efficiency and nurses' attitudes, which may affect retention and recruitment. When nurses are asked to participate in renovation planning or in new expansions, then the environment typically is a more nurse-friendly environment and more patient-oriented nurses understand what is a healing environment. The staff members are the ones who really know what they need to get their work done. Leighty (2003) noted that increased use of private patient rooms (a) decreases requests for transfers, which decreases costs and increases patient satisfaction; (b) increases patient sleep and rest, which affects outcomes and patient satisfaction; (c) along with location of sinks and airflow, decreases nosocomial infections, which affects costs due to complications and outcomes; and (d) can even affect market share because patients want to come to hospitals where they get private rooms. More research needs to be done about environmental factors and how they affect organizational culture. Most would agree that it is much easier to work in a pleasant, attractive environment and that these factors make it easier for patients and families during times of stress, but more information is needed on the effect of these strategies and how they can be improved.

# APPLYING LEADERSHIP AND MANAGEMENT

## MY HOSPITAL UNIT

The goal is to have an effective, creative, and productive workplace. What does this goal mean to you? Make a list of the critical factors that you think your unit and the organization would have to demonstrate to meet this goal. You might share your list in small teams in your class and find out if your views are similar or different from your classmates in their own units. Discuss why there may be differences. What have you listed as factors that describe an organization's culture? Some of the factors that might be found on your list (although there are many more and your list does not have to agree) include the following: clear vision and mission, goals and objectives, vision/mission/goals/objectives that can be demonstrated in your unit's and in the organization's actions, staff trust management and vice versa, clear communication with staff input into decisions, staff care for one another, management cares about staff as individuals, safe work environment is supported, staff feeling loyal to the organization, staff feeling empowered, positive reputation in the community, management is visible and available to staff, and organization demonstrates partnership and collaboration. Describe three strategies you might use in your unit to improve the culture. Remember to consider past decisions you have made about your unit and plans you completed in earlier chapters for your unit. Use the virtual unit site found on the textbook website to record the work that you do in the role of nurse manager for your unit.

## Critical Thinking Questions and Activities

1. Consonant and dissonant cultures can be found in many organizations. It is important to understand the differences between a consonant and a dissonant organization culture in order to improve an organization's culture. Select an organization (a hospital unit, a home care agency, school, or other clinical site that you have worked in as a student or staff, or you might choose your school, other schools attended, organization you belong to, and so on). Determine if the culture of that organization is consonant or dissonant and provide your rationale. When you are doing your assessment, use the characteristics of a dysfunctional or dissonant organization culture identified by Sovie in this chapter. You will also want to consider how members of the organization share values, group behavior norms, and communication methods with new members. Is the organization adaptive, and in what ways? Is it rigid, and what effect does this has on its members (staff)? What is your feeling about the organization? We all get these feelings when we have been in an organization. How comfortable does it feel to be in the organization? What influences your reaction?

2. Interview or ask a member of the human resources department in a local hospital to discuss how diversity in the workforce affects what the human resources department does and its processes.

3. Review the basic concepts on the website Diversity in Health and Illness (http://www .culturediversity.org). Select one of the case studies and discuss how you would apply these concepts in your nursing practice.

4. Listen to the audiotape, Telemedicine Is a Success for Navajos, listed on the website (http://www.npr.org/features/feature.php?wfId=1472515) and describe how you would envision using telemedicine for the underserved populations in your geographic area. How would you overcome problems such as financing, access, and education of the clients in its use?

5. Paint a verbal picture of the culture of your organization as you see it. How does your picture relate to content in this chapter?

6. Review the AONE diversity principles. How do you think these could be applied in a health care organization?

# Media Links

- **URL: http://www.ahrq.gov/qual/qrdr08.htm**
  National Healthcare Disparities Report

- **URL: http://www.hhs.gov/ocr/civilrights/resources/specialtopics/health_disparities/**
  U.S. Department of Health and Human Services: Healthcare Disparities/Nondiscriminatory Quality Healthcare Services

- **URL: http://www.aacn.nche.edu**
  American Association of Colleges of Nursing: Tool Kit of Resources for Cultural Competent Education for Baccalaureate Nurses
  Search for the tool kit, which is in PDF format.

- **URL: http://www.thinkculturalhealth.org**
  Think Cultural Health Website
  Sponsored by the Office of Minority Health (OMH). This website offers the latest resources and tools to promote cultural competency in health care. Users can access free online courses accredited for continuing education credit. The site also provides supplementary tools to help providers and organizations promote respectful, understandable, and effective care to an increasingly diverse patient population.

- **URL: http://www.intlnursemigration.org/**
  International Council of Nurse (ICN): Migration of nurses

**Pearson Nursing Student Resources**
Find additional review materials at
**nursing.pearsonhighered.com**
Prepare for success with additional NCLEX®-style practice questions, interactive assignments and activities, Web links, animations and videos, and more!

# References

Aiken, L., et al. (2001). Nurses' report on hospital care in five countries: The ways in which nurses' work is structured have left nurses among the least satisfied workers, and the problem is getting worse. *Health Affairs, 20*(3), 43–53.

Aiken, L., Clarke, S., Sloane, D., Lake, E., & Cheney, T. (2008). Effects of hospital care environment on patient mortality and nurse outcomes. *JONA, 38*(5), 223–339.

Allen, R., & Kraft, C. (1982). *The organizational unconscious.* Upper Saddle River, NJ: Prentice Hall.

American Association of Colleges of Nursing. (2008). *The essentials of baccalaureate nursing education for professional nursing practice.* Washington, DC: Author.

American Hospital Association. (2002). *In our hands. How hospital leaders can build a thriving workplace.* Chicago, IL: Author.

Armstrong, K., Laschinger, H. & Wong, C. (2009). Workplace empowerment and magnet hospital characteristics as predicators of patient safety climate. *Journal of Nursing Care Quality, 24*(1), 55–62.

Baldwin, D. (2003). Disparities in health care: Focusing efforts to eliminate unequal burdens. *Online Journal of Issues in Nursing, 8*(2), 1–16.

Bates, S. (2003). Creating a credible culture. *Nurse Leader, 1*(1), 37.

Bertholf, L., & Loveless, S. (2001). Baby Boomers and Generation X: Strategies to bridge the gap. *Seminars for Nurse Managers, 9*(3), 169–172.

Braveman, P. (2006). Health Disparities and Health Equity: Concepts and Measurement. *Annual Review of Public Health, 27*, 167–194.

Cameron, K., & Quinn, R. (1994). *PRISM 5: Changing organizational culture: A competing values workbook.* Ann Arbor, MI: University of Michigan.

Carmichael, M. (2008, October 21). ER overload. A new study looks at overcrowding in America's emergency rooms and finds some surprising reasons for those long waits. *Newsweek.* Retrieved October 4, 2009, from http://www.newsweek.com/id/164922

Center for Health Design. (2000). The health care consumer's environmental bill of rights. Retrieved from http://www.healthdesign.org

Collins, K., et al. (2002). *Diverse communities, common concerns: Assessing health care quality for Minority Americans.* (Findings from the Commonwealth Fund 2001 Health Care Quality Survey) New York: The Commonwealth Fund.

Cooke, P., & Rousseau, D. (1988). Behavioral norms and expectations. *Group Organizational Studies, 13*, 245–273.

Cooke, R., & Lafferty, J. (1987). *Organizational culture inventory.* Plymonth, MI: Hanar Synergistics.

Cuilla, J. (2000). *The working life: The promise and betrayal of modern work.* New York: Times Books/Random House.

Curtin, L. (2001). Healing health care's organizational culture. *Seminars for Nurse Managers, 9*(4), 218–227.

Davis, S. (2001). Diversity and generation X. *Seminars for Nurse Managers, 9*(3), 161–163.

De Ruiter, H., & Larsen, K. (2002). Developing a transcultural patient care web site. *Journal of Transcultural Nursing, 13*(1), 61–67.

De Ruiter, H., & Saphiere, D. (2001). Nurse leaders as cultural bridges. *Journal of Nursing Administration, 31*(9), 418–423.

Dessler, G. (2002). *Management.* Upper Saddle River, NJ: Prentice Hall.

DeWalt, C., Berkman, D., Sheridan, kS., Lohr, K., & Pignone, M. (2004). Literacy and health outcomes: A systematic review of the literature. *Journal of General Internal Medicine, 19*(12), 1228–1239.

DeWalt, D. & Pignone, M. (2008). Advocacy and patient literacy: What Health care professionals can do to help patients overcome patient literacy barriers. In J. Earp, E. French, & M. Gilkey (Eds), *Patient advocacy for health care quality* (pp. 215–239). Sudbury, MA: Jones and Bartlett Publishers.

Drenkard, K. (2009). Introduction: The Evidence for Magnet® Status. *JONA, 39*(7/8 Supplement), S1.

Finkelman, A. & Kenner, C. (2009). *Teaching IOM: Implications of the Institute of Medicine reports.* (2nd ed). Silver Spring, MD: American Nurses Association.

Frusti, D., Niesen, K., & Campion, J. (2003). Creating a culturally competent organization. *Journal of Nursing Administration, 33*(1), 31; 38.

Gerke, M. (2001). Understanding and leading the quad matrix: Four generations in the workplace: The traditional generation, boomers, gen-X, nexters. *Seminars for Nurse Managers, 9*(3), 173–181.

Griffin, C. (2002). Embracing diversity. *NurseWeek Midwest/Great Lakes, 2*(12), 12–13.

Guido, G. (2001). *Legal and ethical issues in nursing* (3rd ed.). Upper Saddle River, NJ: Prentice Hall.

Health Resources and Services Administration. (2010). *The registered nurse population: Initial findings from the 2008 national sample survey of registered nurses.* Retrieved May 15, 2010, from http://bhpr.hrsa.gov/healthworkforce/rnsurvey/

The Institute for the Future. (2000). *Health and health care 2010: The forecast, the challenge.* San Francisco: Jossey-Bass.

Institute of Medicine. (2001). *Crossing the quality chasm.* Washington, DC: National Academies Press.

Institute of Medicine. (2002). *Unequal Treatment. What health care providers need to know about racial and ethnic disparities in health care.* Washington, DC: National Academies Press.

Institute of Medicine. (2003a). *Health professions education.* Washington, DC: National Academies Press.

Institute of Medicine. (2003b). *Leadership by example.* Washington, DC: National Academies Press.

Institute of Medicine. (2004). *Health literacy.* Washington, DC: National Academies Press.

International Council of Nurses. (2010). Migration Center. Retrieved March 30, 2010, from http://www.intlnursemigration.org/

Joint Commission. (2007). "What did the doctor say?" Improving health literacy to protect patient safety. Retrieved November 10, 2009, from http://www.jointcommission.org/NewsRoom/PressKits/Health_Literacy

Jones, K., & Redman, R. (2000). Organizational culture and work redesign: Experiences in three organizations. *Journal of Nursing Administration, 30*(12), 604–610.

Kogan, M. (2001). *Bridging the gap.* Retrieved November 15, 2007, from http://cmsreports.com/generation_next

Leighty, J. (2003). Healing by design. *NurseWeek Midwest/Great Lakes, 2*(5), 14–16.

McCullough, C., & Wille, R. (2001). Healing environments. In C. McCullough (Ed.), *Creating responsive solutions to health care change* (pp. 109–134). Indianapolis, IN: Center Nursing Press.

McNeese-Smith, D., & Crook, M. (2003). Nursing values and a changing nurse workforce. *Journal of Nursing Administration, 33*(5), 260–283.

Mead, H., Cartwright-Smith, L., Jones, K., Ramos, C., & Woods, K. (2008, March 13). *Racial and ethnic disparities in U.S. health care: A chartbook.* Retrieved December 3, 2009, from http://www.commonwealthfund.org/Content/Publications/Chartbooks/2008/Mar/Racial-and-Ethnic-Disparities-in-U-S—Health-Care—A-Chartbook.aspx

Milgram, L., Spector, A., & Treger, M. (1999). *Managing smart.* Houston, TX: Cashman Dudley.

National Institutes of Health (NIH) Strategic Research Plan and Budget to Reduce and Ultimately Eliminate Health Disparities. (2002–2006), Vol 1.

National Quality Forum. (2009). Health disparities. Retrieved April 1, 2010, from http://www.qualityforum.org/Topics/Disparities.aspx

Parker, M., & Gadbois, S. (2000). Building community in the health care workplace, Part 3. *Journal of Nursing Administration, 30*(10), 466–473.

Planetree. Retrieved January 10, 2010, from http://www.planetree.org/about.html

Ray, M., Turkel, M., & Marino, F. (2002). The transformative process for nursing in workforce redevelopment. *Nursing Administrative Quarterly, 26*(2), 1–14.

Salimbene, S. (1999). Cultural competence: A priority for performance improvement action. *Journal of Nursing Administration, 13*(3), 23–35.

Salisbury, J. & Byrd, S. (2006). Why diversity matters in health care. Retrieved June 16, 2009, from http://www.csahq.org/pdf/bulletin/issue_12/Diversity.pdf

Santos, S., & Cox, K. (2002). Generational tension among nurses. *American Journal of Nursing, 102*(1), 11. Schein, E. (2004). *Organizational culture and leadership.* Hoboken, NJ: John Wiley and Sons.

Seago, J. (2000). Registered nurses, unlicensed assistive personnel, and organizational culture in hospitals. *Journal of Nursing Administration, 30*(5), 278–286.

Shea-Lewis, A. (2002). Workforce diversity in health care. *Journal of Nursing Administration, 32*(1), 6–7.

Sovie, M. (1993). Hospital culture: Why create one? *Nursing Economics, 11*(2), 69–90.

Sullivan, L. (2004). *Missing persons: Minorities in the health professions, a report of the Sullivan Commission on diversity in health care workforce.* Retrieved January 2, 2010, from http://www.aacn.nche.edu/Media/pdf/SullivanReport.pdf

Sullivan, E., & Decker, P. (2001). *Effective leadership and management in nursing* (5th ed.). Upper Saddle River, NJ: Prentice Hall.

Tornabeni, J. (2001). The competency game: My take on what it really takes to lead. *Nursing Administration Quarterly, 25*(4), 1–13.

Ulrich, B. (2001). Successfully managing multigenerational workforces. *Seminars for Nurse Managers, 9*(3), 147–153.

Werner, R., Goldman, L., & Dudley, R. (2008). Comparison of change in quality of care between safety-net and non-safety-net hospitals *Journal of the American Medical Association, 299*(18), 2180–2187.

Wieck, K., Prydun, M., & Walsh, T. (2002). What the emerging workforce wants in its leaders. *Journal of Nursing Scholarship, 34*(3), 283–288.

Zemke, R., Raines, C., & Filipczak, B. (2000). *Generations at work.* New York: American Management Association.

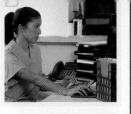

# 9

# Recruitment and Retention: Meeting Staffing Requirements

## CHAPTER OUTLINE

## LEARNING OUTCOMES

Before you begin, take a moment to familiarize yourself with the learning outcomes for this chapter.

- Describe how the human resources department assists the health care organization and employees.
- Describe staff recruitment.
- Explain how a position description is developed.
- Apply the employment process to nursing staff recruitment.
- Apply critical guidelines that a nurse should consider when applying for a position.
- Explain why it is important for nursing staff to be involved in recruitment and how they might do this.
- Analyze the issue of retention and impact on staff and quality care.
- Apply the performance appraisal process.
- Examine strategies that can be used to prevent or decrease stress and passive-aggressive behavior in the work setting.
- Analyze reasons for the nursing shortage.

## KEY TERMS

- Background check
- Competence
- Full-time equivalent
- Human resources department
- Job analysis
- Job stress
- Orientation
- Patient classification system
- Performance appraisal
- Position description
- Reality shock
- Recruitment
- Resume
- Retention
- Screening
- Self-scheduling
- Staff distribution
- Staff mix
- Staffing
- Termination
- Turnover

## WHAT'S AHEAD

The link between recruitment and retention is clear—recruiting the right staff for the right job is the first step in retention of staff. In 2008 it was reported that there was a 27% average voluntary turnover among new graduates (Christmas, 2008). This is a major problem today in health care along with the nursing shortage. The Institute of Medicine (IOM) core health care professions core competencies relate to recruitment and retention of staff. Having qualified staff, in appropriate number, that is satisfied with work conditions impacts effective patient-centered care, interprofessional teamwork, quality improvement, effective use of informatics, and whether or not staff is willing to apply evidence-based practice. Dissatisfied, overworked, and stressed staff is less interested in the improvement of all aspects of care.

The work environment and many other factors also affect retention, as well as the ability to recruit. Recruitment and retention may be seen as functions of human resources; however, it is a wise nurse leader who recognizes that nursing staff need to be involved in this process. Staff needs to help identify factors that drive recruitment and retention. Nurse managers, and in many cases staff, need to be involved in the interview and selection process of staff. Word of mouth can be a critical factor in the community—nurses let other nurses know the best places to work. Nurses in the community know which health care organizations have problems hiring and retaining staff. Organizational culture has a strong effect on recruitment and retention. In many situations nurses in the community can identify the factors that drive recruitment and retention problems, but health care organizations do not always ask for this feedback. This chapter speaks to two perspectives: the health care organization's recruitment and retention efforts from the employer and the candidate/employee perspectives and to the critical problem of the nursing shortage, which affects recruitment and retention. There are many factors that impact staffing levels and shortages, particularly the economy. For example in 2009 it appeared as if the shortage was decreasing in some areas of the country. The poor economy was causing nurses who would retire to postpone retirement due to financial needs and also nurses who had been out of practice or had been working part time wanted more full-time work. This had a negative impact on new graduates getting jobs, particularly if they were unwilling to move from their own communities. However, none of this really eliminates the impending nursing shortage. There are still many nurses who will retire in the next decade, and there are still major problems with having enough clinical sites and faculty to expanding enrollment in nursing programs.

The American Nurses Association (ANA) *Agenda for the Future* (2002) includes a section on recruitment and retention as described in Box 9-1. Recruitment and retention also have an impact on the shortage.

The Institute of Medicine (IOM) has commented on the nursing shortage, retention, and staffing in several of its health care quality reports. In the report on nursing (Institute of Medicine, 2004a) the need to maximize the capability of the workforce is discussed along with the nursing shortage. Maximizing the workforce requires attention to promoting safe staffing levels, supporting knowledge and skills acquisition and clinical decision-making, and fostering interprofessional collaboration. All of this is in line with the IOM five health care core competencies. The report states there is a connection between patient outcomes and these three elements that are needed to maximize the workforce (Aiken, Sloane, Lake, Sochalski, & Weber, 1999; Institute of Medicine, 2004). The Joint Commission agrees with the relationship between nursing staff and outcomes, noting that "inadequate orientation and training is a factor in 58% of serious medication errors. Staffing levels impacted 24% of 1,609 sentinel events over the past five years" (Joint Commission, 2004, p. 1). Given these facts, effective recruitment and retention of competent staff are critical issues. The potential employee also should be aware of the critical facts and issues about recruitment and retention. With the increasing shortage of nursing staff, recruitment, retention, and related staffing activities have become critical functions within health care organizations.

---

**BOX 9-1**　　**ANA'S *AGENDA FOR THE FUTURE* RECRUITMENT AND RETENTION**

Building on work in other domains, professional opportunities will be enhanced to attract and sustain excellent nurses for long, rewarding careers.

### DESIRED FUTURE STATEMENT (VISION)

Nursing is comprised of a diverse body of individuals committed to promoting and sustaining the profession through addressing diversity, image, education, funding, practice models and environments, and professional development.

Five strategies were identified to achieve the vision and one of these was identified as the primary or driving strategy.

They are as follows:

- Professional/career development opportunities cross the career span. (Primary Strategy)
- Funding is secured for creative educational initiatives that support nurses across the career span.
- Nursing is seen as a highly desirable and appealing career choice.
- Nurses develop professional practice models and work environments that ensure career satisfaction.
- Comprehensive recruitment and retention strategies demonstrate nursing's strong public image and appeal to a diverse population.

### OBJECTIVES TO SUPPORT PRIMARY STRATEGY

- Establish national, professional development models for mentoring, leadership, and diversity for nurses across their career trajectory.
- Address diversity issues by obtaining funding to support an increase in minority enrollment, identifying a specific mobility track for nurses of diverse cultures throughout their careers, and creating a specific curriculum to address diversity.
- Develop and distribute promotional and recruitment materials that attract individuals of diverse backgrounds into the variety of nursing career opportunities.
- Recruit retired nurses to form the foundation of a professional mentoring corps.
- Advocate for standardized internships and residencies through partnerships between schools of nursing, professional organizations, and practice sites. Graduates will participate in an individualized mentoring program to socialize them into the profession and enhance their knowledge of clinical practice.
- Negotiate professional development opportunities with employers that are supported through a variety of resources such as paid time off, education days, cost reimbursement, or as part of the scheduled workday.
- Create a website for leadership development activities and templates, and make it available for use by hospitals and nursing organizations.

Source: American Nurses Association. (2002). *Nursing's agenda for the future. A call to the nation.* Washington, DC: Author. Reprinted with permission.

# Recruitment

**Recruitment** focuses on finding the right staff for the right job when needed. Issues that are included in this discussion are the department of human resources' responsibilities, policies and procedures, employment legal issues, job analysis, and the employment process. Nurses are involved in all of these issues as managers, team leaders, staff nurses, new employees, or potential employees.

## Human Resources

The **human resources (HR) department** in a health care organization is responsible for ensuring that staff is recruited, hired, promoted and transferred, retained, and terminated according to the organization's policies, procedures, and relevant laws. The goal is to hire and retain the best staff possible to meet the mission and goals of the organization and its components.

FUNCTIONS AND ACTIVITIES    The Joint Commission, the primary organization for accreditation of health care organizations, includes management of human resources in its standards. The key focus areas are human resources planning; orienting, training, and educating staff; assessing competence, and managing staff requests.

It is not only important to find staff to fill openings, but it is also important to find competent staff. This is difficult to do with new graduates as confirmed by the IOM and also the recent report on nursing education (Institute of Medicine, 2004; Benner, Sutphen, Leonard, & Day, 2010). The IOM emphasized in its report on nursing that "Pre-licensure and pre-employment education cannot provide sufficient frequency and diversity of experiences (and sometimes offer no experience) in the performance of every clinical nursing intervention needed for every clinical condition found in patients, especially as the breadth of knowledge and technology expands. Nurses, therefore, like physicians, come to their initial place of employment as novices, without certain skills and knowledge—their limited skill and expertise reflecting the limitations of time and experience in their academic education" (2004, p. 202). Benner and colleagues recommend that new graduates should have a one-year, high-quality postgraduate residency (2010, p. 31), though this landmark nursing education report recognizes that there is also much more that needs to be done to improve pre-licensure nursing education as does the IOM (2010).

Meeting the goal of hiring competent staff requires planning by leaders to identify guidelines related to qualifications, competencies, and staffing. Competent staff must be provided to ensure that patient care goals are met. Staff competencies need to be assessed, maintained, and improved, which should be an ongoing process. A culture needs to be established in which self-development and learning are supported. When the Joint Commission standards are reviewed, it is clear that human resources does not work in isolation, but rather, the organization's leaders or management set the tone and guide human resources. It takes a coordinated and collaborative effort to ensure that recruitment and retention processes are functioning and effective, and this requires clear communication about the functions and activities to be carried out by human resources and management. Effective human resources departments have strong positive relationships with management, and staff feel that human resources is a support service for them, not a department that acts against them.

HUMAN RESOURCES POLICIES AND PROCEDURES    The human resources department in collaboration with management develops policies and procedures related to employment and staffing. Issues that are typically considered include hiring, promotion, transfers, termination, staffing and scheduling, benefits and staff requests, and other related issues. Procedures to ensure effective communication related to these policies and procedures are a critical concern as communication is a typical problem area. For example, staff may not be informed about a change in policy about work schedules, or a manager may not be informed about the hiring process. Required employment documentation needs to be clearly identified and implemented because this can have serious consequences on staff performance. Monitoring the implementation of policies and procedures is used to determine if standards are met. Health care organizations with labor unions must factor this into the management of their human resources. Labor contracts affect policies and procedures, documentation, monitoring, human resources decision making, and staff involvement.

LEGAL ISSUES   Laws, both federal and state, protect employers and employees. It is important for both the HR staff and management to understand these laws and their implications to the hiring, promotion, and termination processes. It is equally important for employees to understand the implications of these laws, many of which are not explained during orientation. The following descriptions highlight the major laws and how they affect employers and employees.

AMERICANS WITH DISABILITIES ACT (ADA)   The Americans with Disabilities Act of 1990 prohibits discrimination in hiring and job assignments based on disability (Pell, 2000). Reasonable accommodation must be made (for example, equipment for the hearing challenged, ramps for wheelchairs, allowing employees to work in an area of the building that is easier to get to, allowing reasonable time for medical appointments, and so on). Substance abuse is classified as a disability, as is mental illness. A past history of problems in these areas cannot be used to disqualify a qualified person for employment. If, however, the employee is unable to do the job due to absences or errors, or if the employee has a history of this work behavior in a previous position, the employee can be terminated for poor work habits. However, the employee may not be terminated for a disability. The employer can refuse to hire the candidate based on poor work habits, but not a history of substance abuse or mental illness.

EQUAL EMPLOYMENT OPPORTUNITY COMMISSION (EEOC)   The Equal Employment Opportunity Commission is the federal agency that administers the Civil Rights Act/EEO, the Age Discrimination in Employment Act, and the Americans with Disabilities Act. The EEOC is the agency that receives complaints when these laws may be violated. It conducts the investigation, makes the decisions as to fault, and designates the penalties. The EEOC can make an employer keep an employee or hire a candidate, require an employer to pay back pay, and even require that employee/candidate's legal fees are covered by the employer. The EEOC does not have to inform an employer that it is coming to investigate a complaint; however, records should not be turned over without presentation of a subpoena or a search warrant nor should staff be interviewed without legal counsel. Methods for avoiding EEOC problems include use of routine and appropriate management education about the laws and implications, implementation of policies and procedures that comply with the laws, recruitment that does not discriminate, development of standardized interviewing process, use of application forms that meet legal requirements, and maintenance of accurate notes regarding application and hiring, promotions, and terminations.

CIVIL RIGHTS ACT OF 1964   The Civil Rights Act of 1964 and its amendments have had a major effect on the workplace. This law prohibits discrimination in employment on the basis of race, color, sex, religion, or national origin. There is one section of this law, Title VII, that is particularly relevant, and it is referred to as the Equal Employment Opportunity (EEO) law (Pell, 2000). What does this law mean? Businesses with 15 or more employees cannot discriminate on the basis of race, color, or nationality. Questions on applications and during interviews cannot address these factors. Employment tests must be designed so as not to discriminate in these areas. The law also addresses discrimination based on religion, as businesses must now make reasonable accommodation for religious practice (for example, wearing of religious clothing and days off for religious holidays). Allowing for the latter does not mean that the business cannot make the employee use personal leave days for these days off nor are they required to pay them on these days. If meeting this requirement is an undue hardship for the business, then pay does not have to be provided. Businesses, however, can prohibit proselytizing in the workplace. This law also protects against discrimination on the basis of gender. Businesses can identify gender-specific positions; however, they must be clearly defined. Pregnancy cannot be used to discredit a woman for a position.

AFFIRMATIVE ACTION   Despite the fact that the Civil Rights Act of 1964 clearly states an employer cannot discriminate based on race, religion, national origin, or sex, giving preference to special groups continues to be a concern and is a highly controversial issue. Several presidential executive orders, beginning with those issued by President Johnson, require affirmative action for protected classes (African Americans, Hispanics, Asians or Pacific Islanders, Native Americans or Alaskan Natives, and women), which applies to all federal contractors and subcontractors that have contracts of more than $50,000 and have 50 or more employees (Pell, 2000). Executive orders are not laws and only apply to government agencies and organizations that do business with the government. Most health care organizations do business with the federal government, so many must meet these requirements. This business occurs when health care organizations accept Medicare and Medicaid payments for health care services that they provide. What does this mean to the employer? They must hire members from these protected classes "in proportion to the population of people in each class in their community" (Pell, 2000, p. 65). Employers must actively seek candidates from these minority groups. Over the years this effort has also led to accusations of reverse discrimination. In these cases, the complaint is that in giving members of the protected classes preference this denies or discriminates against someone who does not belong to one of the classes but is qualified for the position.

**FAMILY AND MEDICAL LEAVE LAW (FMLA)**   The Family and Medical Leave Law of 1996 applies to employers of 50 or more employees who work within a 75-mile radius. What does it cover? For employees who are eligible (and not all are eligible), it covers 12 weeks of unpaid leave during a 12-month period for medical reasons, which may include the birth or adoption of a child as well as care of a spouse, child, or parent who has a serious medical problem (Danaher, 2001). The medical problem may be mental or emotional illness. This law is complex, and when applied, it requires careful review. The employer may require that the employee submit medical certification of the claimed medical condition. If the employer has concerns about the validity of the certification, the employer can ask for a second medical opinion and even a third, but the employer is responsible for these costs. The employer may select the provider who will give additional medical opinions; however, this health care provider cannot be an employee of the employer (for example, a physician who works in the employer's hospital or clinic). Until all of the opinions are complete, the employee should receive FMLA benefits. For long-term or chronic conditions, the employer can request recertification but not second and third opinions.

**SEXUAL HARASSMENT (EEOC)**   Recent data from a national survey conducted from October 2001 through March 2002 of 7,600 nurses indicated that 19% of them had experienced sexual harassment or a hostile work environment related to other staff, and 19% had experienced harassment from physicians (*NurseWeek*, 2002). What is sexual harassment? First, it is a form of sex discrimination and a violation of the Civil Rights Act of 1964. In 1980, the Equal Employment Opportunity Commission (EEOC) further defined sexual harassment as "(1) unwelcomed sexual advances, (2) requests for sexual favors, (3) verbal conduct of a sexual nature, or (4) physical conduct of a sexual nature. These advances, requests, and types of conduct were considered sexual harassment when they (1) acted as a term or condition of employment, (2) were a criterion for employment decisions, (3) interfered with the victim's job performance, or (4) created a hostile, intimidating, or offensive work environment" (Aiken, 2001, p. 576). When an employee initiates a complaint, the employee must prove that there is a causal connection between the harassment and the job benefit in question or a quid pro quo (Aiken, 2001). This is one type of harassment. A second type is a hostile work environment that interferes with the employee's ability to perform the job. The EEOC decides whether or not the situation qualifies as a hostile environment. Some factors that are considered are (a) type of conduct (verbal, physical), (b) frequency of conduct, (c) whether offensive or hostile, (d) offender category such as supervisor or co-worker, (e) how many employees experienced the conduct, and (f) consistency of victim's conduct (Aiken, 2001). Other types of harassment are verbal, harassment of men, and harassment of homosexuals. Organizations should have a sexual harassment policy that describes how complaints are made. The EEOC has specific guidelines that need to be followed when complaints are filed with the EEOC (for example, there are time limits for filing complaints related to the alleged discriminatory act). Sexual harassment is a very emotional issue. Power over others plays a major role in this type of discrimination. There is abuse of authority, which is frightening. Harassers can be found at all levels and types of staff, in all types of organizations, and can be of either gender. Sexual harassment is extremely serious. "The employer can be held liable if the employer knew or should have known of the harassment and failed to take appropriate and immediate action to correct it" (Aiken, 2001, p. 579).

AGE DISCRIMINATION AND EMPLOYMENT ACT (ADEA) The Age Discrimination and Employment Act of 1967 and its amendments focus on age by prohibiting discrimination against anyone 40 years or older (Pell, 2000). In addition to this federal law, some states have their own laws protecting persons 18 years and older. This law covers businesses with 20 or more employees. As long as the person meets the requirements of the position, persons who fall in this age range cannot be denied the job. Many applications no longer include birth date or age, and most people do not include birth date on their resumes. How do some businesses try to get around this law? They say that the candidate is overqualified, the candidate made more money in his or her last position held than this position offers, or this is a trainee position. Businesses cannot say they will not cover older employees because their benefits will not cover them, because the law requires that the benefit plan, if it is offered, cover all employees. The Older Workers Benefits Protection Act of 1990 established this plan (Pell, 2000).

FEDERAL DRUG-FREE WORKPLACE ACT The Federal Drug-Free Workplace Act of 1988, which covers certain federal contractors and grantees and federal agencies, does not make screening for alcohol and drug use a requirement for employment; however, it does not make these tests illegal. This screening may be done as part of the pre-employment physical exam or at other times. Urine tests are usually used first, and then, if a problem is identified, blood tests may follow. The law does require that all federal contractors with contracts of more than $25,000: (a) Notify all employees in writing of the drug-free policy related to manufacturing, distributing, and using controlled substances, which are prohibited in the workplace (b) Provide a drug-free awareness and education program for employees (c) Provide employees with the policy statement, which employees must agree to follow (d) Violation of the policy must be punished, and employees must participate in rehabilitation, and (e) Establish as a condition of employment that employees must report, within 5 days, any criminal arrest and convictions for drug-related activity in the workplace (Pell, 2000).

WORKERS' COMPENSATION Workers' compensation is a very expensive type of insurance for employers, and its costs increased in the 1980s and early 1990s (Fox, 1998). This insurance is an important part of the national health care delivery system. Workers' compensation provides medical benefits and replacement of lost wages that result from injuries or illnesses that arise from the workplace. When an employee receives these benefits, the employee cannot then sue the employer for the injury. Typically, employees are provided workers' compensation coverage, as mandated by state law, employee medical benefits, and often disability benefits. Workers' compensation is not equivalent to employee medical benefits. Actually, workers' compensation was the first form of social insurance used in the United States. It is a social contract in that it is a form of mutual protection for the employee and the employer and is required by a federal law and delegated to states. The employer must follow state requirements related to benefits and limits. The financial status of the employer is not a factor in determining the type of plan it offers. The state's workers' compensation commission is the authority that supervises these health care services. States, however, do vary in the benefits they require.

Disability costs are an important part of workers' compensation costs. Workers' compensation is not, strictly speaking, health coverage. Most employers offer short-term disability that covers a portion of the worker's pay for up to 3 to 6 months after an incapacitating accident or illness. These policies may cover pregnancy and maternity leaves, usually for 10 weeks. Long-term disability becomes effective when short-term disability insurance coverage is exhausted (Gottlieb, 1998). Why is this insurance important? "For people between the ages of thirty-five and sixty-five, the odds of a disability lasting more than three months are three times greater than the chances of dying" (Gottlieb, 1998, p. 45). Paying for this care without any insurance can be a major financial crisis for most employees. Disability management is critical for most employers because it is used to control costs. Many workers who experience a disability feel a sense of entitlement of the benefit, and some experience a secondary gain from receiving this coverage. The entitlement or the workers' feeling that this benefit is "a right" can lead to workers demanding excessive medical care, and this in turn delays their return to work. As a result, employer costs also increase. Secondary gain comes from the wages the employee receives during the disability period without working.

Keeping workers' compensation separate from the traditional health care delivery system has not always proven to be the most cost-effective method of providing medical care for work-related injuries and illnesses. Workers' compensation is regulated under state laws. States vary in benefit levels, medical reimbursement schedules, and the amount of control that the employer has over employee medical choices. Occupational health nurses play an important role in the prevention of work-related injuries and illnesses as well as providing on-site treatment and follow-up.

WAGNER ACT OF 1935 AND THE TAFT-HARTLEY ACT OF 1948    The Wagner Act of 1935 and the Taft-Hartley Act of 1948, which amended the original law of 1935, cover issues related to employer–union relations (Pell, 2000). These laws prohibit discrimination based on union membership. Employers may not ask candidates if they are members of a union. Employers are no longer required to hire union members, but union contracts may specify that nonunion employees must join the union within a specific time period after they are hired. This is called "union shop." This issue has been taken over by some state laws, known as "right to work" laws, which prohibit "union shop" or fair-employment laws. This is an area that requires careful review of specific state law in addition to federal law.

EQUAL PAY ACT OF 1963    The Equal Pay Act of 1963 prohibits the determination of pay based on gender (Pell, 2000), referred to as "equal pay for equal work." The person must be legally able to work in the United States. Comparable worth is more than equal pay for equal work, and it is more than just addressing appropriate values to the employer. This is complicated and includes job analysis with points assigned to jobs so that even jobs that seem completely different may be of comparable worth based on such factors as education, training, responsibility, and so on.

IMMIGRATION REFORM AND CONTROL ACT OF 1986    The Immigration Reform and Control Act of 1986 prohibits the denial of employment due to nationality. However, there are key responsibilities that must be met when hiring immigrants, such as examining required documentation to prove identity and citizenship, or documents authorizing employment of noncitizens.

HR must be informed on changes in labor laws and share relevant information with management. If a health care organization is unionized, then this information must be factored in and managers must be knowledgeable about the union contract requirements.

## What Is Recruitment?

**Recruitment** is a planned and coordinated effort to ensure that competent and appropriate staff is available to meet the goals and provide the organization's services. The recruitment process includes five steps, which are described in Figure 9-1.

**FIGURE 9-1    The recruitment process.**

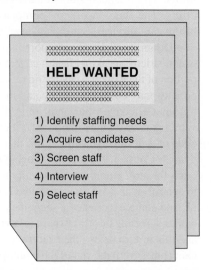

After this process is completed and a candidate accepts employment, then the final steps of admitting the candidate to employment and orientation take place. There is no doubt that recruitment is critical for any organization as without competent staff organizations will not be effective and will not survive. The goal is to hire the right person for the right job at the right time.

How do human resources and management get the right person in the right job at the right time? The first step is to have a clear understanding of the job or position and then develop a position description that meets the needs. Hiring criteria need to be developed to identify the attributes of successful employees, and these can then be used to help make hiring decisions (Hutchison, 2001a). The goal is to hire staff that has a chance of succeeding in order to decrease turnover and of course better ensure high-performance employees. This is not easy to accomplish as sometimes criteria do not effectively address critical characteristics. Hutchison (2001a) states, "Passion never should be overlooked because it is the single most universal trait of success" (p. 53). How can this attribute be evaluated? Interviewers can ask candidates about examples of when they made an extra effort to get something done and were enthusiastic about something at work. What examples can be described to indicate a drive toward success, leadership, and a pattern of growth? Other issues to consider in hiring criteria are (a) education and work experience, (b) problem-solving skills, (c) personal values, (d) specific clinical skills, and (e) cultural fit. Cultural fit with the organization is important as staff tend to stay in organizations where they feel there is a match between their values and the organization's values—staff will be happier when this occurs. Since change is ever present today, asking candidates to describe their experiences with change can be helpful in identifying the right employee for the job by assessing their coping styles when change occurs.

**Job analysis** includes a clear description of responsibilities and skills for a specific job. How does HR arrive at this description? Various methods such as observation of performance, interviews of staff who hold the position, interviews of supervisors/managers, and discussions with team members, and how other organizations describe a similar position, are used to gather data about jobs/positions. The result should be the **position description**, which lays out the job expectations to be used for hiring and performance evaluation. The typical parts of a job or position description include the following:

- **Education**—the type and level required to meet the job requirements (for example, a BSN degree)
- **Skills**—the skills the new employee needs to meet the job requirements (for example, EKG analysis for a cardiac care unit position)
- **Work experience**—what past experiences and duration are related to present job requirements (for example, 2 years as staff nurse in a medical-surgical unit for a home health position)
- **Physical strength or stamina**—what is required to meet the job requirements (for example, heavy lifting)
- **Intelligence**—specific requirements for the job, which may be measured by standardized tests, but is not frequently identified in health care position descriptions
- **Communication skills**—should be specified (for example, ability to lead groups for a position in a mental health clinic)
- **Accuracy of work**—jobs requiring detail and those that must be done right the first time (for example, data entry)
- **Stress level**—what is the level and need for coping skills (for example, ability to handle rapid patient turnover for a position in an Emergency Department)
- **Special factors**—might include fluency in a foreign language, willingness to travel, willingness to work on weekends, or to be on call (Pell, 2000, pp. 24–25)

Each of these specifications must meet any relevant legal requirements.

## The Employment Process

The employment process is long and complex. It, of course, begins with recruitment of candidates. Typical methods used to attract job candidates include (a) print advertising (newspapers, professional journals), (b) Internet, (c) job fairs, and (d) use of nurse recruiters. Word-of-mouth is also an important method. The latter is what has driven the use of incentives that some health care organizations have used to encourage their staff to refer job candidates. To attract nursing students many employers are now meeting with nursing students in schools of nursing. Some schools of nursing have required co-op programs where students spend some time employed in a guided situation as for example at Northeastern University. Another strategy used by some hospitals is nurse internship programs offered to nursing students between their junior and senior year. This is done to get students involved in the organization and to see how they do in the intern role. These students may then be offered positions after graduation. The students are familiar with working in the hospital, which can assist in orientation. After receiving resumes, these candidates then need to be screened. During **screening**, applications are reviewed in more detail, and selections are made for interviews. Preparation for interviews takes time. After the interviews, another selection is made to determine if additional interviews are required, additional candidates should be sought, or who will be offered the position. The offer is then made, and negotiation may take place. It is important to frequently evaluate the process, which is highly dependent on communication that can easily fail.

It is very important to remember that the very first initial contact in the employment process is a potential employee's first impression of the employer. Many potential employees are lost when they are unimpressed with the process and associate this with the organization. When telephone calls go unanswered; staff members do not respond when they say that they will; applications are lost; or staff is rude on the telephone, potential employees may look elsewhere for employment.

SCREENING   The goal of screening is to identify those candidates who should be evaluated further. Screening actually can take place more than once. The first time may be when potential candidates call or e-mail for further information. A second opportunity for screening is after candidates submit resumes and in some cases applications to determine which candidates will be interviewed. The third screening is directly involved in the final decision when choices are made about additional interviews, or a candidate is selected for the position. Sources of data that are used in screening are by telephone and e-mail, application, references, resume, licensure, certification status, and in-person interview contact.

PROS AND CONS OF APPLICATION FORMATS   Applications are important. A candidate may send a resume and then indicate on application, "See resume." Candidates, however, should be required to complete the organization's application. First, this protects the organization legally—the organization is meeting the requirements of employment laws. Applications also provide a standard record of information about candidates that can be used when recruitment is evaluated; when consistent types of data from the applications are needed; and it also provides one consistent source of information about employees. When candidates are compared, then the application is the best source for comparison data.

Despite the fact that applications provide a consistent format for information about candidates, it is important to approach application review with some flexibility. This requires, first, a clear understanding of the position and need. If the position description says the candidate must have 5 years of experience but the candidate only has 3 years, this should be considered with an open mind. In some cases, a candidate may not have the required experience but has some characteristics that indicate the candidate could quickly adapt and learn to meet the job requirements. Reviewing the application form with a rigid eye may lead to missing out on an important candidate. Another problem that can occur is reviewing candidates too quickly because positions need to be filled. When there is a shortage in nursing, it is easy to think any nurse is better than none. In this case, little or no consideration may be given to the job requirements and matching them with the best candidate. This can lead to serious performance problems.

RESUME   In reviewing **resumes**, the format or style does make a difference. The chronological style, the most commonly seen resume, is an easy style to review and provides an overall picture of the candidate with a listing of jobs by dates of employment. The functional style is organized around functions that the candidate performed in previous jobs (for example, direct care, management, and patient education functions). This style may not provide as much detailed information and also may not describe duration of employment, but it does build up experience. Red flags that require further investigation are (a) gaps in dates, (b) more information supplied on earlier positions than more current ones, (c) overemphasis on education and non-job factors, and (d) poor grammar and spelling.

REFERENCES   References are typically requested at some time during the hiring process. Human resources staff contacts references via telephone or request written information. Candidates supply names, telephone numbers, and addresses for their references.

LICENSURE   Licensure is very important to many positions in the health care setting such as registered nurses. Some time during the application process, employers will ask for the nurse's professional license number, renewal date, and the state that issued the license. Typically after the position is accepted, the candidate must show the license and/or submit a copy of it. This is required by state licensure boards to ensure that appropriate staff for example registered nurses are licensed. Checking licensure of a nurse candidate with the state board of nursing may lead to information about professional misconduct. However, the reporting of misconduct and disciplinary action process is not perfect. It is the employer who needs to make the decision about offering employment, but only licensed professionals can hold positions that require licensure.

CERTIFICATION STATUS   Certification is also important for some positions. Probably, the certification that covers many who work in health care is cardiopulmonary resuscitation certification. Candidates may be asked if certified and when hired to show documentation. Other certifications that may be relevant are nursing certifications for specific clinical practice for example for nursing specialties of community health, gerontological, maternal-child, and others; nurse practitioner specialties such as family, adult, pediatric; and clinical specialists. See Media Links for the American Nurses Credentialing Center website.

THE INTERVIEW PROCESS   The interview is a critical step in the hiring process; in fact, it is the most important method used in selecting staff. It is costly and time-consuming, and so must be done with thought, from the selection of the candidates to interview, preparation for the interviews, the interview itself, and then analysis of the interview results so that the best possible decisions can be made.

INTERVIEWER: PLANNING FOR THE INTERVIEW   The interview step begins as soon as candidates are selected for interviews, which will affect the number and types of interviews as well as when they will take place. Interview appointments must be made, frequently requiring coordination of schedules between many people. The candidate needs to be told who will be doing the interviews and their positions, locations, time frames, and any other pertinent information such as parking and information to bring to the interview. All staff who will be involved in the interviews needs to be sent a copy of the candidate's resume and, if available, an application as well as being informed about the time, place, and so on, for the interview. Prior to the interview, those who are interviewing the candidate need to review the candidate's resume and application, if the application has been completed prior to the appointment. Time should be spent in developing questions that will be asked during the interview. Although both the interviewer and interviewee are interviewing one another, the interviewer should be in control of the process. Preparing ahead will better ensure that this control is maintained. There may be more than one interview so, after the first interview, a decision must be made to ask the candidate to return for a second interview. All of this requires planning with multiple people and receipt of their feedback. The interviewee/candidate should be told the steps that follow the interview (for example, when decisions will be made and how the candidate will be informed).

INTERVIEWING GUIDELINES   An interview is a formal discussion, although many approach it more casually. An effective result requires some thought and homework. It is, however, not helpful to have an overly structured interview in which the interviewer does not allow for some flexibility as topics arise. Follow-up is critical during the interview. Effective interviewers are cognizant of the relevant laws and how they impact questions asked in the interview and on the process itself.

Language during the interview is also affected by employment laws—what can be said or not said. Another concern is actually saying too much about the position to the candidate before the candidate is given the opportunity to share information. If this is done, the candidate has more opportunity to formulate responses that match the position requirements, which may or may not be an accurate reflection of the candidate or candidate's experiences.

It is easy for many interviewers to quickly jump to a conclusion about a candidate soon after the interview begins or even in initial telephone conversations. Biases—what is seen or heard— can lead to positive or negative responses to the candidate. This can also work in the reverse, in that the candidate can have biases about the employer and also jump to conclusions before all the facts are known. "It is good to realize that most people are not at their best during an interview. It takes 20 minutes for most candidates to become less tense and open up for the talented intervie- wee to let down her guard" (Hutchison, 2001a, p. 54).

EVALUATION CRITERIA    Evaluation and selection of candidates involves reviewing all the material available on the candidates. All staff members who are involved in the process need to share their feedback in a timely fashion, whether this is written or verbal. Then the hiring criteria are used to make a final determination. The identification of person or persons who will make the final decision should be clear to all involved in the process.

There are structured and unstructured interviews; however, there needs to be some structure in every interview for it to be effective. This is where planning becomes important—considering what needs to be asked and why. There may be a list of standard questions that are routinely asked and then supplemented with more job-specific and individual candidate questions. Having a list of questions better ensures that all questions are asked. Some organizations use group interviews with a group of key staff sitting in on the same interview. In this case, the group should work out procedures about asking questions and follow-up. Again, this is done to ensure that everything is covered. If the interview appears disorganized, the job candidate may then conclude that the staff is disorganized. Candidates should be told if there will be a group interview.

The interview should begin with establishing rapport. Privacy, of course, is important during the entire process. Introductions of all staff members present should be done with some brief statement about their roles. After a few introductory comments to put the candidate at ease, the interview should begin. Most of the questions should be open ended. Box 9-2 provides some sample questions and content to consider.

The interviewer should allow the interviewee/candidate time to respond and not feed the interviewee answers or cut the interviewee off. The interview should stay on task and not wander off. As the interview progresses, information found in the candidate's resume and application should be explored. One technique that is useful is the nondirective approach, which encourages the candidate to expand on ideas (Pell, 2000). This might include "Tell me more about. . . ." Nodding the head and using other methods to indicate interest will lead the candidate on to say more. Health care organizations are using more situational questions by asking nurse candidates what they would do for specific problems or by discussing hypothetical situations. Using real examples instead of hypothetical ones can be more helpful as "people tend to repeat actions" (Hutchison, 2001a, p. 55). When candidates discuss their own experiences this can provide infor- mation about how they might handle similar problems. This allows the interviewer to gauge the interviewee's critical thinking and ability to handle multiple problems. Of course, the interviewer must be knowledgeable about the situation proposed in order to assess the response and ask follow-up questions. Another technique is to end with summarizing questions by asking the can- didate to summarize some aspect of the discussion. The candidate might also be asked about examples of when the candidate was resourceful, received criticism, worked under supervision, and worked with others. The applicant may also be asked to describe him or herself. At the end of the interview, the candidate needs to be given the opportunity to ask additional questions and told about the next steps in the process. During the interview, the interviewer should take notes to ensure that information is not forgotten.

Interviewers can make serious mistakes during the interview that may lead to obtaining inadequate information and to poor decision making. Talking too much can be deadly as it limits time for the candidate to respond. Cutting the candidate off by jumping in too soon with another question or comment is not helpful either. The interviewer does need to be in the control of the interviewer. To accomplish this, the interviewer needs to be clear about the position, know the interview questions that need to be asked, and aware of the content of the candidate's resume and application. Interviewers need to listen and follow-up on questions or important information may be ignored. Throughout the interview the interviewer's body language and communication techniques are important. The candidate will watch for cues and interest. For example, if the interviewer communicates through body language that there is limited interest in the candidate even though this may not be the case (the interviewer may just be tired), the candidate may decide that this is not the organization where he or she wants to work. If there are doubts about the candidate and the particular position or fit with the organization, then the interviewer should comment on this and allow the candidate to respond (Carroll, 2001). This might open up the discussion, allowing the candidate to further expand on experiences and skills, and help in the selection process.

At some point in the application process, it is important to offer the candidate the opportunity to visit units or other worksites. This allows the candidate to see the work environment and staff. As this is time-consuming and costly, since it does take staff time, this visit should be planned with staff accompanying the candidate and should not disturb work or interfere with patient care. With the increasing concern and legal requirements about patient privacy and confidentiality, consideration

## BOX 9-2　SAMPLE JOB INTERVIEW QUESTIONS AND CONTENT

These questions and content areas might be used in a job interview. Candidates for positions should give these some thought prior to interviewing.

### CLINICAL EXPERIENCE

- Discuss your most recent nursing experience.
- Describe your experiences with nursing procedures.
- What are your strengths in nursing skills?
- Discuss the documentation system with which you are most familiar.
- Describe what you feel is an appropriate work schedule.

### NURSING SKILLS

- How would you organize care for a patient? What needs take priority?
- Describe the nursing care you give.
- Describe how you feel about and use nursing care plans.
- Tell me about your best example of patient teaching.
- Describe what skills you have that would benefit this unit.

### LEADERSHIP

- Discuss your concept of "team building" skill and interprofessional work.
- If you had your choice, would you choose primary care, total patient care, functional care with a medication nurse, or team nursing? Why do you prefer this model?
- Tell me how you would conduct a patient care conference.
- Discuss a situation in which you approached a physician concerning a problem with a patient.
- If you were a team leader, how would you handle a problem with a team member's care?

### SELF-ASSESSMENT AND MOTIVATION

- Describe a major accomplishment during your last experience (college, work).
- Discuss how you plan to continue to grow personally and professionally. What are your short-term and long-term goals?
- Explain how this position fits into your career goals 3 to 5 years from now.
- What factors do you wish to avoid in nursing positions?

### HUMAN RELATIONS AND RESPONSIBILITY

- Describe the working relationship between the RN, LPN, and UAP. Provide some examples from your own experience.
- What is your management style? What do you assess in supervising others?
- What factors in your college career were most and least challenging?

needs to be given as to the private information about patients the candidate might view during tours. Staff members who escort the candidate need to be briefed as to their role and should be willing to do this, or it will not provide the most positive view of the organization. However, this should not be a staged experience with the staff member told what to say or not to say to the candidate. The candidate will notice this, and it will not be a positive experience for the candidate. After the tour the staff member can share information with HR or a manager about questions the candidate asked, concerns expressed by the candidate, and the candidate's communication skills.

THE JOB CANDIDATE AND THE INTERVIEW   The job candidate should arrive at least 10 to 15 minutes early to allow time to unwind and collect his or her thoughts before the interview. Parking information and directions should be clarified before going to the interview to avoid getting lost and being late. When entering the room for the interview, it is best to first see if the interviewer offers direction to a specific seat; if this does not occur, the best seat is one that is directly opposite the interviewer. During the interview, sharing of personal information should be limited. It is important to be aware of and avoid behaviors that indicate nervousness such as swinging legs, clinching hands, pencil tapping, knuckle cracking, and chewing gum. Dress should be business attire.

Before the interview, the interviewee should consider personal career goals and experiences. If the job candidate is a new graduate, the candidate should think about clinical experiences from courses taken. These may serve as examples during the interview. Coming to the interview with prepared questions that address critical issues demonstrates an understanding of the position sought. Finding out about the organization, its nursing services, and nursing staff prior to the interview is helpful. It also communicates interest.

The type of position sought is also a consideration that affects questions that might be asked (for example, questions about responsibilities and types of patients and patient problems). Other issues that might be considered are the organization's culture, mission and vision, communication within nursing, interprofessional and organization-wide policies, scheduling, staff development and career advancement, differential for education and certification, and ability to change positions and receive promotions. It is important for the job candidate to listen to the interviewer and to clarify questions that might be confusing before answering them. As the candidate goes through the process, the candidate should consider if this is the place he or she wants to work. The American Nurses Association (2001) developed a Bill of Rights for Registered Nurses, which can be used as a guide to assist in the evaluation of the workplace, as described in Box 9-3.

Interviewing provides experience in how to evaluate organizations and positions. Even an interview for a position that might be of limited interest can give nurses more experience about the process. Some nurses even work for temporary agencies so that they can get into an organization and learn more about it before pursuing a long-term position in the organization.

---

**BOX 9-3**   **BILL OF RIGHTS FOR REGISTERED NURSES**

1. Nurses have the right to practice in a manner that fulfills their obligations to society and to those who receive nursing care.
2. Nurses have the right to practice in environments that allow them to act in accordance with professional standards and legally authorized scopes of practice.
3. Nurses have the right to a work environment that supports and facilitates ethical practice, in accordance with the *Code for Nurses* and its interpretive statements.
4. Nurses have the right to freely and openly advocate for themselves and their patients, without fear of retribution.
5. Nurses have the right to fair compensation for their work, consistent with their knowledge, experience, and professional responsibilities.
6. Nurses have the right to a work environment that is safe for themselves and their patients.
7. Nurses have the right to negotiate the conditions of their employment, either as individuals or collectively, in all practice settings.

Source: American Nurses Association. (2001, September/October). *The American Nurse*, p. 20. Reprinted with permission. All rights reserved.

POST-INTERVIEW AND SELECTION    References should be checked carefully, although responses are frequently vague. When this occurs, the person who calls for references should push for more information. There is only so much that can be done to encourage a past employer to reveal information, as many organizations have been advised by attorneys not to reveal information (Pell, 2000). This does not, however, mean that attempts to obtain this information from references should not be made.

Federal regulations require **background checks** for some health care providers who apply for clinical privileges, such as physicians and dentists (Fiesta, 1999). This information is checked in the National Practitioner Data Bank every 2 years. Long-term care employers are often required by state laws to check their employees, including nursing staff. Some acute care hospitals now do background checks. Initial registered nurse licensure now requires fingerprinting to be used for a background check. Of particular interest in criminal background checks are patient abuse and neglect, rape, and child abuse.

Personnel testing is done for some positions, but this is not as common for nursing positions. Some organizations require a pre-employment physical. Alcohol and drug screening may be included in the physical, but it must meet the requirements of the Federal Drug-Free Workplace Act of 1988. The candidate cannot be discriminated against based on disability.

Selection of candidates for positions must be done thoughtfully. This decision needs to include all staff that had a formal role in the process and all relevant information (the resume, application, information from interviews, and reference information). Many organizations have forms that are used to evaluate candidates based on specific criteria. The staff member who is responsible for making the job offer should be clearly identified, and typically, this is someone in HR. This staff member needs to know what is negotiable and what is not before contacting the candidate. If negotiation is then done, the staff person needs to know who in the organization needs to be consulted about the negotiation with the candidate and kept informed of the progress.

The candidate is involved in the negotiation of the salary, but what should the candidate consider? The first step is a self-assessment of worth. This is also important when a nurse wants an increase in salary. The self-assessment should consider factors such as education, experience, certification, cost of coverage by a temporary agency nurse or outsourcing compared with the employee, and contributions that the nurse has made in previous positions (or in the present position if seeking a promotion rather than a new position). Arguments for the salary need to be clearly made, discussed, and then at the end of the meeting there should be a summarization of the critical reasons used to support the salary change. After the position is accepted, then the candidate is informed about the next steps to take and what the employer will do. If the candidate rejects the position, it is helpful to know the reason as this information may assist in understanding recruitment problems.

WHEN IS THE JOB THE RIGHT JOB?    There are many factors to consider when deciding to accept or reject a job offer. The benefit package is the description of services or additional pay that the employer offers employees, and benefits are important factors when accepting a position. Employers may cover these benefits, or the employee and employer may share the costs for them, often at a reduced rate for the employee. The benefits that are offered vary from employer to employer. Benefits are not required, but they go a long way to attract potential competent employees to accept positions. Labor unions affect the types of benefits offered, as this is part of the negotiated labor contracts; however, not all health care organizations are unionized. Potential employees should evaluate benefits carefully. It is important to understand individual needs, and then evaluate the benefit package based on this information. If information is not clear or there are questions, candidates for positions, new employees, and long-term employees should address these with the organization's human resources staff. During new employee orientation, benefits are typically discussed. If a nurse changes positions, there could be an effect on benefits, so this needs to be addressed. What are some of the benefits that might be offered in a benefit package by health care organizations?

- Insurance: health, life, disability, dental, vision
- Vacation and/or personal leave

- Sick days
- Maternity/paternity leave/family leave
- Paid time off (PTO) shift differential
- Charge nurse differential
- Differential for nurses with advanced degrees
- "On Call" pay
- Credit union
- Recruitment bonus
- Relocation assistance
- Housing assistance
- Uniform allowance
- Flexible scheduling/job sharing
- Orientation, refresher courses, continuing education
- Nurse internships and residencies
- Career ladder
- Education assistance (undergraduate-graduate)
- Reduced fee for gym facilities
- Discounted or free meals in facility cafeteria
- Free or discounted parking
- Child care such as pre-school on site
- Other services such as drop off/pick up cleaning, making appointments for staff, are offered by some health care organizations

Most nurses in their career will work in a variety of settings and hold several different types of positions. Some of this will be due to changes in educational levels, but it is also due to changes in interest and personal requirements such as scheduling and level of responsibility. An advantage of nursing as a profession is there are so many different ways that a nurse can practice and places where that practice can take place. With the variety of positions available, there are a number of job-related factors that the nurse needs to consider when evaluating a new position.

- The nurse applicant will want to decide whether or not the level of work required meets the nurse's personal needs and career goals. This would include (a) working part time or full time, or (b) shifts (day, evening, night, 12-hour shifts, or short shifts, which are used to cover busy times and when there are short staff periods).
- The type of health care organization may make a difference on whether or not the nurse is able to meet individual needs, goals, and skill level. Examples of organizations are (a) community, (b) acute care, (c) long-term care, (d) academic medical centers, (e) smaller community hospitals, (f) schools, (g) home care, and (h) other types of organizations.
- A critical question should be whether or not the position focuses on direct or indirect care. Making this decision will eliminate or clarify which positions to pursue.
- As positions are evaluated, the nursing delivery model that is used may be important. Is primary nursing or a form of team nursing used?
- How are team leaders chosen and how will this affect the applicant's interests?
- If the applicant has no interest in being a team leader at the time and team leadership is rotated among team members, then this may not be the position for the nurse.
- Another area of concern that each nurse should assess is the nurse's strengths and weaknesses. Weaknesses can be changed with education and/or additional experience, but to do this they need to first be acknowledged. The areas that need consideration when identifying strengths and weaknesses are (a) technical skills, (b) interpersonal relationship skills, (c) communication, (d) leadership, and (e) management skills. It is not expected that a nurse be at a high level of functioning in all these areas, but an honest appraisal is helpful. Certain positions require more of some skills than others. Mental health nurses clearly need to be more skillful in interpersonal relationships and communication, although they still need some basic technical skills. A nurse who works in the community needs to have strong skills in interpersonal relationships, communication, epidemiology, leadership, and management, but if the nurse is working in the community as a home health nurse, technical skills will be a critical part of the position competencies.

■ The last consideration is specialty area, something that also may change over time. Specialty positions are also affected by education and certification. Some specialty decisions may be driven by required experience level before employment in that specialty area. Some organizations offer internships to further prepare nurses for work in the specialty, such as in intensive care or the operating room.

What is happening when a lot of effort is made to find a new position, but no offers are coming in (Cardillo, 2002)? If a nurse is getting interviews, but still no offers, it is important to do an assessment of the interviews. Issues to consider are communication, how one is coming across, strengths that are emphasized, and responses to interviewer questions. Clearly, this is not easy to consider as it requires stepping back and taking an objective viewpoint. Obtaining some assistance with interviewing can be helpful. It might be helpful to follow-up with an interviewer who did not offer a job and ask for feedback with the goal of improvement. If a nurse is not getting calls for interviews, then the resume and cover letter may need to be reviewed. Asking others to review the resume and cover letter can provide helpful, objective feedback. It could be that the positions that are sought are just not appropriate to the nurse's education or experience. Networking can be helpful, as can using mentors to help identify possible positions that might be a better fit. Self-assessment is never easy, particularly when there seems to be little success; however, if done well and with as much objectivity as possible, it can lead to some changes that may result in more positive results.

# Retention: Why Is It Important?

Organizations that ignore staff **retention** soon experience problems with quality of care and costs. Staff retention keeps the organization going and meeting its mission and goals. Staff is needed to meet these goals. "The nursing philosophy, standards, rules that determine the working conditions, perception of peer cohesion, administrative support, autonomy, task orientation, work pressure, clarity, control, and innovation all help to develop the organization culture and maintain it" (Finkelman, 1996, p. 2–1:2). When staff does not mesh with the culture, problems occur such as staff frustration, unsatisfactory job performance, and decreased quality of care. (See Chapter 7 for further discussion about an organization's culture.) These all affect staff negatively and can lead to loss of staff. Problems with retention are extremely costly for health care organizations. Every organization has to make a concerted effort to create an environment that helps to retain staff, particularly nursing staff. "The purpose of recruitment is to hire the staff necessary for your agency to provide quality care. Retention is the tool that will allow your recruitment program to meet these goals. If you cannot retain your staff, you will never be able to recruit sufficient staff" (Hutchison, 2001b, p. 15).

## Turnover: Costs, Reasons, Prevention

**Turnover** problems are related to retention, as commented on earlier in this chapter, there are turnover problems particularly with new graduates. The costs of turnover are great, most notably the costs incurred during the recruiting and hiring process, orientation, and maintaining the staff member, such as human resources records, staff development provided, and so on. Turnover costs typically are from $22,000 to more than $64,000 per nurse (Jones & Gates, 2007). The variation in cost depends upon the type of nursing for example the turnover costs for an intensive care nurse is higher due to the need more orientation and training. In addition, turnover causes great strain on work teams. Staff turnover is extremely costly to health care organizations. The first thought when considering turnover costs is it is simple, but it is not. The following are all part of turnover costs:

■ Advertising for new staff
■ Interviewing job candidates (Nursing and human resources departments are involved.)
■ Administrative time in human resources (job posting, position control, referencing, and investigation)
■ Union requirements
■ Terminal pay-outs

- Lost productivity and intellectual property
- Pre-employment physicals and drug screens
- Increased use of per diems and travelers
- Bed and unit closures
- Orientation and training costs
- Preceptor time
- Employment agencies
- Increased overtime
- Increased call-outs
- Elevated weekend rotations
- Elevated shift and floating rotations
- Impact on morale and additional turnover effects
- Increased stress that can lead to medical problems and increased use of health benefits (Colosi, 2002, p. 53)

When new staff must be oriented and become part of the team, this affects a unit's or a team's productivity, decreasing productivity time, which is costly. If the turnover becomes a more extensive problem, the organization as a whole suffers, leading to stress and frustration as more and more staff try to cope with empty positions, orient new staff, and adjust to new team members or temporary staff. Work teams eventually develop communication and methods of working together, but all of this takes time. When this is disturbed, work is disturbed. When there is a variance that disturbs the productivity, turnover rates need to be monitored and analyzed. It is important to identify the reasons for the turnover.

Clearly, there are reasons for turnover that are related to natural life events, such as births, ill family members, spouse job changes and required relocation, a need to stay home with younger children, and a return to school. If a move is required and the health care organization is a state or national organization, encouraging staff to stay in the system can be helpful for the health care system. An example is a nurse who works for the VA system able to transfer to another VA hospital in the system. Employers need to monitor the reasons staff members are leaving their jobs because some of the reasons can be addressed through prevention methods (for example, by providing child care, encouraging nurses to work part time while in school, and supporting them with educational benefits). Staff members view reasons for turnover differently as their personal perspective comes into play. One of the simplest interventions that can be used to help prevent retention problems is to let staff know they are appreciated—recognition and "thank you" is one place to start when addressing retention problems. It is also important for organizations to ask What is good about the organization? What does it offer its staff? What is unique about it? Where does it need to improve? Answers to these questions can help an organization develop an action plan to retain staff. Organizations want to retain their best people, but this takes effort. When management assumes that staff must be satisfied when they are good at their jobs, this may lead to a false sense of security. "But although competence can certainly help a person get hired, its effect is generally short lived. People who are good at their jobs aren't necessarily engaged by them" (Butler & Waldroop, 1999, p. 147). Job sculpting can and should be used by managers to help retain the best. "Job sculpting is the art of matching people to jobs that allow their deeply embedded life interests to be expressed. It is the art of forging a customized career path in order to increase the chance of retaining talented people" (Butler & Waldroop, 1999, p. 146). If this process is turned over to human resources, it will not be effective because it needs to come from management. Listening to staff is the place to begin. What excites a staff member? Using performance review time to discuss those things that make the staff member excited about work can be very useful and involves the staff member in the sculpting. Job sculpting must be done from a realistic stance. What can be done to help the staff member improve? What can be changed in the workplace to assist the staff member in becoming involved in activities that really drive the staff member forward and stimulate interest? It has to be remembered that "when job sculpting requires taking away parts of a job an employee dislikes, it also means finding someone new to take them on. If staffing levels are sufficient, that won't be a problem—an uninteresting part of one person's job may be perfect for someone else" (Butler & Waldroop, 1999, p. 152). However, there are many times when there is no one else who can do the parts of the job that the staff member does not like to do. Managers must be careful about promising too much as this can lead to even greater staff frustration and retention problems. Strategies for retaining staff should focus on providing "a safe and caring work environment, offer a good orientation, create pride, have a forum for open communication, be honest in the expectations of the position, and be competitive in salary and benefits" (Hutchison, 2001b, p. 16).

## Staff Role

Staff plays a major role in retention of other staff. How staff works together can make an important difference in whether or not staff feels comfortable in the work environment. Motivation especially has a major impact. What motivates staff to work? Motivation is complex and very individual. It helps to explain why one staff member works differently or better than another, and this has a direct effect on performance. The typical factors that affect motivation are (a) job design, (b) organizational structure, (c) autonomy and empowerment, (d) staff participation in decision making, (e) communication, (f) leadership style, (g) organizational culture, (h) ethics, and (i) mutual trust between management and staff (Finkelman, 1996). Some assume that job satisfaction and motivation are the same, but they are not, although they are related. "Job satisfaction is a consequence of rewards and punishment related to past performance. Job dissatisfaction leads to decreasing morale, increasing absenteeism, and turnover" (Finkelman, 1996, p. 2–1:7). Motivation may be influenced by the need to have a job, need for another pay level, or a different work schedule. Nurse managers and their actions have an impact on staff motivation. Actions such as providing positive feedback, recognizing work effort, some degree of flexibility, asking staff to take part in decision making, providing resources staff needs to do its jobs, and trying to find the best staff to fill empty positions and retain staff that improves the level of productivity all demonstrate that management is concerned about staff.

Another important factor in staff retention is the efforts that are made in career advancement. Identifying staff with skills and expertise for promotion is an important management responsibility. The "Peter Principle" or promoting past one's ability is not what should be done, but rather staff members who can succeed should be the ones promoted (Peter & Hull, 1969). Organizations must also provide support, training, and opportunities for further education to staff. This can be very effective in retaining staff. Then staff feels recognized and more motivated to remain.

## Orientation: Its Role in Retention and Prevention of Reality Shock

**Orientation** is a key tool for getting staff members ready to do the job they were hired to do and important staff retention. As mentioned earlier, organized postgraduate residencies can be helpful to new graduates. They still complete orientation, but the residency provides them with more intensive support, guided experience, and further education.

A work contract or commitment is established during orientation as new staff gains a greater understanding of the organization and its expectations. Spirit and respect are critical during the orientation process. New staff should get the sense of respect given to staff and the importance of staff input. Commitment to a job tends to decrease if staff members

- Do not feel safe and secure.
- Consider their pay or benefits inadequate.
- Believe their position is not what was presented in the interview and hiring process.
- See their managers as non-responsive.
- Perceive administration as non-responsive (Hutchison, 2001b, p. 16).

Along with orientation, staff development and continuing education are important tools in retention as well as recruitment. A strong program that ensures staff competency will be noticed by candidates for positions and will go a long way to retaining staff.

What is an effective orientation program? First, it must be organized, and orientee feedback needs to be used to evaluate orientation to appropriate changes. Orientation should include up-to-date general information about the organization. Typical content includes the organization's vision, mission, goals, structure, human resources or personnel policies and procedures, benefits, communication, labor union (if applicable), and staff education or development. Specific orientation is given about the worksite or unit including its relevant goals, structure, communication, policies and procedures, and (if applicable) shared governance and career advancement. Preceptors should be assigned to orientees to assist with their orientation. The best preceptors are those who volunteer and can be available to the new staff. Preceptors help new staff, particularly recent graduates, develop the following:

- Increased confidence and competence in the clinical setting
- In-depth understanding of the nurse's role
- Increased ability to problem-solve through critical thinking
- Feelings of belonging and professional nurturance (Diehl-Oplinger & Kaminski, 2000, p. 46)

Orientation is often viewed as boring and approached with dread. Orientation programs that try to make it a more interactive experience, allowing new employees time to get to know one another as well as the other staff, are more effective. The experience should provide new employees with the information and tools that they need to begin a new position in the organization. Orientation is also important for employees who are changing positions, from one area to another or through a promotion, but this orientation is often neglected. When new positions are considered, nurses should ask about preceptors and their use in orientation. Potential employees should ask what is provided to staff that changes positions or is promoted within the organization in these circumstances, as this will demonstrate how the organization values career advancement and change.

## Losing Staff

Losing staff should be an organizational concern. Analyzing the reasons for staff resignations is the place to begin and then, whenever possible, these causes need to be resolved.

Terminating staff is never easy. It needs to be done thoughtfully with a clear understanding about the reasons for the **termination**. Staff is often given the opportunity to resign. A manager may use the time to counsel the staff member, particularly if the manager feels that the position or type of nursing are not the best fit for the staff member. Most staff, however, is usually quite upset and has difficulty hearing this advice. How terminations are handled and why staff is terminated has a tremendous effect on staff morale. Although termination is initiated by the organization this does not mean that the organization should ignore the reasons for the terminations (for example, staff that has been terminated due to an inability to fulfill job requirements). Causes for this should be analyzed. Staff may not be clear about expectations, not know how to do the job, lack continuing education on the job responsibilities, and so on.

Resignation should be carried out in a positive manner even when negative feelings are felt (Cardillo, 2002). The first resource a nurse should consult is the employee policies and procedures, which should describe what is expected of employees at the time of resignation. It is also important that the immediate supervisor be informed before gossip gets to the supervisor about the resignation, which can come from an internal or external source. After verbal notice is given, a written letter of resignation is provided addressed to the immediate supervisor. Copies are sent to the department director and human resources. This letter needs to be clear, well written, and typed on good but plain stationary. It is not appropriate to use the letter as a vent for negative feedback. The letter will be kept in personnel files and thus will be referred to if references are sought. How a nurse terminates from a position can make a difference in obtaining future positions. Following the appropriate process is important "because you never know when you'll need references or a recommendation from your employer or supervisor. And you never know when you'll encounter someone from that facility when you apply for work at another one later on" (Cardillo, 2002, p. 11).

The exit interview is an important tool for gathering information about the work environment and retention. Health care organizations need to consider the reasons staff is leaving. The following questions are important to ask in exit interviews.

- Why did you choose not to stay?
- What did you like most about your position?
- What did you like least?
- What did you like most about the agency/organization? The least?
- What could we have done differently to make your position more fulfilling (Hutchison, 2001b, p. 16)?

The interviewer should not be defensive when hearing negative comments about the organization or the job. The goal is to collect information and to try to arrive at a more positive departure viewpoint. It is important to remember that ex-employees will talk about past employers in the community, which is a public relations concern. Ex-employees who feel efforts have been made to listen to them, even though it may be late in the process, may feel more positive about the organization.

# Performance Appraisal

**Performance appraisal** is part of retention. During the process, management decides if staff is fulfilling job requirements and determine how to improve staff performance; by doing this, they provide guidance that will help to retain staff. All employers have some type of performance appraisal, but performance appraisal may be called by many other terms, such as performance review, performance evaluation, performance assessment, and performance rating. Accreditation organizations require that health care organizations implement a performance evaluation process although there can be great variation in the type and effectiveness of the process. The traditional view of performance appraisal focuses on job competence and areas that need improvement; however, there are other important reasons for conducting a performance appraisal.

- It is an opportunity to provide feedback, direction, and leadership.
- It is a time to show support and encouragement.
- It is a time to initiate a discussion about areas that need improvement.
- It is an opportunity to evaluate accomplishments and to set goals

   Other reasons for performance evaluation are as follows:

- Building team cohesion
- Preventing discrimination problems
- Ensuring compliance with relevant laws
- Assisting with promotion (Milgram, Spector, & Treger, 1999, p. 195)

## APPLYING EVIDENCE-BASED PRACTICE

### Evidence for Leadership and Management

Citation: Newhouse, R., Hoffman, J., Suflita, J., & Hairston, D. (2007). Evaluating an innovative program to improve new nurse graduate socialization into the acute health care setting. *Nursing Administration Quarterly, 31*(1), pp. 50–60.

Overview: There is considerable evidence indicating that transition to practice is stressful and has an impact on nurse retention. This quasi-experimental, posttest only, control group design study tested whether an internship program improves new nurse graduate retention, sense of belonging, organization commitment, and anticipated turnover. Three instruments were used to collect data. The results indicate that transition programs need to include "not only the skills and knowledge needed for novice nurse competence but also the opportunity for socialization into the professional role" (p. 59).

Application: Many nurse internship and residency programs have been developed over the last few years. Studies have tested the effectiveness of these programs. What is the best approach to provide a nurse internship or a nurse residency? Over time more will be learned about best practice for these programs, and which types of programs yield greater retention, competency, and professional role development.

Questions:

1. *After reviewing this particular internship program, what is your opinion of it?*
2. *What do you think needs to be included in a transition program to increase retention, competency, and professional role development post-graduation?*
3. *Would you consider participating in such a program? Why or why not?*

Evaluation is also an opportunity to reinforce the organization's vision, mission, and goals and to draw the employee into the organization's culture. The formal performance appraisal should not be the only time that the supervisor has a discussion with an employee or shares positive feedback. If this is the case, there are 364 days of lost opportunities to ensure staff improvement and growth. Staff will feel disconnected from the organization, and this affects performance, quality of care, safe care, staff dissatisfaction, and workplace stress and burnout. The ultimate result may be loss of staff and major problems with retention and recruitment as the word gets out that the organization or a unit or service is not concerned about its staff.

The idea of doing and participating in performance appraisal, despite its positive attributes, is rarely seen as a positive experience, and many dread it. Managers put off preparing appraisals and see it as an unpleasant task that often they do not feel competent to perform. The process is then conducted quickly with less thought. Employees sense this dissatisfaction with the process, and this then becomes something that just must be done. Feeling inadequate in conducting a performance appraisal is a major problem. Another potential problem is inadequate position descriptions that do not set clear performance standards for employees or for the person conducting the appraisal. If there are inadequate rewards, staff may not see the process as a positive one. Recruitment also plays a role. If staff is hired just to fill positions, then down the road there will be problems with performance appraisal when staff cannot meet the standards of the position, although this does not necessarily mean that the staff member will lose the position. There will be more of a struggle for the appraiser to find reasons to keep the staff member, especially when there are staff shortages. This, in the long run, dilutes the performance appraisal process and its results and has a direct impact on productivity, quality of care, and costs. The major tool that is usually used for appraisal is the appraisal interview; however, before the interview can take place there are other concerns. The goal is to implement an effective performance appraisal that provides honest feedback to the employee and includes the employee in the process to better ensure quality of care, as well as improve staff performance and the organization's goals. What are issues or factors that need to be considered?

## Performance Standards and Position Descriptions

Health care organizations establish performance standards in their position descriptions. The human resources department plays a major role in all personnel issues, including performance appraisal. This department ensures that the process is maintained, keeps records, assists with development and review of standards and position descriptions, and consults with supervisory staff about performance issues and disciplinary concerns. There should be a positive relationship and effective communication between human resources and management. When this is lacking, there are major problems for all concerned.

The position description provides both the appraiser and the employee the standards or competencies that need to be met. This information needs to be given to all employees as they begin a new position. If changes are made in the description, then employees should be informed in writing. Organizations typically use a standard format for their position descriptions. Position descriptions are very important documents, and each staff member should have a copy of the description of his or her position. Typically, the position includes job title, department (if applicable), status of the job (for example, full time, part time, or temporary), reporting relationship or to whom the employee reports (not a specific person but position; e.g., nurse manager), job summary, essential functions of the job or duties, qualifications, any physical requirements, and the date the description was approved. Position descriptions are also important for staff that is supervising other staff. They need to know what staff members can do in their positions. For example, a team leader needs to have an understanding of the job that a UAP is expected to perform.

## Competency-Based Performance Appraisal

**Competence** is a frequently used term today. The National Council of State Boards of Nursing (NCSBN) defines competency as "the application of knowledge and the interpersonal, decision-making, and psychomotor skills expected for the nurse's practice role, within the context of public health, welfare, and safety" (National Council of State Boards of Nursing, 1996; as cited in Mustard, 2002, p. 37). The goal of staff education within health care organizations is to maintain nursing competency throughout employment. Maintaining competency requires evaluation of competency, but this is not easy to accomplish. There needs to be "active reporting and corrective action without establishing a punitive environment" (Mustard, 2002, p. 41). The best approach is a proactive one that helps staff improve and prepare for changes and thus better ensure competency. Nursing organizations also emphasize the need to develop and maintain competencies, as does the Joint Commission and the recent IOM report on nursing (2010).

Who is responsible for staff competency?

- The employer clearly has a responsibility to ensure that patients receive safe, quality care. Performance evaluation is one method that is used to ensure this.
- Regulatory boards such as the state boards of nursing also play a role when they establish the state practice act and scope of practice and monitor licensure because they are entrusted with protecting the health and safety of the public.
- Professional organizations are also involved by developing standards of practice that are used by regulatory boards, employers, and nurses to guide decisions and evaluation. These organizations are now more involved due to their participation in the certification of specialty nurses.
- Colleagues or other nurses have a role to play in peer evaluation and support of one another. The individual nurse has a major responsibility as a professional to meet state licensure requirements, maintain continuing education, participate in ongoing self-evaluation, participate in the employer–employee evaluation process, and assist colleagues through peer evaluation. The *Code for Nurses* (American Nurses Association, 2008) indicates that a nurse is responsible for professional growth and maintenance of competence.

How competency is demonstrated continues to be a problematic issue. The Institute of Medicine report (2001) on quality care indicates that retooling practicing clinicians is critical today, and assessing this is part of performance appraisal. Should nurses be required to take only one exam in a lifetime career to demonstrate competency? How does attendance at continuing education programs demonstrate competency? Certification has been used as one method to demonstrate competency; however, it too has limitations. After the exam is taken for certification, if there are no other exams and only continuing education requirements, is competency demonstrated over time? Should this be left in the hands of professional organizations? There is no universal definition of continuing competence (Whitaker, Carson, & Sawlanski; 2000). This is a highly controversial, complex issue that has yet to be resolved.

The panel recommended that individual nurses develop professional nurse portfolios to document ongoing behaviors that are important in promoting competent practice (Whitaker, Carson, & Sawlanski, 2000). This process should include self-reflection and peer feedback. It is important for employees to understand how the competency-based performance appraisal process is used in their organization. Part of this understanding needs to include the following:

- Who does the evaluation?
- Does that person understand the job that is being evaluated?
- How were the standards identified, and what occurs when they are changed?
- What methods are used to obtain data for evaluations?
- What are the performance evaluation documentation requirements?

Components of a performance management program have been changing, and there are now several new approaches that can be used. Some of these approaches are a greater emphasis on self-appraisal, continuous feedback, peer appraisal, and 360-degree appraisal.

Self-appraisal should be part of every performance management program. Staff needs to assess themselves and to include this information in their performance appraisal. How do they view their own performance? What are its strengths and limitations? What would staff recommend for improvement strategies? It is not easy to do self-evaluation, but it is an important skill to learn. Every nurse should be evaluating his/her performance daily and strive for improvement.

Continuous feedback lets staff members know as soon as they do something positive or need performance improvement. Staff members need to receive clear recognition when their performance goes beyond expectations, improves, and also routinely, if their performance warrants it.

Documenting this performance in the personnel file is important. This form of evaluation also helps to clarify expectations on a regular basis and offers more direct contact with staff. Timing of giving feedback is very important. During a stressful incidence, it is best to give feedback when the situation is calmer. Feedback should be given in private, although it is important to provide public recognition when a staff member accomplishes something special or when a team or group of staff performs effectively. When appointments are made with staff, it is best to state the purpose of the meeting or staff may become concerned and spend time wondering about its purpose—maybe building it out of proportion.

Peer appraisal is used in some organizations, with peers giving feedback to peers about job performance. This can be a very sensitive process that requires trust in peers to provide the constructive feedback objectively. All staff needs to understand what needs to be done and how to do it. This feedback should not be the only method used in the evaluation process, but it can be helpful to know how peers respond to a staff member's performance.

Another method of evaluation is 360-degree evaluation, which includes a variety of people in the feedback loop, thus forming a complete circle. This evaluation includes constructive feedback from supervisors, peers, other subordinates, self, and could include patients, family members, and other customers. All staff needs to understand this method, why it is being used, and how it will be done. The staff member may choose who will do the evaluation, with a specified number of reviewers identified. This feedback should be anonymous. Then feedback needs to be summarized. It is critical that those involved understand the criteria and that the focus is on performance, not personality issues. This type of evaluation should be used for development, not to make critical decisions such as salary increases.

## Legal and Regulatory Issues

Some of the laws that were discussed earlier in this chapter are relevant to the performance appraisal process (for example, Civil Rights Act, Age Discrimination in Employment Act, Americans with Disabilities Act, and Fair Labor Standards Act). Performance appraisal must focus on performance and not individual characteristics such as gender, age, race, or sexual orientation. If any of these factors are used to determine a performance appraisal decision or a decision about salary, promotion, or any other job-related decision, then there is great risk of discrimination and noncompliance with required legal regulations. During the evaluation there needs to be a conscious effort to avoid generalizations, labels, personality issues, gender-based comments, and subjective language. The focus should be on job performance, and clear examples should be provided to the staff member to support feedback comments.

## Performance Appraisal/Evaluation Process

APPRAISER'S ROLE   The appraiser is expected to provide an honest, thorough evaluation of an employee. This should not be viewed as competition among staff but an evaluation of each staff member's performance. Objectivity is critical throughout the process. If the supervisor does not understand or feel competent to evaluate a staff member, then that supervisor is obligated to get direction and assistance with the process. Staff needs to view the process as important and feel respected during the entire process.

Data or information needs to be collected in order to prepare for performance appraisal. Methods that might be used are observation, maintenance of a log of observations, or anecdotal notes. The information should be collected throughout the year. These observations take place as the staff member is providing care, in meetings, during interactions with other staff, during interactions with patients and families, or whenever the job requires. Checklists, particularly for tasks, can be used to structure observation and to keep a record. Rating scales can also be used. Documentation can be reviewed to better ensure accuracy and quality. Quality improvement data may provide helpful data. If information is collected and reviewed throughout the year, the task of the annual performance appraisal should not be viewed as such a heavy burden. After data are collected and reviewed, then the required performance appraisal forms must be completed and should provide clear information about the employee's performance.

Implementation of the following year's performance appraisal process actually begins as the current year's performance appraisal process ends. Goals are established for the next year. Throughout the coming year feedback should be provided before the formal, annual review takes place. Employees do need notice when the annual performance review is due so that they can prepare for it, and they need to know what is expected from them during the appraisal process.

THE APPRAISAL INTERVIEW    The purpose of the interview can be categorized in the following ways.

1. **Probationary**—to determine if the employee has met the job's requirements; typically used for orientation to determine if the new employee meets the competency requirements for the position.
2. **Annual**—to determine the current competency of the employee, provide feedback, and plan for professional goals for the coming year as past year goals are reviewed.
3. **Ongoing–continuous**—performance appraisal should not just occur once a year but should be ongoing. Feedback needs to be given when the employee demonstrates competence or when the employee needs guidance to improve.
4. **Transfer**—if an employee is transferring to another area within the organization or receiving a promotion, a performance appraisal should take place before changing position and after orientation to a new position.
5. **Exit**—if an employee is leaving an organization, a terminal performance appraisal should be done, and as is true with all evaluations, the results should be documented in the employee's personnel file.

The supervisor (e.g., nurse manager) contacts the employee to arrange a time and place for the performance interview. There should be sufficient time for the meeting with no interruptions. Privacy, of course, should be maintained. Both parties should come to the interview prepared to discuss performance. The general format of the interview includes initial comments and greetings, review of expectations, review of previous year's goals, performance data and discussion with input from the employee, and establishment of goals for the coming year. It is easy to conduct the interview by telling the employee what is wrong or right about the employee's performance with limited mutual communication and self-evaluation by the employee; however, this is an ineffective approach. It is important for the employee to be able to use self-evaluation as this is a skill that the employee needs throughout the year. Staff may also be more defensive if the approach is to tell staff what is wrong without allowing staff the opportunity to comment, or to only focus on the negative. Bias based on personal feelings should be avoided during the evaluation process and the interview. This can be difficult sometimes as there are personalities that just do not do well together; however, this needs to be recognized so the parties can work toward a more positive viewpoint. Beginning the interview with positive comments and a clear focus on job performance can get the interview off to a productive start. The interviewer needs to avoid patronizing, doing all the talking, focusing too much on negative feedback, not listening to the employee, answering his or her own questions, and allowing interruptions to occur. Beginning with an open-ended question will draw the staff member into the process quickly, setting the standard of a dialogue instead of a lecture.

Organizations typically use a standard form during the process, and it is reviewed with the employee during the appraisal interview. Appraisal forms indicate that the organization has thought about what should be included in the evaluation process, provide some consistency, and should reflect the organization's philosophy. Regulatory requirements need to be demonstrated in the form's content. Use of a form helps the interviewer remember what should be covered. The form guides the interview; however, the supervisor needs to be flexible, encouraging the employee to participate in all aspects of the interview. If the approach is one of problem solving, identifying problems or issues and then working together to figure out the best strategy for improvement, then this will stimulate more staff development. It is important that both the supervisor and the employee provide specific examples to support comments. The focus should be on behavior and facts, and while doing this, encouraging the employee to contribute comments. Both the supervisor and employee should sign the appraisal form, which only indicates that the employee has read the form but may not necessarily mean that the employee agrees with its content. Some forms have space for employees to make their own comments about the evaluation.

All appraisal interviews must be documented with records kept in the employee's personnel file. The employee should be given a copy of the completed performance appraisal form. The supervisor may keep notes along with data about the employee. A copy of future goals should also be kept.

THE EMPLOYEE'S ROLE    The employee plays an active role in performance appraisal. The Joint Commission requires that employees participate. Preparing for performance appraisal is key for the employee just as it is for the supervisor. It begins with self-evaluation. The employee should review position requirements, past year's goals, last year's evaluation, and ask colleagues for feedback. A portfolio may be developed or updated for the evaluation. This all requires time and should be a thoughtful process, not a hurried one. The idea is to have a positive experience that focuses on improvement and recognizes accomplishments, not to emphasize failures. The performance evaluation may be a time to discuss or negotiate a salary increase, change in positions, promotion, and other job-related matters. Since mutually established goals should be agreed upon in the interview, the employee should develop goals for the coming year in preparation for the performance appraisal interview. These goals need to be clear and specific and relate to the position and professional growth. Examples of content for goals are (a) to improve documentation by describing clinical problems more clearly, (b) to attend one conference in a specialty area, (c) to organize work better so that the employee can leave work at a scheduled time, (d) to develop more specific patient education plans, and so on. Some topics are not appropriate for the performance interview. "It's best not to cloud a discussion of your performance with issues relating to coworkers, systems that don't work, or general gossip. Let the focus be on you and your performance" (Bradley, 2001, p. 74).

## CASE STUDY

### A First Experience with Complicated Performance Appraisal

Six months ago you were promoted to a nurse manager position on a surgical unit. The first six months have been rocky with short staff, high census, high acuity, and several critical incidents such as a medical error that led to a patient being transferred to ICU. You have been trying to learn more about your new role. Staff seems to be accepting of you, but a couple of nurses do not think you have enough experience. You have heard this through the grapevine. Two of these nurses are now up for their annual performance appraisal. The hospital uses competency-based performance appraisal. The following briefly describes the two nurses:

a. Jane has been working on the unit for 8 years longer than you. She has experienced three nurse managers in this time period. Jane has a BSN. When there are staff issues she is the first to lead the charge and can get very emotional. She has had three arguments with physicians in the last 6 months. Jane has also been involved in 4 medication errors over the last eight months. This year her documentation meets required criteria.

b. Sue has worked on the unit for three years. She had an AD but just completed her BSN five months ago. Her behavior has changed in the last five months. She has not worked well with the certified nurse assistants (CNAs) and had an argument with a new nurse. She told this nurse, "You don't know what you are doing." The nurse is ready to leave the job. Sue has never been an effective delegator, but no one has ever addressed this. She has no known errors, but her documentation does not consistently meet required criteria. You wonder if her attaining her BSN has made a difference, and not necessarily a positive difference.

You now have to prepare for Jane's and Sue's performance appraisal.

### Questions:

1. Describe what information you would need to prepare for the interviews—information described here and any additional information.

2. What are the critical issues for each nurse that you think need to be addressed interview and how will you address them?

3. During the meeting with Jane, she says, "I have to tell you that I think you are not an effective nurse manager." How would you respond to her?

4. Sue tells you in the interview that she is better than the other nurses since she got her BSN, particularly the three AD nurses. How would you respond to her?

5. Describe the plan you would recommend to Jane and to Sue to improve in the next year. Include a time line for review.

## Problems with Employees

As with any relationships, there can be problems in the employer–employee relationship. How these problems are handled can affect retention and staffing. Problems may occur during the performance appraisal or throughout the year.

Employees and supervisors may encounter problems with one another. As managers and team leaders supervise staff they may wonder why staff members are not doing what is expected of them. Some of the reasons for the inability to meet expectations may be because staff members

- Do not know what they are supposed to do.
- Do not know how to do it.
- Think the way they are told to do something will not be most effective.
- Think their way of doing a job is better.
- Think something else is more important.
- Anticipate future negative consequences.
- Have personal problems.
- Have personal limits.
- Encounter obstacles beyond their control (Fournies, 1999, p. 131).

It is important to try to understand the causes of these problems. After the job or work begins, staff members may think that they are doing what they are supposed to do. They may not recognize any positive consequences for doing their job. Obstacles beyond their control may get in the way of doing the work. It may be that staff members think there are more important tasks that they should be doing. Sometimes staff members do not do what they are asked to do because they are punished for doing it or they may be rewarded for not doing it. If staff members do not see any negative consequences for poor performance, they may not feel the need to do the job well or to improve. Personal problems, of course, can interfere with job performance at any time. The goal is to prevent these barriers from occurring so the work gets done effectively. Prevention strategies include the following:

- Be clear about what needs to be done (expectations).
- Find out if staff knows how to do what needs to be done.
- Explain why something needs to be done.
- Listen to staff input on how to do the job and evaluate if it is a better way—if not, explain this to staff.
- Openly discuss concerns about negative consequences to clarify fact and fiction.
- When possible, ensure that personal problems will not interfere with work requirements.
- Remove all barriers to getting the job done if at all possible (Fournies, 1999).

These strategies should also be used while the work is being done so that the work can be completed effectively. Just providing negative feedback bluntly can crush employees and does little for including the employee in the process of identifying a positive strategy to resolve the problem and improve performance.

There has also been a growing problem with lateral violence in health care organizations, nurse to nurse, mostly in form of verbal comments, not supporting one another, negativity, and lack of teamwork. Stress plays a big role in this problem. In addition, experienced nurses may not be as supportive and helpful to new staff. This has an impact on job satisfaction of new staff and retention. When staff does not feel welcomed and supported then this can lead to staff leaving.

Not all evaluation interviews go smoothly. The interviewer may know before the evaluation interview that there may be problems during the interview. This is particularly true if the employee's performance has been less than expected. In this case, the appraiser needs to be very careful about preparing for the interview and spend time thinking through the evaluation and how to discuss it. The interviewer should not become defensive but stay on the subject of performance and expectations. Certainly, some positive, honest feedback should be given if at all possible. The employee may express emotion, from happiness, to frustration, to anger. Happiness is not so difficult, but frustration and anger will be stressful for both persons. Giving the staff member some time to get control is important. It allows the interviewer to also gain some composure and not respond with emotion. If the staff member cannot control emotions at the time, the interview may need to be rescheduled, although this is not preferable. If there is any threat of aggression, then the interview should be terminated. Safety is a priority. Workplace violence should never be tolerated. The supervisor may recommend that the employee seek assistance from the Employee Assistance Program (EAP), if one is available. This program provides counseling for emotional problems and substance abuse problems, and many organizations offer this service to their staff. If there is concern before the evaluation interview that the employee might respond with aggression, then the interview should not be conducted alone. Employees who are not meeting expectations need to be treated with respect. The interview should allow time to discuss performance objectively and to work on an improvement plan that includes deadlines and a clear description of what is required to improve performance. The employee needs to understand the plan and feel that it represents a joint effort.

STRESS ON THE JOB     **Job stress** is defined by the National Institute for Occupational Safety and Health Administration (NIOSH) as "the harmful physical and emotional responses that occur when the requirements of the job do not match the capabilities, resources, or needs of the worker" (National Institute for Occupational Safety and Health, 1999). The National Mental Health Association reported that workplace stress causes about 1 million employees to miss work each day (National Mental Health Association, 2005). The health care work environment is no different. Staff is experiencing much change and frustration with staff shortages and reengineering of organizations. Nurses often identify the following as reasons for their stress:

- Staff shortage
- Increasing responsibility with less time
- Excessive and/or redundant paperwork
- Interdisciplinary issues
- Job dissatisfaction
- Working different shifts
- Fatigue and overwork
- Mandatory overtime
- Decreasing quality personal time
- Poor communication
- Ineffective management

Some nurses have described themselves as experiencing chronic guilt from their inability to meet patient needs effectively as staff shortages increase while patient acuity continues to be high (Hemmila, 2002). This type of stress is destructive and can lead to major personal and performance problems. These nurses need to learn how to balance what can be done and what are unrealistic expectations. What are realistic goals? Are there staff or managers who communicate expectations that are too high? Colleagues need to support one another both by pitching in and helping to give someone a break and also by providing emotional support—communicating that we are a team that helps one another. Employers need to be aware of these feelings and assist staff members who are experiencing them because in the long run such stress affects retention.

In some organizations there also seems to be a "disconnect" between staff and managers. Signs and symptoms of this "disconnect" include the following:

- High frustration levels reported from both staff RNs and their managers
- A sense among staff of not being valued (for example, low self-esteem)
- Few RNs who seek a managerial career track
- Adverse incidents that involve patients and staff
- Ongoing misunderstanding between both groups that hurts interprofessional communication, cooperation, and patient care
- An "us against them" mentality that pervades the workplace
- Nurses telling their own patients they are overworked and understaffed
- Poor nurse retention across the board or in particular departments
- Labor unrest
- High vacancy rates resulting in excessive overtime, routine use of agency nurses, or bed closure (Forman, 2001, p. 24MW)

This disconnect is related to stress within the organization.

Since it seems that stress in health care is inevitable, two key questions are what can individual nurses do to decrease their own stress and what can the organization do to decrease staff stress? Individual nurses need to first recognize what causes their own stress and how they respond to stress-producing situations. This personal self-assessment should provide valuable information that can then be used to work out a prevention plan. Strategies that can help a nurse prevent or decrease stress are as follows:

- Set reasonable priorities.
- Ask for help and do not see this as a weakness.
- Do one task at a time.
- Take a few minutes to slow down several times during the day.
- Get sufficient sleep, eat a healthy diet, and exercise.
- Focus on what is happening rather than worrying about what could happen.
- Use appropriate self-assertion.
- View problems as challenges and opportunities.
- Laugh and take time for self.

Another strategy that can be used to learn how to better prevent or decrease stress is to better understand what occurs within oneself that can affect stress (Vernarec, 2001). For example, when a person feels overwhelmed by stress, time should be taken to write down what another person said or did that might have influenced the person's reaction. Faulty beliefs are often behind these responses. Employers can also help staff with stress. One strategy is to work with staff to develop self-care contracts (Ellis, 2000). These contracts are used to help staff members identify how they will care for themselves with a focus on wellness. The contract might contain content about responsibility for self, physical fitness, nutritional awareness, stress reduction, creative activities, and appreciation for the arts. Nurse managers can recommend that the staff develop these contracts.

New graduates are particularly vulnerable to stress as they learn their new professional role. **Reality shock**, which has been defined as "the shock-like reaction that occurs when an individual who has been reared and educated in that subculture of nursing that is promulgated by schools of nursing suddenly discovers that nursing as practiced in the world of work is not the same—it does not operate on the same principles" (Kramer, 1985, p. 291). New graduates need an organized orientation and preceptors who take an interest in them to assist them with transition from the classroom to practice. Staff on the unit can make a difference in how well a new graduate adjusts. It is important for nurses to feel an obligation to assist new nurses in the profession. Reaching out is critical as many new nurses do not feel comfortable reaching out themselves. Patient assignments need to be done with care as new nurses further develop their skills and learn their way around. They need supervision and guidance with "frequent and regular opportunities for 'debriefing' with more experienced or expert nurses" (Nayak, 1991, p. 66). This provides a time for the new nurse to talk through an experience and use critical thinking in a safe environment—one that does not focus on punishment but rather growth. Self-confidence builds slowly; however, when there is a staff shortage, experienced nurses often expect new nurses to gain experience quickly, although this is an unrealistic expectation. The pressure and stress that experienced nurses feel increases their impatience with colleagues. Taking time to help new nurses with the transition and supporting them will go a long way to decrease problems of rapid turnover of this vulnerable staff group, who may change jobs thinking it will get better, or eventually leave the nursing profession.

COPING WITH PASSIVE-AGGRESSIVE BEHAVIOR    Passive-aggressive behavior can be difficult to cope with in the work environment, and sadly it is something that all staff will undoubtedly experience with colleagues. When staff members use passive-aggressive behavior they usually exhibit at least four of the following:

- Passively resist fulfilling routine social and occupational tasks
- Complain of being misunderstood and unappreciated by others

- Appear sullen and argumentative
- Unreasonably criticize and scorn authority
- Express resentment toward those perceived as more fortunate
- Voice exaggerated and persistent complaints of personal misfortune
- Alternate between hostile defiance and contrition (Whitaker, Carson, & Sawlanski, 2000, p. 82)

When coping with a staff member who exhibits this type of behavior, it is important to clarify expectations, particularly those related to assignments. The overall expectation should be that the work will be done. Apologies and excuses will not be enough. When complaints are made, it is important to consider the facts and avoid defensiveness. Seeking the truth and expecting facts will drive performance. This does not mean that a staff member cannot be understanding, but this should not interfere with performance expectations.

# Staffing: The Critical Issue Today

Staffing is a critical concern in all health care organizations as "60 to 80 percent of your budget goes to staffing" (McConnell, 2000, p. 52). With the increasing costs of health care, this is an expense that must be considered daily. It is also important to remember that "staffing is both a process and an outcome. It's inextricably linked to leaders' accountability to stay within budget and control costs, regulatory and legal mandates, staff competency, quality of care, and the versatility of staffing levels and assignments based on census and acuity" (Beyers, 1999, p. 56). The Institute of Medicine includes staffing issues in its report on nursing (2004). The health reform legislation of 2010 addresses the shortage in its provisions. The law establishes a health care Workforce Advisory Committee to develop workforce strategy, and it identifies needs for fund to increase nursing education capacity, support training programs, provide loan repayment and retention grants, and create a career ladder to nursing. This discussion provides some general information about staffing basics and the nursing shortage. Each nurse needs to become familiar with the staffing policies and procedures that are used in the nurse's organization and specific unit or service. During the recruitment process it is important for the nurse candidate to ask about staffing levels, skill mix, and scheduling. All of these issues directly affect all staff, including new staff.

## Staffing Basics

**Staffing** is the method used to ensure that the appropriate staff—qualifications and quantity—are available to provide the care that is needed for patients to meet their needs and thus provide quality, safe care. This is not easy to accomplish with patients changing and the ever unstable nursing workforce. Factors that must be considered in staffing are as follows:

- Types of patients and care required
- Number of patients
- Workload patterns such as when patients are admitted and discharged
- Times of procedures, and other treatment
- Average daily census
- Hours of work (for example, an inpatient unit is operational 24 hours a day, 7 days a week, whereas a clinic may just be operational 5 days a week but may have variable and evening hours)
- Types of nursing staff used (for example, RNs, LPNs, and UAP)
- The use of support staff such as a unit secretary and staff to transfer patients to exams and procedures can make a big difference, as does the communication system (e.g., use of pagers, cellular phones, and handheld computers). The documentation system also is a critical factor, with computerized systems typically providing effective documentation and effective use of time.

What are some of the key terms and issues that nurses need to know to understand scheduling and staffing needs?

- A **full-time equivalent (FTE)** is the term used to designate a position, which is equal to 40 hours of work per week for 52 weeks or 2,080 hours per year. As scheduling is considered, one FTE can be filled by one person or several, with hours divided.
- Another term is **nursing care hours** or the number of hours of patient care provided per unit of time.
- **Staffing mix** is also important, which is the type of staff that is needed to provide the care (for example, RNs and UAP). To determine the staff mix it is important to identify the type of care that is required and who is qualified to provide that care. Staff mix also includes an assessment of staff competency to fulfill the care needs. This becomes important, for example, when staff members are transferred from their usual work environment into a new one, even if temporarily; they must, nonetheless, be competent to carry on the assigned tasks.
- Nurse practice acts and other state regulations must always be met when staffing decisions are made. For example, if the patient requires more activities of daily living care such as would be found in a long-term care facility, then UAP should be included in the staff mix with RNs providing supervision, assessment, and other procedures that require RN competency.
- **Staff distribution** is another important factor that focuses on when staff are needed (for example, if a surgical unit gets most of its admissions on Sunday evening for Monday surgeries or if a unit has medical procedures that are done in the morning, then these factors need to be considered in the schedule).
- Shift hours have changed over the years with 8-, 10-, and 12-hour shifts used. Twelve-hour shifts have become more common; however, a recent Institute of Medicine report indicates that when shift durations exceed 12 hours, errors increase (Institute of Medicine, 2004). It is not yet clear what effect this conclusion will have on practice. Split shifts are also used to provide extra staff for busy times (for example, 7:00 AM to 11:00 AM or 3:00 PM to 7:00 PM). These various shifts, when used in combination, tend to meet patient needs during high workload times, satisfy staff more, and maximize the use of nurses (Sullivan & Decker, 2001).

Scheduling can be a challenge for the scheduler and for staff members who want their schedule needs met. Getting a schedule established that is acceptable to management and staff is the goal, and then it can become cyclical. There will always be times when adjustments need to be made because of staff illness, vacation, and other factors. Some organizations have moved to self-scheduling, which is discussed later in this section. Supplemental staff issues have become of concern with the shortage. Extra staff hours are also needed to cover vacations, illness, and other such situations; cover vacancies; and cover when patient acuity demands it. What do organizations do? Some have their own internal pools of staff that float as needed. Others use agency nurses who are hired per shift. Use of travelers has also become a more frequent intervention. These are nurses who are hired by travel nurse agencies and then contracted to work for specific hospitals and positions for specific time periods through the agency. These nurses move from one community to another. Use of agency nurses and travelers is expensive for health care organizations.

Scheduling also has implications for staff and for patient care outcomes and quality. There is increasing use of scheduling nurses for a mix of shifts on one unit in order to attract or retain staff (Kalisch, Begeny, & Anderson, 2008), for example, to have staff on a single unit working 4-, 6-, 8-, and 12-hour shifts. This means multiple reports and handoffs. In this situation there will be communication problems, errors, and patients who feel like they have no anchor in the staff that changes multiple times in one day. This can also cause staff stress trying to keep up with the rotating staff. What impact does this have on teamwork? This study indicates that consistent staffing has a positive impact on teamwork and the multiple shifts have a negative impact on teamwork. Staff in the study felt that patient safety was improved when teamwork was better.

## The Nursing Shortage

The nursing shortage is the number one topic in nursing and probably also in health care delivery in general. The shortage is compounded by the fact that it will only get worse due to aging baby boomers who will retire and need to be replaced. In addition, enrollment in nursing schools increased, for example enrollment in baccalaureate nursing programs increased by 9.6% in 2008, which will have a positive impact on care delivery (American Association of Colleges of Nursing, 2010). However, the capacity of nursing schools to admit more students continues to be a problem due to an inadequate number of clinical sites and shortage of nursing faculty. In addition, many nursing faculty will also be retiring. Due to these issues almost 40% of all applicants to pre-licensure programs were denied admission in 2008–2009 (National League for Nursing, 2010). Data indicate that there is increased enrollment in doctoral programs that will help increase number of faculty; however, more will be needed (American Association of Colleges of Nursing, 2010). Along with the education problems there is the problem of staff turnover. "Reported turnover rates of Newly Licensed Registered Nurses (NLRNs) vary from 13%–70%" (Pellico, Brewer, & Kovner, 2009, p. 194; Kovner et al., 2007; Squires, 2002). Job burnout and dissatisfaction are causing retention problems, with nurses leaving the profession or taking extended time off from work. This leads to high turnover rates, which affects costs, health care quality and safety, and the image of nursing, leading to problems with attracting people into the profession.

The present, complex shortage is primarily lack of supply (not enough nurses) (Nevidjon & Erickson, 2001). It is believed that past strategies, such as sign-on bonuses and premium packages, only redistribute nurses from employer to employer, rather than increase the number of nurses. In addition to not having enough nurses under usual circumstances, researchers and professional organizations have identified multiple interrelated factors that affect the demand for nurses that still need to be considered. These factors are as follows:

- Cost-containment pressures within health care organizations resulting from managed care and an increasingly competitive health care environment
- Hospital consolidation, downsizing, and reengineering
- Reductions in inpatient hospitalization rates
- Increased acuity of hospital patients
- A shift of outpatient care from hospitals to ambulatory and community-based settings (Peterson, 2001, p. 1)

What are the data that indicate there is a nursing shortage? Tables 9-1 through 9-4 provide information about the shortage and the impact this is having on patient care. There are also shortages in other health professions such as physicians.

All areas of nursing are experiencing some shortages, including hospitals, home care, and long-term care. The ANA developed nursing staffing principles that can be found in Box 9-4. The *Principles for Nurse Staffing* (ANA, 1999) describes a matrix for staffing decision making. It is composed of patients, intensity of unit and care, context, and expertise, and is described in Box 9-5.

The key elements related to *patients* are specific patient characteristics and number of patients for whom care is to be provided. *Intensity* includes "patient intensity; across the unit intensity (taking into account the heterogeneity of settings); variability of care; admissions, discharges, and transfers; volume" (American Nurses Association, 1999, p. 3). *Context* incorporates some other critical elements such as architecture and layout of individual patient rooms and arrangement of the entire patient care unit(s); technology that is used such as beepers, cellular phones, and computers; and same unit or cluster of patients. The fourth element is *expertise* of the staff, which includes staff consistency, continuity and cohesion, use of cross-training, control of practice, involvement in quality improvement, and professional expectations. All these elements affect staffing needs and should be reviewed when staffing schedules are developed.

| **TABLE 9-1** | **REASONS FOR THE CURRENT NURSING SHORTAGE, 2004 AND 2005** |
|---|---|

| Main reasons for the current nursing shortage | RNs 2004 (N=657) Percent | MDs 2004 (N=445) Percent | CNOs 2005 (N=222) Percent | CEOs 2005 (N=142) Percent |
|---|---|---|---|---|
| More career options for women | 32 | 18* | 35 | 33 |
| Faculty shortages in nursing schools | 12 | * | 20 | 23 |
| Salary and benefits | 41 | 21* | 14 | 21* |
| Difficult occupation/high workload/ undesirable hours | 28 | 27 | 26 | 17* |
| Inadequate nursing schools/ programs/seats for students | 12 | 3* | 18 | 17 |
| Nursing not seen as a rewarding career | 26 | - | 6* | 9* |

*Statistically significant different from registered nursed (p≤ 0.05)
-Questions not asked

Source: National surveys of RNs, physicians, and hospital executives as cited in P. Buerhaus, D. Staiger, & D. Auerbach. (2009). *The Future of the Nursing Workforce in the United States*. Boston: Jones and Bartlett Publishers.

| **TABLE 9-2** | **IMPACT OF CURRENT NURSING SHORTAGE ON INSTITUTE OF MEDICINE'S SIX INDICATORS OF HIGH-QUALITY HEALTH CARE SYSTEMS, PERCENT RESPONDING FREQUENT OR OFTEN ADVERSE IMPACT, 2004 AND 2005** |
|---|---|

| Thinking about the criteria for quality of care established by the Institute of Medicine, how often would you say the shortage of nurses has had an adverse impact on the following aspects of patient care? | RNs 2004 (N=657) Frequently or Often Percent | MDs 2004 (N=445) Frequently or Often Percent | CNOs 2005 (N=222) Frequently or Often Percent | CEOs 2005 (N=142) Frequently or Often Percent |
|---|---|---|---|---|
| Patient centered | 74 | 61* | 44* | 44* |
| Effective | 74 | 58* | 34* | 28* |
| Safe | 65 | 36* | 26* | 17* |
| Timely | 84 | 72* | 50* | 41* |
| Efficient | 72 | 55* | 55* | 46* |
| Equitable | 63 | 38* | 23* | 18* |

*Statistically significant different from registered nurses (p≤ 0.05)

Source: Buerhaus, P., Donelan, K., DesRoches, C., Ulrich, D., Norman, L., & Dittus, R. (2007). Impact of the nursing shortage on hospital patient care: Comparative perspectives, *Health Affairs, 26*(3), 853–862; Exhibit 3: Impact of Nurse Shortage on Institute of Medicine's (IOM's) Six Aims for High-Quality Health Care Systems, 2004–2005. The article is copyrighted and published by Project HOPE/*Health Affairs*. The published article is archived and available online at http://www.healthaffairs.org executives as cited in P. Buerhaus, D. Staiger, & D. Auerbach. (2009). *The Future of the Nursing Workforce in the United States*. Boston: Jones and Bartlett Publishers.

The definitions of each aim for improving the quality of the U.S. healthcare system were provided by the Institute of Medicine. (2001). *Crossing the quality chasm: A new health system for the 21st Century*. Committee on Quality Health Care in America, Institute of Medicine. Washington, DC: National Academies Press.

**Patient centered:** Providing care that is respectful of and responsive to individual patient preferences, needs, and values, and ensuring that patient values guide all clinical decisions. **Effective:** Providing services based on scientific knowledge to all who could benefit and refraining from providing services to those to likely to benefit. **Safe:** Avoiding injuries to patients from the care that is intended to help them. **Timely:** Reducing waits and sometimes harmful delays for both those who receive and those who give care. **Efficient:** Avoiding waste, including waste of equipment, supplies, ideas, and energy. **Equitable:** Providing care that does not vary in quality because of personal characteristics such as gender, ethnicity, geographic location, and socioeconomic status.

| TABLE 9-3 | IMPACT OF CURRENT NURSING SHORTAGE ON RNS AND THEIR ABILITY TO PROVIDE PATIENT CARE, PERCENTAGE RESPONDING MAJOR PROBLEM, 2004 AND 2005 |
| --- | --- |

| From what you know, how much of a problem do you think the shortage of nurses has been for . . . ? Major, minor, or no problem. | RNs 2004 (N=657) Major Problem Percent | MDs 2004 (N=445) Major Problem Percent | CNOs 2005 (N=222) Major Problem Percent | CEOs 2005 (N=142) Major Problem Percent |
| --- | --- | --- | --- | --- |
| Quality of patient care | 78 | 61* | 64* | 54* |
| Time for collaboration with teams | 55 | 33* | 56 | 50 |
| Ability of nurses to maintain patient safety | 69 | 21* | 62 | 38* |
| Early detection of complications | 65 | 44* | 60 | 47* |
| Nurses' time for patients | 91 | 78* | 66* | 59* |
| Quality of nurses' work life | 82 | 59* | 76 | 62* |

*Statistically significant different from registered nurses (p≤ 0.05)

Source: Buerhaus, P., Donelan, K., DesRoches, C., Ulrich, D., Norman, L., & Dittus, R. (2007). Impact of the nursing shortage on hospital patient care: Comparative perspectives, *Health Affairs, 26*(3), 853–862; Exhibit 2: Impact of Nurse Shortage on Nurses and Their Ability to Provide Care, 2004–2005. The article is copyrighted and published by Project HOPE/*Health Affairs*. The published article is archived and available online at http://www.healthaffairs.org executives as cited in P. Buerhaus, D. Staiger, & D. Auerbach. (2009). *The Future of the Nursing Workforce in the United States*. Boston: Jones and Bartlett Publishers.

| TABLE 9-4 | IMPACT OF NURSING SHORTAGE ON PROCESSES OF CARE AND HOSPITAL CAPACITY, 2004 AND 2005 |
| --- | --- |

| In the past year have you observed any of the following as a result of nursing shortages in the hospital? | RNs 2004 (N=657) Percent | MDs 2004 (N=445) Percent | CNOs 2005 (N=222) Percent | CEOs 2005 (N=142) Percent |
| --- | --- | --- | --- | --- |
| **Impact on Care Delivery Processes** | | | | |
| Nurses' delayed response to pages or calls | 82 | 67* | 84 | 76* |
| Increased patients' complaints about nursing care | 84 | 74* | 58* | 55* |
| Increased staff communication problems | 85 | 71* | 72* | 69* |
| Increased workload for physicians | 50 | 55 | 29* | 30* |
| **Impact on Hospital Capacity** | | | | |
| Reduced number of available beds | 78 | 64* | 60* | 56* |
| Delayed discharges | 69 | 50* | 60* | 61 |
| Increased patient wait time for surgery or tests | 68 | 45* | 47* | 48* |
| Discontinued/closed patient care programs | 44 | 49 | 20* | 20* |

*Statistically significant different from registered nursed (p≤ 0.05)

Source: Buerhaus, P., Donelan, K., DesRoches, C., Ulrich, D., Norman, L., & Dittus, R. (2007). Impact of the nursing shortage on hospital patient care: Comparative perspectives, *Health Affairs, 26*(3), 853–862; Exhibit 1: Impact of Nurse Shortage on Processes of Care and Hospital Capacity, 2004–2005. The article is copyrighted and published by Project HOPE/*Health Affair*s. The published article is archived and available online at http://www.healthaffairs.org executives as cited in P. Buerhaus, D. Staiger, & D. Auerbach. (2009). *The Future of the Nursing Workforce in the United States*. Boston: Jones and Bartlett Publishers.

---

**BOX 9-4**    **ANA PRINCIPLES FOR NURSE STAFFING**

I. Patient Care Unit Related
  A. Appropriate staffing levels for a patient care unit reflect analysis for individual and aggregate patient needs.
  B. There is a critical need to either retire or seriously question the usefulness of the concept of nursing hours per patient day (HPPD).
  C. Unit functions necessary to support delivery of quality patient care must also be considered in determining staffing levels.

II. Staff Related
  A. The specific needs of various patient populations should determine the appropriate clinical competencies required of the nurse practicing in that area.
  B. Registered nurse must have nursing management support and representation at both the operational level and the executive level.
  C. Clinical support from experienced RNs should be readily available to those RNs with less proficiency.

III. Institution/Organization Related
  A. Organizational policy should reflect an organizational climate that values registered nurses and other employees as strategic assets and exhibit a true commitment to filling budgeted positions in a timely manner.
  B. All institutions should have documented competencies for nursing staff, including agency or supplemental and traveling RNs, for those activities that they have been authorized to perform.
  C. Organizational policies should recognize the myriad needs of both patients and nursing staff.

Source: American Nurses Association. (1999). *Principles for nurse staffing.* Washington, DC: Author. Reprinted with permission "© 1999 By American Nurses Association. Reprinted with permission. All rights reserved."

---

**BOX 9-5**    **MATRIX FOR STAFFING DECISION MAKING**

The American Nurses Association identified four key factors that are part of a matrix for staffing decision making in its publication *Principles for Staffing* (1999).

    Patients
    Intensity of unit and care
    Context
    Expertise

## Strategies to Resolve the Problems

In the fall of 2002, Congress passed and funded the Nurse Reinvestment Act. This legislation addresses the issue of the nursing shortage, both of nursing staff and nursing faculty and there have been other laws passed for support of professional training. Prior to the Nurse Reinvestment Act, a federal law, California adopted a major policy related to nurse-to-patient ratios in general acute care hospitals, acute psychiatric hospitals, and special hospitals by passing a law in 1999 about this issue. This model of nurse staffing policy is called fixed minimum ratios. "Facilities are required to staff to a certain fixed minimum nurse-to-patient ratio" (Robert Wood Johnson Foundation, 2007, p. 3). The California's health services department was mandated to develop regulations that require nursing staff to be based on the following:

- Severity of illness
- Need for specialized equipment and technology
- Complexity of the clinical judgment needed to develop, implement, and evaluate patient care
- Ability of patients to provide self-care
- Licensure of the professional

The law also prohibits assigning nursing functions to UAP, and it requires that certain functions can only be assigned to UAP with supervision. This law was strongly supported by nurses and included major nursing input in California. Since then many states are moving in the same direction. It should be noted that the law itself does not state what the nurse-to-patient ratio must be but rather directs the health services department in the state to develop these regulations based on the criteria identified in the new state law. There have been changes made to the law, and in 2007 there was still no clear indication that this had solved the problems. This type of model has had little research to support its use and does not address the problem of funding for staff; however, a significant study was published in 2010 (Aiken et al.). This study's sample included 22,336 hospital staff nurses in California, Pennsylvania, and New Jersey (2006) and the state hospital discharge databases in these three states. The purpose of the study was to determine whether nurse staffing in California hospitals that had state mandated minimum nurse–patient ratios were different from two states that did not have this mandate and were the differences associated with nurse and patient outcomes. The conclusion from the study is "hospital nurse staffing ratios mandated in California are associated with lower mortality and nurse outcomes predictive of better nurse retention in California and in other states where they occur" (Aiken et al., 2010, p. 904). This model has had an impact on other states. As of September 2009, 14 states and the District of Columbia enacted similar legislation, and 17 other states had introduced legislation (American Nurses Association, 2009). This is not unusual in that states look to see what other states are doing and may then follow with similar policy changes.

Using patient classification systems is another nurse staffing policy (Robert Wood Johnson, 2007). This requires the use of computer software to determine nurse staffing for each shift; requiring nurses to assess patients and input data. The software then calculates the number and type of staff needed. California requires patient classification though there are no standards about what should be used to determine patient classification so hospitals can choose their own methods. Hospital units must provide the minimum staffing required by law (based on type of unit), and then use the classification system to determine if more staff is required. It is important to recognize that patients vary and that this impacts staffing needs; however, these systems are not perfect. There are no universal standards, staff may not know how to use them well, and there are questions as to whether they really put the nurse in the decision-making position. Others wonder if the systems can be manipulated to increase acuity and thus get more staff.

A third model is pay-for-performance. In this model there would be greater reimbursement for care provided based on quality—performance. This is not easy, would not be easy to do, and currently there are more questions than answers about it (Robert Wood Johnson Foundation, 2007). This has also been influenced by the Institute of Medicine (2001) report on quality.

Though many states are trying to get similar laws there are experts who believe that mandatory staffing is not the best approach. It takes years to determine if this type of policy change is effective. Mandatory staffing requires financial support—increase staffing increases costs, and yet just mandating staffing does not address the funding required to meet the staffing levels. Welton (2007) recommends that unbundling nursing care from room and board charges. Currently, hospitals do not specifically identify nursing costs from other costs but rather include these costs in a flat rate for room and board. Using nursing intensity ratings would allow for more specific billing. This would be an incentive to hospitals to improve nurse staffing levels. The hospitals would have a better chance of covering the actual costs of providing nursing care and would then staff for these needs and be paid for the staff.

- In March of 2010 health care legislation was passed that will have a significant impact on staffing. With the passage of the health care reform legislation of 2010 there is now greater need for nurses because more people will obtain insurance who were uninsured in the past. The legislation addresses this by including provisions to establish the Workforce Advisory Committee to develop a national workforce strategy and to also increase workforce supply and support training of health professionals through scholarships and loans. Nurse practitioners will be in greater demand to assist in areas that have medical shortages.
- What are some other strategies that have been tried or could be tried to address the staffing problems? It is clear that there needs to be a multistrategy or multisolution approach. The

following represent some strategies that are used or might be used. Some are more success-ful than others, but most depend upon the environment in which they are used and the sup-port that is given to the strategy.

- Use of **self-scheduling** is an approach that some organizations are using (Hung, 2002). It is well known that scheduling can be an operational nightmare. In this approach nurses in a unit collaborate and coordinate their schedules rather than having the nurse manager do it. Staff has a time period in which to sign up for a schedule, and at the end of the period the nurse manager or a staff designee reviews the schedule to see if all needs are met. This type of scheduling has many benefits. It saves on management time, improves morale and pro-fessionalism, and reduces costs related to staff turnover. Nurses must take on participation, accountability, creativity, and responsibility to make this work.

- Communities are joining together to form task forces to look at the problems with rep-resentatives from health care providers and nursing education. Regional workforce task forces identify common issues and possible strategies to resolve them. This collabora-tion includes nursing education, practice, and consumers, which can lead to effective partnerships.

- Many hospitals and other large health care organizations are using nurse retention special-ists to help with recruitment and retention. The difference between a recruiter and the retention specialist is the focus not only on hiring good staff but also keeping them—retention and recruitment.

- Education and training is a critical strategy that is used in many types of situations. Using creative cross-training to allow staff from medical or surgical units to work in intensive care units (ICU) is one approach (Gilbert & Counsell, 2000; Snyder & Nethersole-Chong, 1999). The benefits from this approach are increased availability of staff that has the skills that are needed in short-term specialty care; provides opportunity for professional develop-ment; and some of the staff may wish to eventually transfer to ICU staff, which then decreases the cost of recruitment and training. Rapid response teams (RRT) are also being used in many hospitals and has an impact of staff satisfaction and quality care. "The Rapid Response Team—known by some as the Medical Emergency Team—is a team of clini-cians who bring critical care expertise to the bedside. Simply put, the purpose of the Rapid Response Team is to bring critical care expertise to the patient bedside (or wherever it's needed)" (Institute of Health Improvement, 2010).

- Another staff approach might be to decrease the per diem pool and create a resource pool that is eligible to receive benefits (Beyers, 1999). The goal is to reduce overtime and use of supplementary staff. In addition, standardizing skill requirements and competencies in these groups will help make them more flexible and more acceptable to staff as they can carry expected responsibilities. This same institution also used SWAT teams or teams of staff that could be called to areas that needed extra assistance for a short time (for example, for 2 hours) may be used to assist with assessments, admissions, procedures, and so on.

- The use of unlicensed assistive personnel has been discussed in this text. This strategy for coping with RN shortages has caused much conflict. Health care organizations have sup-ported it as a strategy to reduce costs, but this must be analyzed carefully in each situation to determine if costs will actually be reduced (Murphy, 1995). It is easy to assume that unlicensed means unskilled or uneducated, but this is not a fair assumption. UAPs can be skilled with the right education, training, and supervision; however, short training periods and lack of follow-up will lead to problems with quality and safety and require even more RN supervisory time—time that is rarely available.

- Teaching staff how to cope with inadequate staffing is a strategy that can be incorporated in any health care organization. There are few, if any, who do not experience shortages. Filipovich (1999) recommends the following. Safety comes first and because of this nurses should (a) assess the situation and define the implications for nursing care, (b) notify the supervisor and describe the specific problem in terms of the standards that can-not be met and the type of assistance that is needed, and (c) document staffing objectives and keep them on file. Nurses also need to conduct research to provide more data about quality indicators.

- Use of float staff is a strategy that is used to respond to staff shortages. One of the major concerns with this strategy is whether or not the nurse is qualified and competent to practice in the clinical area where the nurse is asked to work. Nurses have the right to refuse to go but then should request training and orientation. If, however, this training and orientation is offered and the nurse refuses to attend and then refuses to float, the nurse may be terminated (Gobis, 2001). The nurse needs to know what the state's practice laws and regulations say about performing care for which one is not qualified to do.

- The image of nursing is a critical factor that needs to be addressed. Nurses need to be the drivers of the effort to improve this image. This topic is important in much of this text's content. The ANA and other health care organizations have been working on the image of the health care system. Nursing has tried running television and radio ads as well as using print media. It is important that collaborative efforts are made with other groups to work on the image. Consumers need to know what a nurse is and what a nurse can do. Image also affects recruitment and interest of young people in the profession. Some communities have nurses and nursing students go to high schools to talk about nursing. Recruitment fairs have also become very common.

- Use of mandatory overtime has become a common strategy for handling the staffing shortage, and one that has serious consequences—affecting ability to work, health of staff, retention, quality, and safety. It is a short gap or crisis approach that will not solve the problem long-term. Many states are passing legislation to limit the use of mandatory overtime, and the ANA has pushed for federal legislation in its staffing act. The Fair Labor Standards Act offers some protection. First, it does not mandate that employers provide lunch or rest breaks and does not comment on health care employee mandatory overtime (Overtime pay, 2002). It does, however, require employers to pay overtime wages for assigned hours worked over 40, of which it has knowledge, or of which it should have knowledge, but there may be exempt employees so new staff should clarify this during the hiring process. Nurses need to know what their rights are in relation to overtime pay and should inquire about it and be aware of changes in legislation. This does not, however, resolve the problems of mandatory overtime when nurses have no choice about staying at work after their scheduled time or, if they refuse, risk losing their jobs.

- **Patient classification systems (PCS)** can be used to help identify and quantify patient needs (McConnell, 2000; Seago, 2002). The systems are used to "objectively determine workload requirements and staffing needs" (Sullivan & Decker, 2001, p. 285). There is much in the nursing literature about PCS usage. The following factors are important to consider when using a PCS, factors that can affect the PCS rating and decisions that might be made about scheduling: "(1) the patient's preferences and medical condition, including co-morbidities, (2) time-consuming non-clinical facets such as patient turnover, (3) complex clinical decisions and the intricate interaction of health care's physical, social, ethical, emotional, and financial aspects, (4) nurses' unpredictable multitasking, and (5) caregivers' varying knowledge levels, experience, and clinical and critical thinking skills" (McConnell, 2000, p. 52). There have been criticisms of these systems, particularly the earlier systems. As technology has developed, it is now expected that newer PCS will be more effective in matching caregiver profiles with patient care needs, and caregiver–patient interactions can be tracked and monitored (Malloch & Conovaloff, 1999; Sullivan & Decker, 2001).

- Skill mix is an important aspect of staffing. Nursing skill mix is "the proportion of RNs to the total complement of nursing staff" (Mark, Salyer, & Wan, 2000, p. 552). It is a topic that has been the focus of many research studies.

- Magnet recognition is another strategy that has been used to improve recruitment, retention, and staffing during staff shortages. These hospitals meet certain standards that tend to support staff recruitment and retention.

- Increased compensation will not be enough to solve the problem although it does help some and should not be ignored.

- Job sharing, which has been used in a variety of work settings, is now also used in some health care organizations. It is an innovative approach, but it will not work for all positions.

"An alliance of two nurses in a job-sharing role is one option for successfully meeting the challenges of today's health care, while promoting job satisfaction and personal endeavors" (Gliss, 2000, p. 40). Some key issues are selecting the job that can be done by two people and finding the right staff matches. It requires partnership and sharing. This strategy can attract nurses who want to work part time and still make a contribution.

- Employers need to change their view of staff—moving away from viewing staff as just an expense but also an asset. Strategies to value staff need to be used (Nevidjon & Erikson, 2001). Nursing leaders and managers need to be assertive in communicating the value of nursing to upper level management.
- Providing clinical practice opportunities and responsibility that match the nurse's knowledge and skill can help to retain nurses.
- The *Code for Nurses* (American Nurses Association, 2008) requires that nurses should participate in the development of workplaces so that they are environments in which quality care can be provided. Nurses must advocate for their patients. This type of workplace should help to retain nurses and also to attract nurses—decreasing job dissatisfaction.
- Nurses need more assistance with developing delegation skills because delegation is required more and more with the increased use of non-RN caregivers. "Nurses must know what tasks are appropriate to 'give away,' how to manage the workload and be accountable for outcomes, and how to provide for the growth and development of non-RN caregivers and other support staff. Nurses sometimes feel less valued when they must delegate tasks to a non-nurse. However, nursing can consider delegation, along with shared governance, as another form of empowerment" (Andreoli, 1992; as cited in Nevidjon & Erickson, 2001, p. 10).
- The decreasing number of nursing faculty is a serious problem. Attracting more nurses into teaching is critical. There is now more funding available for graduate education. Schools of nursing need to develop programs to educate future faculty to develop alternative effective strategies for coping with the faculty shortage.
- Nursing curricula need to be current. Graduates must be prepared to practice. If they are not, there is a risk of losing the new nurse early in the career track, as noted in the 2010 nursing education report (Benner, Sutphen, Leonard, & Day, 2010).
- Greater attention needs to be given to orientation, preceptorships, internships and residencies, and other creative methods to assist in helping new graduates adjust to the workplace and retain them (Benner, Sutphen, Leonard, & Day, 2010; IOM, 2010).
- The recruitment of foreign nurses, a strategy that has been used in past nursing shortages, is increasing again. These nurses need to be able to pass the NCLEX exam, speak English, and provide assistance with culture adjustment. Some ethical issues with this strategy should be considered. Many countries are experiencing shortages, so the United States is taking nurses from some countries that need them, too (Pearson & Peels, 2001). The International Council of Nurses (ICN) "condemns the practice of recruitment of nurses to countries where governments and other relevant authorities have failed to address deficiencies known to cause nurses to leave the profession" (Steefel, 2001, p. 36). The Rural and Urban Health Care Act of 2001 proposed an expansion of the H-1C category to allow all hospitals to hire nurses on temporary visas and allow them to stay in the United States for up to 6 years. The goal was to reduce barriers in getting these nurses to come to the United States. Addressing the nursing shortage with this approach will not have a long-term impact on the problem and includes regulatory and legislative issues.
- As hospitals begin to realize that they must figure out how to deliver quality care more effectively despite the shortage, they have arrived at a number of staffing strategies. One strategy looks at the delivery system. "The delivery system determines the way that nursing care will be delivered" (Manthey, 2001, p. 424). One of these is a core incremental staffing plan (Manthey, 2001). This plan has two major components (a) experienced, full-time staff that manages and/or delivers care and (b) part-time, short-term, transitional regular employees and supplemental staff (agency and travelers), that delivers most of the daily care activities. The first level of staff is the senior staff. This level would include the

appropriate skill mix for the patient acuity level. The staffing plan is part of the system as is the care delivery model (for example, team nursing, primary care nursing, Synergy model, and so on). The risk with this approach is creating a class system by communicating that one level of staff is better than the other. The real focus should be that some RNs have chosen different lifestyles and career interests (e.g., travelers and agency nurses) and want the flexibility. The core staff is responsible for continuity of care.

- Regulatory and policy issues may be a factor affecting the shortage (Nevidjon & Erickson, 2001). One particular area is documentation that is often affected by regulations. Documentation is complex and time-consuming. It can be very repetitive, and staff may not see the value in the documentation. Documentation needs to be streamlined, standardized, and must take advantage of computers. In addition, state boards of nursing should review their policies and procedures and determine what is contemporary or out-of-date as these policies and procedures may not be helpful in retaining nurses. The electronic medical record and other electronic methods may assist in making work more efficient and safer. (See Chapter 18.)

- Organizations need to explore how staff spends its time and if there are better ways of doing things to decrease activities that could be better done by someone else. Nurses spend more time than they need to on non-nursing tasks. Over the years these tasks have only increased. Effective management requires that work be allocated according to who is the best person to do the work. As this problem area is explored, it is important to consider trends such as patient population, staffing patterns, workload, and care practices (Hader & Clandio, 2002). All of this should be directed at effective staff utilization and allocation of limited resources (Institute of Medicine, 2004).

- Some health care organizations are using their own staff to increase the pool of RNs. They are identifying nonprofessional staff that might be interested and have the ability to pursue nursing education (Fox & Brooks, 2000). This is an excellent example of an organization supporting career advancement. In addition, many organizations are supporting RN efforts to obtain a BSN degree. Support can be in the form of tuition reimbursement, scheduling flexibility, and other types of services to make it easier to go back to school. Some organizations have partnered with nursing schools to conduct courses onsite or to develop online programs. These efforts indicate that the organizations really do want to help staff develop themselves.

# APPLYING LEADERSHIP AND MANAGEMENT

## MY HOSPITAL UNIT

Your hospital and your unit have been experiencing major problems with staffing. You do not feel you have a good relationship with human resources. In reviewing your staffing data for the past 2 years you notice that new graduates are not staying long, with an average of 6–7 months. This impacts your budget, staff morale with complaints of constantly orienting new staff, and patient outcomes. The latter is of concern as there are documentation errors, medication errors, and patients complain that staff is not tuned into their needs. This is a major challenge for you. What do you need to do? Develop a plan to address this problem given the facts you have here and based on previous decisions you have made about your unit. Use the virtual unit site found on the textbook website to record the work that you do in the role of nurse manager for your unit.

## Critical Thinking Questions and Activities

1. What does it feel like to be an interviewer or an interviewee for a position? This exercise should be done in small teams of four. Get a copy of the local newspaper (the Sunday edition is usually best for this exercise). Review the employment section and select several ads for RN positions to use in the exercise. Two members of the team should role-play a job interview, one as interviewer and the other as interviewee. Use the information found in this chapter to guide the role-play. The other two members should observe and critique the interview. Then those observing can do a role-play for a different jobs, switching roles. As you role-play you should consider the questions suggested in this content and add others that you think about. Effectiveness of communication is also important to observe. How comfortable did the interviewer and interviewee feel doing the role-play? Which role was easier to do and why do you think so? What can you learn from this exercise to help you improve your interviewing skills? Going on interviews even if not really interested in taking a position can help you learn more about interviewing, just as role-playing can help you.

2. There are some important questions that should be asked by the interviewee. The following are questions that could be asked in an interview for a position in a health care organization. Review the questions, then select a health care organization and see how much of the information you can find out about the organization. This exercise might be done in small teams. It is best to select a number of different types of organizations as well as some that are the same (for example, several acute care hospitals) so that you can compare and contrast the data.
   - What are the goals of the organization for the next 5 years? What are the goals of patient services or nursing services?
   - What has been the nurse turnover rate for the last 2 years?
   - What is the nurse–patient ratio? It is best to clarify the department or services as ratios can vary. What is the staff mix? What is the scheduling method used?
   - Do they use competency-based performance appraisal?
   - What is the leadership style of nursing management? Ask for examples.
   - How does management view staff suggestions? Ask for a recent example and what happened with the suggestion.
   - What is the staff satisfaction rate?
   - Does nursing services use a specific care model, and if so, what model? How effective has it been?
   - Is there shared governance? Ask for a description.
   - Is there a clinical ladder or something similar, and what is it like?

- What is done for employees in relationship to safety on the job?
- Is mandatory overtime used?
- What is the organizational structure, and to whom does the particular position sought report?

Your answers to these questions will depend upon the individual organizations that you select. After the information is collected, compare and contrast it and then consider what would be important for you to consider in your job search. Discuss these with your class-mates to understand different viewpoints. Not everyone looks for the same factors in a job or an employer.

3. What is the status of nursing shortage in your local area? What strategies are health care organizations using to recruit staff? Are they effective? What do you think should be done to decrease the nursing shortage? Does your state or local area have a workforce group, and if so, what can you find out about it?

4. Do a literature search on patient acuity classification systems. What can you learn about them? Does a hospital in your area use a system, and if so, what can you find out about it?

## Media Links

- **URL: http://www.nursingworld.org**
  American Nurses Association
- **URL: http://www.aacn.nche.edu**
  American Association of College of Nursing
- **URL: http://www.bls.gov**
  Bureau of Labor Statistics
- **URL: http://www.dhhs.gov**
  Department of Health and Human Services
- **URL: http://www.nln.org**
  National League of Nursing
- **URL: http://www.hrsa.gov**
  Health Resources Services Agency
- **URL: http://www.nursecredentialing.org/certification.aspx**
  American Nurses Credentialing Center

---

**Pearson Nursing Student Resources**

Find additional review materials at
**nursing.pearsonhighered.com**

Prepare for success with additional NCLEX®-style practice questions, interactive assignments and activities, Web links, animations and videos, and more!

---

## References

Aiken, L., Sloane, D., Lake, E., Sochalski, J. & Weber, A. (1999). Organization and outcomes of inpatient AIDS care. *Medical Care, 37*(8), 760–772.

Aiken, T. (2001). Sexual harassment. In J. Dochterman & H. Grace (Eds.), *Current issues in nursing* (6th ed., pp. 576–582). St. Louis, MO: Mosby, Inc.

Aiken, L., et al. (2010). Implications of the California nurse staffing mandate for other states. *Health Services Research, 45*(4), 904–921.

American Association of Colleges of Nursing. (2010). Press release: Amid calls for more highly education nurses, AACN data show impressive growth in doctoral nursing programs. Final data from AACN's 2009 survey indicate ninth year of enrollment and admissions increases in entry-level baccalaureate nursing programs. Retrieved from http://www.aacn.nche.edu

American Nurses Association. (1999). *Principles for nurse staffing.* Washington, DC: Author.

American Nurses Association. (2001). *Code for nurses with interpretation and application.* Washington, DC: Nursing Publishing, Inc.

American Organization of Nurse Executives. (1999). *Nurse staffing survey: February 23, 1999.* Chicago, IL: American Hospital Association.

Andreoli, K. (1992). Primary nursing for the 1990s and beyond. *Journal of Professional Nursing, 8*(4), 24.

Benner, P., Sutphen, M., Leonard, V., & Day, L. (2010). *Educating nurses.* San Francisco: Jossey-Bass Publishers.

Beyers, M. (1999). About how to reduce overtime and use of per diem staff. *Nursing Management, 30*(12), 56.

Bradley, C. (2001). A response to California's mandated nursing ratios. *Journal of Nursing Scholarship* (second quarter), 179–184.

Butler, T., & Waldroop, J. (1999). Job sculpting: The art of retaining your best people. *Harvard Business Review, 87*(September–October), 143–152.

Cardillo, D. (2002). How to resign in style. *Nursing Spectrum Metro Edition, 3*(2), 11.

Carroll, P. (2001). Questions to avoid when conducting interviews. Retrieved April 28, 2001, from http://www.nurses.com/content...12-11D5-A770-D0B7694F32} &Bucket=Columns

Christmas, K. (2008). How work environment impacts retention. *Nursing Economics, 26*(5), 316–318.

Colosi, M. (2002). Rules of engagement for the nursing shortage. *JONA Health care Law, Ethics, and Regulation, 4*(3), 50–54.

Danaher, M. (2001). Medical leave under the family and medical leave act: Understanding the impact of the act's interpretive guidance. *Journal of Legal Nurse Consultants, 12*(3), 3–6.

Diehl-Oplinger, L., & Kaminski, M. (2000). Need critical care nurses? Inquire within. Use preceptors to orient your facility's nurses to critical care. *Nursing Management, 31*(3), 44, 46.

Ellis, L. (2000, March). Have you and your staff signed self-care contracts? *Nursing Management,* 47–48.

Fiesta, J. (1999). Greater need for background checks. *Nursing management, 30*(11), 26.

Filipovich, C. (1999). Teach nurses effective ways to deal with inadequate staffing. *Nursing Management, 30*(12), 38.

Finkelman, A. (1996). *Psychiatric nursing administration manual.* Gaithersburg, MD: Aspen Publishers.

Forman, H. (2001). Diagnosis: Disconnect. *Nursing Spectrum Midwest Region, 2*(9), 24–25MW.

Fournies, F. (1999). *Why employees don't do what they're supposed to do.* New York: McGraw-Hill.

Fox, D., & Brooks, M. (2000). The professional nurse education program. A work force development model. *Journal of Nursing Administration, 30*(10), 490–496.

Fox, K. (1998). Workers' compensation and managed care. NCSL LegisBrief. *National Conference of State Legislatures, 6*(31), 1–2.

Gilbert, M., & Counsell, C. (2000). Intensive care unit cross training: Saving dollars while retraining staff. *Journal of Nursing Administration, 30*(6), 308, 324.

Gliss, R. (2000). Job sharing: An option for professional nurses. *Nursing Economics, 18*(1), 40–41.

Gobis, L. (2001). The perils of floating. *American Journal of Nursing, 101*(9), 78.

Gottlieb, M. (1998). *The confused consumer's guide to choosing a health care plan.* New York: Hyperion.

Hader, R., & Clandio, T. (2002). Seven methods to effectively manage patient care labor resources. *Journal of Nursing Administration, 32*(2), 66–68.

Hemmila, D. (2002). When helping hurts. *Nurse Week. Great Lakes Region, 2*(2), 7.

Hung, R. (2002). A note on nurse self-scheduling. *Nursing Economics, 20*(1), 37–39.

Hutchison, P. (2001a). Strategies for recruiting and retaining health care professionals. Part 1. *Home Care Provider, 6*(2), 53–55.

Hutchison, P. (2001b). Strategies for recruiting and retaining health care professionals. Part 2: The right candidate. *Home Care Provider, 6*(4), 14–17.

Institute for Health Improvement. (2010). *Establish a rapid response team.* Retrieved May 23, 2010, from http://www.ihi.org/IHI/Topics/CriticalCare/IntensiveCare/Changes/EstablishaRapidResponseTeam.htm.

Institute of Medicine. (2001). *Crossing the quality chasm.* Washington, DC: National Academies Press.

Institute of Medicine. (2004). *Keeping patients safe.* Washington, DC: National Academies Press.

Institute of medicine. (2010). The future of nursing: Leading change, advancing health. Washington, DC: National Academies Press.

Joint Commission. (2004). *The Joint Commission Press Kit.* Retrieved October 7, 2007, from http://www.jointcommission.org/NewsRoom/Press/Kits/

Jones, C. & Gates, M. (2007). The costs and benefits of nurse turnover: A business case for nurse retention. *Online Journal of Issues in Nursing, 12*(3). Retrieved from http://www.nursingworld.org

Kalisch, B., Begeny, S., & Anderson, C. (2008). The effect of consistent nursing shifts on teamwork and continuity of care. *Journal of Nursing Administration, 38*(3), 132–137.

Kovner, C., et al. (2007). Newly licensed RNs' characteristics, work attitudes, and intentions to work. *American Journal of Nursing, 107*, 58–70.

Kramer, M. (1985). Why does reality shock continue? In J. McCloskey & H. Grace (Eds.), *Current issues in nursing* (pp. 891–903). Boston, MA: Blackwell Scientific Publication.

Malloch, K., & Conovaloff, A. (1999). Patient classification systems, Part 1: The third generation. *Journal of Nursing Administration, 29*(7/8), 49–56.

Manthey, M. (2001). A core incremental staffing plan. *Journal of Nursing Administration, 31*(9), 424–425.

Mark, B., Salyer, J., & Wan, T. (2000). Market, hospital, and nursing unit characteristics as predictors of nursing unit skill mix. *Journal of Nursing Administration, 30*(11), 552–560.

McConnell, E. (2000). Staffing and scheduling at your fingertips. *Nursing Management, 31*(3), 52–53.

Milgram, L., Spector, A., & Treger, M. (1999). *Managing smart.* Houston, TX: Gulf Publishing Company.

Murphy, E. (1995). Unsubstantiated assumptions about unlicensed assistive personnel obscure the challenge of delivering quality care. *AORN, 62*(7), 8, 10.

Mustard, L. (2002). Caring and competence. *JONA's Health care Law, Ethics, and Regulation, 4*(2), 36–43.

National Council of State Boards of Nursing. (1996). *Definition of competence and standards for competence.* Chicago: Author.

National Institute for Occupational Safety and Health. (1999) *Stress at work.* Washington, DC: Department of Health and Human Services.

National League for Nursing. (2010). Press release: Findings form latest NLN annual survey of schools of nursing administered October through December 2009 confirm reported trends.

National Mental Health Association. Promoting mental health in the workplace. Retrieved March 10, 2005, from http://www.nmha.org

Nayak, S. (1991, March/April). Strategies to support the new nurse in practice. *Journal of Nursing Staff Development,* 64–66.

Nevidjon, B., & Erickson, J. (2001). The nursing shortage: Solutions for the short and long term. *Online Journal of Issues in Nursing, 6*(1). Retrieved June 6, 2001, from http://www.nursingworld.org/ojin

Nurse Reinvestment Act, H.R.3487ENR, 107th Congress. (2002). Retrieved on December 8, 2002, from http:// www.access.gpo.gov/nara/publaw/ 107publ.html

Overtime pay. (2002). *Ohio Nurses Review,* July 6.

Pearson, A., & Peels, S. (2001). A global view of nursing in the new millennium— 2: The nursing workforce. *International Journal of Nursing Practice, 7*(S5–S10), 55–59.

Pellico, L., Brewer, C., & Kovner, C. (2009). What newly licensed registered nurses have to say about their first experiences. *Nursing Outlook, 57*(4), 194–203.

Pell, A. (2000). *The complete idiot's guide to recruiting the right stuff.* Indianapolis, IN: Alpha Books.

Peter, L., & Hull, R. (1969). *The Peter Principle: Why things go wrong.* New York: William Morrow.

Peterson, C. (2001). Nursing shortage: Not a simple problem—no easy answers. *Online Journal of Issues in Nursing, 6*(1). Retrieved June 6, 2001, from http://www .nursingworld.org/ojin

Robert Wood Johnson Foundation. (October, 2007). *Charting nursing's future. Reports on policies that can transform patient care.* Retrieved April 1, 2010, from http:// www.rwjf.org

Seago, J. (2002). A comparison of two patient classification instruments in an acute care hospital. *Journal of Nursing Administration, 32*(5), 243–249.

Snyder, J., & Nethersole-Chong, D. (1999). Is cross-training medical/surgical RNs to ICU the answer? *Nursing Management, 30*(2), 58–60.

Squires, A. (2002). New graduate orientation in the rural community hospital. *Journal of Continuing Education in Nursing, 33,* 203–209.

Steefel, L. (2001, May). Hands from abroad shore up nursing shortages. *Nursing Spectrum Metro Edition,* 35–36.

Steinbrook, R. (2002). Nursing in the crossfire. *New England Journal of Medicine, 346*(22), 1757–1766.

Sullivan, E., & Decker, P. (2001). *Effective leadership and management in nursing.* Upper Saddle River, NJ: Prentice Hall.

Vernarec, E. (2001). How to cope with job stress. *RN, 64*(3), 244–246.

Welton, J. (2007). Mandatory hospital nurse to patient staffing rations: Time to take a different approach. *The Online Journal of Nursing, 12*(3).

Whitaker, C., Carson, D. & Sawlanski, J. (2000). Dealing with difficult behavior. *Nursing 2000, 30*(6), 81–82.

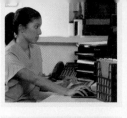
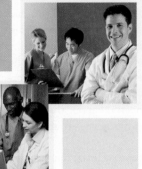

# 10

# Consumers and Nurses

## CHAPTER OUTLINE

## LEARNING OUTCOMES

Before you begin, take a moment to familiarize yourself with the learning outcomes for this chapter.

- Examine the history of health care consumerism and its impact on health care. Assess the relationship between public policy and the health care consumer.
- Compare and contrast the consumer implications of *Healthy People* and the Institute of Medicine reports (*Quality Chasm* series).
- Assess how technology plays a role in consumer health care information.
- Examine the relationship between patient education and health care consumerism.
- Critique how consumers are involved in evaluating the quality of care.
- Apply patient advocacy in your role as a nurse.

## KEY TERMS

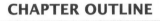

- Advocacy
- Consumerism
- Macroconsumer
- Microconsumer

The consumer's role has changed as health care has undergone major changes and managed care became the dominant approach to health care reimbursement. This chapter addresses the role of the consumer or the patient in the health care delivery system. By its very nature the nursing process places both the patient and the patient's family in a major role. The recent work by the Institute of Medicine (IOM) also emphasizes patient-centered care—which is a consumer-oriented approach. Viewing patients as consumers of health care services has been gaining strength as consumers speak out about their health care. They are concerned about the quality of care and its cost. Nurses have had a role in this as well, as patient advocacy is an important component of nursing care.

There is no doubt that the patient is paying more for care as employers pay less. Premiums are higher, as are co-payments and deductibles. Recognition of consumer priorities and understanding the criteria that consumers use as they evaluate their health care services are critical to maintaining a positive relationship with the health care consumer. Health care delivery organizations, providers, and insurers need to know more about consumer issues: What does the patient want? Is the outcome what the patient wanted? With the greater focus on interprofessional teams, the patient is viewed as part of the team (Institute of Medicine, 2003). Consumer rights and protection are front page news as health care legislation on the state and federal levels escalates. Legislation, however, may lead to more problems, and thus must be considered carefully. A balance needs to exist in meeting the needs of all consumers, patients/enrollees/employees, employers, the government, providers, and insurers. Patients are turning more to nurses and asking questions about their health care and health delivery, so nurses need to be prepared to answer their questions or know how to help patients seek the answers about health care. Customer- or patient-centered health care means the nurse must be more aware of customer/patient needs. This chapter discusses consumerism, the role of the consumer or patient in health care policy, health care information and consumers, patient evaluation of health care, and the nurse as patient advocate.

# The Consumer and Health Care

## Who Is the Consumer?

Consumers can be described in a variety of ways. A **macroconsumer** is a large purchaser of health care services (e.g., employers, government). The macroconsumer may also be called the customer. Clearly, this type of consumer has a major voice in health care decisions due to its size and acts as a liaison between the insurers and employees. A **microconsumer** is the employee, the employee's family, and people who buy insurance as individuals rather than through an employer. They are the users of the health care services or patients. All consumers, whether macro or micro, make decisions about the purchase of health care coverage, but the microconsumer is involved in more decisions about health care services that directly affect them. Choice is an important aspect of health care, and some consumers feel that their choices have diminished (e.g., choice of health plan has decreased as employers offer fewer plans and more tightly control the types of plans; the choice of provider and when the provider can be consulted have been affected; and in some cases the choice of using specialty care has diminished). As health care reimbursement has changed, choice has become an important health care consumer issue and one that is integral in many consumer complaints about their health care.

## History of Health Care Consumerism

**Consumerism** has been evolving over many years. With the development of managed care, consumerism became even more important, and we see even more involvement today with the development of health care reform of 2010. What is the history of health care consumerism? How did it evolve? In the 1970s, consumers were informed and assertive about their active participation in health care (Armer, 1998). During that time, the focus was on patient satisfaction and utilization of health care services. A 1971 study found that 75% of the families sampled believed that there was a crisis in health care, but only 10% said they were dissatisfied with the quality of their care (Andersen, Kravits, & Anderson, 1971). This is a confusing result; despite the fact that a high percentage felt that the health care system was in a crisis, few were critical of that care's quality. Patient satisfaction is a very complex issue, and it is not always easy to know what a patient is responding to during a satisfaction survey. Quality is also difficult to define, and the perspective of the person defining quality has a major impact on the definition.

In the 1980s, the focus of consumer and provider concerns changed to the cost of health care (Boston, 1990; Sovie, 1990). In addition, accessing health care is important and particularly in rural areas, the poor, the elderly, and minorities as discussed in Chapter 8 on health care disparities. Quality and access to services have been important issues throughout the health care consumer movement, and these issues are even more important today.

As managed care became the dominant player in the health care system in the 1990s, a change developed regarding health care consumerism. Consumers were not as active in the early 1990s as they became by the end of the decade. Managed care developed on the West Coast and then moved to the East Coast. Then managed care slowly moved across the country, with some areas not feeling its effect until the mid-1990s. As this was occurring, managed care did not affect enough consumers to cause them to organize and protest against it. The media were not as cognizant of the changes, so it was not a front-page news item. However, as more consumers were affected by managed care, consumers became stronger and made a major impact on health care delivery. Consumers finally became concerned when the problems affected their personal care. Consumers reached a point of dissatisfaction to say "Enough!" This cry came from the soon-to-be-seniors generation. The baby boomers, in contrast, are not new to protesting and being assertive. They had an impact on managed care, which has now lost much of its influence in health care; however, managed care strategies were adopted by many third-party payers and integrated into all types of health insurance plans. Consumers are now addressing their concerns about health care delivery. An example is the role of consumers in the health care reform process of 2009–2010. Proponents for different approaches reached out to consumers via ads, television, radio, and the Internet. Consumers had an active voice through their representatives in Congress. Sometimes these issues became very emotional. Members of Congress used patient or consumer experiences to make their points. There is no doubt that as consumers experience problems with health care, they often criticize health care and have been successful just as they demanded changes in managed care and other aspects of reimbursement. There are, however, positive aspects of managed care that should not be ignored, such as its gradual increased emphasis on preventive care, health promotion, and continuity. Nonetheless, it is easy to lose sight of the positive aspects of managed care. Emotions sometimes undermine rational policy changes and criticism. If the goal is to control costs, provide quality care, and increase care delivery to those who cannot afford care, it is critical to find a balance and identify the strengths and limitations of managed care, while building on its strengths.

Health care providers and third-party payers recognize the need to listen more to consumer criticisms and are more willing to make some changes that address these criticisms. Today, *patient centered* is a frequently heard term, although it does not always significantly affect health care in practical changes. More effort has been made to provide the consumer with information. In 2010 pre-existing conditions was a critical issue that was addressed during health care reform legislation so that pre-existing conditions cannot be used to exclude persons from insurance coverage. This was a key consumer issue. Insurers did not want this to be part of the legislation.

Nurses have long supported a more consumer-based approach, but why would health care organizations and insurers be interested? Health care organizations are increasingly aware of the need to develop satisfied consumers who participate in their care. This does affect costs in that insurers want to hear that their enrollees are satisfied with the health care they receive. Certainly, the need to obtain contracts from employers is one driving force. Insurers also want consumers to have more understanding about their health care needs in order to be informed purchasers of care and informed users of health care services. They believe that an informed health care consumer will reduce health care costs. At the same time, consumers are turning more to government and legislation to influence health care policy making and get their needs met.

# Public Policy and the Health Care Consumer

"Only through better understanding of the consumers' perceptions of the current system and their expectations for future health care delivery can policy makers and health care providers develop responsive health care programs that will meet local and national health care needs and be acceptable to consumers in the decades ahead" (Armer, 1998, p. 515). This need for understanding is still relevant today. The Institute of Medicine strongly supports this need with its emphasis on patient-centered care. Health care reform of 2010 legislation was influenced by the IOM reports and the need for patient-centered, quality care. Nursing organizations have a responsibility to advocate for the consumer and partner with consumer groups, and they frequently do this because collaboration can result in a win-win outcome. More, however, could be done. The examples of health care fraud and abuse found in Chapter 2 indicate that nurses do get involved in situations when the consumer needs strong nurses who will take risks for them. This can be very difficult for nurses, but situations like these can demonstrate nurses' leadership skills.

The consumer must also become involved in the development of health care public policy. This is usually done through organizations such as the American Diabetes Association, National Alliance for the Mentally Ill, the American Association of Retired Persons, the Arthritis Foundation, the Susan G. Komen Breast Cancer Foundation, and other organizations that advocate for specific policies while representing their membership. Frequently, these organizations also have health care professional members who participate in policy advocacy. Individual consumers also go directly to their legislators, on both the state and federal levels, to have a voice in policy decision making. Television, the Internet, and newspapers keep the public informed on health care policy issues and are good resources for identifying current policy issues. Nurses can be supportive of consumer involvement by ensuring that consumers get accurate information by acting as consultants, through serving as experts while writing letters to editors, and keeping up with media content. Typically, the media turns to physicians for comments about health care, but nurses are also good resources for this information. This means that nurses have to let the media know that they are competent and available to do this. Nursing organizations usually let the media know that they have representatives who are willing to be interviewed.

In late 2009 the U.S. Preventive Services Task Force reversed its recommendation about the use of mammography screening for women 40 and older in addition to changes in recommendation for cervical cancer screening. The task force based this decision on evidence-based practice after a review of current research. Consumers, primarily women, were angry about the decision and concerned that this would mean insurers would no longer cover this screening at the age of 40 but rather only cover based on the age recommended, 50 years old. This decision was a very important topic on news channels, newspapers, and so on with consumers expressing their concerns (Aronowitz, 2009; Grady, 2009; Kolata, 2009; U.S. Preventive Services Task Force, 2009). This decision was complex and struck a negative cord with consumers, particularly women. There is greater emphasis on basing medical decisions on evidence, which is also an IOM recommendation (2008). In this case, however, when the evidence was reviewed and indicated a need for change, consumers did not agree with the change. This will not be the only medical decision issue that arises when more evidence-based practice is implemented. Consumers know how to voice their opinions, and in this case they did—through the media, their government officials, and their health care providers.

## Consumer Rights

Consumer rights have slowly become a major issue in health care policy, particularly due to dissatisfaction with managed care. States are active in establishing requirements related to information that the insurer must supply to the consumer and to identify grievance and appeal requirements. The Patient Self-Determination Act of 1990 (PDSA) is a law that applies to all health care organizations (hospitals, long-term care facilities, and home health agencies) that participate in Medicare or Medicaid by receiving reimbursement from these government sources (American Cancer Society, 2008). What does this law require? All facilities that receive Medicare and Medicaid funding must provide their patients with information about patients' rights, which are typically referred to as a Patient's Bill of Rights. In reality, this means all health care facilities as few do not receive this federal funding through reimbursement. Some of the rights that organizations typically develop relate to (a) confidentiality, (b) consent, (c) right to make medical decisions, (d) right to be informed about diagnosis and treatment, (e) right to refuse treatment, and (f) use of advance directives.

The consumer rights issue is highly controversial. If too many consumer rights are recognized, how will this affect the ability of insurers to meet their goals to reduce health care costs? Reducing costs is a concern for all, not just the insurers. What effect will patient rights have on health care provider organizations? For example, changes in patient privacy protection are costly to implement and yet they represent a consumer issue. Consumers also want costs lowered; however, the critical factor is what must be given up to reach this goal. Health care organizations such as hospitals, clinics, long-term care facilities, and home care agencies must consider how particular patient's rights might impact care and costs. Although probably initiated by dissatisfaction with managed care, many of the consumer driven changes had little to do directly with managed care and really focused more on health care in general, leading to demands for a more patient-centered health care delivery system today and health care reform.

The Consumer Assessment of Healthcare Providers and Systems (CAHPS) is a public-private program that develops patient surveys to assess patient perspectives of their ambulatory and facility level care (Consumer Assessment of Healthcare Providers and Systems, 2009). CAHPS is funded and administered through the Agency for Healthcare Research and Quality (AHRQ). The goals of this program are to assess patient-centeredness, compare contract performance, and improve quality of care. The data provide benchmarking opportunities for comparison of health plans (commercial plans, Medicare, and Medicaid), clinician groups, and hospitals. The CAHPS website is a valuable resource about consumer views of their health care. The site provides an interactive benchmarking database. A quality improvement process is described on the site that includes content related to plan strategy, development and testing of strategy, monitoring strategy, and reassessment and response. The level of content and resources this site provides indicates that consumer viewpoints about their health care are much more important than they were ten years ago.

The end of the 1990s brought major efforts to pass additional federal legislation to establish a greater patient or consumer protection bill of rights. There have been many proposals in Congress, and in the fall of 1999, the Senate and the House passed two very different bills, requiring compromises on their parts; however, no patient's rights legislation has been passed.

The consumer rights issue is highly controversial. If too many consumer rights are recognized, how will this affect the ability of insurers to meet their goals of reducing health care costs? Reducing costs is a concern for all, not just the insurers. What effect will it have on health care provider organizations? For example, the changes in patient privacy protection are costly to implement and yet they represent a consumer issue. Consumers also want costs lowered; however, the critical factor is what must be given up to reach this goal. Health care organizations such as hospitals, clinics, long-term care facilities, and home health care agencies need to consider how particular patient's rights might impact care and costs.

All of this activity indicates how the late 1980s and the 1990s were an active time for patient consumerism. Although probably initiated by dissatisfaction with managed care, many of the changes had little to do directly with managed care and really focused more on health care in general. HIPPA legislation discussed earlier in the text is a consumer rights law in that it addresses privacy and confidentiality.

## Special Reports and Initiatives: Implications for Health Care Consumers

*Healthy People* and the Institute of Medicine reports on quality in the health care delivery system are very important for the consumer. These reports and initiatives, one led by the government and the second by a non-governmental agency that serves in an advisory capacity for the government, have had a major influence on health care professions, the delivery system, and health care professions education.

### Healthy People

*Healthy People* is a national prevention initiative that identifies opportunities to improve the health of all Americans by identifying goals and objectives that are used by the U.S. Department of Health and Human Services (DHHS), as well as many health care organizations and institutions, to promote health and disease and illness prevention (U.S. Department of Health and Human Services, 2010). The DHHS identified the first objectives in 1979, and then additional sets in 1990, 2000, and 2010.

A major goal of the *Healthy People* national initiative is to eliminate health disparities. This is a difficult goal to meet, as it requires improved access to care for all persons as well as new knowledge about the determinants of disease and effective interventions. With the large number of uninsured in the United States, this has been a challenge. Socioeconomic disparities, demographic changes, education-related differences, race, and ethnicity are significant barriers to the success of this goal. The Institute of Medicine report on disparities further clarified major problems in health care disparities (2002). This initiative is also the United States' contribution to the World Health Organization's "Health for All" strategy. *Healthy People 2020* program will be implemented over the next 10 years as has been done with the other *Healthy People* initiatives. It is based on work done with *Healthy People 2010* and its outcomes. The *Healthy People* website provides current information about 2010 final outcomes and changes in process for 2020 version of this important initiative. *Healthy People 2020* goals and objectives, which is the next time period for the initiative, can be found on the *Healthy People* website (see Media Links). Why does the *Healthy People* initiative have relevance to this chapter's content? *Healthy People* is an example of health policy, and it provides methods to improve the health status of individual consumers and communities. One of its major overall goals is to improve the quality of health-related decisions through effective communication. Interwoven into its other goals and their objectives is the need for consumer education, advocacy, and self-management of illness via health promotion and disease and illness prevention, all of which are supported by the IOM quality reports.

## The Institute of Medicine Reports on Quality Care

The Institute of Medicine reports on quality care have been discussed in most chapters in this text. The IOM strongly recommends the need for patient-centered care, collaboration, care coordination, and advocacy. Patients as consumers need to play an active role in their treatment and are members of the interprofessional team. Self-management is an important part of the IOM recommended changes (2003). Along with this emphasis, the matrix used to collect data and assess the status of health care quality annually includes two dimensions, one of which is "consumer perspectives of health care needs"—including staying healthy, getting better, living with illness or disability, and coping with the end of life (2001, p. 61). What does each of these elements mean?

- *Staying healthy:* the individual needs to get health care to stay well and avoid illness.
- *Getting better:* the individual requires care to reach recovery.
- *Living with illness or disability:* the individual needs assistance in learning how to manage and cope long-term.
- *Coping with end of life:* the individual needs support and care during terminal stages of illness.

Families and caregivers need to be involved in each of these elements of the consumer dimension. This quality improvement matrix draws the patient directly into the quality improvement process. Patients and their families can assist in identifying near misses, catching errors before they occur, by asking questions and being informed about their care and need to participate in evaluating care, at a minimum on the four elements of the consumer dimension.

## Information Resources and the Consumer

Technology has revolutionized consumer access to information. For example (Medical Library Association, 2009):

- More than 60 million people have used the Web to look for health information.
- Sixty percent of all Americans have access to the Web.
- Sixty-seven percent of Americans expect to find reliable health information on the Web.

There is no doubt that these numbers are increasing. Interactive technology has certainly changed the availability of information, particularly electronic mail, websites, intranets, interactive voice response systems, mobile phones, and smartphones. These new technologies offer additional ways to communicate with patients and to collect, manage, and utilize health care information. Who uses this technology and for what reasons? Patients use the information to learn more about their own health.

Technology opens up new roles for the nurse in health care organizations. Nurses may play an active role in the development and maintenance of these sites for providers and for insurers who want to make them available to members. Content needs to be accurate and useful, and nurses have the clinical expertise and ability to develop this content for consumers. Health care provider organizations need to use more nurses in the development of their websites. This is something that nursing management needs to be assertive about to gain more nursing input. Nurses who participate in these projects need to understand the basics of reimbursement, clinical needs, educational principles, and the use of technology to provide information. They must also be creative. Computer expertise is a plus, but in most cases, it is not required. Most providers and insurers that develop sites have computer experts to assist in this aspect of the project. Many consumer Internet sites provide information for consumers, and these are identified in Box 10-1.

National organizations and the government often provide the most accurate patient information. Information and education play vital roles in promoting health; preventing, managing, and coping with disease; and supporting appropriate decisions across the spectrum of health care. For individuals, effective health communication can help raise awareness of health risks, provide motivation and skills to reduce them, bring helpful connections to others in similar situations, and offer information about difficult choices, such as health plans and providers, treatments, and long-term care. For the wider community, health communication can set the public and social agenda, advocate for healthy policies and programs, promote positive changes in the socioeconomic environment and health infrastructure, and encourage social norms that benefit health and quality of life (U.S. Department of Health and Human Services, 2000).

## Patient Satisfaction and Quality

In today's highly competitive health care delivery environment, patient satisfaction and quality have become more important (Institute of Medicine, 2001). This text discusses many aspects of leadership and management, and yet sometimes it is difficult to see how this all relates to patient care. Do the health care environment and culture, services, satisfaction, staff retention,

---

| BOX 10-1 | CONSUMER INTERNET INFORMATION |
| --- | --- |

1. Consumer information is found on many Internet sites. The following are examples of sites: http://www.healthfinder.gov, http://familydoctor.org. Who sponsors the site? What information does each site provide? Is it helpful for the consumer? Is the information easy to access? Can you search for specific information? Is the information accurate? As a health care professional, how might you use the site? Can you find any information related to managed care, reimbursement, health care delivery, quality care, or patient rights? Why is the site's content related to this chapter's content?

2. http://www.ahcpr.gov. Visit this site and click on "Consumer Health." What information is available for consumers as they choose their health plans? Use the checklist to determine the health plan that is best for you.

3. http://www.aarp.org. What is this organization? What group of consumers does it serve and what are some of its services?

4. http://www.ncqa.org. Visit this site and click on "Health Care Organization." What is CAHPS? Does it provide helpful information? How might an MCO use this information? How might a health care professional or organization use this information?

5. http://www.medicare.gov. Visit this site and discover the types of consumer information that the government provides for Medicare beneficiaries.

## APPLYING EVIDENCE-BASED PRACTICE
### Evidence for Effective Leadership and Management

**Citation:** *Barriers and Drivers of Health Technology Use for the Elderly, Chronically Ill, and Underserved.* November, 2008. Agency for Healthcare Research and Quality. Rockville, MD. http://www.ahrq.gov/clinic/tp/hitbartp.htm. (Full report available at the government website.)

**Overview:** This is a systematic review of 563 full-text articles including 129 articles for abstraction. Few of the studies were specifically designed to compare the elderly, chronically ill, or underserved with the general population. Of the studies that reported the impact of the interactive consumer health information technology (IT) on health outcomes, a consistent finding was that these systems tended to have a positive effect when they provided a complete feedback loop that included the following:

a. Monitoring of current patient status
b. Interpretation of data in light of established, often individualized, treatment goals
c. Adjustment of the management plan as needed
d. Communication back to the patient with tailored recommendations or advice
e. Repetition of this cycle at appropriate intervals

The most common factor influencing the successful use of the interactive technology by these specific populations is that the consumers' perceived a benefit from using the system. Convenience is an important factor. Effective data entry is not cumbersome and the intervention needs to fit into the user's daily routine. Clinicians who respond in a timely and frequent manner increase use and user satisfaction. The researchers identify questions that need further examination.

**Application:** The consumer's perception of benefit, convenience, and integration into daily activities facilitates effective use of the interactive technologies for the elderly, chronically ill, and underserved. Nurses who are involved in the development and/or implementation of consumer health technology should be aware of research results to improve consumer health technology.

**Questions:**

1. *What is meant by a complete feedback loop in this systematic review?*
2. *How would you see the feedback loop impacting nursing care, and what types of settings might this be particularly helpful?*
3. *What is your opinion of the three questions that are mentioned in the conclusion? How might these questions relate to nursing and nurses?*

and type of organizational structure matter to patients? Do they just go through the system untouched by it? Patient satisfaction outcomes seem to indicate that patients are affected by all of these factors (Stumpf, 2001). Patients do report greater satisfaction with their care in shared governance organizations, which tend to have greater staff retention and work satisfaction. So the contexts in which staff work and patients receive their care are interrelated and affect patients' views of their care.

However, some problems do exist with patient satisfaction. "The customer satisfaction bandwagon, rampant in the business world throughout the 1990s, has now been joined by health care. Fortunately the days when health care personnel could have an attitude of 'just be grateful that we are here' are gone. In the search to improve both humanistic caring and profitability, however, many have allowed the pendulum to swing too far. They have adopted a misguided *excessive* and *exclusive* focus on customer satisfaction as the measurement of quality patient care. Making customer satisfaction the supreme goal has major inherent flaws, particularly when used in the health care arena for 'patient' customers" (Zimmermann, 2001, p. 255). Several myths related to patient satisfaction have been identified.

1. *Customer satisfaction is objective and straightforward.* This is not true. Surveys are difficult to develop, and they are often poorly designed.

2. *Customer satisfaction is easily measured.*   Satisfaction is complex and not easily measured. Patient expectations play a major role in the process, and there are many factors that can affect patient responses.
3. *Customer satisfaction is accurately and precisely measured.*   This is not possible at this time. Attitudes are being measured.
4. *Customer satisfaction is quickly and easily changed.*   This does not occur. In fact, "The best care may actually be accomplished by *preventing* the customer patients' return."
5. *It is obvious who the customer is.*   The tendency is to classify all customers as patients when there are many different customers related to a health care organization; for example, insurers, physicians, and internal customers. (Staff members within the organization become customers to other staff; e.g., laboratory provides services to the units and thus staff members on the units are the laboratory's customers.) All groups of customers need to be considered when customer satisfaction is assessed (Zimmermann, 2001, pp. 255–256).

Besides addressing difficulties in determining satisfaction, other issues need to be considered. One issue that comes up is whether the patient, as a health care consumer, is able to judge what is quality care? This question tends to generate strong feelings on both sides—the patient and the provider. How does the patient's illness affect the patient's impression of the treatment, and how does the patient express the evaluation? This is an important consideration during assessment—finding out about the patient's past experiences. This may reveal potential problems and concerns that need to be addressed to prevent patient satisfaction problems. Along with this issue, Zimmermann (2001) also notes that the patients who complete surveys are patients who are able to do this—alert, typically English-speaking, and often younger. This eliminates many other patients. As is true for many problems that may be identified in the evaluation process, staff tends to trivialize complaints by saying the patient was annoying or a constant complainer. This is a way of avoiding complaints and not working on improvement.

"Despite extensive research on defining and measuring quality of care, less attention has been given to consumers' views" (Oermann, Dillon, & Templin, 2000, p. 9). A study conducted on indicators of quality of care in clinics recognized that both providers and consumers are interested in assessing quality of care, but they have different views of quality (Oermann, Dillon, & Templin, 2000). What indicators are important in determining the quality of health care and nursing care? This study included a sample of 119 clinic patients in an urban ambulatory care facility. The results indicate that the most important quality indicators for health care were as follows:

- Getting better
- Getting care and services when needed
- Having diagnoses and treatment options

Nursing care indicators were different and included the following:

- Communicating with the nurse
- Being treated with respect
- Being cared for by nurses who were up-to-date
- Teaching by the nurse
- Not being rushed through the visit

The indicators for nursing care appear to be more specific than those of health care quality, although clearly they are all interrelated. "Patient satisfaction studies have consistently demonstrated the importance of patients' communication with the clinician and education during hospitalization and in ambulatory care. . . . People with chronic illnesses also valued instruction by the nurse more than did other patients" (Oermann, Dillon, & Templin, 2000, p. 11). What is important to note here is the recognition of education, communication, and interpersonal relationships. At the same time that these are identified as key factors to patient satisfaction and patients' views of quality care, health care organizations and nurses are experiencing less time to provide care, which limits their time for communication and education with patients. This is a grave concern with staffing shortages and increased workplace stress.

Acute care is also no exception when comparing provider and consumer viewpoints. Shannon, Mitchell, and Cain (2002) conducted a study to compare patient, nurse, and physician assessments of quality of care and patient satisfaction in selected critical care units. The sample included 25 units in 14 hospitals, 489 patients, 518 nurses, and 515 physicians. Standardized instruments were used to collect the data. The results indicated that physicians rated quality of care higher than either the patients or the nurses and tended to overestimate patient satisfaction. Nurses and patients had similar ratings for quality of care. There was, however, great variation within and between units for all three groups. The study concluded that physicians, nurses, and patients view patient satisfaction and quality of care differently, and it supports the need to avoid assuming that if health care professionals have positive views of quality of care and patient satisfaction that the patient will agree. The views of all three groups need to be considered. In another study of patient's perceptions of hospital care used data from the Hospital Consumer Assessment of Healthcare Providers and Systems (HCAHPS) (Jha, Orav, Zheng, & Epstein, 2008). The data included hospital performance data related to quality care. There was a high correlation between high performing hospitals on quality indicators and patient satisfaction with their experiences. The results also indicate that "there is preliminary evidence that a higher ratio of nurses to patient-days may be associated with somewhat better performance with respect to certain interpersonal aspects of patient care. Whether this relationship is causal or a marker of the hospitals' commitment to better service is not clear" (p. 1926).

Patient satisfaction data are also an important component of report cards. As more is learned about the type of data that are really helpful, the report cards should become more useful and reliable for the patient, employer, all types of providers, and insurers. It is important to recognize that the variables of satisfaction need to be identified by the patient, not the health care professional. This presents a problem. "Health care professionals tend to define the elements of patient satisfaction as mainly service components such as waiting time, courtesy, and food quality. The movement by both macroconsumers and microconsumers, however, is toward a far more complete and sophisticated inventory of both process and outcome measures that concern the quality of care along with the styles of care delivery. It is now widely recognized, if not happily embraced by providers and insurers, that care cannot be high quality unless the consumer recognizes it as satisfactory" (Sullivan, 1998, p. 573). Patient satisfaction is a core element of quality of care. A government survey of patient satisfaction that examined data from 2006–2007 indicated that patients were not fully satisfied with their hospital care (U.S. Department of Health and Human Services, 2008). Though 65% agreed that they would refer others to the hospital, the results also indicated that the patients did not feel that nurses and physicians treated them with respect; they received inadequate post-surgery pain medication; and they did not get the discharge information they felt they needed. Twenty-five percent felt that nurse–patient communication was infective. These are serious concerns, and all of them are related to the need for more effective patient-centered care.

## CASE STUDY

### Consumer Satisfaction Is Not My Problem!

A community health center received its annual patient satisfaction data, a summary provided to staff from patient satisfaction surveys that are mailed to all current patients by an external organization. The return rate this year was 40% of surveys mailed, which was up from 20% the previous year. The center has a new director who has asked staff to respond to the data. Staff members are rather surprised as in the past they were lucky if they even saw the data. Many staff members do not feel it is their job to make the center better or solve consumer problems. This is management's job. Over the past year more patients and their families have been verbal about their complaints to staff. Some of the complaints, which also showed up in the summarized data, included (a) increased wait times for getting an appointment, (b) longer wait times when arriving for appointments, (c) staff attitude (rude, abrupt, non-caring), (d) little patient education, (e) inadequate parking, and (f) confusion over payment.

### Questions:

1. Why is it important for staff to be involved in improving consumer satisfaction?
2. Who are the consumers in this case?

3. What type of structure would be most effective to make a plan for improvement? Consider who should participate, size, purpose, and so on.

4. After considering the major complaints highlighted, how might the center respond to improve consumer satisfaction? (Be specific in the interventions that might be taken.)

# The Nurse as Patient Advocate

**Advocacy** has always been a major aspect of the nursing role with the consumer. Nursing standards developed by the American Nurses Association (ANA), nursing specialty organizations, and health care institutions, as well as those developed by accrediting organizations and other health care professional organizations, support many of the critical aspects of advocacy and consumerism. The ANA *Nursing: Scope and Standards of Practice* (2004) includes advocacy in the ethics standard by identifying that the registered nurse "serves as a patient advocate assisting patients in developing sills for self advocacy" (p. 39). This standard is patient oriented. The ANA standards for nursing administration expands on advocacy and discusses the nurse administrator role in advocating for staff and for a healthy work environment, which is also supported by the American Organization of Nurse Executives (2009). Box 10-2 describes the ANA nursing administration standard on advocacy. Patient education, patient satisfaction and complaint process, quality improvement, patient participation in health care decision making, and all components of advocacy and consumerism are found in both of the ANA standards.

There are two important components of advocacy: (1) providing information that is useful to the patient and (2) supporting the patient's decision, which may not be the decision the nurse thinks is best but nonetheless must be supported. To be successful, collaboration must be part of this process. The nurse provides services through a collaborative relationship with the patient and the patient's family and advocates for the patient. To be an advocate, the nurse needs to be persuasive with the patient and with others with whom the nurse may interact on behalf of the patient. Advocacy does not mean that the nurse takes over for the patient, but rather that the nurse

| BOX 10-2 | AMERICAN NURSES ASSOCIATION SCOPE AND STANDARDS ADVOCACY: ADMINISTRATION |

**The nurse administrator advocates for the protections and rights of individuals, families, communities, populations, health care providers, nursing and other professions, and institutions and organizations, especially related to health and safety.**

*Measurement Criteria:*

The nurse administrator

- Supports the involvement of individuals in their own care.
- Supports access by individuals to their own personal health information and development of awareness of how that information may be used and accessed by others.
- Supports the individual's right and ability to supplement, request correction of, and share their personal health data and information.
- Evaluates factors related to privacy, security, and confidentiality in the use and handling of health information.

- Integrates advocacy into the design, implementation, and evaluation of policies, programs and services, and systems.
- Demonstrates skill in advocating before providers, public representatives and decision-makers, and other stakeholders.
- Exhibits fiscal responsibility and integrity in policy development and advocacy activities and processes.
- Strives to resolved conflicting expectations from populations, providers, and other stakeholders to promote safety, guard their best interests, and to preserve the professional integrity of the nurse.
- Serves as an expert for peers, populations, providers, and other stakeholders in promoting and implementing health policies.

Source: American Nurses Association. (2009). *Nursing Administration: Scope and Standards of Practice.* Silver Springs, MD.

helps the patient to be more independent, recognizing that the patient is a stakeholder in the care process. Changes in reimbursement such as the expansion of managed care has certainly also affected physician–patient relationships. An advocate must also recognize limits and refer patients to appropriate resources.

Advocacy needs to be part of practice. A perspective of advocacy described by Gilkey, Earp, and French (2008) describes advocacy as a continuum.

- The individual level focuses on informing patients, and considers "interventions that target the personal beliefs, attitudes, and knowledge needed to achieve health" (p. 17). This would include self-management and patient education. Chronic illness, discussed earlier in this book, is a critical concern. E-health has become more and more important as consumers turn to the Internet for information.
- The next level is the interpersonal level focusing on supporting and empowering patients. Interventions such as "advice giving, emotional support, and provision of resources and other help" (p. 18) are an integral part of this level, and all require interpersonal interactions. Families and significant others need to be brought into this process.
- The third level is the organizational and community levels focusing on transforming culture. What are organizations and communities doing to support patient advocacy?
- The fourth level is the policy level focusing on translating consumer voice into policy and laws. "In patient advocacy, important policies are those that (1) control access to patient care; (2) regulate health care organizations, especially with regard to patient safety surveillance; and (3) protect health care consumers" (Gilkey, Earp, & French, p. 21).

Managed care approaches to health insurance have had an impact on health care advocacy. In many situations the physician may be involved in making decisions based on financial issues rather than as an advocate for the patient's needs. How has it affected the nurse's role as advocate? Nurses working in hospitals and home health care frequently face issues with patients about reimbursement, decisions that limit the care patients receive. Nurses then feel frustrated when there is nothing they can do to assist the patient. Advanced practice nurses experience many of the same conflicts as physicians.

What can the nurse do to assist the patient and advocate for the patient? Ensuring that the nursing process is complete and includes active patient and family/significant other participation is the critical first step. Built into the process are individualized care, patient rights, respect for the patient, and patient education. The nurse also needs to empower the patient with information and support the patient and the family as health care choices are made. Accessing care, which includes services, supplies, and medical equipment, is not always easy today. Doing this today in a health care environment in which patients have shortened lengths-of-stay or do not come in for care early enough is very difficult. Patient education takes time. More and more of this load is shifting to the community. It takes commitment on the part of the nurses to ensure that it happens and that the patient education is appropriate to meet the needs of the patient. Nurses will have to be more creative in meeting the needs, probably by turning more to technology. Care, however, does need to be taken to ensure that individual needs and human contact are still present. The nurse can help the patient understand the complex health care system and reimbursement issues related to the system in order to receive care when it is needed. Prevention is important in today's health care environment, and helping the patient understand the need for prevention and how it can benefit the individual patient is part of the nurse–patient relationship.

# APPLYING LEADERSHIP AND MANAGEMENT

## MY HOSPITAL UNIT

Your hospital has an initiative to increase consumer involvement in hospital activities and services. Today you are meeting with your staff to discuss how consumerism impacts the unit and what can be done to improve consumer or patient-centered care. Remember that families and significant others should also be involved. How would you (1) determine the current status of patient involvement, (2) identify what needs to change, (3) plan for change, and (4) evaluate the outcomes? Who should be involved? Use the virtual unit site found on the textbook website to record the work that you do in the role of nurse manager for your unit.

## Critical Thinking Questions and Activities

1. This is a good time to assess health care consumerism in your community. What are the health care consumer groups? What do they do? How effective are they? Are nurses involved in any of these groups and in what ways? Is your school of nursing or students involved in any of these groups? What could be done to increase this involvement? It might be helpful to first develop a list of consumer organizations in your class and then divide the organizations for further research by smaller teams or individual students. Then information can be shared.

2. Working in small teams, determine how you might get information about the nurse as a patient advocate in your community. Consider the data you would want to collect and where you might obtain the data. What methods are you going to use?

3. Select an example of health communication such as a television ad, pamphlet, Internet health site, and so on. Using the attributes related to health communication discussed in this chapter, assess the example. This could be done in class so that students can share their examples and assessments.

4. Find out more information about how a local health care organization evaluates patient satisfaction. Consider the content, frequency, analysis of the data, and who gets the information. Has the assessment of patient satisfaction made a difference and how?

5. Visit the Agency for Healthcare Research and Quality (AHRQ) site section that focuses on talking to patients about health care quality: http://www.talkingquality.gov/. How might you use this information with patients and planning communication for groups of patients.

6. Nurses need to be aware of the *Healthy People* report and incorporate its goals and objectives into the program planning and care provided to all patients. Visit http://www.healthypeople.gov. Check the most current status of the new version—*Healthy People 2020*. Information about the report and related information are readily available on the Internet and in publications. This information is used as health care policy issues, as well as educational needs of health care professionals.

7. The *Healthy People* site has current results on outcomes related to the goals and objectives in the report (http://www.healthypeople.gov). These data help in tracking the success of the goals and objectives. It is important to remember, however, that these goals and objectives are not required. Health care organizations and individual providers choose to use them. This is a major drawback as one cannot really say that they accurately reflect health care in the United States when there are many who do not even know what *Healthy People* is or apply it. The government is doing much to increase its usage. How might you apply this information to nursing management in acute care and community care?

## Media Links

- **URL: http://www.dhhs.gov**
  U.S. Department of Health and Human Services
- **URL: http://www.familiesUSA.org**
  FamiliesUSA

- **URL: http://www.healthfinder.gov**
  HealthFinder
- **URL: http://www.medicarerights.org**
  Medicare Rights Center
- **URL: http://www.pressganey.com**
  Press Ganey Associates: Satisfaction Measurement
- **URL: http://ahrq.gov**
  Agency for Healthcare Quality and Research: For Your Health
- **URL: http://www.hospitalcompare.hhs.gov/Hospital/Search/Welcome.asp?version= default&browser=IE%7C7%7CWinXP&language=English&defaultstatus= 0&pagelist=Home**
  U.S. Department of Health and Human Services: Hospital Compare
- **URL: https://www.cahps.ahrq.gov/default.asp**
  Consumer Assessment of Healthcare Providers and Systems (CAHPS)
- **URL: http://www.hcahpsonline.org/home.aspx**
  Hospital Consumer Assessment of Healthcare Providers and Systems (HCAHPS)

**Pearson Nursing Student Resources**

Find additional review materials at
**nursing.pearsonhighered.com**

Prepare for success with additional NCLEX®-style practice questions, interactive assignments and activities, Web links, animations and videos, and more!

# References

American Cancer Society. (2008). The Patient Self-Determination Act. Retrieved June 20, 2009, from http://www.cancer.org/docroot/MIT/content/MIT_3_2X_The_Patient_Self-Determination_Act.asp?sitearea=MIT

American Nurses Association. (2003). *Nursing's social policy statement.* Silver Spring, MD: American Nurses Publishing.

American Nurses Association. (2004). *Scope and standards of practice.* Silver Spring, MD: American Nurses Publishing.

American Nurses Association. (2009). *Nursing administration: Scope and standards of practice.* Silver Spring, MD: American Nurses Publishing.

Andersen, R., Kravits, J., & Anderson, O. (1971). The public's view of the crisis in medical care: An impetus for changing delivery systems? *Economic and Business Bulletin, 24,* 44–52.

Armer, J. (1998). Consumers as allies or partners in care. In T. Sullivan (Ed.), *Collaboration: A health care imperative* (pp. 515–533). New York: McGraw-Hill.

Aronowitz, R. (2009, November 20). Addicted to mammograms. *New York Times.*

Boston, C. (1990). Health care reform. *Journal of Nursing Administration, 20*(7/8), 8–9.

Consumer Assessment of Health care Providers and Systems. (CAHPS). Consumer Assessment. (2009). Retrieved August 20, 2009, from https://www.cahps.ahrq.gov/default.asp

Gilkey, M., Earp, J., & French, E. (2008). What is patient advocacy? In J. Earp, E. French, & M. Gilkey, *Patient advocacy for health care quality,* pp. 3–28.

Grady, D. (2009, November 20). Guidelines push back age for cervical cancer tests. *New York Times.*

Institute of Medicine. (2002). *Unequal treatment.* Washington, DC: National Academies Press.

Institute of Medicine. (2003). *Health professions education.* Washington, DC: National Academies Press.

Institute of Medicine. (2008). *Knowing what works in health care.* Washington, DC: National Academies Press.

Jha, A., Orav, E., Zheng, J. & Epstein, A. (2008). Patients' perception of hospital care in the United States. *New England Journal of Medicine, 359*(18), 1921–1931.

Kolata, G. (2009, November 17). Panel urges Mammograms at 50, not 40. *New York Times,* p. 74.

Medical Library Association. (2009). Medical Information on the Internet. Retrieved December 17, 2009, from http://www.mlanet.org/resources/hlth_tutorial/mod6.html

Oermann, M., Dillon, S., & Templin, T. (2000). Indicators of quality care in clinics: Patient's perspectives. *Journal of Health Care Quality, 22*(6), 9–11.

Shannon, S., Mitchell, P., & Cain, K. (2002). Patients, nurses, and physicians have differing views of quality of critical care. *Journal of Nursing Scholarship,* second quarter, 173–179.

Sherman, B. (1998). How non-profits can benefit from marketing research. *Association Forum, 28*(2), 22–23.

Sovie, M. (1990). Redesigning our future: Whose responsibility is it? *Nursing Economics, 8*(1), 21–26.

Stumpf, L. (2001). A comparison of governance types and patient satisfaction outcomes. *Journal of Nursing Administration, 31*(4), 196–202.

Sullivan, T. (1998). Consumers in health care, part II: Expert viewpoints. In T. Sullivan (Ed.), *Collaboration: A health care imperative* (pp. 561–590). New York: McGraw-Hill.

U.S. Department of Health and Human Services. (2010). *Healthy People 2020.* Washington, DC: U.S. Government Printing Office.

U.S. Preventive Task Force. (2009). Screening for breast cancer: U.S. Preventive Services Task Force recommendation statement. *Annals of Internal Medicine, 151*(10), 716–726.

Zimmermann, P. (2001). The problems with health care customer satisfaction surveys. In J. Dochterman & H. Grace (Eds.), *Current issues in nursing* (6th ed., pp. 255–260). St. Louis: Mosby, Inc.

# 11

# Developing Interprofessional and Intraprofessional Teams

## CHAPTER OUTLINE

## LEARNING OUTCOMES

Before you begin, take a moment to familiarize yourself with the learning outcomes for this chapter.

- Discuss the importance of teams in the health care delivery system.
- Compare and contrast the different types of teams.
- Assess team leader characteristics and how these relate to the team leader's tasks and responsibilities.
- Explain the important considerations related to team building.
- Compare and contrast a nursing team and an interprofessional team.
- Apply the stages of team development.
- Explain motivation and its relationship to teamwork.
- Use three strategies that might be used to improve motivation.

## KEY TERMS

- Cross-functional project team
- Empowerment
- Followers
- Followship
- Formal team
- Forming
- Groupthink
- Informal team

- Interdisciplinary/ interprofessional team
- Motivation
- Multidisciplinary team
- Norming
- Performing
- Power
- Self-directed work teams (SDWTs)

- Storming
- Team
- Team building
- Team functions
- Team leader
- Teamwork

## WHAT'S AHEAD

With an increasing outcome-oriented health care delivery system, synergy from teams can work to the health system's benefit. Synergy requires good communication, particularly through listening and clarifying; supporting and encouraging one another; use of differing and confronting skills; a commitment to quality; acceptance of the value of teams and their collective contributions; and use of constructive feedback for the betterment of the team and outcomes. In addition to increased use of teams in practice settings, nursing education has experienced an increase use of collaborative learning experiences for students. One reason for this is it can improve learning, but another reason is it facilitates student learning about teams—how teams function, roles and responsibilities, setting an agenda, and evaluation. It helps students appreciate that multiple views and knowledge is better than just one (Michaelsen, Knight, & Fink, 2008). The content in this text is related to teams, how they function, and how they impact health care supporting the Institute of Medicine's (IOM) recommendation for more effective teams. This chapter specifically provides information about critical team elements and the team's functioning, or the structure process of teams that are important for nurses. Content in Chapter 12 continues the discussion on teams.

# Teams in Today's Health Care Environment

No one person can do it all. This fact is even more relevant in today's health care environment with its dynamic and frequent changes. The information explosion has made it impossible for any one person to know it all. Expertise is developed over time, and some staff have different types of expertise. The Institute of Medicine has emphasized that teams improve skills, communication, participation, and effectiveness (2003) and includes use of interprofessional teams as one of the key five core health care professions competencies. The IOM report on nursing identifies six major concerns about direct care and nursing with the sixth concern described as integration and coordination of care (2004). Teams play a critical role in ensuring integration and coordination of care. All organizations desire to perform effectively, although clearly many do not. The IOM has commented in their reports that the health care system is not working effectively—it is dysfunctional. There is a lack of continuity and coordination and poor communication (2001, 2003). "An interdisciplinary [interprofessional] team is composed of members from different professions and occupations with varied and specialized knowledge, skills, and methods. The team members integrate their observations, bodies of expertise, and spheres of decision making to coordinate, collaborate, and communicate with one another in order to optimize care for a patient or a group of patients" (Institute of Medicine, 2003, p. 54). Interprofessional teams can improve care and reduce costs (Institute of Medicine, 2003, p. 55). Salmon (2007) stated, "I must say I have grown tired of us saying that we are making major strides in collaboration and partnership with others beyond nursing. I worry that we in nursing have fought so hard for our professional identity and autonomy that we see being separate from others as a condition for future success. I see our separateness as antithetical to our most basic professional values. How can we reconcile our commitment to providing the best possible care when we still grapple with the place that nursing assistants, technicians, and others have in relation to our work" (p. 117). Achieving the competence of using interprofessional teams is not easy to accomplish, and developing and maintaining teamwork has been a long-term issue in health care.

## Teams, Groups, and Teamwork

What is the difference between teams and teamwork? "The team is a means rather than an end, while teamwork is about performance and how to achieve the primary objective" (McCallin, 2001, p. 422). Based on this definition a team is the structure and teamwork is the function, how the team works together. Shared governance, discussed in Chapter 4, might be confused with use of teams; however, it is different though teams play critical role in shared governance. A health care organization may not use the model of shared governance and yet still will use teams in the clinical area, to support management functions, and to develop and implement projects.

Another area of confusion comes from comparing teams and groups. Most assume that teams and groups are synonymous, but they are not. In health care organizations the more common term is teams. It is rare for staff to refer to its "work group" as a group but rather refer to it as a team. A group is more commonly viewed as less organized than a team. For example, a group of people may get together for social activities, but a team is structured. It should have clear goals and purpose, membership requirements, leader and follower responsibilities, and evaluate its work. There is less emphasis on a shared vision and mission with a group as compared to a team. Teams typically feel committed to one another. Teams have operating guidelines, decision-making processes, and a defined relationship with other parts of an organization. For example, a patient unit may have several nursing staff teams that cover the care of the patients, or there may interprofessional teams of nurses, physicians, social workers, and other health care providers. Sharing, acceptance, collaboration, and communication are critical elements of effective team functioning.

## Types of Teams

Teams have been classified in many different ways, although two broad common categories for classifying teams within organizations are formal and informal. **Formal teams** are created by the organization with a specific purpose in mind, and the team may be permanent or temporary. Examples of formal teams are clinical teams, policy committees, nurses' councils, and quality improvement committees. **Informal teams** or groups are quite different in that the members form these teams, and typically members share something in common. There is less structure, and the team would not really be recognized as a team by the organization. An informal team may simply be a social or support group, but it can also serve as a real resource to resolve problems or provide a service. Formal teams can be formed for different reasons. The most common is the patient care team that is assigned specific patients and ensures that the care is provided. Health care organizations (HCOs) may form teams to work on special projects such as a project to change to an electronic medical record. Other teams may work on long-term projects such as policy and procedures and in this case may be called a committee.

There have been many changes in how teams are formed and how they are used in health care organizations. **Self-directed work teams (SDWTs)** often are associated with patient-centered care (McCullough & Sanders, 2000). This approach focuses on the patient, decentralized services, and use of a more efficient worker skill mix while maintaining or improving patient satisfaction. The goal is to move services as close to the patient as possible. Health care organizations that use this model—which can be found in acute care as well as community health organizations such as ambulatory care—bring services to the patient. For example, laboratory services are provided at the bedside whenever possible, and if the organization is a clinic, these services would be provided onsite so that patients do not have to go to another site. It is thought that SDWTs decrease bureaucracy and improve staff motivation (McCullough & Sanders, 2000). With the greater emphasis on patient-centered care there is more emphasis on patient-centered teams—the patient is the center with the team focusing on ensuring that patient needs are met (Spitzer, 2008).

How is the SDWT model different from team nursing? In team nursing, teams are composed of nonprofessional nursing staff that provides most of the direct care with an RN team leader directing the team. The team leader plans and supervises the care delivered to a group of patients, which means the team leader probably spends less time providing direct care. SDWTs are different from team nursing in that "employees are expected to be responsible for creating significant change in the way patient care is delivered and in the cost to the institution for the care delivered" (McCullough & Sanders, 2000, p. 93). These teams tend to accomplish more positive outcomes related to (a) patient, staff, and physician satisfaction; (b) patient outcomes; (c) decreased costs with increased resource effectiveness; and (d) staff retention and productivity. The critical assumptions related to the SDWT model are as follows:

- All team members are responsible for fulfilling their portion of the care.
- All team members understand what is expected of them.
- Managers relinquish control.
- There are boundaries regarding autonomy.
- Managers are responsible for the environment and culture that determine, in part, the success of the team (McCullough & Sanders, 2000, p. 94).

In addition to these assumptions, the team culture of SDWTs requires that the team have some characteristics that may not be typically found in health care teams.

- The team defines specific responsibilities and boundaries for team members.
- Roles within the team change because teams are structured around an entire process and everyone is equally responsible for the outcomes.
- Education of the team members focuses on the technical, administrative, and interpersonal skills necessary for people to function within the SDWT.
- Teams evolve into groups that work with less and less dependence on managers or other leadership.
- Teams define their own performance measures to identify growth and accomplishments within the teams.

If management does not support the concept of SDWTs and their decisions, then this model will fail. It is also true that if team members do not accept the concept and their own responsibilities, these teams will also fail. The team and its members must learn how to set goals for the team and evaluate its performance. Teams need training and education so that they can be effective and obtain the skills that are needed to work together. Role transition may be very difficult and takes time. Over time, however, most teams develop into cohesive units.

## The Team Leader

The **team leader** is very important to a team's effectiveness. RNs are the team leaders on many health care teams. Their leadership and management skills assist the team as it works toward its goals. This is a leadership role that new graduates typically assume early on in their careers: Who is the team leader, how does the leader function, and what are some issues that affect the team leader?

### Team Leader Characteristics

In most organizations the team leader has less formal authority than those individuals in management staff; however, a team leader should have the necessary authority to meet the position requirements. Self-confidence and the ability to act as a role model for team members are important characteristics. Team leaders often must act as the "cheerleader" to move the team along with enthusiasm, but this should be done appropriately. No one wants to work with someone who is always "cheery." Team leaders need to demonstrate facilitative leadership, although how this is implemented may vary. This means that the leader leads with a vision and is willing to become a learner. Coaching is an important part of team leadership by supporting and encouraging team members. If the leader is effective, the leader gradually relinquishes control as the team gains strength though may not transfer all control or decisions to the team.

The leader's role changes over time as the team develops, and the leader gradually relinquishes direct control and becomes a facilitator. Not all teams become fully developed. This means the team leader needs to assess team performance over time and provide guidance as needed. Less experienced RNs who are developing their leadership and management skills usually have more difficulty recognizing when a team is ready to be more independent due to a lack of self-confidence, lack of trust, and fear that something will go wrong if they do not make all decisions for the team. They also have greater difficulty communicating, delegating, and assessing team members. With time, experience, and mentoring, less experienced RNs can further develop these important competencies.

The team leader focuses on the team's process as well as on its outcomes. Process is how the team works together. The facilitative leadership approach offers coaching and development to members. Team leaders, as is true with other types of leaders, need to have an understanding of communication, psychology, change, problem solving and decision making, motivation, and systems. It is important to encourage team members to give honest feedback and to provide an environment in which members can feel comfortable and safe in doing so. By establishing open communication when the team meets, the team leader sets the stage for a comfortable work environment. In addition, the team leader moves the team from the use of first-person singular to words that focus on the team as a group with joint responsibilities; for example, "we" and "let us" to emphasize the team and interdependence rather than "I" and "me." Team leaders provide praise to the team and, during stressful times, support. This does not mean, however, that individual members should never be praised as there are clearly times when an individual team member shines through in the team. "There's no 'I' in 'team.' Health care is a team sport, but too often practitioners act as individual players" (Weinstock, 2010).

## Tasks and Responsibilities

Team leaders who approach the position with an attitude that they are different from team members or above the team members will not be successful. Effective leaders must jump in and work too, although they must continue to see the whole—what needs to be done and how best to accomplish it. Guiding from above will not be effective, but guiding from within the team will. The organization needs to be clear about the decision-making boundaries for its teams. Competiveness between teams is not uncommon, but under most circumstances this is not helpful in developing a positive organization culture of collaboration. The key tasks and responsibilities of the team leader are to do the following:

- Guide the team by helping to establish goals and objectives.
- Provide an environment where team members are active in all stages of team planning and feel comfortable in this role.
- Reinforce the focus on the patient, if that is the focus of the team.
- Ensure that the team's tasks are clear, planned, and accomplished in a timely manner.
- Ensure that standards and rules are established, and encourage team members to monitor their use.
- Link the team to key resources and with others in the organization.
- Assist the team to stay on task.
- Challenge the team to improve and develop.
- Remove barriers to collaboration.
- Follow-up on problems in a timely manner.
- Recognize and value contributions from team members.
- Minimize micromanaging, and encourage team members to assist in management issues.
- Use conflict management to benefit the team and help it reach its outcomes.
- Ensure that team self-evaluation occurs with an emphasis on outcomes.
- Accept feedback from team members.
- Provide appropriate and timely evaluation of team members' performance and team effectiveness.

## CASE STUDY

### So You Are the Team Leader Now

The unit you are working on had an opening for a team leader position. You applied and to your surprise you get the position. You begin the new position next week. After the excitement dies down, you begin to get nervous about the new position. Can you really do this job? You know that the team includes two RNs, one LPN/LVN, and two CNAs. You have worked with all of the members, but you don't know any of them well. Your nurse manager tells you that one of the RNs has a reputation of being quiet and passive and the other is "pushy." He has made most team leaders wish he would go away. The LPN has worked on the unit longer than any of the other team members and is a hard worker. The two CNAs also have a lot of experience. Now what do you do?

### Questions:

1. What information about teams do you need to consider?
2. Describe the type of team leader you want to be and how this might impact decisions you need to make now.
3. What additional information about the team members might you ask the nurse manager?
4. What would be the expected phases of team development?
5. How will you build team cohesiveness? Consider the barriers and strategies to address.

## Gender Issues and Team Leadership

There can be no doubt that literature about leadership and theories of leadership have been more interested in masculine leadership than feminine leadership. Some of this can be understood in that historically women did not hold many leadership positions. Today, however, this is not true. Women are found in leadership positions in all major types of organizations, although clearly more are needed, as the majority of women are found in the lower ranks and in lower management positions. Health care is no exception.

How are masculine and feminine leaders described? In a study of women leaders in 19 different businesses including health care women were found to have difference characteristics than men (Caliper, 2005). Female leaders usually prefer a more participatory approach to leadership and encourage others to be involved. They are more empathetic, flexible, and more willing to take risks than men. Men also scored high in these areas but not as high as women. Sharing power is seen as a positive characteristic, as is sharing information to reach the goals. Improving staff perceptions of themselves can improve the work environment and performance. Often female leaders focus more on process than on "the bottom line." They are concerned with broader issues. It is important to recognize that this description of female leaders can become a stereotypical viewpoint. The approach should also not be viewed as a negative or ineffective approach just because it is more commonly found in women. Notably, these characteristics are emphasized more in current leadership theory and styles such as transformational leadership. There are certainly men in leadership positions who have these characteristics, and there are female leaders who do not. Focusing too much on gender issues ignores the importance of individual differences in leaders regardless of gender.

## Followership: A Critical Concept

Team leaders must recognize that teams do not exist without **followers**, the team members. Followers are critical to the success of any organization. "There can be no leaders without followers, and there can be no followers without leaders" (Grossman & Valiga, 2000, p. 44). Followers have become more important as leadership theory has turned more and more to a participatory approach. Leadership means that followers are developed. Despite the importance of understanding this concept, it is still not a critical topic in many management and leadership publications, where the emphasis has been on leadership (Grossman & Valiga, 2000). In many publications, there is a direct and indirect message that **followship** is negative; however, when this is seriously considered, how could this be? Without followers there would be no work done and no need for leaders.

What does it take to be an effective follower? Every new graduate should consider this question, as it is a role that all will play. Even leaders experience situations when they are followers. It takes energy to be a follower, although some may think that following is just an automatic response. To be effective, it is not automatic nor is it a passive role that does not involve thinking. It requires use of expertise, development of expertise, sharing, understanding of problems and others, effective communication, and collaboration. "Followership also involves knowing when and how to assume the role of leadership when necessary" (Grossman & Valiga, 2000, p. 48). It is important, however, to understand that followers do not exist just to become leaders. They exist because they are needed and have a critical role to play.

Not all followers are alike. One description of followers identifies four major types: effective or exemplary followers, alienated followers, "yes" people, and sheep (Grossman & Valiga, 2000).

1. Effective or exemplary followers are able to function independently and use critical thinking. They are not followers who simply do what they are told, but rather they add their own ideas to the process. They are engaged.
2. Alienated followers may use critical thinking but are not active. Passivity is common, and some may appear angry. Sometimes they are described as complainers, unhappy, and not involved. They do not like to invest energy.
3. "Yes" people will do what they are told with enthusiasm and support the leader. These followers do not like being in a position of decision making, preferring instead to complete tasks with little input. They like structure and are not the ones to suggest new ideas.
4. Some followers called "sheep" may sound like they would be "yes" people, but sheep are even more passive, dependent, and just do as told. This type of follower is the one that others can manipulate. They do not take initiative and must be given clear directions.

The last two types of followers are not team members who will challenge others, take on new projects, ask questions, or go beyond assignments. It is important for leaders to understand the types of followers when they are on the team. It is also important for followers to understand their co-workers and themselves.

There are other followership styles that are used in the work situation. Typical styles are partner, contributor, politician, and subordinate. What are some differences in these styles? The partner style demonstrates "positive, reciprocal relationships with leaders" (Grossman & Valiga, 2000, p. 50). Partners often become leaders later. Contributors are active in the work process and add to the process, working well with co-workers. When compared with partners, contributors do not align as closely with leaders or work to ensure that the leader's vision is met. The politician approach focuses on interpersonal skills and communication, but may not demonstrate the highest level of general work performance. The fourth style is subordinate. Here the focus is on doing the job but not necessarily with a strong commitment to improving. Considering the types and styles of followers, who are the effective followers? It may be surprising to note that the characteristics of effective followers are remarkably similar to the characteristics of effective leaders. The following are some of the characteristics of effective followers.

- Strength and independence
- Critical thinking
- An ability and willingness to think for themselves
- An ability to give honest feedback and constructive criticism, particularly in a timely fashion
- A willingness to be one's own person
- Innovativeness and creativity
- Cooperativeness and collaborativeness
- A tendency to be a self-starter
- A tendency to "go above and beyond the call of duty" to go beyond job assignments
- A willingness to assume ownership

- A tendency to take initiative
- An attentiveness to what is happening in the environment
- A tendency to "hold up our end of the bargain"
- A sense of being energized by work and the organization (Grossman & Valiga, 2000, pp. 52–53)

Followers who are contributing to the team or the work environment are eager to add their ideas to the process, to participate actively in decision making, and to feel committed to the process and the vision. These followers trust the leader and recognize the importance of sharing feelings and concerns. They also feel comfortable discussing their own limitations. One should not view followers as insignificant or invisible because if they are, they are not effective followers. "Leaders and followers are therefore interdependent" (Grossman & Valiga, 2000, p. 54). It is important for leaders to develop trust in their relationships. Strategies that increase followers' trust in leaders are keeping promises, and when promises cannot be kept offer explanations, give and encourage honest feedback, and reward followers. All of these strategies build mutual trust.

# Team Structure and Process

Teams do not just appear as fully functioning effective teams; rather, they develop through team leadership and team members who are committed to team goals. The team's structure and processes are gradually developed. Team leaders need to assess the individual team members and the team as a whole, considering styles of followers, communication team purpose, roles, and so on, to determine what needs to be improved to make the team even more effective. Effective teams require members (health care professionals) who do the following (Institute of Medicine, 2003):

- Learn about other team members' expertise, knowledge, and values.
- Learn individual roles and processes required to work collaboratively.
- Demonstrate basic group skills, including communication, negotiation, delegation, time management, and assessment of team dynamics.
- Ensure that accurate and timely information reaches those who need it at the appropriate time.
- Customize care and manage smooth transition across settings and over time, even when the team members are in entirely different physical locations.
- Coordinate and integrate care processes to ensure excellence, continuity, and reliability of the care provided.
- Resolve conflicts with other members of the team.
- Communicate with other members of the team in a shared language, even when the members are in entirely different physical locations.

## Team Tasks and Functions

Typical service roles in teams besides the leader role are participant and service roles such as recorder, observer, resource person, and timekeeper. Participants are the real team workers when they focus on doing the job, whatever it might be. The leader is the team guide who facilitates the work of all members of the team. To ensure that there is documentation of team activities, the recorder or secretary records minutes from team meetings. Some teams also have an observer, who observes the process and shares this information with the team; a timekeeper to watch the time for specific discussions and meetings; and a resource person who provides specific content or expertise. The latter three roles are typically used for specific tasks or periods of time. An example might be when a team must produce a particular report or a team is having a thorough discussion that is conflictual. Clinical teams usually do not have all of these service roles, and the leader may have a more formal role defined in a specific organizational position description.

Teams that develop an identity are more successful. "Effective teams have a culture that fosters openness, collaboration, teamwork, and learning from mistakes" (Institute of Medicine, 2001, p. 132). The team leader and members may actively move toward developing this identity.

Some methods for developing identification are matching coffee mugs, t-shirts, and use of a team name. These may appear to be unimportant, but they do support the idea that "we are in this together." Informal interaction helps teams become more effective as they get to know one another and develop relationships (McCallin, 2001). Teams begin to develop inside jokes and stories that mean something to them. All of this develops team spirit, which affects outcomes and how team members pitch in to help one another. They will be more tolerant of one another and more able to recognize when team members need help. Team members will also feel more comfortable asking for help. Sharing knowledge and skills then becomes the norm in the team because the team feels connected and has a team identity. Teams exist to get a job done, and they need to be active. This involves both talking and doing. The major **team function** is to complete the assigned task(s). This task can vary from planning and development to actually completing tasks such as delivering patient care. The team needs to clearly understand its purpose(s), timeline, and relationship to other parts of the organization. Effective team function also means that members need to be committed to improvement—both in how they work together and in their outcomes. Delegation is also a critical skill for team leaders and those team members who will be delegating (see Chapter 14). It can make a key difference in the effectiveness of the team.

The type of team affects its tasks and functions. A clinical team provides care, and thus, tasks and functions are centered on patient care. A team that is formed to complete a specific project such as change in documentation would include tasks and functions related to literature research and contacting other health care organizations to learn about their documentation review, development of forms and methods for ensuring that standards are met, planning staff orientation, and planning a pilot.

## Team Size and Composition

Team size is a common concern when teams are developed. In some situations, such as a clinical one, the size may be predetermined based on the number and types of staff required to provide care for a specific number of patients. A general principle related to size is that the team should include the smallest number necessary to do the assigned task. Size is directly related to team effectiveness. Seven or more members becomes difficult to manage. Another issue that is related to team composition is whether or not participation in the team is voluntary or involuntary. Again, in a clinical situation if the team model is the delivery model then all clinical staff, such as RNs, LPNs, UAP, and so on, would be assigned to teams. Volunteer team membership can be found in some organizational committees, while staff may be assigned to project teams or to committees. In these situations, volunteer membership is better as staff will hopefully then feel more committed, although this is not always clear. For example, a nurse may be told that participation on a committee will improve chances for a promotion, although the nurse may select which committee team to join. Professional organizations are, for the most part, run by volunteers through committees. Again, this fact may not be so clear. A nurse may volunteer for a committee because this will "look good" on the nurse's resume, but commitment to the committee's work may be variable and not known.

## Examples: The Nursing Team and the Interprofessional Team

Nursing teams have been organized in a variety of ways over the years, and the typical method has been to organize according to function. Understanding some of the history of the development of nursing teams is helpful to appreciate the current status of teams. This type of work team might include a medication nurse, treatment nurse, and UAP. Team members see patients based on the patients' need and related tasks. If no one staff member reviews the patients' total care needs this approach can lead to segmented care that is not patient-centered and may result in inadequate coordination. Total patient care is a second approach to organizing nursing teams. Most if not all UAP are removed from the team, which then is composed of RNs, who provide all the care. The primary care team model was similar to this model but added an associate nurse to assist the primary nurse, and then they cared for all of their assigned primary care patients. The primary care nurse was responsible for 24-hour plans of patient care—although not providing all of the direct care for 24 hours. Primary nursing, which began in the 1980s, had a major impact on changing how nurses interacted with other professionals. This included altering interprofessional interactions from one of the physicians, always deciding what should be done and how it should be done, and making decisions in the background to one of more active nurse leadership (Lyon, 1993). In the 1990s, there was further development of these models and recognition of the need for greater teamwork (Minnen et al., 1993). It is important to note that just decentralizing an organization will not automatically make different health care professionals more inclined to collaborate and work effectively on teams. It takes much more than this organizational change.

Today there is a greater need to move to interprofessional teams (Institute of Medicine, 2003). In the literature, **interdisciplinary/interprofessional** teams and **multidisciplinary** teams are teams that can sometimes be confusing and used interchangeably. Interprofessional "refers to people with distinct disciplinary training working together for a common purpose, as they make different, complementary contributions to patient-focused care" (McCallin, 2001, p. 419). Multidisciplinary is "a team or collaborative process where members of different disciplines assess or treat patients independently and then share information with each other" (McCallin, 2001, p. 420). When the interprofessional approach is used, the focus is more on tasks that are part of an individual's profession and then blending these tasks with others. The interprofessional approach considers a more collective action and is process oriented (Finkelman & Kenner, 2010). This is the approach that the IOM recommends. The Magnet Forces of Magnetism also recognizes need for interdisciplinary/interprofessional relationships: "Collaborative working relationships within and among the disciplines are valued. Mutual respect is based on the premise that all members of the health care team make essential and meaningful contributions in the achievement of clinical outcomes. Conflict management strategies are in place and are used effectively, when indicated" (American Nurses Credentialing Center, 2009). What are the advantages of using interprofessional teams (Finkelman & Kenner, 2010, p. 337)?

- Decreased fragmentation in a complex care system
- Effective use of multiple expertise (e.g., medicine, nursing, pharmacy, allied health, social work, and so on)
- Decreased utilization of repetitive or duplicate services
- Increased creative and innovative solutions to complex problems
- Increased learning for team members about different roles and responsibilities, communication and coordination, and how to better plan care
- Provides motivation and increased self-esteem in team and individual performances
- Greater sharing of responsibility
- Empowers others to speak up

Another approach to a clinical team is to view it as a microsystem (Nelson et al., 2008). "A microsystem in health care delivery can be defined as a small group of people who work together on a regular basis to provide care to discrete subpopulations including the patients. It has clinical and business aims, linked processes, shared information environment, and produces performance outcomes. They evolve over time and are (often) embedded in larger organizations. As a type of complex adaptive system, they must (1) do the work, (2) meet staff needs, (3) maintain themselves as a clinical unit. Clinical microsystems are the front-line units that provide most health care to most people. They are the places where patients, families, and care teams meet. Microsystems also include support staff, processes, technology and recurring patterns of information, behavior, and results. Central to every clinical microsystem is the patient. The microsystem is the place where

- Care is made.
- Quality, safety, reliability, efficiency and innovation are made.
- Staff morale and patient satisfaction are made.

Microsystems are the building blocks that form hospitals" (Dartmouth College, 2010). Microsystems as well as mesosytems and macrosystems were discussed in Chapter 4, and this view focuses on patient-centered care.

# Effective Teams

What is an effective team? Various characteristics have been used to describe effective teams, including the following tips for effective team functioning include the following (Institute of Medicine, 2003, p. 56):

- Learn about other team members' expertise, background, knowledge, and values
- Learn individual roles and processes required to work collaboratively
- Demonstrate basic group skills, including communication, negotiation, delegation, time management, and assessment of group dynamics
- Ensure that accurate and timely information reaches those who need it at the appropriate time
- Customize care and manage smooth transitions across settings and over time, even when the team members are in entirely different physical locations
- Coordinate and integrate care processes to ensure excellence, continuity, and reliability of the care provided
- Resolve conflicts with other members of the team

Communicate with other members of the team in a shared language, even when the members are in entirely different physical locations.

## Stages of Team Development

In 1965, Tuckman, a psychologist developed a method for describing team development, which is easy to apply to teams (MindTools, 2010). These stages are highlighted in Box 11-1.

1. **Forming or the initial orientation**   During the first stage, **forming**, the team is learning about one another, and trust is not likely to be high at this time. If the task(s) is complex or unclear, anxiety may be experienced. As the team meets, it will focus on developing trust and team member working relationships, although this may not actually be stated. Team members begin assessing their roles in the context of the team. A leader is identified or may be identified prior to the first meeting. For a clinical team there is typically an identified person or position who is always the formal leader, such as the nurse team leader. Informal leaders, however, may develop within the team as time goes by.

2. **Storming or the stage of conflict and confusion**   At the time of the second stage, **storming**, team members see themselves as individuals and will want to respond to the task in the manner that they would respond to tasks as individuals. Some members may be reluctant to really work as a team, and others will be restless with the need to get through the **team building** activities to the task. It may be noticed at this time that some members attempt to control the team and its communication. Other team members should step in to avert this move so that the team can function as a group. Conflict can arise from this process. As this stage begins to change into **norming**, the next stage, the team will formulate team rules that will guide team members in their performance, interaction, decision making, and how they accomplish their goals (MindTools, 2010). Ideally, these rules are developed during the norming stage; however, during the storming stage these rules may be revised and then solidified. When rules are considered, one needs to factor in the organization's requirements that may affect team rules such as meeting requirements, minutes, and attendance. What might be included in these team rules?
   - Definition of purpose
   - Meeting schedule, days, time, and place
   - Documentation requirements for meetings
   - Attendance at meetings, requirements, and what happens if one does not attend
   - Confidentiality
   - Roles and responsibilities
   - Assignment of tasks
   - Sharing of information
   - Collaboration and assisting one another
   - Consensus process and decision making
   - Evaluation of work

| **BOX 11-1** | **STAGES OF TEAM DEVELOPMENT** |

1. Forming                         3. Norming
2. Storming                        4. Performing

3. **Norming or the stage of consolidation around tasks**    As team members begin to work together, establish their roles, and help one another to see value in this, team cohesion develops. At this point, members must appreciate one another's strengths and limitations.
4. **Performing or the stage of teamwork and performance**    When work is getting done, and the team feels positive about this, the **performing** stage has arrived. If interpersonal issues arise they can be worked through within the team. An important part of this stage is consensus building that occurs as decisions are made. Time is an important issue, which is dependent on the nature of the decisions that need to be made. Clinical decisions typically have the highest pressure for decision making. Many clinical decisions do not require consensus, or the consensus may be decided outside the team (for example, a clinical pathway has been developed that the team needs to apply). The team then decides when to use the clinical pathway, which is a tool developed by a team through research and consensus. Individual team members may need to make some decisions (for example, a physician may need to order a medical procedure or medication). Other issues that the patient may encounter, such as discharge problems, may be something the treatment team discusses before reaching a consensus to determine the best approach.

   As the team members suggest ideas and approaches for the team to take there are some factors that need to be considered. When suggestions are made the reasons behind the suggestions and opinions should also be provided. It is important to ask others for information and their opinions. This would, of course, be other team members, but it may also mean seeking out others outside the team who have specific expertise. As one presents a suggestion or opinion, the team should be open to ideas and contributions made by others to make the team's work even better.

   Conflict can arise when consensus is developed. However, this is not necessarily a negative situation as long as the conflict addresses the issues and does not focus on personalities of team members. The latter situation will be destructive to the team's work. Team members have the responsibility for suggesting alternatives when they disagree with other team members (MindTools, 2010). Consensus is also not a unanimous agreement but rather a general agreement. All team members must agree to support the decision although all may not totally agree with it. All feelings or reactions to the decision should then be expressed appropriately. Box 11-2 identifies examples of strategies to build team performance.

| **BOX 11-2** | **BUILDING TEAM PERFORMANCE** |

- Seek employee input
- Establish urgent, demanding performance standards
- Select members for skill and skill potential
- Pay special attention to first meetings and actions
- Set clear rules of behavior
- Move from "boss" to "coach"
- Set a few immediate performance-oriented tasks and goals
- Challenge the group regularly with fresh facts and information

- Use the power of positive feedback
- Shoot for the right team size
- Choose people who like teamwork
- Train, train, train
- Cross-train for flexibility
- Emphasize the task's importance
- Assign whole tasks
- Encourage social support
- Provide the necessary material support

Source: Dessler, G. (2002). *Management*. Upper Saddle River, NJ: Prentice Hall, pp. 288–289. Reprinted with permission.

## Motivation

It is difficult to discuss any work issue without considering motivation. Motivation relates to individual staff members, teams, management, components of the organization (units, divisions, departments), and the organization as a whole. Theories of leadership and management often address motivation. If one is a team leader or a team member, motivation will be important because it will affect whether or not the team works effectively. Given this, it is important to understand motivation. What is motivation, and how does it affect work? Figure 11-1 provides an overview of the motivation process.

MOTIVATION THEORIES    The willingness to work and the ability to work go hand-in-hand. Knowledge about what drives a person to work is key for all who hold any leadership position and for those who work on teams. Motivation is related to behavior, performance, satisfaction, and rewards. Mobilizing the team to meet the outcomes is an important role for the team leader. "**Motivation** is the intensity of a person's desire to engage in some activity" (Dessler, 2002, p. 229). As was true with the theories discussed in Chapter 1 about leadership and management, theories about motivation vary, and there is no one correct or universally accepted motivation theory. The following is a brief historical review of some of the major motivation theories and their impact on management.

### Maslow

Maslow's theory of motivation focuses on a need hierarchy (Maslow, 1943). These needs are physiological (the lowest level); safety and security; belongingness, social, and love; esteem; and self-actualization. People attempt to satisfy the lower needs first. His theory emphasizes that once a need is met then it no longer motivates the person. If a need is not satisfied, the person may feel stress, frustration, and conflict, which can affect performance.

### Herzberg

Herzberg's two-factor theory of motivation, extrinsic (dissatisfiers) and intrinsic (satisfiers) (Herzberg, Mausner, & Snyderman, 1959) was originally based on research of engineers and accountants. It was thought to oversimplify the nature of job satisfaction, as it did not look at unconscious factors that might affect motivation.

### McClelland

McClelland's learned needs theory focuses on three needs: (a) the need for achievement, (b) the need for affiliation, and (c) the need for power (McClelland, 1962). The achievement need encourages a person to set goals, challenging one to achieve those goals. The affiliation need

**FIGURE 11-1    The Motivation Process.**

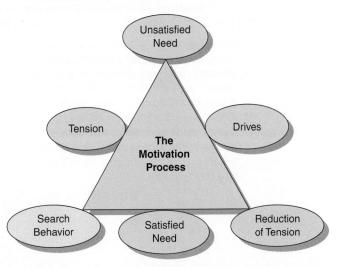

Source: Robbins, Stephen P.; Decenzo, David A., *Fundamentals of management: Essential concepts and applications*, 3rd, © 2001. Printed and Electronically reproduced by permission of Pearson Education, Inc., Upper Saddle River, New Jersey.

pushes a person toward social interaction, which affects motivation as few things can be achieved without others. The need for power focuses on the person's efforts to obtain and exercise power and authority. The theory supports the idea that people learn about these needs as they learn to cope with their environment. If they are learned, then behavior that is rewarded will probably increase. This theory is different from Maslow's and McClelland's in that it focuses on socially acquired needs.

### Skinner

Skinner's theory identifies reinforcement as its key factor. By accepting the importance of reinforcement, one can accept that behavior will continue if it is rewarded. Specific behavior will stop if punishment is received for the behavior (Dessler, 2002).

### Equity theory

Equity theory emphasizes that staff make comparisons of their own efforts and rewards with those of others who work in similar jobs or situations. The critical question for the employees is "Are they equivalent" (Adams, 1963)? If inequity is felt, then staff tension rises, which affects motivation. This tension, however may work one of two ways. The staff member may feel that less work is required because some staff may be getting the same reward but with less effort. The staff members may also feel that more work or effort are required if they recognize that others are working at a higher level and receiving additional rewards. This is a theory that most staff can probably relate to easily.

### Theory X and Y and Theory Z

Theory X and Y and Theory Z are related and are theories that are mentioned when motivation is discussed. Box 11-3 highlights key issues with these motivation theories.

## Assessment of the Motivational Climate

Understanding a person's motivation is helpful in developing strategies to increase a person's motivation and to better understand the team's motivation. The critical questions are what makes a person work and also want to improve work performance? Methods that might be used to increase motivation include observation, asking staff, and comparing and contrasting outcome

---

**BOX 11-3    THEORY X AND THEORY Y PREMISES**

**THEORY X**
A manager who views employees from a Theory X (negative) perspective believes the following:

1. Employees inherently dislike work and, whenever possible, will attempt to avoid it.
2. Because employees dislike work, they must be coerced, controlled, or threatened with punishment to achieve desired goals.
3. Employees will shirk responsibilities and seek formal direction whenever possible.
4. Most workers place security above all other factors associated with work and will display little ambition.

**THEORY Y**
A manager who views employees from a Theory Y (positive) perspective believes the following:

1. Employees can view work as being as natural as rest or play.
2. Men and women will exercise self-direction and self-control it they are committed to the objectives.
3. The average person can learn to accept, even seek, responsibility.
4. The ability to make good decisions is widely dispersed throughout the population and is not necessarily the sole province of managers.

Source: Robbins, Stephen P.; Decenzo, David A., *Fundamentals of management: Essential concepts and applications*, 3rd, © 2001. Printed and Electronically reproduced by permission of Pearson Education, Inc., Upper Saddle River, New Jersey.

results with rewards that staff receives. When people are identified as having poor motivation, how are they usually described? Typical descriptors are lack of energy, lack of initiative, poor communicator, lack of follow-through, low socialization at work, and no "get up and go." It is helpful to watch for changes in self and others. Motivation at work is also affected by personal problems and thus may interfere with staff motivation.

STRATEGIES TO IMPROVE MOTIVATION   Rewarding team members for achieved outcomes and effective performance is critical in developing the team and improving and supporting motivation. Recognizing effort should never be taken for granted. There will be times when team members or the team as a whole will excel, and it is particularly important to recognize these times. There will also be times when things do not go well, and these times cannot be ignored. The focus should be on improvement and moving forward, not on dwelling on errors (although they do need to be analyzed if improvement is to take place). The most common strategies used to motivate staff are pay for performance; merit raises; spot rewards; skill-based pay; recognition awards; job redesign that results in greater job satisfaction; empowerment; goal setting, because when people set goals they are more motivated to reach them; positive reinforcement; and lifelong learning that improves skills and demonstrates that the organization is committed to the employees (Dessler, 2002). The decision to use the reward method depends on the individual, situation, policies and procedures, roles and responsibilities, and timing.

## Building Team Power and Spirit

The development of effective teams does not just happen nor is there an end point as teams are always evolving and developing. One cannot just put a group of staff members together, call them a team, and then assume that they will function as a team with very little change. As described in the stages of team development, it takes time and effort to really build a team. Empowerment is also relevant to team functioning. When people work together, such as on a team, power issues do arise. There are different agendas, personal and team, that may conflict. Teams and individual team members can feel powerlessness when they feel like their ideas are not considered or no one is listening. **Power** means you can influence others and influence decisions. To empower is to enable to act. **Empowerment**, however, means that some may lose power and prestige. In organizations that truly practice shared participation in decision making, middle management tends to lose the most, turning over power and authority to teams. Now, a key question that those who are empowered often ask and should ask is, "What am I empowered to do?" If this is not clear, then more questions need to be asked. Muddled empowerment is worse than no empowerment because this often increases errors, frustration, and conflict.

Empowered teams are involved in a process of self-control and feel a responsibility for the team's performance. Empowerment does not mean telling someone or a team exactly what he or she must do but rather giving some direction when required and giving the team authority to do the task(s) without having to wait for approval and other management control methods. More content about continuous quality improvement is found in Chapters 16 and 17, but quality is also related to teamwork and empowerment. What happens to a team that feels empowered? An empowered team feels confident to make decisions and to assess its own work. The team recognizes its role and responsibilities and knows it will get the support needed to get the job done.

The development of team relationships is critical. Developing team spirit and a concern for one another will go a long way in setting up an environment in which the team can function effectively. Crowell (2000) developed a five-stage process to build spirited teams.

1. *Initiating*, the first stage, is when team members get to know one another. It is important for the members to understand their differences and appreciate what each can offer as different individuals and different professionals. Members need to learn more about the rules of behavior and values of the different members. Positive results are a sense of belonging and trust rather than disorientation, alienation, and mistrust.
2. *Visioning*, with the focus on sharing meaning and mission, is the second stage. At this time, the team will identify assumptions, which can be anxiety provoking, but this will help the team members to understand each other's work. From this will come a shared vision for the team.

3. *Claiming*, the third stage, is where the focus is on doing the work. These stages build on one another as it takes trust and a shared vision to help the team to do its work effectively. The positive results are establishment of goals, organizational support, and competence rather than incompetence and inability to reach outcomes.

4. *Celebrating*, the fourth stage, focuses on recognition, awards, and rewards. Taking things for granted is never helpful. The team and its members need to know they are valued and have been successful.

5. The last stage is *letting go* or really communicating. Team members may spend so much time trying to prove their point that they do not listen to one another or they are not open with feedback. It is particularly important that team members give feedback as they evaluate contributions given by one another. This may be done directly or indirectly. Subjective feedback often leads to negative feelings and may be destructive to the team. Objective feedback helps the team grow and do its job. Generalities and personal comments are not helpful. Emotions need to be experienced, identified correctly, and communicated. This relates to what was discussed in Chapter 1 about Emotional Intelligence leadership. It is important to be in tune with one's own feelings as well as those of others. Team members do not have to always agree, and in fact, if this is so, then someone is not being open and honest. It is, however, important for members to listen and try to understand other members. Providing feedback within the team requires consideration of others and should focus on the issue and avoid personal attack. Each team member needs to ask: What is it we are trying to do? Then base feedback on this issue or task. If a team member is angry, it is best to get oneself in control before approaching the problem and discussing it. Praising other team members when appropriate also helps to build trust within the team and develops open channels of communication so that when a problem occurs team members are better able to handle it. (See Chapter 12 for further content on conflict.)

## Barriers to Team Success

As teams improve their functioning, which needs to be continuous improvement, teams do encounter barriers. Teams must address these barriers to become more effective, and this too should be a continuous process. Barriers come and go and are affected by many factors. Ineffective teams may be focused on just an individual team or system-wide problems with implementing effective teams. When nursing staff is not prepared or does not understand teams and teamwork this has a major impact. Inadequate intrapersonal skills and communication competency are barriers. If nursing staff is unwilling to take on leadership roles and ownership of work this leads to problems within teams. Shared governance relies heavily on teams, but if the organization supports shared governance in name only and not in action then teams are not empowered. Ineffective communication throughout an organization will interfere with team communication and what happens with communication as it moves outside the team. If staff is not given time to complete work required for the team functions then many staff members will be passive about team work and team assignments. It takes time for a team to form and become productive, and sometimes administration does not recognize this and even team members do not. This leads to frustration and "giving up" before the team can really function. Other factors to consider are the following:

■ Lack of leadership.
■ Lack of power: If the team is not given the authority it needs to do the task then the work will not get done in the manner expected.
■ Poor communication. Any time communication is weak staff and work are affected.
■ Territoriality and cliques. Staff members who feel they "own" some responsibility are likely to interfere with team functioning.
■ Role conflict. Understanding roles is part of effective team and staff collaboration.
■ Sex-role stereotyping: Gender hierarchies, such as believing physicians are more important than nurses or nurses having the stereotype that all physicians are not collaborative (McCallin, 2001). It is important to note that generally today in most colleges of medicine

more than 50% of the students are women. Nursing, however, still has few male students. Stereotyping or making assumptions about others can interfere with effective teams and communication. Separate educational experiences between nurses and physicians have led to increasing problems in this area and working in silos with little sharing and collaboration.

- Conflict between the team leader and the team members. This leads to barriers to effective team decision making.
- Supervisor resistance: This may be in the form of resistance or disagreement and is often based on the purpose of the team; concern about loss of power and prestige; and inability to provide effective direction for the team. Managers need to offer support to teams and provide resources for the team to do its work. In addition, managers need to help staff develop skills to assist them in participating in teamwork.
- Collaboration vs. conflict among team members or with other teams (see Chapter 12 for further content).
- Lack of clearly defined purpose so that the team does not know what they are supposed to do or they feel unnecessary.
- Inability of team to incorporate new members effectively, which disturbs group cohesion and prevents the team from using each member's skills.
- Personnel issues: Common issues include wrong staff on the team, lack of specific expertise that is needed, and staff reluctance to participate on the team.
- Inadequate coping with difficult team members: Typical responses are use of scapegoating, denial of problems, anger, and conflict.

A team typically recognizes when it is not meeting its goals. Every team needs to take time to assess its outcomes and use this information and process to improve. This is no different than evaluating patient care for an individual patient. A nurse knows there are problems with the patient's care when the patient outcomes are not met. Another indicator of unproductive teams is cautious or guarded communication, which indicates a low level of trust among team members or inadequate team communication with others in the organization. Lack of disagreement can also be used to evaluate a team, as it is not healthy. People do need to disagree sometimes, but it should not be frequent or interface with work.

**Groupthink** can be another barrier to effective team functioning. This occurs when the team members reach a unanimous agreement that is based on the pressure to conform. This limits the team from considering options that might actually be a better solution (Baron, 2005). Why does this happen? The common reasons are as follows:

- There is team pressure on each member to agree with everyone else.
- The group feels separated from the consequences of its actions.
- General closed-mindedness prevails.
- The team ignores suggestions, and its thinking is irrational.
- Members censor thoughts that go against group team ideas.

This type of approach to decision making leads the team to poor judgment because the team is unable to effectively consider alternative courses of action. To prevent groupthink, it is important to recognize the value of disagreement and the need for all team members to stretch themselves and consider alternatives.

Dysfunctional meetings can indicate a lack of enthusiasm, inability to reach decisions, control by some team members, or unclear communication. How might a staff nurse evaluate a team meeting? A meeting should have a clear purpose(s) that is stated so that everyone who attends the meeting knows the purpose. Minutes of previous meetings should be available. The team leader should set an agenda and ensure that it is followed. If the discussion varies off the agenda the team needs to be pulled back on track. Maybe the topic needs to be added to another agenda. All members should be respected and allow one another to express opinions. Some teams develop rules for their meetings. Everyone should agree to follow the rules. The team leader or whoever is leading the meetings should not dominate the discussion or cut off team members. There may be times, however, when the leader indicates it is time to conclude a discussion in relationship to the agenda. At the end of the meeting there should be a short summary of what was accomplished—identifying next steps, responsibilities, and timelines. Having a lively discussion does not mean the meeting is dysfunctional as long as the discussion stays on the planned agenda. Team members need to be engaged as this is a sign of commitment plus there will be sharing of more ideas. If a team member dreads going to a meeting and feels nothing is accomplished, then there are problems in the team meeting. The best approach is to discuss this with the team.

## Getting the Job Done

Using teams to better ensure effective care can lead to the following (Fabre, 2005). Workload can be distributed so that staff is not overburdened. This can decrease the risk of errors and staff fatigue, stress, and frustration. Teams build on synergy so that more is accomplished. "Synergy occurs when a group (team) achieves more together than the sum of what the group/team members could have accomplished individually" (Fabre, 2005, p. 117). Working together using the best that each member has to offer leads to better use of everyone's intellectual capacity and experience. This should provide for improved patient care. Teams promote accountability and staff retention. If a team thinks as one this can be a disadvantage. Yes, consensus is needed for decisions, but there are times when first it is best to explore multiple solutions and then select the best. Team members need to value diversity, think critically and use clinical reasoning and judgment, and use synergy. Each member needs to build self-esteem. Clear communication is critical to getting the job done effectively. (See Chapter 12.)

## The Charge Nurse or Shift Manager and the Team

Methods used for selecting charge nurses or shift managers vary from one organization to another. Common methods are permanent charge nurses per shift (who may be assistant nurse managers) or rotating charge nurses per shift. The charge nurse is typically not the nurse manager. The major responsibility of the charge nurse is to ensure that the unit is managed effectively and patient care is delivered in a quality, safe manner for a specific shift. A charge nurse needs to understand the organization, job responsibilities, and those who are supervised, and must also demonstrate clinical and managerial competencies. The charge nurse considers the broad unit perspective, and the team leaders focus on their individual group of patients. All nurses who hold the positions of charge nurse or team leader either permanently or temporarily need to practice self-evaluation. Nurses who are charge nurses or team leaders should be able to assess themselves by considering the following questions whether or not they are listening to staff, trust staff, consistent, communicate clearly, and guide rather dictate to staff.

Both the charge nurse and the team leader must spend a lot of time making decisions and ensuring that work gets done. Typically, a charge nurse is responsible for several teams that are providing care, and each team has a team leader. If teams are not used, the charge nurse supervises a large number of staff that has individual assignments. As has been pointed out in this text, the work will be easier and more effective if the charge nurse cultivates staff participation in decision making and encourages collaboration. Working with several teams requires the nurse manager and charge nurse to understand team strengths and limitations, share appropriate timely information with the teams, and assist teams by providing needed resources whenever possible. The latter requires an awareness of team needs and also asking teams what resources they need. Interpersonal skills are constantly tested as work is assigned, evaluated, and staff coordinates care; therefore, it is important for nurses who hold either of these positions to be competent in these areas just as it is for a team leader. Both the charge nurse and team leaders hold similar positions with related required competencies; however, the charge nurse carries a larger responsibility for the unit or service during a specific shift while the team leader focuses on part of that unit or service.

Teams are also used to address quality care issues in health care organizations. One of the methods used is TeamSTEPPS, which was developed by the government. This process is described in Box 11-4. It is a structured approach to team analysis and development of solutions for a health are quality concern.

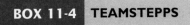

## BOX 11-4   TEAMSTEPPS

### ABOUT TEAMSTEPPS

TeamSTEPPS is a teamwork system designed for health care professionals that is

- A powerful solution to improving patient safety within your organization.
- An evidence-based teamwork system to improve communication and teamwork skills among health care professionals.
- A source for ready-to-use materials and a training curriculum to successfully integrate teamwork principles into all areas of your health care system.
- Scientifically rooted in more than 20 years of research and lessons from the application of teamwork principles.
- Developed by the Department of Defense's Patient Safety Program in collaboration with the Agency for Healthcare Research and Quality.

TeamSTEPPS provides higher quality, safer patient care by

- Producing highly effective medical teams that optimize the use of information, people, and resources to achieve the best clinical outcomes for patients.
- Increasing team awareness and clarifying team roles and responsibilities.
- Resolving conflicts and improving information sharing.
- Eliminating barriers to quality and safety.

TeamSTEPPS has a three-phased process aimed at creating and sustaining a culture of safety with

- A pretraining assessment for site readiness.
- Training for onsite trainers and health care staff.
- Implementation and sustainment.

The TeamSTEPPS curriculum is an easy-to-use comprehensive multimedia kit that contains

- Fundamentals modules in text and presentation format.
- A pocket guide that corresponds with the essentials version of the course.
- Video vignettes to illustrate key concepts.
- Workshop materials, including a supporting CD and DVD, on change management, coaching, and implementation.

### THREE PHASES OF THE TEAMSTEPPS DELIVERY SYSTEM

The three phases of TeamSTEPPS are based on lessons learned, existing master trainer or change agent experience, the literature of quality and patient safety, and culture change. A successful TeamSTEPPS initiative requires a thorough assessment of the organization and its processes and a carefully developed implementation and sustainment plan.

**Phase 1—Assess the Need**

The goal of Phase 1 is to determine an organization's readiness for undertaking a TeamSTEPPS-based initiative. Such practice is typically referred to as a training needs analysis, which is a necessary first step to implementing a teamwork initiative. For more information about conducting a needs assessment see the website.

**Phase 2—Planning, Training, and Implementation**

Phase 2 is the planning and execution segment of the TeamSTEPPS initiative. Because TeamSTEPPS was designed to be tailored to the organization, options in this phase include implementation of all tools and strategies in the entire organization, a phased-in approach that targets specific units or departments, or selection of individual tools introduced at specific intervals (called a "dosing strategy" in TeamSTEPPS parlance). As long as the primary learning objectives are maintained, the TeamSTEPPS materials are extremely adaptable. For more information about planning, training, and implementing TeamSTEPPS see the website.

**Phase 3—Sustainment**

The goal of Phase 3 is to sustain and spread improvements in teamwork performance, clinical processes, and outcomes resulting from the TeamSTEPPS initiative. The key objective is to ensure opportunities exist to implement the tools and strategies taught, practice and receive feedback on skills, and provide continual reinforcement of the TeamSTEPPS principles on the unit or within the department. For more information on sustaining TeamSTEPPS initiatives see the website.

### DETAILS OF A SITE ASSESSMENT

A site assessment entails identifying opportunities for improvement; determining the readiness of the institution, such as leadership support; identifying potential barriers to implementing change; and deciding whether resources are in place to successfully support the initiative. Each part of the Phase 1 assessment is described below.

*(continued)*

## BOX 11-4   TEAMSTEPPS (CONTINUED)

1. Establish an organizational-level change team.
   - The organizational-level change team should consist of a multidisciplinary group that represents the breadth of health care professionals within the organization. Successful change teams are comprised of organizational leaders who are committed to changing the current culture.
2. Conduct a site assessment.
   - A site assessment, also called team training needs analysis, is a process for systematically identifying teamwork deficiencies so training programs can be developed to address those deficiencies. This information is then used to identify critical training and develop training objectives.
3. Define the problem, challenge, or opportunity for improvement.
   - The team must identify the recurring problem that threatens patient safety and then determine how this problem results from existing processes and procedures. The team should devise a flowchart or map of the process during which the problem occurs. With information and processes properly mapped, it becomes clear what interventions are needed, what the objective of these interventions should be, and how ready the organization is to engage in these interventions.
4. Define the goal of your intervention.
   - List the goals that will reduce or eliminate the risk to safe patient care. For each goal, state in one sentence what will be achieved, who will be involved (whose behavior will change), and when and where the change will occur. Ideally, a team process goal, a team outcome goal, and a clinical outcome goal will be defined.

### DETAILS FOR PLANNING, TRAINING, AND IMPLEMENTATION OF TEAMSTEPPS

The tools and strategies needed to address opportunities for improvement in an organization will be determined by the Phase 1 assessment. The next step is to develop a customized Implementation and Action Plan, followed by training and implementation. Below is a brief description of steps for planning, training, and implementation.

1. Define the TeamSTEPPS intervention.
   - Decide whether "whole training" (all the tools in one sitting) or "dosing" (specific tools targeted to specific interventions) is the best intervention tactic. Whole training optimizes teamwork but does not maximize learning. It can also lead to overload or uncertainty about which tools best fit improvement opportunities. Dosing is the recommended approach because it allows for direct linking of tools and strategies with specific opportunities for improvement to minimize training fatigue and overload.
2. Develop a plan for determining the intervention's effectiveness.
   - There are a variety of ways to evaluate the impact of training. The plan should assess whether trainees have acquired new knowledge, skills, or attitudes at the end of training; if individuals are taking their learning back to the workplace and using it on the job; and organizational outcomes.
3. Develop an implementation plan.
   - Assess what groups will be trained, the order in which they will be trained (if not together and all at once), and what level of training they will receive. Include in the plan who will conduct training and where and when training will take place.
4. Gain leadership commitment to the plan.
   - Inform leaders of all facets of the plan, including how much time will be used for training and the desired resources to support it. Leadership commitment often yields plan refinement. The key is to know what elements of the plan cannot be altered.
5. Develop a communication plan.
   - Develop a plan for communicating what will be done and how the goal will be achieved. Leaders (both designated and situational) should provide information to all those in their departments or units about the initiative. It is crucial to tie together all activities that will take place with the overall goal for the initiative (i.e., improved patient safety).
6. Prepare the institution.
   - For any initiative to be fully successful, transfer of training must be achieved. Transfer is achieved by ensuring new knowledge or skills are learned and applied in the work environment. The change team must ensure the work environment is prepared to foster transfer of training so new tools and strategies are applied on the job.

BOX 11-4   TEAMSTEPPS (CONTINUED)

7. Implement training.
   - The most effective strategy for delivering the training initiative is one that involves teams of trainers that include physicians, nursing staff, and support staff. A combination of the curricula is recommended when training different sets of staff independently. The TeamSTEPPS system includes three different medical team training curricula and a complete suite of multimedia course materials:
     1. **Train-the-Trainer.** This 2.5-day training course is designed to create a cadre of teamwork instructors with the skills to train and coach other staff members.
     2. **TeamSTEPPS Fundamentals.** This curriculum includes 4 to 6 hours of interactive workshops for direct patient care providers.
     3. **TeamSTEPPS Essentials.** This curriculum is a 1- to 2-hour condensed version of the Fundamentals Course and is specifically designed for nonclinical support staff.

## DETAILS FOR SUSTAINING A TEAMSTEPPS INTERVENTION

The designated change team manages sustaining interventions through coaching and observing team performance. An effective sustainment plan should account for ongoing assessment of the effectiveness of the intervention, sustainment of positive changes, and identification of opportunities for further improvements. Below is a brief description of the steps to include in a TeamSTEPPS sustainment plan.

1. Provide opportunities to practice.
   - Any TeamSTEPPS-based initiative will be much more successful if the change team accounts for opportunities to practice these behaviors. It is important to embed opportunities for practice in day-to-day functions.
2. Ensure leaders emphasize new skills.
   - Leaders play a critical role in sustainment because they are responsible for emphasizing daily the skills learned in TeamSTEPPS training. The goal is for leaders to engage in activities that will ensure continuous involvement in teamwork.
3. Provide regular feedback and coaching.
   - Regular feedback and coaching are key to ensuring interventions are sustained. Change team members, champions from the unit, and leaders should develop and use a coaching and feedback plan that allows for sufficient observation and feedback opportunities.
4. Celebrate wins.
   - Celebrating wins bolsters further sustainment and engagement in teamwork. When using a TeamSTEPPS-based initiative, it is critical to celebrate successes for two reasons. First, it recognizes the efforts of those who were engaged from the beginning, and second, it provides detractors or laggards a tangible example of how teamwork has improved the current operations.
5. Measure success.
   - The change team should measure success by demonstrating satisfaction with training, learning, the effective use of tools and strategies on the job, and changes in processes and outcomes. It is useful to ensure that measurement of pretraining factors is parallel with post-training factors so changes can be assessed.
6. Update the plan.
   - The final stage in any TeamSTEPPS-based intervention is to revise the plan as the organization's needs change. The change team should determine when organizational needs have changed and ensure the sustainment plan continues to focus on the needs of the organization or unit where the intervention has been implemented.

Source: Agency for Healthcare Research and Quality. About TeamSTEPPS. Retrieved May 20, 2010, from http://teamstepps.ahrq.gov/about-2cl_3.htm

## APPLYING EVIDENCE-BASED PRACTICE

### Evidence for Effective Leadership and Management

**Citation:** Kalisch, B. & Lee, H. (2009). Nursing teamwork, staff characteristics, works schedules, and staffing. *Health Care Management Review*, 34(4), 323–333.

**Overview:** This cross-sectional study explored whether and how staff characteristics, staffing, and scheduling variables are associated with the level of nursing staff teamwork. The sample included staff (77.4% RNs and LPNs; 11.9% assistive personnel; 7.9% unit secretaries) in two hospitals and 38 patient care units. The participants completed the Nursing Teamwork Survey. The conclusions indicate that there is a difference in certain characteristics and effective teamwork. Service type makes a difference in that the highest scores were on pediatrics and maternity and lowest scores in medical-surgical and emergency. Higher teamwork scores are seen in staff with less than 6-months experience, worked 8- to 10-hour shifts instead of 12-hour or combination 8- and 12-hour shifts, part-time staff, and those who worked night shift and limited overtime, and higher perception of the adequacy of staffing and fewer patients assigned.

**Application:** Teamwork is part of everyday practice in health care. A greater understanding of the processes and effectiveness of teams is still needed. The Institute of Medicine in its report on health care professions' education identifies a need for greater interprofessional teamwork; however, though this is very important nursing staff teams provide much of patient care. We need to understand more about both types of teams. This study focuses on nursing teams.

### Questions:

1. *Explain why you think each of the staff characteristics identified with higher teamwork scores received higher scores? Did you think any of them would have been lower and why?*

2. *Why is team functioning so important today in health care delivery?*

3. *If you were a chief nurse executive, how might you use the information from this study?*

# APPLYING LEADERSHIP AND MANAGEMENT

## MY HOSPITAL UNIT

You are developing your annual plan for your unit. From data you have received from staff, other care providers, patients and families, and quality improvement you recognize that the unit does not use teams effectively. The entire organization is moving to interprofessional teams. Develop your plan to move your unit to interprofessional teams including how you would work with other health care providers on the unit. The plan should be clear and identify steps you will take and who you will involve in the process. How will you evaluate whether or not you have met your goals? This is your unit so past decisions you have made may impact current decisions. Use the virtual unit site found on the textbook website to record the work that you do in the role of nurse manager for your unit.

## Critical Thinking Questions and Activities

1. Attend a team meeting in a clinical site. Do not participate but simply observe the interactions. Describe the team as to size and composition. Consider the following when you write up your analysis. What were the key team tasks for that meeting? Was the leader clearly identified? What role did the leader take? How did team members interact between themselves and the leader? Did you notice differences in team members based on their position or discipline? If so, what did you observe? How would you evaluate the effectiveness of the team based on the meeting you attended?

2. If you have an opportunity to lead a team or group meeting, do so. You may belong to groups or organizations where you are in a leadership position or there are opportunities to do this. Then self-evaluate your experience. What would you include in your self-evaluation?

3. Self-directed work teams (SDWTs) are used to increase patient-centered care. Consider your clinical group in one of your clinical courses. Would you describe it as a self-directed work team? Back up your decision with a rationale that is formulated from your experience and content in this chapter. You should include information about the goal of the team. Compare and contrast the difference in this type of team and team nursing and the types of outcomes that are typically accomplished such as improved patient, staff, and physician satisfaction and patient outcomes, cost-effective delivery of care, and better staff retention and productivity. Identify critical assumptions such as team member responsibility, amount of manager (in this case, faculty) control, boundaries and autonomy, and how roles are defined and performed. What is the dependency of the members (students) on the leader (faculty)?

4. How do you function in a team? Team members need to practice self-evaluation of their own participation as a team member or performance as a team member or follower. What might be included in this self-evaluation? A member might begin by keeping a log for a specified period of time of contributions to the team as well as those ideas that were not contributed but were considered by the individual staff member. At the end of the time period, what was the members' overall impact on the team? What was contributed, and what was its value? What was the knowledge level, interest in the topic, willingness to listen to others, and comfort level in participating? Attitudes and behaviors demonstrated in the team should also be considered. Besides the log and evaluation of its content, a team member might ask a co-worker or the team leader to critique team participation. Reasons behind effectiveness or ineffectiveness should be analyzed. The final step is to develop a plan of action that addresses improvement areas. This process is the same as that used for any self-assessment process.

5. Do you think the team approach is effective, based on your own experience? Provide rationale and examples for your response.

6. Review the material on TeamSTEPPS provided in the chapter and go to the TeamSTEPPS website http://teamstepps.ahrq.gov/. Analyze how the information on TeamSTEPPS relates to content in this chapter with a team of students. What is the team's opinion of this method?

7. Review the website MindTools provided in the Media Links section of this chapter and discuss with your peer discussion group. This site provides more information on some of the topics found in this chapter.

8. How might you envision using SBAR? (See Media Links.) How does SBAR relate to teams?

## Media Links

- **URL: http://www.accel-team.com/**
  Team Building: Tools for building strong teams, plus useful links and articles
- **URL: http://www.abacon.com/commstudies/groups/groupthink.html**
  Groupthink: Learn how to identify conditions, negative outcomes, and solutions to groupthink.
- **URL: http://www.au.af.mil/au/awc/awcgate/ndu/strat-ldr-dm/pt3ch10.html**
  Strategic Leadership and Decision Making: Read about how to create and manage teams.
- **URL: http://emotionalliteracyeducation.com/abraham-maslow-theory-human-motivation.shtml**
  Abraham Maslow's Theory of Human Motivation
- **URL: http://www.accel-team.com/motivation/**
  Motivation at Work: Read about how to motivate your employees.
- **URL: http://www.mindtools.com/pages/main/ThemedIndex.htm**
  MindTools: See list of articles and resources on Team Tools
- **URL: http://www.mindtools.com/pages/article/newLDR_86.htm**
  MindTools: Forming, Storming, Norming, and Performing
- **URL: http://www.mindtools.com/pages/article/newLDR_82.htm**
  MindTools: Avoiding Groupthink
- **URL: http://www.ihi.org**
  Institute for Health Improvement: Teams
- **URL: http://teamstepps.ahrq.gov/**
  Agency for Healthcare Research and Quality: TeamSTEPPS
- **URL: http://www.ihi.org/IHI/Topics/PatientSafety/SafetyGeneral/Tools/SBARTrainingScenariosandCompetencyAssessment.htm**
  Institute for Health Improvement: SBAR

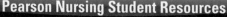

**Pearson Nursing Student Resources**

Find additional review materials at
**nursing.pearsonhighered.com**

Prepare for success with additional NCLEX®-style practice questions, interactive assignments and activities, Web links, animations and videos, and more!

# References

Adams, J. (1963, November). Toward an understanding of inequity. *Journal of Abnormal and Social Psychology*, 422–436.

American Nurses Credentialing Center. (2009). Magnet forces of magnetism. Retrieved November 12, 2009, from http://www.nursecredentialing.org/ Magnet/ProgramOverview/ ForcesofMagnetism.aspx

Baron, R. (2005). So right it's wrong: Groupthink and the ubiquitous nature of polarizsed group decision making. In M. Zanna (ed.) *Advances in experimental social psychology*, Vol. 37 (pp. 219–253). San Diego: Elsevier Academic Press.

Caliper. (2005). *The qualities that distinguish women leaders*. Princeton, NJ: Author.

Crowell, D. (2000). Building spirited multidisciplinary teams. *Journal of PeriAnesthesia Nursing*, *15*(2), 108–114.

Dartmouth College. (2010). Clinical Microsystems. Retrieved May 5, 2010, from http://dms.dartmouth.edu/cms/

Dessler, G. (2002). *Management*. Upper Saddle River, NJ: Prentice Hall.

Fabre, J. (2005). *Smart nursing*. NY: Springer Publishing Company.

Finkelman, A. & Kenner, C. (2010). *Professional nursing concepts. Competencies for quality leadership*. Boston: Jones and Bartlett Publishers.

Grossman, S., & Valiga, T. (2000). *The new leadership challenge: Creating the future of nursing*. Philadelphia: F. A. Davis Company.

Herzberg, F., Mausner, B., & Snyderman, B. (1959). *The motivation to work*. New York: John Wiley and Sons.

Institute of Medicine. (2001). *Crossing the quality chasm*. Washington, DC: National Academies Press.

Institute of Medicine. (2003). *Health professions education*. Washington, DC: National Academies of Sciences.

Institute of Medicine. (2004). *Keeping patients safe: Transforming the work environment for nurses*. Washington, D.C.: National Academies Press.

Lyon, J. (1993). Models of nursing care delivery and case management: Clarification of terms. *Nursing Economics, 11*(3), 163–169.

Maslow, A. (1943, July). A theory of human motivation. *Psychological Review*, 370–396.

McCallin, A. (2001). Interdisciplinary practice—a matter of teamwork: An integrated literature review. *Journal of Clinical Nursing, 10*, 419–428.

McClelland, D. (1962 July–August). Business drive and national achievement. *Harvard Business Review*, 99–112.

McCullough, C., & Sanders, D. (2000). Building self-directed work teams. In F. Bower (Ed.), *Nurses taking the lead* (pp. 89–118). Philadelphia: W.B. Saunders Company.

Michaelsen, L., et al. (2008). *Team-based learning* for health professions education: *A guide to using small groups for improving learning*. Sterling, VA: Stylus Publishers, Inc.

MindTools. (2010). Forming, storming, norming, and performing. Retrieved May 5, 2010, from http://www.mindtools .com/pages/article/newLDR_86.htm

Minnen, T., et al. (1993). Sustaining work redesign innovation through shared governance. *Journal of Nursing Administration, 23*, 35–40.

Nelson, C., et al. (2008). Clinical Microsystems, Part 1: The building blocks of health systems. *The Joint Commission Journal on Quality and Patient Safety, 34*(7), 367–378.

Salmon, M. (2007). Guest editorial: Care quality and safety: Same old? *Nursing Outlook, 55*(3), 117–119.

Spitzer, R. (2008). Teamwork, teams, and reality. *Nurse Leader, 6*(6), 6, 49.

Tuckman, B. (1965). Development sequence in small groups. *Psychological Bulletin, 63*(6), 334–399.

Weinstock, M. (March 3, 2010). There's no "I" in team. *H&HN*. Retrieved March 22, 2010, from http://www.hhnmag.com

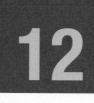

# 12

# Improving Teamwork: Collaboration, Coordination, and Conflict Resolution

## CHAPTER OUTLINE

## LEARNING OUTCOMES

Before you begin, take a moment to familiarize yourself with the learning outcomes for this chapter.

- Analyze key aspects related to collaboration.
- Examine barriers to achieving effective collaboration.
- Discuss the skills and strategies that are needed to improve collaboration.
- Explain the impact collaboration has on nursing staff and interprofessional interactions.
- Analyze key aspects related to coordination.
- Examine barriers to achieving effective coordination.
- Discuss the skills and strategies that are needed to improve coordination.
- Discuss the impact coordination has on nursing staff and interprofessional interactions.
- Apply methods to prevent conflict.
- Discuss how individuals respond to conflict.
- Explain conflict management and strategies that might be used.
- Examine the impact conflict has on nursing staff and interprofessional interactions.

## WHAT'S AHEAD

This chapter continues the discussion about teams focusing on collaboration, coordination, and conflict resolution as critical skills needed by every nurse regardless of the specialty or type of setting where the nurse works. These skills are directly related to effective leadership and management and teamwork. Health care organizations in which staff members collaborate with one another, work together to coordinate care delivery, and strive to resolve conflicts that inevitably will occur will be successful in meeting their goal—to provide quality, safe care. This chapter discusses these three critical competencies that are needed by each nurse.

# Collaboration

The American Nurses Association (ANA) defines **collaboration** as "recognition of the expertise of others within and outside the profession, and referral to those other providers when appropriate. Collaboration involves some shared functions and a common focus on the same overall mission" (2003, p. 8). This is a critical competency required to practice in any health care setting today or to participate in any aspect of health care delivery—critical for effective patient-centered, quality care. The increased emphasis on using interprofessional teams to meet the patient's needs across the continuum of care requires collaboration. Team members and different health care providers must be able to work together, recognize strengths and limitations, respect individual responsibilities, and maintain open communication.

Nurses who have long worked on teams should be familiar with teamwork. Despite this, there continues to be a separation between physicians and nurses, who often work in silos. Nurses and physicians can work together to ensure that the patient receives the care that is required when it is required. Collaboration requires cooperative effort among all health care providers providing care for a patient, and this will result in more effective decision making. All health care professionals need to work together to accomplish the identified goals and reach identified outcomes. This is not easy to do. There are professional issues, territory issues, conflicting goals, inadequate communication, and multiple differences; however, despite all of this, effective and efficient care requires collaboration. The system is just too complex to function well without collaboration. The nurse is often the person who must lead the effort to ensure collaboration occurs.

## Key Definitions

Collaboration is a cooperative effort that focuses on a win-win strategy. To collaborate, each individual needs to recognize the perspective of others who are involved and eventually reach a **consensus** of a common goal(s). The ANA states that "collaboration among health care professionals involves recognition of the expertise of others within and outside the profession, and referral to those other providers when appropriate. Collaboration involves some shared functions and a common focus on the same overall mission" (2003, p. 8). The American Nurses Association's *Nursing: Scope and Standards of Practice* (2004) and the *Nursing Administration Scope and Standards of Practice* (2009) also identify the need for collaboration, emphasizing that all nurses are expected to collaborate. Box 12-1 compares these two standards. Clearly, collaboration is important for practice, but how does one develop this competency and use it effectively?

| BOX 12-1 | COMPARING NURSING AND NURSING ADMINISTRATION STANDARDS ON COLLABORATION |

### NURSING: SCOPE AND STANDARDS OF PRACTICE

**Standard VI. Collaboration**
The registered nurse collaborates with the patient, family, and other health care providers in the conduct of nursing practice.

*Measurement Criteria:*

**The registered nurse**
- Communicates with the patient, family, and health care providers regarding patient care and the nurse's role in the provision of that care.
- Collaborates in creating a documented plan, focused on outcomes and decisions related to care and delivery of services, that indicates communication with patients, families, and others.
- Partners with others to effect change and generate positive outcomes through knowledge of the patient or situation.
- Documents referrals, including provisions for continuity of care.

### NURSING ADMINISTRATION SCOPE AND STANDARDS OF PRACTICE

**Standard 11. Collaboration**

*Measurement Criteria:*

**The nurse administrator**
- Communicates with health care providers and other stakeholders regarding care and services and the nurse's role in the provision of care.
- Collaborates in creating a documented plan focused on outcomes and decisions related to care and delivery of services.
- Partners with others to enhance health care and employee satisfaction through interprofessional activities such as education, consultation, management, technological development, or research opportunities.
- Models an interprofessional process with other members of the health care team.
- Documents plans, communications, rationales for plan changes, and collaborative discussions.

Source: Nursing Scope and Standards of Practice – Standard 13. Collaboration. From *Nursing: Scope and standards of practice*, 2nd ed. © 2010 By American Nurses Association. Reprinted with permission. All rights reserved.

Key concepts related to collaboration are (a) partnership, (b) interdependence, and (c) collective ownership and responsibility. Considering these concepts and those identified by Tahan helps us to understand the impact of collaboration. Collaboration is also a process. It is not stagnant but rather changes, which requires staff to make adjustments as situations change in order to collaborate with others. The American Association of Critical Care Nurses' standards for healthy work environments that is associated with their model of nursing practice emphasizes the need for true collaboration, which is an ongoing process built on mutual trust and respect (2005). Most people can remember experiences when working with others where the work just seemed to flow with less stress and good communication. This probably means that the people working together were collaborating.

Collaboration should be a positive experience, but this is not always the case. If it is not positive, it will not be effective. If a group of nurses were surveyed, it would be surprising to get a consensus that collaboration was always a positive experience. Often attempts at collaboration mean struggle, conflict, and sometimes, ineffective results. Some research has been conducted to assess the effectiveness of collaboration. A review of 100 studies, however, indicates that studies of collaboration have not always been scientifically rigorous enough to prove that collaboration improves care (Dechairo-Marino, Jordan-Marsh, Traiger, & Saulo, 2001). The Institute of Medicine recognizes the importance of collaboration in its rules to guide behavior in the 21st century health care system (2001). The tenth rule is cooperation among clinicians emphasizing that "cooperation in patient care is more important than professional prerogatives and roles" (p. 93). To meet this rule health care staff needs to collaborate and use effective teamwork, which is weak in the health care delivery system.

## Barriers to Effective Collaboration

As noted by the IOM, working in isolation with only concern for your own profession is not effective; however, nursing also has much work to do to improve the image of nursing and nursing leadership. Salmon (2007) noted that "Improvements in care quality and safety will simply not happen with nurses working by themselves. To take it a step beyond what may seem obvious, it can't happen just by adding physicians to the equation. It's going to take the partnered engagement of other clinicians, health administrators, and, ultimately, the public" (p. 117). Given these issues how does the nursing profession arrive at the right balance, one that focuses on nursing and its professional role and needs, while simultaneously developing nurses who can work collaboratively with others to meet patient outcomes? Collaboration requires an interactive process. If staff is not willing to interact or have any other barrier to interaction, collaboration cannot take place. Lack of understanding about the roles and responsibilities of others and lack of respect for what others contribute interferes with effective collaboration. How much do nurses know about what physicians do and vice versa, or social workers and nurses, or physical therapists and nurses, and so on? If there is distrust, collaboration is hindered because distrust affects willingness to share information, which is an integral component in the collaborative relationship. Disch (2001) suggests an analogy to support her recommendation for greater interprofessional collaboration, "A violinist needs to develop expertise and be the best violinist possible. But when working in a group/team, the violinist must weave his or her melodies into making the string quartet the most impressive it can be" (p. 275). This analogy demonstrates how collaboration can result in an effective or ineffective team. If each violinist continues to play as if he or she was the only one present, ignoring the others, the music will not come together. Although each nurse must develop individual expertise, this expertise must come together with others' expertise. Few nurses really can work effectively in isolation. Nursing is a profession that requires contact with others—patients, other nursing staff, other health care professionals, families, community members, and so on.

There is conflict between professions, but there is also conflict within the nursing profession and with co-workers. In these situations, staff members may attack one another by asserting their position or by attacking ideas. In some cases, they attack one another personally. The first response typically is to attack back, which acts as an additional barrier to effective collaboration. When this occurs, it is best to step back and take some time to de-escalate and then discuss the problem in a private setting. In some situations it may be useful to have a third party present, but all staff involved needs to agree to the addition of a third party. The goal is to break down the barrier by avoiding counterattacking and focusing on common interests and resolutions.

Collaboration often is used to reach an agreement during a conflict. This is often true with nurse–physician collaboration, though ideally collaboration should be part of all of their interactions. Nurse–physician relationships are complex. There is overlapping of focus in that both are concerned about the patient though maybe from different points-of-view, and this is not always understood or appreciated. There is also some confusion about roles, which can lead to problems. In some cases there is a certain amount of competition, which really is a sad statement as the goal should be focused on what is best for the patient.

## Skills and Strategies to Achieve Effective Collaboration

Collaboration is a critical competency required to practice in any health care setting. The increased emphasis on interprofessional teams to meet the patient's needs across the continuum of care requires effective use of collaboration. The very nature of a team implies that there is more than one idea or approach and not all can usually be accomplished. Decisions need to be made, and this is where collaboration comes into play. It is important to remember that collaboration is also a critical factor in the nurse–patient relationship. Nurses need to actively pursue patient collaboration to ensure that patients are involved in their own care—patient-centered care. The nursing profession has long emphasized patient participation in planning care and in patient education. Collaboration is also important in the development of effective management.

To be effective in collaboration, staff requires a number of skills.

- Communication skills are critical. Verbal skills are the focus; however, in some instances written communication is also important as information and process are described in written format.
- Staff members also need to be aware of their own feelings, as was discussed in some of the leadership theories such as Emotional Intelligence.
- Staff needs to be able to make decisions to solve problems effectively.
- As is discussed in this chapter, coordination is also important when collaborating with others.
- Conflicts will arise, which may interfere with collaboration. Staff needs to develop negotiation skills to be used in resolving difficult conflicts.
- Assessment skills are needed to collect information and analyze as relationships as collaboration is developed. Box 12-2 highlights these skills.

Collaborative care is central to the success of efficient, outcome-driven care. With the complex health care system, specialization of many health care professionals, variety of health care settings, complex reimbursement systems, technology, and new drugs, collaboration is the only way that patients will receive quality, cost-effective care. Today, the health care system is an interdependent system with multiple settings and a variety of health care professionals, who are dependent on one another. Delivery of care in the complex delivery system requires sharing of information, analysis, clear communication, and ability to use team problem solving. These activities are integral to successful care as the nurse works with many different health care providers, within many different health care settings, and with the patient and family to ensure quality, cost-effective care for the patient.

**Collaborative planning**, or joining together to form alliances or partnerships (coalitions), is an important method used to address the following (Puetz & Shinn, 2002):

1. Maximize resources such as funding, equipment and supplies, space, and staff.
2. Minimize duplication of work.
3. Improve relationships.

This type of planning also recognizes that collaboration has a positive effect on achieving patient outcomes (Institute of Medicine, 2001). Collaborative planning requires that all parties agree on the mission and goals of the partnership so that they have common expectations. All members of the effort need to commit to open and honest communication, which is essential to sharing. This can be difficult in some organizations, components of an organization such as specific units or departments, and for some individuals. Those who fear competition and are concerned about power will struggle with the need to share.

Regular evaluation needs to be built into collaborative planning. This evaluation should not only focus on the content of the planning but also on the process—how is the collaborative relationship working? This is something that is often neglected. Power, which is discussed later in this chapter, plays an important role in collaboration. Usually some of the partners in a relationship have more power than others. "Any imbalance in capacity and capability can be smoothed out by the establishment of mutually agreed-upon goals and expectations. Clarity about outcomes and inputs can help build trust and buy-in from the outset" (Puetz & Shinn, 2002, p. 183).

---

## BOX 12-2    COLLABORATION: SKILLS NEEDED

- Communication
- Awareness of personal feelings
- Problem solving

- Negotiation
- Assessment

When partners work through the collaborative planning process, some issues may interfere with the process. These may include the following:

- Preconditions
- Lack of commitment
- Changing players in midstream
- Saboteurs and rumors
- Diversions from the timeline (Puetz & Shinn, 2002)

Recognizing these potential issues should be a priority to prevent barriers to success. What can be done to prevent them? Clear communication about purpose, particularly identifying issues from the past that may affect the collaborative planning, can help to clear up misconceptions. Team members need to accept the importance of effort and commit to it. All efforts should be made to keep team membership committed. Evaluation data about the collaborative effort can help to improve team functioning.

## Application of Collaboration

What is gained from collaboration? The complex health care delivery system requires many competencies, and no one health care profession has all of the necessary competencies to provide all the care that is required. Interprofessional teams and effective collaboration are critical. The Institute of Medicine (IOM) (2004) report on nursing identifies practices that have an impact on the delivery system, and these practices require collaboration to be effective. The practices are to create and maintain trust throughout the organization, deploy staff in adequate numbers, create a culture of openness so that errors are reported, involve staff in decision making pertaining to work design and work flow, and actively manage the change process (Institute of Medicine, 2004).

The Magnet Hospital Recognition Program® also considers the impact of collaborative relationships on care and the work environment for nurses by assessing the presence of collaboration when determining if a hospital meets criteria for excellence in nursing. (See Chapter 6 for more information on Magnet hospitals.) By including collaboration, Magnet recognition establishes that collaboration is a critical component in the delivery of care.

How do health care professionals develop the skills necessary for effective collaboration? There is a great need to incorporate more interprofessional educational experiences in all health care professional education, including nursing. Students from the various health care professions need to have some experiences learning together in the same classroom and participating in clinical experiences together. Learning separately makes it very difficult to expect that at the time of graduation new health care professionals will easily collaborate when they have had limited collaborative experience with other health care professional students or health care professionals. They do not understand or respect the knowledge and learning experiences of other students, or their roles and typical communication methods and processes. They may not even value or respect what other health care professionals offer to the team and to the patient. This causes serious problems as new health care professionals begin to work and are then confronted with working with one another. In addition, nurses need to have a positive understanding of their own roles and responsibilities—what they have to offer is valuable—so that they can approach collaboration while understanding that they have important knowledge and competencies to add to the collaboration. This, however, must be accomplished *not* from the perspective of "I am better than you" but rather "How can we bring our respective skills and knowledge together to provide comprehensive, consistent care?"

Interprofessional relationships and activities can result in positive, collaborative outcomes; however, it is not easy to establish these relationships and maintain them over time. It takes time to develop an effective interprofessional environment. Other recommendations are to set realistic goals with commitment from all involved disciplines to these goals; negotiate the means to meet the goals; avoid battles that only serve as barriers such as turf battles; and measure success based on established goals.

If the idea is to improve interprofessional and collaborative relationships, what might be the results? Cody summarizes possible desired outcomes that can result from collaborative interprofessional relationships and activities described in the literature. These outcomes include the following:

- Professionals will be more familiar with one another's activities and roles, thereby improving interprofessional communication.
- Professionals will be better able to work collaboratively, thereby improving care.
- Professionals will have broader repertoires of knowledge and skills, thereby in effect increasing access to care for the people.
- Professionals will have more career mobility as health care systems change.
- With larger, more diverse research teams, research productivity on issues of importance in health care will increase.
- Cross-disciplinary peer review and critique of practice and research will be more available and more intellectually sound.
- Cross-fertilization with creative ideas from many sectors will enhance and accelerate innovations in health care (Cody, 2001, p. 276).

If these results or outcomes can be reached, the working environment will be improved.

# Coordination

The IOM identifies care coordination as one of the critical priority areas of care that need be monitored and improved. The purpose of care coordination is "to establish and support a continuous healing relationship, enabled by an integrated clinical environment and characterized by a proactive delivery of evidence-based care and follow-up" (Institute of Medicine, 2003a, p. 49). Care coordination and patient-centered care were discussed in Chapter 7; however, patient-centered care is an important theme throughout this text. There needs to be greater attention on how care is coordinated across people, functions, activities, and sites so that the outcome is effective and efficient care that meets the patient's specific outcomes. How the pieces are put together to reach desired outcomes is an important part of case management. Coordination

## APPLYING EVIDENCE-BASED PRACTICE

### Evidence for Effective Leadership and Management

Citation: Dougherty, M. & Larson, E. (2010). The nurse–nurse collaboration scale. JONA, 40F(1), 17–25.

Overview: This study focused on the development of a new measurement tool, the nurse–nurse collaboration (NNC) scale, to determine if it was a reliable and valid instrument. Measurement tools or instruments are developed using a research process, and then these instruments may be used in studies to collect and measure data related to a variety of research questions. To develop the instrument a comprehensive review of literature provided information for the instrument content. The five domains used were problem solving, communication, coordination, shared process, and professionalism. The scale was pilot tested with 76 staff nurses in one hospital. Statistical analysis was completed, and reliability and validity were demonstrated.

Application: As noted by the Institute of Medicine (IOM) collaboration is important in reducing errors and improving care and has an impact on nurses' job satisfaction. Collaboration may be interprofessional or nurse-to-nurse or nursing staff (e.g., RNs, LPNs, UAP).

Questions:

1. *What is your opinion of the process used to develop this instrument?*
2. *Why do you think the five domains would be important in measuring nurse–nurse collaboration?*
3. *In what way is collaboration important in improving care and reducing errors?*

requires that the nurse understands patient needs and the resources that are available to meet these needs. An awareness of the association of costs and services is part of coordinating patient care. The health care delivery system has become more complex, which has made communication and coordination more complex, all of which leads to increased errors. There is greater need for interprofessional teams. Team members may not always view the patient, problems, or priorities in the same way, and yet it is critical that the team find a way to work collaboratively to provide coordinated patient care. Team members need to have a better understanding of individual responsibilities and stress in order to appreciate each other and develop more realistic working relationships. As noted by the IOM health care core competency, all health care professionals need to know how to work in interprofessional teams (Institute of Medicine, 2003b). Recognizing this will make coordination less frustrating.

## Key Definitions

**Coordination** is the process of working to see that "the pieces and activities fit together and flow as they should" (Finkelman & Kenner, 2010, p. 347). Effective coordination requires working across services that are complementary—may be across clinicians or settings—to ensure quality care across patient conditions, services, and settings over time (Institute of Medicine, 2001). Examples might be physicians, nurses, social workers, pharmacists, informatic specialists, and administrators working together to improve documentation through an electronic medical record or staff from a hospital and an ambulatory care center working together to coordinate better care for patients. Coordination is related to collaboration, and in fact, it is very difficult to do one without the other. When considering patient care, however, there is a critical difference between the two. Collaboration with a patient requires a direct interaction with the patient. Coordination of care usually takes place before or after patient care is provided or interwoven in the care. In the latter situation a nurse may ensure that all the plans for the patient's discharge are complete or that the various treatment and exam procedures are scheduled appropriately for the patient's needs. Coordination does not mean that the patient is not involved because patient input is critical to achieve patient-centered care, but the nurse may do the coordination such as calling for supplies or making sure a treatment is scheduled when not in the presence of the patient or while providing direct care. Both coordination and collaboration are also found daily in staff–staff interactions. Collaboration focuses on solving a problem with two or more people working toward this goal. Coordination is done to ensure that something happens such as the provision of services. The ANA *Nursing Administration Scope and Standards of Practice* (2009) includes a standard on coordination: "The nurse administrator coordinates the implementation and other associated process" (p. 30). The measurement criteria for this standard includes the nurse administrator doing the following:

- Coordinates implementation of the plan and associated activities.
- Coordinates human, capital, system, and community resources and measures, including environmental modifications, necessary to implement the plan.
- Provides leadership in the coordination of multidisciplinary health care resources for integrated delivery of care and services.
- Promotes communication systems for an open and transparent organization.

## Barriers to Effective Coordination

As health care organizations and services become more complex and they use more interprofessional teams, team members may not always have the same view of the patient, problems, or priorities, and yet it is critical that the team find a way to work collaboratively to provide coordinated patient care and prevent errors, disorganized care, and care that does not reach effective outcomes. Team members need to have a better understanding of individual responsibilities and their own stress in order to appreciate each other and develop more realistic working relationships. Coordination is also more effective when those involved have a better understanding of their respective roles and work stresses. Recognizing this will make coordination less frustrating. If resources are not available when and in the manner required, this will act as a barrier to coordination. Staff that is not willing to listen and include others will find that coordination may not be as successful as planned. Other barriers are a lack of interprofessional understanding, lack of resources, and inadequate communication. Ineffective problem solving is also a critical barrier. Coordination needs to include the patient and when appropriate the family. If this is not present, it is a major barrier.

### Skills and Strategies to Achieve Effective Coordination

For staff to provide effective coordination, they need to make decisions to solve problems, plan, use the abilities of other staff, identify resources required, communicate, and be willing to collaborate. Delegation often is required, so delegation skills are important. (See Chapter 14 for more discussion on delegation.) The nurse also needs to develop evaluation skills to determine if outcomes are met as well as when to change course or make adjustments. The skills required for coordination are the same ones required for collaboration with the primary goal of working together to reach agreed upon goals. Box 12-3 highlights the skills needed for effective coordination.

### Application of Coordination

Coordination is integral to daily operations, short- and long-range planning, and the daily care process. All of these activities require coordination of clinical and administrative resources. The following strategies are helpful in improving coordination (Finkelman & Kenner, 2010).

- All staff needs to understand the importance of coordination.
- All staff should have a clear understanding of purpose and goals.
- All staff should have knowledge of policies and procedures with an understanding of what has to be done, by whom, and how it will help to facilitate coordination.
- Improved organizational performance will depend on coordination at all levels in the organization.
- Communication needs to be clear and timely. (See Chapter 13.)
- Orientation and staff development programs should emphasize the importance of coordination and how to use it.
- Coordination requires effective communication and collaboration.
- Staff/team members need to appreciate the expertise of team members.
- Delegation needs to be used as needed. (See Chapter 14.)

Health care uses many tools that focus on coordination of care to ensure patient-centered care. Some of these are case management, clinical pathways, practice guidelines, and disease management. (See Chapter 7.) To be successful and meet expected outcomes, these tools or methods also require collaboration with the patient, patient's families and significant others, and other health care staff, and they are very useful when coordination is required. With insurers emphasizing more effective and efficient care, coordination plays a major role in reaching this goal. Coordination requires that the nurse understand patient needs and the resources that are available to meet these needs. An awareness of the association of costs and services is part of coordinating patient care. In addition, coordination is a very important part of management within the health care delivery system. This system has become more complex, which has made communication and coordination more complex. Coordination is required to get resources, schedule staff, plan work activities, implement quality improvement, and perform all types of management functions. With the growth of informatics in documentation and decision-making tools, additional methods are now available and new ones will be developed. (See Chapter 18.)

---

**BOX 12-3 COORDINATION: SKILLS NEEDED**

- Problem solving
- Plan
- Use abilities of others
- Identify needed resources
- Communication
- Collaboration
- Delegation
- Evaluation

# Negotiation and Conflict Resolution

Conflict can never be eliminated in organizations; however, conflict can be managed. Typically, conflict arises when people feel strongly about something. Conflicts may take place between individual staff, within a unit, or within a department. They may be inter-unit and interdepartmental, affect the entire organization, or even occur between multiple organizations, between or within teams or units, or between an organization and the community. **Conflict** is the "tension arising from compatible needs, in which the actions of one frustrate the ability of the other to achieve a goal" (Boggs, 2003, p. 366).

## Key Definitions

There are three types of conflict: individual, interpersonal, and intergroup/organizational (Dessler, 2002). The most common type of individual conflict in the workplace is role conflict, which occurs when there is incompatibility between one or more role expectations. When staff does not understand the roles of other staff this can be very stressful for the individual and does affect work. Staff may be critical of each other for not doing some work activity when in reality it is not part of the role and responsibilities of that staff member, or staff members may feel that another staff member is doing some activity that really is not his or her responsibility.

Interpersonal conflict occurs between people. Sometimes this is due to differences and/or personalities, competition, or concern about territory, control, or loss.

Conflict also occurs between groups (e.g., units, services, teams, health care professional groups, agencies, community and a health care provider organization, and so on). When conflict occurs something is out of sync, usually due to a lack of clear understanding of one another's roles and responsibilities. "Conflict can be overt or covert, and both can lead to problems as well as opportunities. However, covert conflict processes, obviously, tend to be fluid and difficult to describe. It is in behaviors between individuals and groups, as well as individual behaviors that are observable. These behaviors can be categorized as reactive, repressive, or avoidant. Reactive behaviors include high levels of competition, inefficiency, 'yesing' people with no real attempt to understand, whining, complaining, destructive behavior, counter organization moves, and passive-aggressive behaviors such as escapist drinking, irregular output, or frequent expression of low job satisfaction. In workplaces that are ripe with unacknowledged conflict, rumor mills flourish. Repressive behaviors include absenteeism, whereas avoidant behaviors can include withholding information, avoidance of contact with managers or other team members, or 'hiding out' on the job" (Clement, 2001, p. 212).

Everyone has experienced covert conflict. It never feels good and increases stress quickly. Distrust and confusion about the best response are also experienced. Acknowledging covert conflict is not easy, and staff will have different perceptions of the conflict since it is not clear and below the surface. Overt conflict is obvious, at least to most people, and thus coping with it is usually easier. It is easier to arrive at an agreement when conflict is present and easier to arrive at a description of the conflict.

The common assumption about conflict is that it is destructive, and it certainly can be. There is, however, another view of conflict. "Despite its adverse effects, conflict is viewed by most experts today as potentially useful because it can, if properly channeled, be an engine of innovation and change. This view explicitly encourages a certain amount of controlled conflict in organizations because lack of active debate can permit the status quo or mediocre ideas to prevail" (Dessler, 2002, p. 315). In reality, staff really cannot avoid conflict because some conflict is inevitable. The following quote speaks to the need to recognize most conflict as opportunity. "When I speak of celebrating conflict, others often look at me as if I have just stepped over the credibility line. As nurses, we have been socialized to avoid conflict. Our *modus operandi* has been to smooth over at all costs, particularly if the dynamic involves individuals representing roles that have significant power differences in the organization. Be advised that well-functioning transdisciplinary teams will encounter conflict-laden situations. It is inevitable. The role of the leader is to use conflicting perspectives to highlight and hone the rich diversity that is present within the team. Conflict also provides opportunities for individuals to present divergent yet equally valid views that allow all team members to gain an understanding of their contributions to the process. Respect for each team member's standpoint comes only after the team has explored fully and learned to appreciate the diversity of its membership" (Weaver, 2001, p. 83). This is a very positive view of conflict, which on the surface may appear negative. If one asked nurses if they wanted to experience conflict, they would say no. Probably behind their response is the fact that they do not know how to handle conflict and feel uncomfortable with it. However, if you asked staff, "Would you like to work in an environment where staff at all levels could be direct without concern of repercussions and could actively dialogue about issues and problems without others taking comments personally" then many staff would most likely see this as positive and not conflict. Avoidance of conflict, however, usually means that it will catch up with the person again, and then it may be more difficult to resolve. There may then be more emotions attached to it, making it more difficult to resolve.

## Causes of Conflict

Effective resolution of conflict requires an understanding of the cause of the conflict; however, some conflicts may have more than one cause. It is easy to jump to conclusions without doing a thorough assessment. Some of the typical causes of conflict between individuals and between groups are "whether resources are shared equitably; insufficient explanation of expectations, leading to performance being questioned; unexplained changes that disturb routines and process and that team members are not prepared for; and to stress resulting from changes that team members do not understand and may see as threatening" (Finkelman & Kenner, 2010, p. 359). Other causes are ambiguous jurisdiction, conflict of interest, communication confusion, and unresolved conflicts (Hansten & Jackson, 2008).

Two predictors of conflict are the existence of competition for resources or inadequate communication. It is rare that a major change on a unit or in a health care organization does not result in competition for resources (staff, financial, space, supplies) so conflicts will arise between units or between those who may or may not receive the resources or may lose resources. As has been demonstrated in some of the examples, causes of conflict can be varied. An understanding of a conflict requires as thorough an assessment as possible. Along with the assessment, it is important to understand the stages of conflict.

## Stages of Conflict

There are four stages of conflict that help describe the process of conflict development (Marquis & Huston, 2009).

1. **Latent conflict.**   This stage involves the anticipation of conflict. Competition for resources or inadequate communication can be predictors of conflict. Anticipating conflict can increase tension. This is when staff may verbalize, "We know we are going to have a hassle with this" or may feel this internally. The anticipation of conflict can occur between units that accept one another's patients when one unit does not think that the staff members on the other unit is very competent and yet they must accept orders and patient plans from them.
2. **Perceived conflict.**   This stage requires recognition or awareness that conflict exists at a particular time. It may not be discussed but only felt. Perception is very important as it can affect whether or not there really is a conflict, what is known about the conflict, and how it might be resolved.
3. **Felt conflict.**   This occurs when individuals begin to have feelings about the conflict such as anxiety or anger. Staff feels stress at this time. If avoidance is used at this time, it may prevent the conflict from moving to the next stage. Avoidance may be appropriate in some circumstances, but sometimes it just covers over the conflict and does not resolve it. In this case, the conflict may come up again and be more complicated. Trust plays a role here. How much does staff trust that the situation will be resolved effectively? How comfortable do staff members feel in being open with their feelings and opinions?
4. **Manifest conflict.**   This is overt conflict. At this time the conflict can be constructive or destructive. Examples of destructive behavior related to the conflict are (a) ignoring a policy, (b) denying a problem, (c) avoiding a staff member, or (d) discussing staff in public with negative terms. Examples of constructive responses to the conflict are (a) encouraging the group to identify and solve the problem, (b) expressing appropriate feelings, or (c) offering to help out a staff member (Figure 12-1 highlights the stages of conflict).

**FIGURE 12-1  Stages of conflict.**

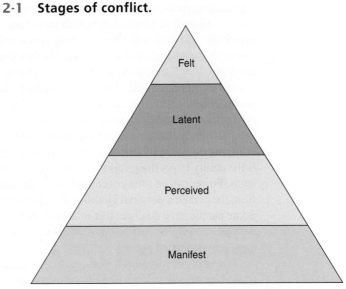

## Prevention of Conflict

Some conflict can be prevented so it is important to take preventive steps whenever possible to correct a problem before it develops into a conflict. A staff team or organization that says it has no conflicts is either not aware of conflict or prefers not to acknowledge it. Prevention of conflict should focus on the typical causes of conflict that have been identified in this chapter. Clear communication, known expectations, appropriate allocation of resources, and delineation of roles and responsibilities will go a long way toward preventing conflict. If the goal is to eliminate all conflict this will not be successful, because it cannot be done.

Since not all conflict can be prevented, staff and managers need to know how to manage conflict and resolve conflict when it exists. It is important to identify potential barriers that can make it more likely that a situation will turn into a conflict or will act as barriers to conflict resolution. First and foremost, if all staff makes an effort to decrease their tension or stress level, this will go a long way in preventing or resolving conflict. In addition to this strategy, it is important to improve communication, recognize team members as members with expertise, listen and compromise to get to the most effective decision given the available data, understand the roles and responsibilities of team/staff members, and be willing to evaluate practice and team functioning.

## Conflict Management: Issues and Strategies

Conflict management is critical in any organization. When conflicts arise then managers and staff need to understand conflict management issues and strategies. The major goals of conflict management are as follows:

1. To eliminate or decrease the conflict
2. To meet the needs of the patient, family/significant others, and the organization
3. To ensure that all parties feel positive about the resolution so that future work together can be productive

### POWERLESSNESS AND EMPOWERMENT

When staff experiences conflict, powerlessness and empowerment, as well as aggressiveness and passive-aggressiveness, become important.

1. **Power and powerlessness**

    When staff members feel that they are not recognized, appreciated, or paid attention to, then they feel **powerlessness**. What happens in a work environment when staff feels powerlessness? First, staff members do not feel that they can make an impact—they are unable to change situations that they feel need to be changed. Staff members will not be as creative in approaching problems. They may feel that they are responsible for tasks and yet have no control or power to affect change with these tasks. The team community will be affected negatively, and eventually the team may feel it cannot make change happen. Staff may make any of the following comments: "Don't bother trying to make a difference," "I can't make a difference here," and "Who listens to us?" Morale deteriorates as staff feels more and more powerless. New staff will soon pick up on the feeling of powerlessness. In some respects, the powerlessness really does diminish any effort for change. As was discussed in Chapter 3, responding to change effectively is very important today. In addition when staff feels powerless this greatly impacts the organizational culture.

**Power** is about influencing decisions, controlling resources, and affecting behavior. It is the ability to get things done—access resources and information, and use it to make decisions. Power can be used constructively or destructively. The power a person has originates from the person's personal qualities and characteristics, as well as the person's position. Some people have qualities that make others turn to them—people trust them, consider their advice helpful, and so on. A person's position, such as a team leader or nurse manager, has associated power.

Power is not stagnant. It changes as it is affected by the situation. There are a number of sources of power. Each one can be useful depending on the circumstances and the goal. An individual may have several sources of power; for example, a team leader may have legitimate power due to the position held, expert power due to team members' recognition of the team leader's expertise in care of oncology patients, and persuasive power because the team leader is able to convince team members the best steps to take to solve a problem. The common sources of power include the following.

- **Legitimate power.**   This power is what one typically thinks of in relation to power. It is power that comes from having a formal position in an organization such as a nurse manager, team leader, or vice president of patient services. These positions give the person who holds one of them the right to influence staff and expect staff to follow requests. Staff members recognize that they have tasks to accomplish and job requirements.
- **Reward power.**   A person's power comes from the ability to reward others when they comply. Examples of reward power include money (such as an increase in salary level), desired schedule or assignment, providing a space to work, or recognition of accomplishment.
- **Coercive power.**   This type of power is based on punishment when a person does not do as expected or directed. Examples of this type include denial of a pay raise, termination, and poor schedule or assignment. This type of power leads to an unpleasant work situation. Staff will not respond positively to coercive power, and this type of power has a strong negative effect on staff morale.
- **Referent power.**   This informal power comes from others recognizing that an individual has special qualities and is admired. This person then has influence over others because they want to follow the person due to the person's charisma. Staff feels valued and accepted.
- **Expert power.**   When a person has an expertise the person can have power over others who respect that expertise. When this type of power is present, the expert is able to provide sound advice and direction.
- **Informational power.**   This type of power arises from the ability to access and share information, which is critical in the Information Age.
- **Persuasive power.**   This type of power influences others by providing an effective point-of-view or argument (Finkelman & Kenner, 2010). (Box 12-4 highlights the types of power.)

It is important to note that a leader must have legitimate power. "A mugger on the street may have a gun and power to threaten your life, but not qualify as a leader, because leading means influencing people to work *willingly* toward achieving your objectives. That is not to say that a little fear can't be a good thing, at least occasionally" (Dessler, 2002, p. 212).

| BOX 12-4 | TYPES OF POWER |
|---|---|

| | |
|---|---|
| Legitimate | Expert |
| Reward | Informational |
| Coercive | Persuasive |
| Referent | |

This is a critical concept to understand about leadership and power. However, it takes more than power to be an effective leader and manager. "If you have the traits and you have the power, then you have the *potential* to be a leader" (Dessler, 2002, p. 212).

All organizations experience their own brand of "politics." Some staff and managers find themselves maneuvering to acquire power within the organization. This is directly influenced by the goals that people feel are important to them. These goals may come in conflict with the goals of others, and when this happens, holding greater power may make a difference in who "wins." Political power maneuvering can become unpleasant for staff and managers and can also damage the organization's culture. Trust may decrease, along with effective communication, coordination, collaboration, and resolution of conflicts. This is not to say that all political power in the organization is negative, but it is a slippery slope and needs to be carefully observed. Part of this process is the need to identify where the power is coming from and to learn how to access the power to meet goals (Marrelli, 2004). As has been said, power can be used negatively, and this can also lead to the unethical use of power or not doing the right thing with the power. Chapter 2 discusses examples of ethical issues. There is no doubt that there are managers who use their power to control staff, as well as staff who use power to control other staff, but this is not a healthy use of power. Rather, it is a misuse of power and does not demonstrate nursing leadership.

A self-appraisal of a person's personal view of power allows the individual to better understand how the person uses power and how it then affects the person's decisions and relationships. This can lead to more effective responses to change during planning and decision making, coping with conflict, and the ability to collaborate and coordinate.

2. **Empowerment**

**Empowerment** is often viewed as the sharing of power; however, it is more than this. "To empower is to enable to act" (Finkelman & Kenner, 2010, pp. 108). Power must be more than words, but rather it must be demonstrated. Participative decision making empowers staff, but only if staff really do have the opportunity to participate and influence decisions. Recognizing that one's participation is accepted makes a difference. True empowerment gives the staff the right to choose how to address issues with the manager.

Should all staff be empowered? A critical issue to answer this question is whether or not staff can handle decision making. This implies that staff members need leadership qualities and skills to make sound decisions and participate together collaboratively. They need to be able to use communication effectively. When staff members are selected, all these factors become important. Empowerment is not gained just by being a member of the staff, but rather staff members become empowered because they are able to handle it. Management that wants to empower staff must transfer power over to the staff, but management must first feel confident that staff can handle empowerment.

When staff is empowered some limits or boundaries need to be set or conflict may develop. Some of these boundaries are established by the organization's policies, procedures, and position descriptions, education and experience, and by laws and regulations (for example, nurse practice acts). The manager must be aware of these boundaries and establish any others that may be required (for example, direct involvement of staff in the selection process for new equipment). If staff members are involved in the decision making, then they should first be given a list of several possible equipment choices that meet the budgetary requirements from which to choose. It is critical that the manager make clear the boundaries, or staff members will feel like their efforts are useless if their suggestions are rejected because they were not given the boundaries. What does this mean? Roles and responsibilities need to be clearly described, and if they change, they need to be discussed. At the same time the nurse manager or the team leader must not control, domineer, or overpower staff. This type of response is usually seen in new nurse managers or team leaders who feel insecure. Ineffective use of empowerment can be just as problematic as a lack of empowerment.

Although empowering one's self may seem like an unusual concept, it is an important one. The amount of power a person has in a relationship is determined by the degree to which someone else needs what the other person has. Anger is related to expectations that are not met, and when these expectations are not met, the person may act out to gain power. It is the responsibility of the nursing profession to communicate what nurses have to offer to patient care and to the health care delivery system, but individual nurses also need to understand what they have to offer as nurses. To have an impact this communication and development must be ongoing. Empowerment can be positive if the strategies that are used to gain empowerment are constructive (for example, gaining new skills, speaking out constructively, networking, using political advocacy, increasing involvement in planning and decision making, getting more nurses on key organization committees, improving image through a positive image campaign, and developing and implementing assertiveness skill). There are many other strategies that can result in empowerment that improves the workplace and the nurse's self-perception.

AGGRESSIVE AND PASSIVE-AGGRESSIVE BEHAVIOR    Aggressive and passive-aggressive behavior can interfere with successful conflict resolution and might even be the cause of conflict. When staff members are hostile to one another, the team leader, or the nurse manager, anxiety rises. Hostile behavior can be a response to conflict. It is important to recognize personal feelings. The first response should be to get under control and communicate control to the hostile staff member. The nurse manager or team leader may be the one who is hostile, which makes it even more complex and requires assistance from higher level management. Hopefully, someone will recognize the need to bring the situation under control and try to move to a private place. Demonstrations of open conflict with hostility should not take place in patient or public areas. If the suggestion to move to a private area does not work and the situation continues to escalate, simply walking away may help set some boundaries. Cool down time is definitely needed.

There are many times when more information is really required before a response can be given. If this is the case, everyone concerned needs to be told that when information is gathered the issue or problem will then be discussed. No one should be pressured to respond with inadequate information as this will lead to ineffective decision making and may lead to further hostility. It is critical that after further assessment is completed that there be additional discussion and a conclusion. "Unless the behavior of a difficult person is physically threatening, try ignoring it. Deal only with the heart of the matter. Focus your attention on the issue and work at refocusing your 'opponent's' attention. Repeatedly use his or her name. State and restate the problem. Try to defuse emotion—yours first, because ultimately the only person you really control is yourself" (Forman, 2001, p. 13). These are methods that can help move a negative situation into a positive one.

When there are problems with patients and families, what is the best way to cope? Many of the same strategies mentioned earlier can be used. Safety is the first issue, as it must be maintained. It is never appropriate to allow patients or families to demonstrate anger inappropriately. When this occurs, someone needs to set reasonable limits that are based on an assessment of the situation. There may be many reasons for anger and inappropriate behavior, such as pain, medications, fear and anxiety, psychosis, dysfunctional communication, and so on. Staff needs to avoid taking things personally, as this will interfere with thoughtful problem solving. When one gets defensive or emotional, interventions taken to resolve a conflict may not be effective. Active listening is critical to cope with emotions. If a different culture is involved, then this factor needs to be considered (for example, some cultures consider it appropriate to be very emotional and others do not). In the long term, clear communication is critical during the entire process.

**HOW DO INDIVIDUAL STAFF MEMBERS COPE WITH CONFLICT?** Not everyone responds to conflict in the same way, and individuals may vary in how they respond dependent upon the circumstances. Four typical responses to conflict are avoidance, accommodation, competition, and collaboration (Boggs, 2003).

- Avoidance occurs when a person is very uncomfortable and cannot cope with the anxiety effectively. This person will withdraw from the situation to avoid it. There are times when this may be the most effective response, particularly when the situation may lead to negative results, but in many situations this will not be effective in the long term. This response might occur when a staff member is in conflict with a manager and disagrees with the manager. The staff member must consider whether it is worth it to disagree publicly. Typically, avoidance occurs when one side is perceived as more powerful than the other. It is a helpful approach when more information is needed, or when the issue is not worth what might be lost.

- A second response is accommodation. How does this occur? The person tries to make the situation better by cooperating. The critical issue may not be resolved, or not be resolved to the fullest satisfaction. The goal is just to eliminate the conflict as quickly as possible. Accommodation works best when one person or team is less interested in the issue than the other. It can be advantageous as it does develop harmony, and it can provide power in future conflict since one party was more willing to let the conflict deflate. Later interaction may require that the other party cooperate.

- A third response is competition. How does this work? Power is used to stop the conflict. A manager might say, "This is the way it will be." This closes further efforts from others who may be in conflict with the manager.

- Collaboration is the fourth response, which has been discussed in this chapter. This is a positive approach, with all parties attempting to reach an acceptable solution, and in the end both sides feel that they won something. Collaboration often involves some compromise, which is a method used to respond to conflict.

Using the best conflict resolution style can make a difference in success. There are many ways that a conflict can be resolved. When conflict occurs each person involved has a personal perspective of the issue and conflict. Today there is more conflict in the health care delivery environment with increased workplace stress that may lead to misunderstandings, ineffective communication, and reduced productivity and dysfunctional organizations as noted in the Institute of Medicine reports (2001; 2004).

**GENDER ISSUES** Are there differences in the way that women and men negotiate? There are differences in how women and men approach leadership issues such as conflict (Caliper, 2004). Men tend to negotiate to win while women focus more on what is fair. It is believed that this is related to the way children play through sports and activities. Women will make an effort to reach win-win solutions. Men will test the limits that have been set more overtly than women, so it is important for women to ensure that limits are set and maintained. It is important, despite the differences described, to avoid stereotyping. (See Chapter 8 for additional gender differences.)

**NURSE–PHYSICIAN RELATIONSHIPS** Though the nurse–physician relationship should be the strongest relationship that nurses have in order to meet the needs of the patient, it frequently is not. Both sides of the relationship play a role in the inadequacies of this relationship. Conflict does occur, and this conflict can act as a barrier to effective patient care. Literature about Magnet hospitals distinguishes between collegial and collaborative relationships and between nurses and physicians (Kramer & Schmalenberg, 2002). Collegial relationships are those where there is equality of power. This power is different but equal power and knowledge. In contrast, collaborative relationships between nurses and physicians focus on mutual power, but the physician's power is greater. The nurse's power is based on the nurse's extended time with patients, experience, and knowledge. In addition to power, this relationship requires respect and trust between the nurse and physician. Due to these factors, it is a complex relationship.

Nurses have long worked on teams, mostly with other nursing staff. However, the nurse–physician relationships have become more important in the changing health care environment with the greater emphasis on interprofessional teams. Nurse–physician interactions and communication have been discussed for a long time in health care literature.

A study that explored the impact of nurse–physician relationships on nurse satisfaction and retention, conducted by a physician, was reported in 2002 (Rosenstein, 2002). The results of the 1,200 nurses, physicians, and hospital executive survey "suggest that daily interactions between nurses and physicians strongly influence nurses' morale (Rosenstein, 2002, p. 26). Overall, 96% of the nurses had witnessed or experienced disruptive physician behavior, including yelling or raising the voice, disrespect, condescension, berating colleagues, berating patients, and use of abusive language. The survey found 344 nurses who knew of other nurses who had left the hospital due to disruptive behavior. These nurses did not feel that the administration supported the resolution of conflict between nurses and physicians. This study recommended the following improvement strategies, which could apply to most health care organizations, which continue to be important strategies to improve the nurse–physician relationship.

- Create more opportunities for collaboration and communication through open forums, group discussions, and collaborative relationships.
- Increase availability of training and educational programs for nurses and physicians that focus on improving teamwork and working relationships (for example, sensitivity training, assertiveness training, conflict management, time management, and phone etiquette, with emphasis on courtesy, respect, promptness, and preparation).
- Improve organizational processes by requiring administrators to take a more proactive approach to avoiding potential confrontations related to staffing, scheduling, and equipment.
- Establish a zero-tolerance policy for disruptive behavior, holding nurses and physicians more accountable for their actions.
- Disseminate code-of-conduct policies and reporting guidelines to both nurses and physicians, and apply policies consistently and quickly, providing feedback to all involved.
- Ensure appropriate nurse competencies.
- Have physicians sign a code-of-conduct policy when they are credentialed or re-credentialed.
- Appoint a physician leader who will take charge of training and education programs.
- Provide an ongoing forum to increase physician awareness of the issues addressed in this survey and raise awareness of other factors that increase nurses' stress levels.
- Place physicians on nurse recruitment teams, enabling them to gain a better understanding and appreciation of the factors that are important to nurses as they consider employment opportunities.
- Provide a case study or conduct role-play exercises that allow physicians a firsthand understanding of nurses' responsibilities and work flow (Rosenstein, 2002, pp. 32–33).

Other studies have examined work relationships and patient outcomes. Rosenstein and O'Daniel (2005) surveyed 1,500 nurses and physicians about the impact of disruptive behavior on job satisfaction and retention. Disruptive behavior included verbal abuse. In this study nurses were perceived as being disruptive as much as physicians. Nurses and physicians surveyed felt that disruptive behavior had a negative impact on stress levels, relationships, communication, collaboration, and transfer of information leading to problems with quality of care and patient satisfaction. Lower (2007) uses the following descriptors for disruptive behavior: verbal abuse, negative behavior, and physical abuse (e.g., profanity, innuendo, demeaning comments), reprimanding or insulting another in public, threatening, telling racial or ethnic jokes, undermining team cohesion, scapegoating, silence (not speaking to a team member), assaulting another, throwing objects, and outbursts of rage. In a study of 20 medical and surgical residents nurse–physician relationships were reviewed from the perspective of relational coordination (Weinberg, Miner, & Rivlin, 2009), which is a theory that views high-quality relationships and communication among participants in the work process as important for effective outcomes (Gittell, 2001). The results of this qualitative study are disturbing though the study was small and had other limitations. Positive relationships depended on whether the resident viewed the nurse as cooperative and competent. Most communication was motivated by the need to tell the nurses something, not necessarily looking for professional feedback from the nurse. The physicians had limited knowledge of the various nursing degrees or which nurses had which degrees and also did not differentiate from RNs, LPNs, or unlicensed assistive personnel. Physicians, however, are not the only health care providers that nurses must work with while they provide care (for example, nurses work with other nursing staff, social workers, support staff, laboratory technicians, physical therapists, pharmacists, and many others). There are also other members joining the health care team such as alternative therapists (massage therapists, herbal therapists, acupuncturists, etc.), case managers, more actively involved insurers, and so forth. The future will probably bring other new members into the health care delivery system. Nurses need to develop the skills necessary to participate effectively on the team, which requires collaboration, communication, coordination, delegation, and negotiation. Communication and delegation are discussed in other chapters. It is difficult to practice today in any health care setting without experiencing interprofessional interactions such as nurse–physician. As teams work together, effective teams

- Work together (collaborate).
- Recognize strengths and limitations.
- Respect individual responsibilities.
- Maintain open communication.

## CASE STUDY

### A Verbal Explosion Leads to Confrontation of a Problem

As a nurse manager in a busy OR you have to ensure that all staff is collaborating and communicating well. In the last six months you have noticed more problems with poor communication between nurses and physicians, some of which have impacted the quality of care. Nurses are also frequently complaining that they are "second-class citizens" in the department. The number of last minute call-ins has increased by 25% over the last 6 months causing last minute staffing problems. Today was the last straw when a nurse and a surgical resident had a shouting match in the hallway. The nurse left the encounter crying, and the resident said he would not work with the nurse anymore. The nurse manager went into the OR medical director's office. They have had a positive collaborative relationship over several years. She went in and said, "We have a problem!" As she described the problems, he said, "I was unaware there was so much tension and lack of collaboration. Why didn't you tell me this earlier?"

### Questions:

1. How would you respond to the medical director's question?
2. What do you and the medical director need to do?
3. How can you avoid this being a "we–they" situation?
4. How will you involve all staff?
5. What can you do about the powerlessness the nurses feel?

Positive professional communication is critical. Both sides should initiate positive dialogue rather than adversarial positions. Cooperation and collaboration are also integral to the success of this relationship. A frequent question discussed in the literature is "Why is there conflict between nurses and physicians?" The structure of work is different for physicians and for nurses, and this has an impact on understanding, communicating, collaborating, and coordinating. This perspective identifies the key elements as sense of time, sense of resources, unit of analysis, sense of mastery, and type of rewards as described by the following.

- The nurse is focused on shorter periods of time, and time is usually short, with frequent interruptions. The physician's sense of time focuses on the course of illness.
- If a physician gives a stat order, the physician has problems understanding what might interfere with the nurse making this a priority. There is a lack of understanding of the nurse's work structure.
- Physicians often are not concerned with resources, though this is certainly changing as physicians do recognize that there is a shortage of staff as well as issues about costs and reimbursement for care. They, however, may not be willing to accept these factors as relevant when their patients need something. There are, of course, other resources such as equipment availability, supplies, and funds that can cause problems and conflicts. Nurses are typically more aware of the effect that these factors have on daily care.
- Unit of analysis is another factor; for example, nurses are caring for groups of patients even though care is supposed to be individualized. Physicians may not have an understanding of this if they have only a few patients in the hospital.
- Physicians also do not have an understanding of nursing delivery models, and often nurses themselves are not clear about them. This affects nurses' ability to explain how they work.
- The sense of reward is different. Nurses work in a task-oriented environment and typically get paid an hourly rate. Most physicians are not salaried and are independent practitioners though some are employees of the organization (hospital, clinic, and so on).

Conflict and verbal abuse are related. Verbal abuse occurs in health care settings between patients and staff, nurses and other nurses, physicians and nurses, and all other staff relationships. This abuse can consist of statements made directly to a staff member or about a staff member to others. A common complaint from nurses regards verbal abuse from physicians. "Some nurses, particularly new ones, allow physicians to verbally abuse them because they are insecure about their knowledge base" (Parks, 2001, p. 20MW). Verbal abuse affects turnover rates and contributes to the nursing shortage so it is has serious consequences. "Poor physician–nurse interaction also compromises patient care" (Stringer, 2001, p. 7).

How can this problem be improved? A critical step is to gain better understanding of each profession's viewpoint and demonstrate less automatic acceptance of inappropriate behavior. This requires that management become proactive in eliminating negative communication and behavior. Some hospitals have tried a number of strategies to deal with verbal abuse. Some of these are (a) encouraging staff to report abuse by allowing anonymity, (b) using physician–nurse counseling teams to act as liaisons with employees, (c) encouraging staff to speak firmly and address abuse, and (d) introducing staff to new physicians and encouraging them to come for assistance (Stringer, 2001). The IOM recommends increased interprofessional approaches to care delivery and the need for increased interprofessional health professions education so that all health professions are prepared to work together on teams (2003). What can nurses do about this? One suggestion is to improve their own knowledge base and thus develop more self-confidence. "Remind yourself that you have many valuable skills, and you don't deserve to be verbally abused. These efforts will help decrease the feelings of intimidation" (Parks, 2001, p. 20MW). Another problem is that nurses think they must resolve all problems and "make things" work correctly when this may not be realistic. The nurses then become scapegoats. Verbal abuse, no matter who is doing it, physician or nurse, should not be tolerated. Those involved need to be approached in private to identify the need for a change in behavior. Staff needs to be respected. The AONE *Guiding Principles for Excellence in Nurse-Physician Relationships* is found in Box 12-5.

| BOX 12-5 | AONE GUIDING PRINCIPLES FOR EXCELLENCE IN NURSE–PHYSICIAN RELATIONSHIPS |
|---|---|

## INTRODUCTION TO THE GUIDING PRINCIPLES

Excellent working relationships between nurses and physicians are key to creating a productive, safe, and satisfying practice environment. The patient and the patient's family benefit from care delivered by a team practicing within this environment.

Senior leadership in health care organizations must support the development of excellent relationships and, more importantly, create an environment that sustains and nurtures these critical relationships.

## GUIDING PRINCIPLES FOR EXCELLENCE IN NURSE–PHYSICIAN RELATIONSHIPS

*Institutions that are committed to establishing and maintaining environments that promote excellence in the nurse–physician relationship adhere to the following principles.*

1. Interprofessional collaborative relationships are promoted, nurtured, and sustained.
2. This requires that practitioners be proficient in communication skills, leadership skills, problem solving, conflict management, utilizing their emotional intelligence, and functioning within a team culture.
3. Excellence in relationship building begins with hiring, continues with learning and developing together, and is reinforced over time.
4. The organization has specific systems for reward, recognition, and celebration.
5. The organization supports the "Platinum Rule" with a specific Professional Code of Conduct that includes a system to support it. A "No Tolerance" standard exists for those unable to adhere to the Code.
6. The organization creates and supports a "Just & Fair" environment.
7. The work of all professional caregivers is seen as interdependent and collegial.
8. Cross-discipline job discovery is supported and encouraged.
9. Patient-focused care and better patient outcomes are the organizing force behind creating a collaborative environment.

## IMPLEMENTATION GUIDELINES

*Interprofessional collaborative relationships are promoted, nurtured, and sustained.*

1. Nurses and physicians are given formal training in communication skills, leadership development, problem solving, conflict management, development of emotional intelligence, and team functions. Education and training is provided to nurse–physician teams and is not discipline specific.
2. Specific education is provided in team building.
3. Organization-governing bodies and committees have representative members from all disciplines.
4. Nurse–physician leadership teams are identified to lead the work at the unit level (Microsystem Management).
5. All organizational task forces include representatives from those stakeholders closest to the issue.
6. Interprofessional collaborative relationships are assessed, unit-by-unit. Each unit has a development and improvement plan for continued growth of the relationship.
7. Teams develop common values for their interprofessional collaboration.
8. Teams develop common language for their interprofessional collaboration.
9. Nurse–physician collaborative champions are identified at the hospital and unit level.

*Excellence in relationship building begins with hiring, continues with learning and developing together, and is reinforced over time together and is reinforced over time.*

1. Nurses and physicians work collaboratively to identify the behaviors that they want in team members.
2. Employees, both nurse and physician, are hired using behavioral interviewing to ascertain a good fit with the organization, teams, values, culture, and behavioral expectations.
3. Nurses and physicians do 360-degree performance reviews.
4. Credentialing criteria includes behavioral attributes and expectations, as well as clinical skills.
5. The Graduate Medical Education competencies are used as hiring criteria and for performance review.
6. Education and team training is done in work teams, as described in the Institute of Medicine reports.
7. Personal accountability for demonstrating team behaviors is rewarded.

*The organization has specific systems for reward, recognition, and celebration.*

1. There is alignment of purpose among the disciplines regarding reward, recognition, and celebration.

*(continued)*

| BOX 12-5 | AONE GUIDING PRINCIPLES FOR EXCELLENCE IN NURSE–PHYSICIAN RELATIONSHIPS (CONTINUED) |
|---|---|

2. Mechanisms for reward and recognition are easy to access.

3. Performance appraisal is linked to patient satisfaction measurements.

4. Awards, recognition, and celebration are public and visible and across disciplines and teams. Example: Physicians identify the Nurse of the Year; Nurses identify the Physician of the Year.

5. Rewards and Recognition programs promote team accomplishments.

*The organization supports the "Platinum Rule" with a specific Professional Code of Conduct that includes a system to support it. A "No Tolerance" standard exists for those unable to adhere to the Code.*

1. The Golden Rule states: "Do unto others as you would have them do unto you." The Platinum Rule states: "Do unto others as they would have you do for/unto them." Thus, this principle speaks to treating others as they want to be treated, not necessarily how you would want to be treated.

2. Code of Conduct Guidelines/Policies exists for all professionals that outline behavioral expectations.

3. Work improvement plans and measures hold the team accountable, not just individual.

4. Individual professional codes of ethics/conduct are known and honored.

5. Contacts and processes/procedures for the impaired professional are easily accessible to all staff.

6. There are identified coaches and mentors for the professionals on site in the hospital to help with performance issues.

7. All professionals receive team training that focuses on communication skills and processes.

8. Processes exist to identify and address conflict situations before they become a crisis and/or deteriorate.

*The organization creates and supports a "Just & Fair" environment.*

1. There is a systems approach to management and decision making.

2. Internal trends and reporting processes are multidisciplinary.

3. Language for reporting and safety is analyzed to assure that it is "Just & Fair."

4. Processes exist for multidisciplinary critical incident debriefing.

5. Decision-making tools are used that support the "Just & Fair" processes, such as the "Just Model."

6. The processes outlined in the patient-safety literature that creates cultures of safety are used as blue prints for culture changes.

7. Remedial training is offered when needed.

*The work of all professional caregivers is seen as interdependent and collegial.*

1. The culture of team includes all disciplines providing care on a unit.

2. Behavioral expectations are defined for all disciplines.

*Cross-discipline job discovery is supported and encouraged.*

1. All disciplines are educated in the role/responsibility of their colleagues.

2. Opportunities for shadowing different professions are encouraged.

*Patient-focused care and better patient outcomes are the organizing force behind creating a collaborative environment.*

1. Work is directed toward identifying and measuring those outcomes that are sensitive to the function of collaboration.

2. Patients and families are appointed to internal committees.

3. Patient-centeredness is a key focus for processes.

Source: American Organization of Nurse Executives. *Guiding principles for excellence in nurse-physician relationships.* Chicago, IL: Author. Reprinted with permission.

## Application of Negotiation to Conflict Resolution

**Negotiation** is the critical element in making conflict a nightmare or an opportunity. Negotiation can be used to resolve a conflict, and some types of negotiation, such as mediation, can be very structured. When two or more people or organizations disagree or have opposing views about a problem or solution, a conflict exists. To resolve the conflict, the involved people need to discuss resolution in a manner that is acceptable to all of those involved. Although it does not have to take long, in some cases it may be very long, such as what might occur in a union–employer negotiation for a contract. Conflict resolution includes the use of a variety of skills and strategies. Key skills and strategies are communication, listening, and respecting different points-of-view. Four needs are clarification, performance, questioning, and expectations (Marrelli, 2004). As the process begins it is important to *clarify* all of the issues and parties who are involved in the conflict. *Performance* or potential outcomes should be established early in the process. *Questioning* is important throughout resolution. For example, it is important to ask about behaviors that started the conflict and how to avoid them in the future. Management needs to be clear about *expectations* and provide these in writing, which helps to decrease conflict over critical issues.

What strategies might be used to resolve specific conflicts?

- Help involved parties settle their differences themselves whenever possible rather than stepping in and taking over.
- Maintain an objective approach.
- Communicate trust to the staff members and communicate that it is believed that they can resolve problems.
- Avoid criticizing or denying feelings.
- Use a problem-solving approach.
- Provide privacy for sensitive discussions.
- Identify staff members who chronically complain and work with them to adapt their behavior as this behavior can increase the risk of conflict and interfere with resolving it when it does occur.
- Listen with understanding rather than judgment. This is important throughout the resolution process and can also assist with prevention of conflict.
- Provide opportunities for all staff members to improve their problem-solving and communication skills (Marrell, 2004).

Since conflict is inevitable, all staff nurses will encounter it. Knowing how to manage conflict will be of great benefit to the individual nurse as well as improve the working environment and ability to better reach patient outcomes.

Why is negotiation identified as a critical skill for nurses in the health care environment? Patients should not become part of staff or organizational conflicts, and there is risk that this may occur. These conflicts need to be resolved or patient care may suffer negative consequences. Consider these examples:

- The interprofessional team cannot agree on a treatment approach and must do this by the end of the team meeting.
- A patient's insurer refuses to allow the patient to stay two more days in the hospital. As the hospital's nurse case manager you must work with the insurer representative to reach a compromise.
- Staffing in a hospital is being reduced, and the nurses are convinced that the new staffing level will be unsafe for patients. Something must be done to resolve this issue.
- A home health care agency has learned that the Medicare contract has decided that specific patients will receive fewer visits.

How can these examples be resolved satisfactorily so that the quality of care does not suffer? Finding a mentor to discuss the process as well as vent feelings may be very helpful. Developing negotiation skills makes conflicts easier to handle and less stressful. Nurses who become involved in unions will find that negotiation skills are also very important. If negotiation is not used effectively, all of these conflict examples can lead to major problems for the patient and/or staff.

When approaching conflict resolution, it is important to recognize that both sides contributed to the conflict. One side cannot have a conflict by itself; it takes at least two. Consider how each side has contributed to the conflict. Another critical issue is to carefully consider if this is the time and place to address the conflict. When the environment is too emotional, conflict resolution will be difficult. Stepping back or taking a break may be the best position to take. The following are strategies that can be used to effectively negotiate.

- Negotiate for agreements—not winning or losing. Clearly state that your desire is to find a solution and to work together.
- Separate people from positions.
- Establish mutual trust and respect.
- Avoid one-sided or personal gains.
- Allow time for expressing the interests of each side/party.
- Listen actively during the process, and acknowledge what is being said; avoid defending or explaining yourself.
- Use data/evidence to strengthen your position.
- Focus on patient care interests.
- Always remember that the process is a problem-solving one, and the benefit is for the patient and family.
- Clearly identify the priority and arrive at common goal(s).
- Avoid using pressure.
- Identify and understand the real reasons underlying the problem.
- Be knowledgeable about organizational policies, procedures, systems, standards, and the law, applying this knowledge as needed.
- Try to understand the other side, and ask questions and seek clarification when unsure or uncertain; understanding the other side first before explaining yours increases effectiveness.
- Avoid emotional outbursts and overreacting if the other party exhibits such behavior; depersonalize the conflict.
- Avoid premature judgments, blame, and inflammatory comments.
- Be concrete and flexible when presenting your position.
- Be reasonable and fair (Gebelein et al., 2000).

MEDIATION    There are some conflicts that will require a third-party negotiator to reach a more effective resolution. This is needed when there is no opportunity for cooperative problem solving and objectivity is required. "**Mediation** is a form of dispute resolution that has been used in many cultures throughout history. . . . Mediation is a problem-solving process in which a neutral third party (who has no stake in the outcome of the process) helps people who have a disagreement or dispute reach a mutually satisfactory resolution." (Gebelein, p. 56, 2000). Mediators are facilitators, not decision makers (as in the case of arbitrators). In mediation, the people with the dispute have an opportunity to tell their story and to be understood, as well as to listen to and understand the story of the other party. A key factor in mediation is the need for all parties to willingly participate in the process. The mediator guides the process and discussion. Certain guidelines are established for the discussion that all parties must follow throughout the process (for example, allowing each party time to speak and complete a statement without interruption, calling for a break when needed, enforcing time limited meetings, substantiating comments with facts, and so on). With these guidelines and the presence of a mediator, this type of negotiation can result in positive outcomes. It provides protection for both sides.

# APPLYING LEADERSHIP AND MANAGEMENT

## MY HOSPITAL UNIT

When you arrive at work today you are confronted with staff members that are upset that work is not being done effectively, particularly with other departments. Successful coordination requires identification of barriers and strategies to resolve barriers to coordination. Coordination also requires collaboration. Identify the barriers to effective coordination and collaboration. Clearly describe them. Then consider what strategies could be used to prevent the barriers or to decrease the barriers on your unit. Your strategies need to be applicable to your unit as you have designed it. Use the virtual unit site found on the textbook website to record the work that you do as the role of nurse manager for your unit.

## Critical Thinking Questions and Activities

1. What do nurses in practice think? Select one of the following issues to discuss with RNs. Students should not all choose the same questions so that when data are discussed there will be different issues described. (1) Is collaboration with other health care professionals part of your practice? If so, describe some examples. If not, why do you think collaboration does not exist? (2) How is coordination used in your practice? (3) How might you and others where you work improve coordination? (4) Describe your worst experience with conflict at work and how it was resolved or not resolved. (5) What were the long-term consequences of conflict? (6) Do you feel empowered at work? Why or why not? How do you think the situation could be improved?

2. The examples of strategies to improve nurse–physician relationships are broad. What do you think about them? Divide into teams and have each team take one of the strategies. Discuss the advantages and disadvantages of the strategy. How would you respond to the strategy? Have you experienced or observed any abusive behavior among staff or with you? Do you think one of these strategies might prevent this type of behavior? Each team should explore the strategy. How would it work? Would it be offensive to staff (nurses or physicians)? It is important to look at both sides, nurses' and physicians'.

3. Conflict is complex and yet there are guidelines for understanding it. Select an example of a conflict, which can be one you experienced or observed. Describe the conflict, identify the type of conflict, and explain your rationale for selecting the type. Apply the four stages of conflict described in the chapter to your example. What resulted from the conflict?

4. Visit the website http://www.mapnp.org/library/grp_skll/grp_dec/grp_dec.htm and read about decision making and teams. How might you use this information?

5. Visit the website http://www.livestrong.com/article/14683-handling-conflict/ and learn more about handling conflicts. How might you use this information?

6. Visit the website http://www.cnr.berkeley.edu/ucce50/ag-labor/7labor/13.htm and explore conflict management skills. How might you use this information?

## Media Links

- **URL: http://www.nursingworld.org/MainMenuCategories/ANAMarketplace/ANAPeriodicals/OJIN/TableofContents/Volume102005/No1Jan05/tpc26_416011.aspx**
  Nurse–physician collaboration
- **URL: http://www.accel-team.com/**
  Team Building: Tools for building strong teams, plus useful links and articles
- **URL: http://www.au.af.mil/au/awc/awcgate/ndu/strat-ldr-dm/pt3ch10.html**
  Strategic Leadership and Decision Making: Read about how to create and manage teams
- **URL: http://www.ihi.org**
  Institute for Health Improvement: Teams

- **URL: http://teamstepps.ahrq.gov/**
  Agency for Healthcare Research and Quality: TeamSTEPPS
- **URL: http://www.mindtools.com/pages/article/newLDR_81.htm**
  MindTools: Conflict Resolution
- **URL: http://www.mindtools.com/pages/article/newTMM_53.htm**
  MindTools: How to Be a Good Team Player
- **URL: http://www.ihi.org/IHI/Topics/PatientSafety/SafetyGeneral/Tools/CommunicationCollaborativeSurveyPhysicianAttitudes.htm**
  Institute for Health Improvement Communication/Collaboration Survey

**Pearson Nursing Student Resources**

Find additional review materials at
**nursing.pearsonhighered.com**

Prepare for success with additional NCLEX®-style practice questions, interactive assignments and activities, Web links, animations and videos, and more!

# References

American Nurses Association. (ANA). (2003). *Nursing's social policy statement.* (2nd ed.). Silver Springs, MD: Author.

American Nurses Association. (ANA). (2004). *Nursing: scope and standards of practice.* Silver Springs, MD: Author.

American Nurses Association. (ANA). (2009). *Nursing administration scope and standards of practice.* Silver Springs, MD: Author.

American Association of Critical-Care Nurses. (2005). *AACN standards for establishing and sustaining healthy work environments.* Aliso Viejo, CA: Author.

Boggs, K. (2003). Resolving conflict between nurse and client. In E. Arnold & K. Boggs (Eds.), *Interpersonal relationships: Professional communication skills for nurses* (4th ed., pp. 368–388). Philadelphia: W.B. Saunders Company.

Caliper. (2005). *The qualities that distinguish women leaders.* Princeton, NJ: Author.

Clement, J. (2001). The leadership imperative: Managing conflict and resolving disputes creatively. *Seminars for Nurse Managers, 9*(4), 211–217.

Cody, W. (2001). Interdisciplinarity and nursing: "Everything is everything," or is it? *Nursing Science Quarterly, 14*(4), 274–280.

Dechairo-Marino, A., Jordan-Marsh, M., Traiger, G., & Saulo, M. (2001). Nurse/physician collaboration. *Journal of Nursing Administration, 31*(5), 223–232.

Dessler, G. (2002). *Management: Leading people and organizations in the 21st century.* Upper Saddle River, NJ: Prentice Hall.

Disch, J. (2001). Strengthening nursing and interdisciplinary collaboration. *Journal of Professional Nursing, 17*(6), 275.

Finkelman, A. & Kenner, C. (2010). *Professional nursing concepts. Competencies for quality leadership.* Boston: Jones and Bartlett Publishers.

Forman, H. (2001). Difficult people? What's the problem? *Nursing Spectrum Metro Edition,* August, 12–13.

Gebelein, S., et al. (2000). *Successful manager's handbook.* Minneapolis, MN: Personnel Decisions International Corporation.

Gittell, J. (2001). Supervisory span, relational coordination, and flight departure performance: A reassessment of postbureaucracy theory. *Organizational Science, 12*(4), 468–483.

Hansten, R. & Jackson, M. (2008). Know how to resolve conflict: Getting coworkers to work together as a team. In R. Hansten & M. Jackson (Eds.) *Clinical delegation skills* (pp. 255–284). Boston: Jones and Bartlett Publishers.

Institute of Medicine. (2001). *Crossing the quality chasm.* Washington, DC: National Academies Press.

Institute of Medicine. (2003a). *Priority areas for national action.* Washington, DC: National Academies Press.

Institute of Medicine. (2003b). *Health professions education.* Washington, DC: National Academies Press.

Institute of Medicine. (2004). *Keeping patients safe: Transforming the work environment of nurses.* Washington, DC: National Academies Press.

Kramer, M., & Schmalenberg, C. (2002). Staff nurses identify essentials of magnetism. In M. McClure & A. Hinshaw (Eds.), *Magnet hospitals revisited. Attraction and retention of professional nurses* (pp. 25–59). Washington, DC: American Nurses Publishing, Inc.

Marquis, B. & Huston, C. (2009). *Leadership roles and management functions in nursing.* Philadelphia: Lippincott Williams & Wilkins.

Lower, J. (September 2007). Creating a culture of civility in the workplace. *American Nurse Today, 2*(9), 49–52.

Marrelli, T. (2004). *The nurse manager's survival guide.* St. Louis, MO: Mosby-Year Book, Inc.

Parks, S. (2001, August). Silence verbal abuse. *Nursing Spectrum Metro Edition,* 20MW–21MW.

Puetz, B., & Shinn, L. (2002). Strategic partnerships. *Journal of Nursing Administration, 32*(4), 182–184.

Rosenstein, A. (2002). Nurse–physician relationships: Impact on nurse satisfaction and retention. *American Journal of Nursing, 102*(6), 26–34.

Rosenstein, A. H., & O'Daniel, M. (2005). Disruptive behavior and clinical outcomes: Perceptions of nurses and physicians. *American Journal of Nursing,* 105, 1, 54–64.

Salmon, M. (2007). Guest editorial: Care quality and safety: Same old. *Nursing Outlook, 55*(3), 117–119.

Stringer, H. (2001). Raging bullies. *Nursing Week, 1*(2), 6–7.

Tahan, J. (2001). A story from the bedside: The primary nurse as an integral health care team member. *Seminars for Nurse Managers, 9*(2), 68–72.

Weaver, D. (2001). Transdisciplinary teams: Very important leadership stuff. *Seminars for Nurse Managers, 9*(2), 79–84.

Weinburg, D., Miner, D., & Rivlin, L. (2009). 'It Depends': Medical residents' perspectives on working with nurses. *AJN, 109*(7), 34–43.

Wyatt, D. (2000). Negotiation savvy: Level the playing field by understanding sex differences. *Dimensions of Critical Care Nursing, 19*(1), 43–45.

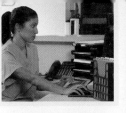

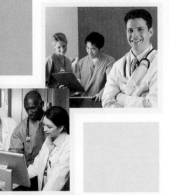

# 13

# Effective Staff Communication and Working Relationships

## CHAPTER OUTLINE

## LEARNING OUTCOMES

Before you begin, take a moment to familiarize yourself with the learning outcomes for this chapter.

- Describe the critical elements of communication.
- Distinguish between the four lines of communication.
- Describe the communication process.
- Assess a team's communication.
- Examine barriers to communication and how to resolve them.
- Compare the four communication methods, including the most effective use of the method.
- Apply two strategies for resolving communication problems.
- Assess your own communication style.

## KEY TERMS

- Active listening
- Communication
- Communication process
- Complementary relationship
- Context
- Decoding
- Diagonal communication

- Downward communication
- Encoding
- Feedback
- Lateral (horizontal) communication
- Medium
- Message

- Metacommunication
- Selective listening
- Sender
- Storytelling
- Symmetrical relationship
- Upward communication
- Videoconferencing

## WHAT'S AHEAD

Communication is part of everything that is done within the health care system. It can appear as staff-to-staff communication and patient-to-staff communication. Communication includes verbal, nonverbal, written, and electronic communication. The major goal of staff communication is the effective exchange of information that assists staff in meeting outcomes. The survival of each organization is dependent upon the transfer of information and actions taken based on information or communication; therefore, this process serves to integrate the organization's activities. Critical to effective communication is respect for another's values, feelings, opinions, and trust. Typically, when a team or teams work together one of the first signs that productivity is down will be an increase in communication problems. Decreasing communication has a direct negative effect on decision making, collaboration, coordination, and prevention of conflict. Communication is expensive as it consumes staff time and affects the organization and patient outcomes. When outcomes are not met, this affects costs. New information technology, such as computer hardware, software, information specialists, maintenance, repair and upgrade of hardware and software, and staff training in use of information technology (IT), is very costly. This chapter discusses many of these issues concerning communication, and how communication affects the work environment and outcomes. It is discussed more fully in Chapter 18.

## Communication: What Is It?

Communication, a key to successful teamwork, is a complex process that should never be ignored. Nurses need this skill daily in their work as they communicate with patients, families, co-workers, physicians and other health care providers, administrators and managers, support staff, case managers, utilization management staff, community agencies, and so on. The American Nurses Association (ANA) nursing standards include communication as an important part of nursing practice (2004), and the ANA nursing administration standards integrate the need for effective communication (2009). Although communication cannot be avoided, nurses can provide inadequate or ineffective communication. The Joint Commission stated that "ineffective communication is the most cited category of root causes of sentinel events" (2007, p. 2).

**Communication** is a two-way process that is used to convey a message or an idea between two or more people. This process is used to share thoughts, attitudes, information, and feelings. Effective care, which should be the goal, requires a focused exchange of ideas, feelings, and attitudes. Communication is best described as a complementary process with sender and receiver roles and, as such, is a process that happens between people and within people. Organizations must exert considerable effort in ensuring that effective communication occurs within the organization, with other external organizations, and with people who are important to the organization. Key issues are (a) who says what, (b) to whom, (c) in what way, (d) when, and (e) with what effect. Even after focusing on these key issues it is still important to remember that "Interpretation plays a major role; Sometimes interpretation confuses or changes the original message" (Finkelman & Kenner, 2010, p. 343).

Nurses need to understand the **communication process** and use it to benefit patient care and the work that needs to be done to reach identified outcomes. With the greater interest on patient-centered care much of communication needs to be focused on the patient. The Institute of Medicine includes information about communication in its discussion about the core competency to provide patient-centered care: "Communicate with patients in a shared and fully open manner. Allow patients to have unfettered access to the information contained in their medical records. Communicate accurately in a language that patients can understand. Offer patients' preferred communication channels (e.g., face-to-face, e-mail, other Web-based communication technologies). Explore a patient's main reason for a visit, associated concerns, and need for information" (Institute of Medicine, 2003a, pp. 52–53). As staff members communicate, they become involved in discussions and in dialogue mostly about patients but also about the work effort related to patient care. There is also personal conversation that takes place among co-workers. This personal conversation is very important in building teamwork—members feel more connected to one another. Effective communication broadens an individual's and a team's view of issues and how best to work with one another. The result should be better outcomes for patients and the organization.

## Communication Systems and Lines of Communication

Typically, communication is thought of as taking place in a straight line, from the sender to receiver; however, in most situations communication is much more complex. Its direction can be downward, upward, lateral, or diagonal. "Downward communications go from superior to subordinate, and consist of messages regarding things like corporate vision, what a job entails, procedures and practices to be followed, and performance appraisals. Lateral, or horizontal, communications go between departments or between people in the same department. Upward communication (from subordinates to superiors) provides management with insights into the company and its employees and competitors" (Dessler, 2002, p. 260). What do these descriptors really mean to nurses?

DOWNWARD COMMUNICATION    Communication is downward when a team leader tells a team member that a specific task must be done. Lines of communication typically relate to the organizational structure. The organizational chart provides the best illustration of these lines of communication. Top level staff communicates to staff in lower levels and so on. **Downward communication** is the most typical communication flow and is found in the traditional bureaucratic organization, although it is used in many types of structures at some time or another. In line with this type of organization, this communication is directive and used primarily to coordinate activities to ensure that outcomes are reached. Downward communication might be used when there are issues related to the organization's (a) policies and procedures, (b) position descriptions, (c) employee rules and regulations, (d) written communication from administration, and (e) other forms of organizational communication that come from above. Performance evaluations traditionally have been primarily downward; however, this type of performance evaluation is less effective, as was discussed in Chapter 9. Most organizations now require that staff participate in its own performance evaluation, thereby changing this communication line.

Changing organizational structures and leadership approaches have required changes in communication. Consider what was discussed about Transformational Leadership in Chapter 1. Dictating from above or downward communication is not a communication approach that supports this type of leadership. As a consequence of leadership change, downward communication is becoming less common as more staff is encouraged to participate in organizational decisions and be innovative and initiate changes. This would encourage more upward communication and other communication forms in which staff interacts in a participatory environment such as shared governance.

Downward communication is also not as effective as other communication lines. Why is this so? Communication really is the act of the message's receiver. If there is no active receiver, does communication really occur? Downward communication can only send commands or directions. Communication needs to begin with the intended receiver rather than the sender. Downward communication comes after upward communication has been successful. It is a reaction rather than an action, or response rather than an initiative.

UPWARD COMMUNICATION   Communication is upward for example when a staff nurse tells a nurse manager that the schedule for the month does not meet the staff nurse's needs or when staff is involved in decision making at the unit level. Examples of **upward communication**, which are increasing in most health care organizations, include staff meetings, staff-to-staff or staff-to-manager communication, and communication that occurs on a daily basis in the work setting. Other examples are a manager's use of an "open door" policy so that staff can feel free to come to the manager with issues or concerns, shift reports, team or project communication and written reports, grievance procedures, staff development evaluation feedback, exit interviews, use of a suggestion box, staff satisfaction surveys, union communication, and the grapevine. Shared governance, a form of organizational process and structure discussed in Chapter 4, requires that staff participates actively in organizational decision making, which is upward communication; however, if there is limited lateral and diagonal communication, this still limits active staff participation in communication and decision making. Downward and upward communication are similar in that communication goes from one level to another, but only in a different direction from bottom to top or the reverse. Those who receive the message last may not receive the exact original message that was sent. This can be a disadvantage as it is critical that the message is received as sent. This can be an advantage if the message's content has been improved with the creative process of the ideas of more than one staff member, but this still means that not all staff received the same message. The issues of perception and expectations will always be factors in limiting consistent communication.

LATERAL COMMUNICATION   **Lateral** or **horizontal communication** is typically used to coordinate activities. This type of communication takes place between staff that is in the same or similar hierarchical level or departmental level in that one does not have formal power over the other (for example, between a staff nurse and another staff nurse or between two nurse managers, one from the cardiac care unit and the other from a medical unit). Typically, this communication is informal and might involve sharing information about patients, committee communication, and communication among team members, interprofessional, and work team project members. As organizations begin to incorporate more teamwork and emphasize the value of working in teams, this type of communication develops and becomes critical for success.

DIAGONAL COMMUNICATION   **Diagonal communication**, another form of communication, is informal. This communication typically occurs when staff members who are from different hierarchical levels are working on a project together, but when they work on the project, they are equal. This form of communication is increasing because more staff from different departments or units are working together increasing collaboration. It also applies to the relationship between a nurse and a physician or a nurse and a patient. For example, if a health care organization is developing a new admission procedure, the project's team ideally should include a physician, several nurse managers, several staff nurses, a patient transportation supervisor, the director of medical records, the director of information system management, a patient representative, an ombudsman or patient advocate, an admission department representative, an administrator, and the chief financial officer. In some organizations a patient representative may be included. This team has representatives from different departments, units within departments, management, administration, and an insurer representative; different hierarchical levels; consumers; and external representatives. The goal of diagonal communication is to improve communication so that all can work together to meet the team's goal.

There is also increasing evidence suggesting that clinical errors are often related to ineffective communication patterns between members of the health care team and miscommunication. The Institute of Medicine report, *To Err Is Human*, discusses the problem of increasing errors in health care (Institute of Medicine, 1999). (See Chapter 16.) The report defines an error as "the failure of a planned action to be completed as intended or the use of a wrong plan to achieve an aim" (Institute of Medicine, 1999, p. 3). Considering this definition, it is difficult to exclude communication as a major factor in errors. Ineffective communication, problems with communication flow, poor feedback, and difficulty in getting relevant patient information are all mentioned in the report. The Joint Commission has also commented on communication and errors: "Given that noncommunication or miscommunication is to blame in many common errors, the central person with whom health providers need to communicate—the patient—should be the first priority. Many times, historical information on the patient is incomplete and does not include detailed information on a patient's allergies, previous diagnoses and lab results, or other medicines that are being taken, including vitamins, herbs and over-the-counter medication" (Mansur, 2010).

### The Communication Process

The transmission of information and understanding of that information in the message takes place on many different levels: individual-to-individual, in small teams, in large organizations, and between organizations. Each level of the process is described in Figure 13-1 and includes the following:

1. **Encoding** or translation of the communicator's ideas into language
2. **Message** or the result of the encoding process
3. **Medium** or the carrier of the message (e.g., face-to-face, memo, medical record, team meeting, computer, policy statement); it can be an unintended message that is sent by silence or inaction
4. **Decoding** or the process the receiver goes through to receive and interpret the message
5. **Feedback**, an important component of two-way communication

The communication process is made up of five elements. It is important to recognize the use of the term *process*, which indicates that communication is a dynamic interaction. The following are the five elements.

1. The **sender** is the individual who initiates the message, which may be verbal and/or non-verbal. Communication may also be written. Verbal communication always includes non-verbal communication. There are many factors that affect the sender and the message (e.g., the sender's attitude toward self and toward the receiver, the situation in which the message is sent, timing, and purpose of the message). The sender uses encoding when decisions are made about what to include in the message and how to transmit the message. Then the message is sent.
2. The message includes both verbal and nonverbal information as well as the sender's attitude toward self, receiver, and the message.
3. The receiver is the person(s) to whom the message is sent. The receiver decodes the message so that it can be fully understood. This includes the actions necessary to understand the message (for example, listening, reading a memo or an e-mail message, or reviewing a chart of data).

**FIGURE 13-1** **Communication process.**

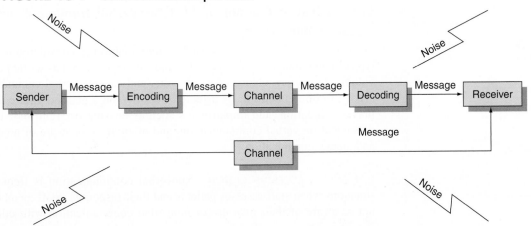

Source: Robbins, S., & Decenzo, D. (20010). *Fundamentals of management.* Upper Saddle River, NJ: Prentice Hall Health, p. 377. Reprinted with permission.

4. The feedback is the message or response that the receiver may send back to the sender. Feedback may be verbal, nonverbal, or both. Clearly, the receiver's feelings, attitudes, experiences, relationship with the sender, the communication climate, cultural factors, and so on affect the decision to respond—the message and method chosen for the response. As discussed earlier, the receiver's perception and expectations are important. This is often referred to as "noise" or that which might interfere with communication. If response occurs, then the process turns around with the receiver becoming the sender and the original sender becoming the receiver. The receiver may also then communicate with other receivers. Two-way communication has then occurred.

5. The **context** is the situation or environment in which the communication takes place (for example, the nurse's station, patient's room, patient's home, the hallway, the clinic, the school nurse's office, staff meeting, or during shift report). This aspect of the process is very important and takes into consideration factors such as noise, number of people present, stress level, emergency or routine, presence of management or supervisors, privacy in the patient care area, organizational culture, morale, ethics and legal requirements, technology and information systems, and so on (Finkelman, 1996, p. 1–1:10; Dessler, 2002).

Why should one be concerned about this process? First, the process can be used to analyze communication. Where was communication effective or ineffective? Was there a problem when the message was developed by the communicator? For example, if a nurse is too tired to be clear when giving directions to an unlicensed assistive personnel (UAP), this then affects the message—instead of telling the UAP to take blood pressures on four patients, one patient is forgotten. Sometimes a less effective medium is chosen; for example, a memo may be sent when it would have been better to call the person to get more immediate feedback. Taking a part in communication by using these levels and elements of the communication process as a framework of analysis can help to identify where the communication process needs to be improved.

The communication process is affected by many factors that are external to the environment in which the communication may take place. Managed care health insurance is one of these factors as it has made communication in health care even more complex. Sometimes just trying to get approval for a patient procedure can strain a staff member's patience. There may need to be telephone calls, written documentation of needs, and in some cases, actual face-to-face contact, and the result may still be unsatisfying. Some external factors cannot be controlled. An example is state health departments require the reporting of all cases of child abuse. If there is a breakdown in this legally mandated communication, the child may suffer physically, and the health care organization may suffer severe consequences such as fines and discipline of specific health care providers. In this situation, the health care organization has no choice but to build in a communication process to ensure that this information is communicated.

## Communication Component Systems: Verbal, Nonverbal, and Metacommunication

VERBAL COMMUNICATION    Verbal communication is considered to be the most common type of communication. It is complex and can be described as written or oral, tone, language, volume, frequency, choice of words, rate, and accent. Verbal communication, like all other types of communication, is affected by a person's gender, age, culture, stereotypes and biases, education, and impairments such as hearing or sight loss. Individuals are highly dependent on verbal communication, and often are less aware of nonverbal communication and metacommunication.

NONVERBAL COMMUNICATION    Nonverbal communication is frequently used in clinical situations when staff assesses patients and their responses. Staff members, however, are often not as aware of their own use of nonverbal communication with other staff, patients, and families. The major functions of nonverbal communication are expression of emotion; expression of interpersonal attitudes; maintenance of rituals; support of verbal communication; establishment, development, and maintenance of relationships; and self-presentation. Nonverbal communication is not something that is always in the awareness or control of the individual. To improve communication a person needs to increase awareness of the impact of nonverbal communication and increase assessment of nonverbal communication during the communication process. Nonverbal communication can consist of facial expressions, body movements or posture, gestures, volume of speech, tone of voice, gait, and physical appearance. Body language typically includes facial expression, eye movements, body movements, posture, gestures, and proxemics, or distance between individuals. This assessment must not only include the nonverbal communication that the other party uses but also self-assessment of nonverbal communication. It is more difficult to be aware of how one is using nonverbal communication while one is using verbal communication. For example, when a nurse is discussing a procedure with a patient is the nurse aware of personal facial expressions, body language, and tone of voice, or is the nurse just focused on the procedure and not the patient's nonverbal communication? Some nonverbal factors that are important to consider are as follows:

- Maintain eye contact and a relaxed manner as this communicates sincerity.
- Smile if it is appropriate to the content, but do not smile constantly because this tends to make the receiver distrust the sender and the message.
- A neutral environment might be useful in circumstances in which meeting in one's office or on one's own territory might make the other person feel uncomfortable.
- If a person stands over or leans over another, it can make that person uncomfortable and feel a loss of power.
- Pulling away or appearing too casual may communicate superiority or disinterest.

Cultural issues are also important because there is great variation in nonverbal communication among different cultures and interpretation of nonverbals. Examples of questions to consider with different cultures are (a) Do men look directly at women who are not their wives? (b) How do people greet one another? (c) Does the husband speak for the wife? Answers to these questions and many others are important to know if a nurse is trying to teach a woman and her husband is present. The Institute of Medicine supports the need for the importance of cultural communications factors in all communication with patients, families, and staff (workforce diversity): "Sociocultural differences between patient and provider influence communication and clinical decision making" (Institute of Medicine, 2003b, p. 214).

Nonverbal communication frequently causes problems because it is often difficult to assess and interpret. This communication includes anything other than the spoken word. It can be deliberate or unintentional, and when it is unintentional, it is out of the control of the sender or the receiver. When there is doubt about the interpretation, the best approach is to ask for clarification about the meaning; however, this is not always easy to do. The receiver may be hesitant, feel incompetent, may be concerned that asking for information may be threatening, or may not know how or what to ask. Comparing the nonverbal with the verbal may assist in greater understanding, but this is not always the case as a person's nonverbal communication may be different from the verbal. Nurses tend to use comparison of verbal and nonverbal communication more during their communication with patients than with co-workers. Nonverbal communication, however, is very important in work-related communication and should not be ignored. Delegation is a time when asking for clarification is critical; both from perspective of delegator and delegatee. (See Chapter 14.)

## Assessment of Communication Effectiveness

Communicators want to have productive communication when the sender sends a message. The goal is that the message will be received and understood as sent. Productive communication can lead to many positive benefits for individual staff, teams, structural units within the organization, the organization, the community, and for the patient and family. Some of these benefits are as follows:

- A team spirit with a common understanding and staff working toward common goals
- Participative management providing the staff with the opportunity to express different points of view and develop the best approach to problems
- Quick resolution of misunderstandings
- A comfortable environment that supports a motivational climate
- More creative thinking by nursing management and nursing staff

- Less staff turnover
- Less evidence of a rumor mill
- Clarification of responsibilities (Finkelman, 1996, pp. 1–1:13–14)

Team leaders, charge nurses, and nurse managers need to periodically evaluate the effectiveness of the communication—their own communication, individual staff members, and team communication, which could be a team, unit, department, or entire organization.

- What might be some indicators of staff communication problems?
- Do staff members feel comfortable expressing their feelings and opinions?
- Are some staff members trying to get on the good side of the nurse manager or leader and not communicating effectively?
- During meetings or in shift report, does staff ask questions?
- Do staff members contribute their ideas to the discussion when there are problems? Silence may be positive as it can allow time for thinking before responding; however, if staff is silent for long periods without contributing to the discussion, this can be an indicator of a communication problem.
- What happens when messages do not seem to be understood or are misinterpreted?

These questions represent some of the many aspects that need to be considered when communication is evaluated.

Staff–staff communication provides the critical framework in which care occurs. Imagine how a nurse might provide care without using communication. The care would have to occur on an isolated island, and even in that situation, the nurse would still have to communicate with the patient. Problems, however, do occur even in the best communication situations. The following are some examples:

- Discussing patients and their care is part of staff responsibilities. This takes time and needs to be considered a critical aspect of each staff member's role. This is not to say that in some cases too much time can be spent talking about care rather than providing care. Undoubtedly, every nurse encounters staff members who seem to talk too much, neglect work, interrupt others' work, and cause tension. This may mean that the team leader or nurse manager will need to talk to the staff member and determine the reason for this type of communication problem, discuss how it interferes with the work and care of patients, and arrive at strategies to improve the staff member's communication and reduce the interruptions. Other staff may even discuss it with the staff member; however, this should be offered as positive criticism and in private.
- Competition among staff can interfere with productive communication. It can lead to withholding of information, distortion of information, and poor morale. Why would staff be competitive? They might be seeking recognition for work, better assignments, better work schedules, or feel that some staff members are treated differently. Clearly, this indicates that there are major problems in the work environment that need to be addressed so that communication can improve.
- Confidentiality is an ever present need in all clinical setting interactions. This has been reinforced by the HIPAA law related to privacy and confidentiality. (See Chapter 2.) Discussing staff and patient issues where others who should not hear about them might hear the conversation is very easy to do. Staff gets involved and forgets; however, the problems that can occur from this can be very serious. Staff members are busy and so they "reach out" to other staff for these discussions when they can (for example, in the hallway, elevator, cafeteria, etc.). These are not private areas. Even the nursing station must be considered an open area unless it is enclosed. Telephone conversations can also be easily overheard. Many health care organizations now give staff cellular telephones to use in the clinical setting. These telephones are frequently used where conversations may be overheard. Nurses who work in the community must be particularly aware of this as they frequently use cellular telephones where the public can overhear confidential information or misinterpret what might be said by a health care professional (for example, taking calls while taking a lunch break in a public restaurant or telephoning a patient while in another patient's home making a home visit).

- There needs to be greater consideration of staff feelings in the workplace. With heavy workloads it is easy to forget about the feelings of co-workers. Dashing around, communicating in short sentences, and moving on creates an environment in which staff forgets to connect and to listen. A critical element of positive communication is the comfort level. Does staff feel comfortable saying "I need help?" "I am overwhelmed?" or does staff feel that this will be seen only in a negative light? Staff communication may be sharp and caustic, leading to hurt feelings or anger, setting up barriers to future effective communication.

- Medical records and documentation are very important parts of communication in the health care delivery system. This form of communication must be clear and provide critical information that is required. Requirements come from the nursing profession, state boards of nursing, standards, state and federal laws and regulations, insurers, legal cases, and the organization's policies, procedures, and quality improvement program. Assessment of this type of communication must include these regulations. It is particularly important today to follow insurer requirements, particularly when describing patient problems, plan of care, and outcomes. This information affects decisions that are made and changes that are instituted, directs care evaluation, communicates responsibilities, identifies outcomes that should be met and (if they are met) determines reimbursement, and guides staff. The common response to medical malpractice issues, "If it is not documented, it did not happen," says much about the importance of this documentation. If a list was made of health care communication concerns, documentation would be a top priority.

- When a staff member does not understand something or what needs to be done, it is important to ask to have the information or instruction repeated or explained. If it is something that makes the staff member feel uncomfortable, these feelings should be discussed. This is very important in delegation, as is discussed in Chapter 14.

- Mutual trust is something that is not easy to accomplish or assess today. Poor or inconsistent communication, inadequate staff input during the change process, and fears such as job loss or change can damage trust. This trust is a critical component of communication. Developing strategies to build mutual trust is important. Effective timing is something that should be considered for an important communication and assessment of the communication process. Box 13-1 identifies some techniques to promote trust.

- At times there seem to be several different "stories" or different versions of information from different staff. This causes major communication and morale problems. Getting facts from the source and discussing them openly helps to resolve this problem.

- Intuition is used by many people, often unconsciously, and when it is used it may predict what will happen within communication or within a situation. This may or may not be helpful as it may cause the sender or receiver to make the wrong assumption.

- Sometimes it is difficult to know when to use face-to-face communication and when to use the telephone or e-mail. Telephone and e-mail communication usually take less time, but if it is important to have a face-to-face conversation, then time needs to be taken for this.

---

### BOX 13-1　TECHNIQUES DESIGNED TO PROMOTE TRUST

- Convey respect
- Consider the person's uniqueness
- Show warmth and caring
- Use active listening
- Give sufficient time to answer questions
- Maintain confidentiality
- Show congruence between verbal and non-verbal behaviors
- Use a warm friendly voice
- Use appropriate eye contact
- Smile appropriately

- Be flexible
- Be honest and open
- Give complete information
- Provide consistency
- Plan schedules
- Control distractions
- Set limits
- Follow through on commitments
- Use an attending posture: arms, legs, and body relaxed, leaning slightly forward
- Confirm responses

When there is major conflict and miscommunication then blasting with a lot of e-mails is not effective. This is the time for a face-to-face meeting. Telephone and e-mail offer more control: The sender selects the time when it is done; the time it takes is usually shorter; it is easier to take notes while in the middle of the communication; and e-mail provides more time to think about what will be said. Although physical nonverbal communication cannot be observed with these methods, tone and use of words communicated in an e-mail can communicate some aspects of nonverbal communication.

- Staff should not be left hanging. Feedback and follow-up are necessary for the development and maintenance of trust and to encourage two-way communication. It takes time to provide feedback, but it is time well spent.

- Interdepartmental/unit communication helps the nurse manager and staff see problems from the other department/unit's point of view. Without this communication, it is easy to be isolated and only see one viewpoint.

- There are times when communication in the nursing station, desk area, or the work area (such as in a clinic) is impossible or undesirable. If it is very busy, the message may be lost amid the confusion. If a sensitive topic needs to be discussed, this location is too public. Never assume that this area is private.

- Selecting the appropriate time to discuss a sensitive issue or even to communicate daily work-related information can make a critical difference. If a staff member is busy with patient care or documentation, this is not the best time. There are times, such as immediately after a critical clinical incident, that staff is not able to discuss fully what has occurred due to emotions or fatigue. Often the first response is to discuss the situation; however, the best approach is to identify another time within a reasonable time frame to discuss the incident. Putting off a discussion is not always negative if it is done thoughtfully and follow-up action is actually taken (Finkelman, 1996, p. 1–1:14–15).

**BARRIERS TO COMMUNICATION**     The exchange of information and transmission of meaning among several individuals or teams throughout the organization or communication is not always successful. There are many barriers to communication that an organization, its management, and staff need to be aware of that affect short-term and long-term activities. The following list is far from complete, but it provides many critical examples of these barriers.

- **Failing to listen to others and not recognizing them:**     This leads to negative feelings and responses. Active listening can improve this problem.

- **Using selective listening so that one hears only what one wants to hear:**     This is often due to the inability to recognize the needs and problems of others. Active listening and gaining more understanding of others' expectations can also improve this problem.

- **Failing to probe or inquire further when encountering vague information, obtaining inadequate answers, reaching a confusing interpretation, or following procedures and standards so closely that the message is missed:**     Using open questions will make a difference with this problem.

- **Making overly judgmental statements:**     This often occurs when the receiver decides what is the overall value of the message (e.g., a staff member who always complains may not be heard when there is legitimate need for complaint). Active listening, trying to understand other viewpoints, and stopping before responding may decrease this barrier.

- **Expressing opinions while intentionally or unintentionally intimidating others:**     Asking for feedback can be helpful so that steps can be taken to improve. Being direct rather than aggressive avoids setting up barriers.

- **Overusing reassuring statements and rejecting statements:**     These types of statements cut off communication. More open communication that respects the other person can limit this barrier.

- **Using a defensive stance stops open communication:**     The communicator needs to be more open and recognize that there is more than one point of view.

- **Making a false inference:**     This often occurs when someone jumps to a conclusion without enough information. Getting more information before responding or communicating can limit this barrier.

- **Using personal criticism, profanity, and crudity:** These act only as barriers to effective communication and also are very destructive to the communication climate. Respecting others is critical in communication and can help to limit this barrier.
- **Responding to spatial issues:** Space can be a barrier—if too close, people may feel uncomfortable, particularly if a person crosses too far into the safe zone. If there is a lot of space, people may feel distant from one another. Important spatial factors that can make a difference are (a) How close are the receiver and sender? (b) Has one of them crossed into personal space that makes the other person uncomfortable? (c) What are the cultural issues related to space? (d) What is the space between the staff and the patient? (e) In a team meeting what is the arrangement of the seating area: at a table, in a circle, and so on? (f) What is the distance between them? (g) Is it easy to have eye contact?
- **Keeping secrets:** Secrecy is very destructive to communication and to organizations. It decreases staff trust and interferes with team building. This leads to ineffective communication. Communicating fully and openly will increase effective communication, and keeps the channels of communication open. It is not easy to develop and maintain a culture in which open communication is valued. Chapter 1 emphasizes the importance of this type of communication in leadership theories such as Emotional Intelligence.

In an open communication environment staff knows that its ideas are respected and should be shared. Effective management openly discusses communication and actively pursues greater communication with staff. Communication is considered when organizational goals are evaluated—assessment of the organization's communication is integrated into the process. Leaders and managers advocate that each staff member has a responsibility to contribute ideas and opinions, and they ask staff to contribute and give them time to respond. Communication should be part of performance evaluation for each staff member throughout the organization.

INFORMATION OVERLOAD    Today, in most organizations, it is very easy for staff to experience information overload. Information is coming from multiple sources at one time. It is difficult to decide what is important, and it seems that everyone feels that their needs are more important and require an immediate response. With the growth of information technology there is now an increased burden of too much communication, often with less real people contact. E-mails, faxes, the Internet, memos, letters, reports, and more are added to the pile. Medical record documentation also increases the amount of information that nurses have to cope with today. With the increase in quantity there is also increased speed—staff gets information faster and then feels compelled to respond faster. This increasing speed of communication receipt has also spoiled staff to expect information quickly, and when it does not come quickly, staff experiences stress.

What are the critical issues with information overload? Staff needs to consider the following questions: What information is important, and what is extraneous? How quickly is a response expected, and what is a realistic response time? What is the purpose of the information? Does the information need to be saved? How should it be saved? Is this the end point of the information or should it be sent on to another? If so, to whom and why? What is the quality of the information? Who sent the information? What is the source of the information? It is very helpful when the sender indicates a time frame for response. This simple intervention can do much to decrease the stress of feeling compelled to respond quickly.

IMPORTANCE OF FEEDBACK: GIVING AND RECEIVING FEEDBACK    Feedback is a part of all communication. To become an effective communicator nurses need to learn how to give and receive feedback. First and foremost, feedback should not be described as something that is negative. Most staff immediately assumes that feedback means "bad news." Positive feedback, what has been done well and so on, is critical. There are several types of feedback: oral, unspoken or nonverbal, substantiated, and perceptive (Milgram, Spector, & Treger, 1999).

- Oral feedback is also referred to as interactive feedback in that a person asks another or a team for clarification, and interpretation is shared.
- Unspoken or nonverbal feedback includes any form of nonverbal communication that indicates how one person is responding to the communication from another. A person might

## APPLYING EVIDENCE-BASED PRACTICE

### Evidence for Effective Leadership and Management

**Citation:**  Capitulo, K. (2009). Addressing disruptive behavior by implementing a code of professionalism to transform hospital culture. *Nurse Leader*, April, 38–43.

**Overview:**  Capitulo examines pilot projects in two hospitals (one unionized and one not unionized) that implemented a code of professionalism, particularly addressing disruptive behavior. "There is a direct link between disruptive behavior and a negative culture of blame and intimidation, which decreases communication, teamwork, and ultimately, patient safety. When staff are yelled at by physicians, superiors, or colleagues, they fear retribution and often stop communicating, leading to errors and decreasing patient safety. Disruptive behavior can occur between and among all levels of staff, e.g., nurse–nurse, physician–nurse, secretary–nurse, and manager–staff" (p. 39). The two pilot organizations used the Agency for Healthcare Research and Quality's (AHRQ) Survey on Patient Safety Culture as an assessment tool. The author provides extensive content on disruptive behavior, a Code of Professionalism, and methods used to reduce disruptive behavior. The pilots did make a difference in reducing staff disruptive behavior.

**Application:**  Disruptive behavior in health care professionals is a growing problem. As noted in this article, the Institute of Medicine describes a quality and safety problem and need for improvement. The Joint Commission identifies disruptive behavior as a barrier to effective, safe care. Every nurse needs to know how to improve communication and also cope with difficult relationships in the work environment.

**Questions:**

1. *Have you observed disruptive or intimidating behavior in a clinical situation? If so, what did you observe and how does it relate to content in this article?*

2. *What do you think about these two pilots and their results?*

3. *Why would it be important to include unionized and non-unionized organizations?*

4. *Do you have suggestions for other strategies to prevent disruptive behavior and to cope with disruptive behavior that might occur in the clinical setting?*

appear uninterested, taking steps out of the office, looking at his or her watch, smiling and moving forward in a move of acceptance, raising one's voice, and so on. Sometimes the unspoken feedback sends a message that is different from the verbal message and may be viewed as the most important part of the message. For example, a nurse is very upset about information that the nurse manager is giving in a meeting. The nurse says, "I agree with what you are saying." At the same time, the nurse appears anxious, taking steps toward the door, and the tone of voice is tight.

- Substantiated feedback is used to obtain accurate and specific data, and to ensure that the message is understood.
- Perceptive feedback concerns whether or not the message behind the words is understood. This gets to the "why" behind the message and "what" the sender or receiver really thinks. Empathy plays a role in the process; however, this type of feedback is difficult to discern. Feedback that is rarely used will soon send a negative message. Likely responses to this lack of interest will be decreased feedback. This may lead to decreased interaction, anger, decreased morale, and criticism, which may be given indirectly via gossip and the grapevine.

Feedback should flow in four directions in health care organizations: (a) from manager to staff, (b) from staff to managers, (c) from staff to staff, and (d) from staff to patients and families/significant others. The first type, between managers and staff, can be difficult, especially if staff feels uncomfortable and threatened in the work setting. How can organizations encourage staff to give feedback to managers so that it is not just manager to staff? Typical methods that are used to increase staff feedback are managers asking directly for feedback, allowing time in staff meetings for feedback, suggestion boxes, surveys, informal meetings such as at lunch or during break time, problem solving or project teams, an open door policy when the manager has open office hours, and walk-around management in which the manager is present on the clinical units and staff can approach the manager with comments and issues. When feedback can be given freely and received without undue stress, the work environment is a much more positive environment. Feedback should focus on performance and outcomes with clear description of the issues. Staff needs time to respond to the feedback and to ask questions.

How should staff respond to supervisory feedback? The most common response is to jump to a defensive response, but the better approach is to carefully consider what is shared. Listening is just as important in this type of communication as in other types. The tendency is to immediately try to explain actions or become defensive rather than to first listen. Sometimes a supervisor is only offering an alternative solution that needs to be thought about. If managers or supervisors do not offer feedback, staff needs to ask for it. Staff sometimes thinks that supervisory feedback means that all of the co-workers think the same thing as the nurse manager. Supervisory feedback should represent the manager's opinion. Though every organization should have a formal performance review for all staff, this does not mean that feedback should not be shared at other times or that staff should not ask for feedback.

Improving feedback communication can be done by using several techniques and considering some factors related to feedback (Milgram, Spector, & Treger, 1999).

- Definitions can make a difference in effective and ineffective communication. What do the words and phrases mean? Different people may use different definitions. Jargon and unfamiliar terms can confuse conversation requiring feedback for clarification.
- Simple and clear language is always better. It is easy to make assumptions about communication (for example, what the sender meant, what the feelings and attitudes are behind the message, or whether or not the sender really wanted to communicate).
- Feedback can be used to avoid the dangers of assumptions.
- Questions can also be used to clarify and to stimulate feedback.
- Observation plays an important role in the communication process, and nonverbal feedback is part of this process. What is the nonverbal feedback indicating? Is the message clear? Does the recipient appear involved, bored, angry, uncomfortable, and so on? Is more feedback required?
- A team leader or a nurse manager often must give team members or staff direct one-to-one feedback. This may be difficult, but the best approach is to focus on the behavior rather than making it personal. All feedback needs to be approached from a constructive perspective with a healthy positive attitude. Downgrading and making remarks that are hurtful are not effective feedback.
- Follow-up is also an important technique to improve communication. In the busy clinical setting it is easy to forget to follow-up. Nurses use various methods such as notebooks with lists to remind themselves. Even computer methods can be utilized as computers are smaller such as personal digital assistants (PDAs), smartphones, and so on.
- Empathy is important. It means that the sender needs to be receiver oriented, or have a greater understanding of the receiver, to be in the place of the receiver. This is closely related to the need for mutual trust between the sender and receiver. Those who use empathy recognize that it is important to understand another person. Questioning and active listening improve empathy. This process requires that the person focus on what is happening and avoid thinking of other things or allowing one's mind to wander.
- Sometimes the sender may find it helpful to repeat information in order to ensure that it was received as sent. Typical situations when information may need to be repeated are during delegation, orientation of new staff, training programs, and working with students (e.g., nursing, medical, and so on).

As team leaders, nurses must give feedback to team members. What is the best way to do this? If this type of communication is new to the team leader, the leader may be hesitant to give feedback, but team members nonetheless expect to receive feedback. In summary, the following guidelines about feedback can be helpful.

- Use specific examples and focus on behavior, not personal criticism.
- Provide feedback that is as immediate as possible to the situation.
- Give honest feedback in a simple and direct manner.
- If feedback is always positive, it probably means that the whole truth is not shared.
- Discuss the effects of positive and negative behavior on patient care, the unit, the clinic, the department, co-workers, nursing, the organization, and so on.
- Tell team members what is expected of them.
- Give positive and negative feedback as it is easy to forget to tell team members that they have done a great job or it was a tough day and they got through it.
- Reinforce positive behavior.
- Ask the team member for strategies to improve.
- Allow team members to give feedback to the team leader.
- Solicit feedback rather than waiting for it to come (Milgram, Spector, & Treger, 1999).

Box 13-2 provides some guidelines for giving and receiving criticism.

## CASE STUDY

### Exchanging Information across Shifts

The ICU has been having problems with communication between shifts, particularly on the weekends. This problem is brought up in the monthly staff meeting. A nurse says, "I think the night shift has not shared important patient information. It has led to serious errors, and I don't want to be held responsible for these errors." Silence follows this statement. As the nurse manager you know you need to respond so you say, "What is going on?"

### Questions:

1. What do you think of the nurse manager's response?
2. What information do you need?
3. What is the best way to frame the problem?
4. How might you go about assessing the unit's communication?
5. What are strategies you might use to resolve the communication problems?

GRAPEVINE: IS IT GOOD OR BAD?    The grapevine is present in every organization, within its service areas, units, and departments. The grapevine can be positive or negative. Clearly, information can be distorted in the grapevine, individual feelings can be hurt, and information can be very difficult to control. The grapevine can affect staff morale when information that should not be communicated is shared; when communication is distorted and its meaning causes damage; or when staff feels left out. Efforts to eliminate the grapevine will undoubtedly fail as grapevines seem to be ingrained in all organizations and have a life of their own. Managers need to learn how to use the grapevine to their advantage. However, using the grapevine can be risky as once a message is put into the grapevine one loses control of the message and how it is presented. If the manager wants to get a message out quickly, the grapevine can be used if the leader knows how to access the grapevine. In addition, corrected information can be put into the grapevine. Given this information about the grapevine, what is the best way to decrease the damage that the grapevine can cause? The best approach is keeping staff informed. This is particularly important when there are critical issues (for example, budget, staffing, and plans for change). Staff needs to also be careful with the grapevine, recognizing that factual information may not always be found in communication that is received via the grapevine.

## BOX 13-2  GIVING AND RECEIVING CRITICISM

### GIVING CONSTRUCTIVE CRITICISM

When you offer criticism, use the following steps to communicate clearly and effectively:

*Criticize the behavior rather than the person.* In addition, make sure the behavior you intend to criticize is changeable. Chronic lateness can be changed; a physical inability to perform a task cannot.

*Define specifically the behavior you want to change.* Try not to drag any side issues into the conversation.

*Balance criticism with positive words.* Alternate critical comments with praise in other performance.

*Stay calm and be brief.* Avoid threats, ultimatums, or accusations. Use "I" messages; choose positive, non-threatening words so the person knows that your intentions are positive.

*Explain the effects caused by the behavior that warrants the criticism.* Help the person understand why a change needs to happen, and talk about options in detail. Compare and contrast the effects of the current behavior with the effects of a potential change.

*Offer help in changing the behavior.* Lead by example.

### RECEIVING CRITICISM

When you find yourself on the receiving end of criticism, use these coping techniques:

*Listen to the criticism before you speak up.* Resist the desire to defend yourself until you've heard all the details. Decide if the criticism is offered in a constructive or unconstructive manner.

*Think the criticism through critically.* Evaluate it carefully. While some criticism may come from a desire to help, other comments may have less honorable origins. People often criticize others out of jealousy, anger, frustration, or displaced feelings. In cases like those, it is best (though not always easy) to let the criticism wash right over you.

*If it is unconstructive, you may not want to respond at that moment.* Unconstructive criticism can inspire anger that might be destructive to express. Wait until you cool down and think about the criticism to see if there is anything important hiding under how it was presented. Then, tell the person that you see the value of the criticism, but also communicate to him or her how the delivery of the criticism made you feel. If he or she is willing to talk in a more constructive manner, continue with the following steps below. If not, your best bet may be to consider the case closed and move on.

*If it is constructive, ask for suggestions of how to change the criticized behavior.* You could ask, "How would you handle this if you were in my place?"

*Before the conversation ends, summarize the criticism and your response to it.* Repeat it back to the person who offered it. Make sure both of you understand the situation in the same way.

*If you feel that the criticism is valid, plan a specific strategy for correcting the behavior.* Think over what you might learn from changing behavior. If you do not agree with the criticism even after the whole conversation, explain your behavior from your point of view.

Source: Katz, J. (2001). *Keys to nursing success* (pp. 272–273). Upper Saddle River, NJ: Prentice Hall. Reprinted with permission.

# Communication Methods

There are four common communication methods that are used by staff and management: written communication, face-to-face communication, storytelling, and information technology and communication. With each of these methods, timing needs to be considered. What is the best time to use a particular communication method? Sometimes it is better to talk to someone face-to-face while at other times an e-mail will be just as effective. The time it takes to complete the communication is another concern. How quickly does the communication need to occur? Today, with the technology that is available communication can be delivered quickly. This may or may not be a positive outcome. What is the best time to initiate communication? The situation, the sender, the receiver, stress, energy level, and support that might be needed are some of the factors to consider. "Many opportunities for successful communication have been lost because of timing" (Sullivan, 2004, p. 57). Each of the following communication methods is important for nurses in their daily practice.

## Written Communication

With so many communication options available today it is often difficult to know when to use each method. Written communication provides a paper trail; documentation of the communication, which for some communication is important. It is particularly important to use this method when a record needs to be kept (e.g., document an important one-to-one meeting; minutes of a team, staff, or project meeting; disciplinary meeting; performance evaluation; reimbursements; and so on). It is important to remember that longer messages do not necessarily include more useful information. Time is important so messages need to get to the point and include required information.

Effective written communication requires thought from the sender. There are two types of messages, direct and indirect. The latter is typically used when the sender expects the receiver to have a negative response to the message. This is the message that begins with general comments, and the bad news is buried near the end. An example might be the letter that comes after a job interview with an introduction describing the wonderful candidates who applied and how difficult the decision was to make, and is followed by the section that says someone else got the job. A direct message gets right to the point, and this type is used when the receiver is expected to respond positively to the information. This does not mean, however, that bad news should not be communicated with a more direct style. Often the sender's comfort level determines the method. Breaking bad news gently seems to make it less bad or less difficult for the sender. Written communication needs to be reviewed and edited before sending. A timely response is always appreciated. This communication method, as is true of all communication, needs to be adapted for the audience. Graphics and other visuals may be appropriate and added to written communication, but they should augment the message, not detract from it.

Written communication can be sent in several ways: hard copy via interdepartmental mail, e-mail, fax, U.S. postal service, non-U.S. postal service delivery companies, or hand delivered by the sender. The form that this type of communication takes can also vary: an informal note, memorandum (memo), formal letter, minutes, policy or procedure, surveys, data collecting tools, or performance evaluation. Most organizations have specific forms or formats that need to be used for memos, emails, minutes, policies, procedures, and performance evaluation. Memos need to follow the organization's format with a clear identification of the subject or topic. Careful consideration needs to be given as to who should receive the memo. Content should be concise and relevant. A memo is not a lengthy report, but rather short and to the point. Clearly, all patient care documentation is a critical component of written communication.

## Face-to-Face Communication

Face-to-face communication is one of the most frequently used communication methods; however, electronic communication has had a major impact on a move away from less face-to-face communication. There are times, however, when face-to-face communication is the preferred method, particularly when personal sensitive information needs to be discussed. When a dialogue is needed with greater give and take, in-person communication is better. If in-person communication cannot be done and is needed, then the next choice is the telephone or, when possible, synchronous online conversation. Some health care organizations, especially large health care networks, have equipment for videoconferencing, which is discussed later in this chapter. This is another alternative to in-person communication. Box 13-3 shows examples of communication techniques.

**Active listening**, a technique that is critical for effective communication, means listening for the message's full meaning and ensuring that judgment of interpretations does not interfere with the understanding of the message. This takes concentration and involvement on the part of the listener. Listening also means that the person is willing to listen even when it means that what is heard may be negative or unpleasant. Seeking out information sometimes means taking risks. It is not uncommon for staff to tell nurse managers what they think the nurse manager wants to hear rather than providing a full disclosure. This does not demonstrate a staff that feels empowered, and it is not productive communication. Staff members want to feel that managers and other staff are communicating *with* them, not *to* them, and the presence of listening increases the chance that communication will be a joint endeavor. Barriers to effective listening include making assumptions before one hears the communication; non-interest in the topic or issue; history

| BOX 13-3 | COMMUNICATION TECHNIQUES |
|---|---|

- Listening
- Silence
- Establish guidelines
- Giving broad openings
- Reducing distance
- Questions: closed, open, circular
- Acknowledgment
- Touch

- Restating
- Clarification
- Consensual validation
- Focusing
- Summarizing and planning
- Paraphrasing
- Reflection

of problems with the sender; and feeling as if the sender is dictating to the receiver. Another barrier today can be electronic communication when staff members are looking at their cell phones to read and send e-mails, text message, or using their laptops in meetings for more than note taking. These tools have improved communication, but they can also interfere with active listening as staff members multitask their way through meetings and as they work. Why is listening important other than to say it improves communication (McConnell, 2001; Fabre, 2005)?

- Listening helps us identify problems.
- Listening exposes feelings—those invaluable but sometimes inconvenient traits that make us human. We need to manage our feelings and give them a positive focus instead of denying them.
- Listening jump-starts the solution process because answers pop up during candid conversations.
- Listening relieves stress. Bottling up thoughts and feelings only depletes our energy.
- Active listening is more than hearing; it requires communicating to the other person that you are listening.
- Saying "yes" and "no" is not active listening.
- Paraphrasing communicates that you have listened; you share back what you have heard to make sure the message is clear.

Questioning can help to resolve some communication problems to get more information and open up the communication. An open-ended question is a question that requires a more extensive answer that a simple "yes," "no," or "I agree." Why is this type of question more effective in most cases than the closed question? Mainly because it expands and facilitates the dialogue between the sender and the receiver, allowing for greater exchange of information.

## Storytelling

**Storytelling** is a useful communication technique that can be used to clarify a confusing message, inspire others, and make communication more interesting. As Denning (2001) describes storytelling, he emphasizes that it is a way to get inside the minds of an organization's individuals and affect "how they think, worry, wonder, agonize, and dream about themselves and in the process create—and re-create—their organization" (p. xiv). Storytelling can be used in many situations, but it is particularly effective during times of change when innovation is needed. It supplements analytical thinking in organizations. Springboard stories are used to enable staff to move to the next level of understanding. As Denning notes, not all stories result in this type of effect. Typically, stories that have the perspective of a single protagonist who is in a predicament that is prototypical of the organization are the most successful. It needs to be familiar to the staff for it to be effective, and yet it must get their attention. When stories are told, they need to be brief and get to the point. Storytelling can be difficult, particularly if the audience is skeptical, but even under normal circumstances the storyteller, just like any sender of a message, must consider the situation, the receiver, and the nature of the message. It is to understand the purpose of communication, choose the right method and time while considering contextual factors, and above all adapt when cues are picked up indicating that the communication is not effective.

Storytelling is associated with Knowledge Management theory. With staff that is learning on the job; identification of knowledge gaps; staff research and analysis; and staff searching for knowledge from outside sources, there is a greater need for Knowledge Management, and then knowledge must be applied in the clinical setting. Storytelling can be used in the first phase of the creation of "cutting edge" knowledge, in the Knowledge Management system, and in the application of knowledge, which are all critical in today's health care environment.

## Information Technology and Communication

Information technology has become important in health care communication. It is used for organization, staff-staff, and staff-to-patient communication. This is done through the organization website, e-mail, and other methods such as smartphones. Hand-held devices are used in many hospitals to assist with communication. With the increased development of communication technology, there has also been an increase in problems that are encountered with this type of communication (for example, hackers, viruses, and multitasking). The information highway grows, and those who want to interfere with communication and productivity increase. Hackers who interfere with computer transmission and can break into secure information are of major concern for health care providers due to the need of maintaining records and patient information confidentiality. In addition, viruses can also destroy software and crucial databases of patient and organization information. Health care providers, like all who use or interact with computers, have experienced times when the "system was down" or inaccessible. This is a major problem in health care organizations when clinical staff needs this information and access to interactive communication to provide care. Back-up plans are clearly critical for every health care organization. Staff needs to be informed about these plans and when they should be used. Information technology has radically changed communication—personal and work-related. (See Chapter 18 for more information on technology and communication.)

TELEPHONE    The telephone is certainly the most basic of the technology options available today, and yet it continues to be a very important one. Use of cellular telephones is now the norm with growth in use of smartphones that have Internet connection and text messaging. Hospitals are giving their staff cell phones to use while at work so that they can be reached, working around paging systems. There are some simple reminders to improve the telephone communication method.

- Answer the phone with your name and title.
- When taking a message, repeat the information for the caller.
- With the increasing use of voice message systems, be prepared to leave a message.
- Keep emotions under control. Some callers may not be doing this and may say things that increase emotions. Stick to the point and get the information you need. If you do not have the answer, tell the caller you will return the call by a certain date/time or ask someone else to call.
- When you conclude a conversation that requires action, summarize the key issues and actions to be taken.
- Health care staff frequently receives calls that must be transferred. Check the number you are transferring to and tell the caller this number.

Voice mail has become so much a part of the workplace that it is easy to get frustrated when someone does not have voice mail or it is not working. This method can be used to send routine information and information that does not require a response. It can be used at any time and, in fact, is a method that is often used when the sender does not really want to talk to the receiver but rather just wants to get the message sent. When a message is left, clearly identify who is calling; from what location or organization, if relevant; date/time; purpose of call; and, if response is required, provide suggested times and method for a return communication. Callers need to speak slowly, repeating numbers and e-mail addresses. Some thought needs to be given to the message's content so that the caller does not appear confused and the message remains clear. Long messages should be avoided. If possible, identify good times to return the call. Confidentiality is important, so it is important to consider the message that is left and the nature of the message, which may be heard by others.

E-MAIL    Some organizations have e-mail policies and procedures, and these policies need to be communicated to staff members when they receive their e-mail addresses. One can never assume that work-related e-mail systems are private as the employer has the right to review e-mails in its e-mail system. E-mail etiquette has been developing over the years. It is easy to forget in the world of rapid-fire messaging that there are important legal and confidentiality issues that need to be considered. Use of patient names and other significant personal information or identifiers should not be used. Care needs to be taken when sending copyrighted material. As this requires permission, policies and procedures should be followed. Security within the organization's e-mail system is an important concern. Using passwords, not sharing passwords, and remembering that even when messages are deleted they may stay on the server and thus are accessible are factors that need to be reviewed with all staff. Organizations have policies about who may access sensitive information, and these policies must be followed. Some organizations have policies about using the organization's e-mail system for personal messages. Thought needs to be taken when writing messages, remembering that once they are sent they cannot be retrieved. E-mail is a good method for sending routine messages. The following are some e-mail etiquette guidelines.

- Remember that e-mail may not be read quickly so when the message is urgent a telephone call may be a better method. At a minimum, indicate the message is "urgent" or "priority" and request receipt reply.
- E-mail should be used thoughtfully. Sending too many messages that are unimportant may mean that important messages are ignored.
- Specify the subject in the subject line.
- It has become more acceptable to attach formal letters or resumes to an e-mail, but the sender should first inquire if this is acceptable such as contracts.
- Acronyms and emoticons (symbols) should not be used in business e-mails.
- Break up content by using paragraphing. This makes it easier to read. Use bulleting or numbering to highlight information. Put the most important information at the beginning of the message to ensure that it is read.
- Color can also be used for emphasis, but it should be used carefully. Some colors do not show up well on the screen. When printed, the message probably will be printed in black and white. Complex graphics should be avoided as they take longer to download such as graphic letterheads.
- When forwarding messages, include only relevant information from the original message to reduce the amount of reading required and length of time for receiving the message. The forwarded message should be clearly distinguished from the original message. When a message is forwarded consideration should be given as to who are the appropriate people to receive the message. The sender may not have intended for the message to be sent to others.
- When using reply, check to make sure that the reply message should go to all recipients automatically or just one recipient. A common error is to click "reply all" when really one only wants the message to go to one sender.
- There are times when a recipient may need more time to respond to a message; for example, to obtain more information. When this occurs, the recipient should acknowledge receipt of the message and indicate when a more detailed message will be sent.
- Not all messages sent via e-mail are received, and messages stating that there was a problem sending the message are not always sent. It is a good idea to ask the recipient to acknowledge receipt of important messages so that the sender can be sure the message was received.
- Use of virus protection is critical. Downloading messages, attachments, and information from the Internet is a good way for an entire system to get a virus, so it is important to make it a practice to check for viruses first.
- When an attachment is sent, double-check to see if the correct attachment is attached before hitting the send button. Another common problem is to say a document is attached and then forgetting to attach it. Extremely long attachments should be avoided unless the receiver has been consulted about the length.
- There is a tendency to ignore grammar, spelling, and so on in e-mails, but this should be considered in business related e-mails.
- Do not use all caps, as this indicates shouting (Milgram, Spector, & Treger, 1999).

**VIDEOCONFERENCING, WEBINAR, AND OTHER WEB-BASED CONFERENCING**   The advantage to **videoconferencing** is it is a live interaction with visual images while the communication takes place. It also can reduce costs and time as staff do not have to travel to another physical location. However, the initial cost of the equipment must be considered. Staff requires some training in the use of the equipment, but it is not difficult. Videoconferencing is also used in telehealth. One example of its use is in providing medical consultations between rural health care providers and academic medical centers. More common uses are for meetings and educational programs. Webinars and other types of Internet-based group communication systems are important today. They can save travel time and costs and yet keep staff and others in contact and able to work collaboratively.

WEB PAGES    Web pages are very common today; most organizations have them. They are used by organizations to communicate to a broad audience such as staff, patients, families, health care providers, consumers, the public, and so on. They need to be designed carefully with consideration given to ease of use, accuracy, timeliness and current information, level of information that might require secure entry, ethics of advertising on the page, and graphics and audio, which often take time to open. Nursing staff should be involved in the development of web pages and consider what should be included that would be helpful to the nursing staff and the care they provide. Pages can be useful in sharing patient and family health prevention education material, contact information for questions and further information, guidance for admission preparation, links to reliable websites that can provide additional information, and support information (for example, related to cancer, diabetes, arthritis, new mothers, breastfeeding, and many other health issues). It is critical that the Web page is monitored and updated. Responsibility for the monitoring needs to be clearly defined. If information is not current, this acts as a barrier to effective communication.

SOCIAL NETWORKING    There is rapid growth of social networking methods through the Internet. Facebook and other types of methods are used by participants to post information and connect with others who have similar interests. How this will be used in work settings is still unknown but no doubt will be used more. Twitter is another type of short Internet communicating method that has grown rapidly. Staff needs to be careful about using work-related content on social networking websites as this is not acceptable and can lead to problems.

## Resolving Communication Problems and Improving Communication

The nurse manager plays a critical role in setting the tone for communication and maintaining open communication channels so that staff can do its work and patient care outcomes can be reached. The manager must continuously assess the communication climate to ensure that it supports effective communication. Marrelli (2004) identifies the manager's role in defining values and setting goals, including the following:

- Initiating and facilitating discussion to elicit clarification of values
- Recording written value statements, seeking staff feedback, and incorporating revisions into the organizational review process
- Initiating discussion of goals at the unit and individual levels with the staff that the manager directly supervises
- Bringing pertinent directives, regulations, accreditation standards, or other factors needing consideration to the discussion
- Recording written goals and action plans for achieving them
- Maintaining momentum of progress toward goals, giving positive and constructive feedback to promote progress toward meeting deadlines
- Communicating to staff the progress toward goals through the use of visual tools

Asking others for feedback about their communication needs is helpful, and this information should be considered carefully. Include an assessment of nonverbal communication as it can make the difference between effective and non-effective communication. Specific methods that can be used to improve communication when it occurs are increased use of paraphrasing, reflection, and summarization. When paraphrasing is used, a person restates what another person has said and asks for confirmation of what was said. The focus is on facts, and the statement should be short. Reflection focuses on the speaker's feelings, and the receiver of the message restates what the receiver thinks are the feelings expressed. Again, this is done for confirmation. Summarization combines content and feelings, by restating both of these elements for confirmation. Additional strategies that can be used to improve staff communication include the following:

- Communicate the "why" behind the "what."
- Realize that effective communication takes time.

- Accept negative news as information and do not take it personally.
- Respond non-defensively when people express differing or contradictory ideas and views.
- Report situations as accurately as possible and avoid downplaying negative factors.
- Send important organizational messages by at least two methods (for example, e-mail and a written memo or verbally and written).
- Do not rely so much on written communication as people often do not read it.
- Use active listening in all conversations.
- Select the location for discussing sensitive issues carefully.
- Say what you mean; avoid assumptions and ensure that the receiver has less need to turn to assumptions.
- Validate to ensure that what has been said has been heard and understood.
- Stress can interfere with communication, while managing stress can improve communication.
- Use appropriate eye contact.
- State information clearly backed up with research to get to the facts.
- Think before speaking.
- State that you do not have the information you need and that you will look for the information and follow up.
- Summarize at the end of a lengthy conversation and ask for confirmation from the other party.
- Use "I" statements, which are more effective than "you" statements and tend to put the other person on the offensive.
- Thank others for their feedback and suggestions as this recognizes they have been heard and supports further communication.
- Provide credible information; trust can make or break how a message is received and interpreted.
- Select the time to communicate carefully when difficult questions must be asked or there is a difficult discussion; a time when the other person (receiver) might be more receptive.

Different people have different ways or styles of communication. Box 13-4 provides information about aggressive, passive, and assertive styles of communication. Recognizing ones style will help to improve communication and to use the most effective approach to communication.

Communication is complex and requires that staff use a thoughtful process to communicate effectively. It is something that is used daily in practice and management, and often is not viewed as important until there is a problem with it. Throughout this text, communication is a driving element for effective managers who are leaders.

---

## BOX 13-4    AGGRESSIVE, PASSIVE, AND ASSERTIVE STYLES

### AGGRESSIVE

- Loud, heated, arguing
- Physically violent encounters
- Blaming, name-calling, and verbal insults
- Walking out of arguments before they are resolved
- Being demanding: "Do this"

### PASSIVE

- Concealing one's own feelings
- Denying one's own anger
- Feeling that one has no right to express anger
- Avoiding arguments
- Being noncommittal: "You don't have to do this unless you really want to . . ."

### ASSERTIVE

- Expressing feelings without being nasty or overbearing
- Acknowledge emotions but staying open to discussion
- Expressing self and giving others the chance to express themselves equally
- Using "I" statements to defuse arguments
- Asking and giving reasons: "I would appreciate it if you would do this, and here's why . . ."

Source: Katz, J. (2001). *Keys to nursing success.* Upper Saddle River, NJ: Prentice Hall, p. 267. Reprinted with permission.

# APPLYING LEADERSHIP AND MANAGEMENT

### MY HOSPITAL UNIT

You are concerned as several staff has complained that there is poor communication on your unit. They do not feel that staff is sharing and that there is poor communication among nurses and the interprofessional teams. You had not noticed this and are concerned that you missed the signals of a problem. What might you do to better ensure that you are on top of and ahead of problems like this in the future? What can you do to improve this situation? Describe the steps you would take. Consider how you would involve staff. Use the virtual unit site found on the textbook website to record the work that you do in the role of nurse manager for your unit.

## Critical Thinking Questions and Activities

1. When communication problems are analyzed, it is important to look at all of the process's components: the sender, the message, the receiver, feedback, and the context. Assessment of communication should include these factors with the understanding that communication is rarely perfect. This chapter has discussed many of the elements associated with the communication process. If you were a team leader, what might you routinely include in your assessment of the team's communication? Develop a checklist of critical elements to assess.

2. How might you apply the guidelines found in Box 13-2? Reflect on an experience that you have had with feedback. Describe whether or not the guidelines for giving constructive criticism or feedback were used. Describe whether or not you used any of the coping techniques. If not, how did you cope?

3. To determine whether you are primarily passive, aggressive, or assertive, read the following sentences and list the ones that sound like something you would say to a peer (Katz, 2001).

> *Get me the keys.*
> *Would you mind if I stepped out just for a second?*
> *Don't slam the door.*
> *I'd appreciate it if you would have this done by two o'clock.*
> *I think maybe it needs a little work just at the end, but I'm not sure.*
> *Please take this back to the library.*
> *You will have a good time if you join us.*
> *Your loss.*
> *I don't know, if you think so. I'll try it.*
> *Let me know what you want me to do.*
> *Turn it this way and see what happens.*
> *We'll try both our ideas and see what happens.*
> *I want it on my desk by the end of the day.*
> *Just do what I told you.*
> *If this isn't how you wanted it to look, I can change it. Just tell me and I'll do it.*

Now check out how these statements would be classified. Are you surprised by any of the classifications and why?

1. Aggressive communicators would be likely to use sentences 1, 3, 8, 13, and 14.
2. Passive communicators would probably opt for sentences 2, 5, 9, 10, and 15.
3. Assertive communicators would probably choose sentences 4, 6, 7, 11, and 12.

4. Errors in health care delivery are a serious concern as has been noted in the Institute of Medicine report, *To Err Is Human* (1999). Interview a nurse team leader or a nurse manager and ask for examples of errors that have occurred. What are they? Are the examples related to ineffective communication? If so, in what way? How could future similar errors be prevented? What is the health care organization doing to improve communication?

## Media Links

- **URL: http://www.nwlink.com/~Donclark/leader/leadcom.html**
  Communication and Leadership
- **URL: http://www.aachonline.org/**
  American Academy on Healthcare Communication
- **URL: http://www.ihi.org/IHI/Topics/PerinatalCare/PerinatalCareGeneral/ EmergingContent/SBARTechniqueforCommunication.htm**
  SBAR Technique for Communication
- **URL: http://www.healthypeople.gov/document/HTML/Volume1/11HealthCom.htm**
  *Healthy People* and Communication

**Pearson Nursing Student Resources**

Find additional review materials at
**nursing.pearsonhighered.com**

Prepare for success with additional NCLEX®-style practice questions, interactive assignments and activities, Web links, animations and videos, and more!

## References

American Nurses Association. (2004). *Nursing: Scope and standards of practice.* Silver Spring, MD: Author.

American Nurses Association. (2009). *Nursing ADMINISTRATION: Scope and standards of practice.* Silver Spring, MD: Author.

Denning, S. (2001). *The springboard. How storytelling ignites action in knowledge-era organizations.* Boston: Butterworth-Heinemann.

Dessler, G. (2002). *Management.* Upper Saddle River, NJ: Prentice Hall.

Fabre, J. (2005). *Smart nursing.* NY: Springer.

Finkelman, A. (1996). *Psychiatric nursing administration manual.* Gaithersburg, MD: Aspen Publishers, Inc.

Finkelman, A., & Kenner, C. (2010). *Professional nursing concepts. Competencies for quality leadership.* Boston: Jones and Bartlett Publishers.

Gebelein, S., et al. (2000). *Successful manager's handbook.* Minneapolis, MN: Personnel Decisions International Corp.

Institute of Medicine. (1999). *To err is human.* Washington, DC: National Academies Press.

Institute of Medicine. (2003a). *Health professions education.* Washington, DC: National Academies Press.

Institute of Medicine. (2003b). *Unequal treatment.* Washington, DC: National Academies Press.

Joint Commission. (2007). "What did the doctor say?" Improving health literacy to protect patient safety. Retrieved September 5, 2009, from http://www .jointcommission.org/NewsRoom/ PressKits/Health_Literacy/

Katz, J. (2001). *Keys to nursing success.* Upper Saddle River, NJ: Prentice Hall.

Mansur, J. (2010). Enhanced medication safety. Retrieved May 30, 2010, from http://www .jcrinc.com/Enhanced-Medication-Safety/

McConnell, E. (2001, April). *About communicating clearly.* Retrieved April 6, 2010, from http://www.findarticles.com/ cf_0/m3231/4_31/74091631/pring.jhtml

Marrelli, T. (2004). *The nurse manager's survival guide.* St. Louis, MO: Mosby-Year Book, Inc.

Milgram, L., Spector, A., & Treger, M. (1999). *Managing smart.* Houston, TX: Cashman Dudley.

Robbins, S., & Decenzo, D. (2001). *Fundamentals of Management.* Upper Saddle River, NJ: Prentice Hall.

Sullivan, E. (2004). *Becoming influential. A guide for nurses.* Upper Saddle River, NJ: Prentice Hall.

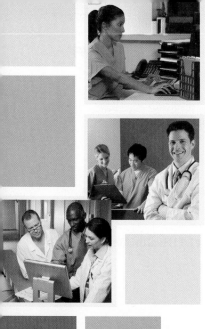

# 14

# Delegation for Effective Outcomes

## CHAPTER OUTLINE

## LEARNING OUTCOMES

Before you begin, take a moment to familiarize yourself with the learning outcomes for this chapter.

- Define delegation.
- Critique the benefits of using delegation.
- Examine key legal issues related to delegation.
- Compare and contrast responsibility, authority, and accountability as they apply to delegation.
- Apply the delegation process in clinical situations when unlicensed assistive personnel are used.
- Assess methods to monitor and improve delegation to reach effective patient outcomes.

## KEY TERMS

- Accountability
- Assignment
- Authority
- Competent
- Delegatee
- Delegation
- Delegator
- Perform
- Standards of practice
- Supervision
- Unlicensed assistive personnel (UAP)
- Vicarious liability/ Respondeat superior

**WHAT'S AHEAD**

With today's emphasis on teams, collaboration, and coordination in the health care system (Institute of Medicine 2001; 2003) and a more diverse workforce, any type of leadership position eventually requires the use of delegation to ensure that the job gets done and that effective patient outcomes are met. Delegation should be focused on the patient—what is best to ensure quality patient care. Not only do nurse managers need to use delegation, but nurses in staff positions must also use delegation daily. Delegation makes the best use of the talents and expertise of all staff as it facilitates the organization's work. To perform delegation effectively, nurses need to develop competencies in delegation and supervision. As has been discussed in several chapters in this text, no one person can do it all. Delegation is essential to productive organizations, and every manager has to delegate. However, all registered nurses delegate as a part of their practice to ensure that care is effective and efficient.

# Delegation: What Is It?

It seems like there should be a simple definition for delegation, but it is not a simple process. First, delegation can relate to assigning a specific task, a range of tasks, a major job such as a project, or leadership of a team. The American Nurses Association (ANA) definition of delegation is "The transfer of responsibility for the performance of a task from one individual to another while retaining accountability for the outcome. Example: the RN, in delegating a task to an assistive individual, transfers the responsibility for the performance of the task but retains professional accountability for the overall care" (American Nurses Association, 2005, p. 4). Registered nurses must consider delegation carefully in their roles to protect patients and advocate for them (American Nurses Association, 2004).

Typically, what drives a leader or a staff nurse to use delegation is simply that he or she cannot do it all. "Delegation, in one sense, is a paradox: The manager who delegates and develops employees to make and take responsibility for decisions begins the process of eliminating the need for a manager" although typically it never gets to the point of no management (Grohar-Murray & DiCroce, 2003, p. 173). The nursing process is the domain of the RN; the following describes how this impacts delegation related to what part of the process can be delegated (American Nurses Association, 2005):

- Assessment: No, because input is solicited
- Diagnosis: No, because this requires professional nursing knowledge and experience
- Planning: No, because input is solicited
- Intervention: Yes, with supervision
- Evaluation: No, because input is solicited

Some key terms are important to consider as one discusses delegation (American Nurses Association, 2005). The **delegator** is the person who does the delegation, and the **delegatee** is the person who receives the delegation. **Supervision** plays a major role in delegation. This involves guidance or direction, including evaluation and follow-up provided by the delegator to the delegatee. Although delegation may include delegation to many different types of staff including the **unlicensed assistive personnel (UAP)**, much of this discussion will focus on delegation to UAP who are "individuals who are trained to function in an assistive role to the licensed registered nurse in providing patient care activities as delegated by the RN regardless of the title of the individual to whom nursing tasks are delegated. The term includes, but is not limited to, nurses' aides, medication aides, orderlies and attendants or technicians" (American Nurses Association, 2005, p. 4).

## Benefits of Delegation

Delegation offers many benefits to the organization and to the staff. "Delegation is a process that, used appropriately, can result in safe and effective nursing care. Delegation can free the nurse for attending more complex patient care needs, develop the skills of nursing assistive personnel and promote cost containment for the healthcare organization" (American Nurses Association and the National Council of State Boards of Nursing, 2005, p. 4). Cost-effectiveness is one benefit when resources, including staff, are used appropriately. There is a potential cost savings. Clearly, there can be time-savings as activities are allocated among others; thereby, multiplying the ability to get work done more efficiently. Professional growth can occur when staff members are challenged to develop new skills as they take on new opportunities. The delegator, who might be a manager, team leader, or staff nurse, has the opportunity to grow as new skills are learned, more time is available to do other activities, and so on. When delegation is done in a thoughtful manner, the environment is typically one in which staff feels valued and trusted.

Delegation has always been present in nursing and, at different points in its history, it has been more important than others. With the increasing use of UAP, delegation is now a skill that every nurse must have and use effectively. This includes newly licensed nurses, as it is difficult even for new nurses to avoid delegation in any health care setting. **Delegation** is *"transferring* to a *competent* individual *authority* to *perform* a selected nursing task in a *selected* situation. The nurse retains accountability for the delegation" (National Council of State Boards of Nursing, 2005, p. 4). The italicized words in this definition are key to successful delegation. *Transferring* implies a process as well as indicates that it is something the nurse would do but is giving the responsibility to someone else. **Competent** means the person who will do the task has the required skills and experience. The nurse must be able to determine that the staff member can do the task. **Authority** or the power to act is given to the staff person. **Perform** means that some action must take place, and this action is described as a selected nursing task in a selected situation. The nurse must tell the staff member what is to be done. It is important that the RN delegate with thought—considering what needs to be delegated and who is qualified to complete the task or activity. The RN will most likely not be present when the work is done.

## Legal Issues Related to Delegation

Decisions the nurse makes must be consistent with law, for example the nurse cannot delegate a task to another if that staff member is not allowed by law to perform that task (American Nurses Association, 2005). The state practice act is the legal guide for RNs and delegation.

Critical legal issues and factors that impact delegation are state boards of nursing, scope of practice and nurse practice acts, labor unions, and standards of care. Each one of these issues affects the "who," "what," "when," and "how" of delegation. Every nurse is responsible for knowing how these factors might affect delegation. The legal authority for delegation comes from state laws and regulations. State statute or law establishes the state board of nursing.

The nursing board in each state is the governing body that ensures the safe practice of nursing is provided to its citizens. Note that the focus is on the patient, not the nurse. The board in each state is also involved in approving the schools of nursing and granting and revoking licenses. Both of these functions are done to ensure the safe practice of nursing. The board regulates nursing practice, although states vary in how this is implemented. The critical issue is the state's nurse practice act. Disciplinary process and related actions are also taken by boards to ensure safe practice. The National Council for State Boards of Nursing (NCSBN), as the umbrella organization for all state boards, is also involved in delegation. It provides guidance to the state boards on practice issues such as delegation. The nurse practice act of each state and its associated rules and regulations represent the law that every nurse needs to know. The law's associated rules and regulations are also important. The scope of practice is described in the practice act, providing the "legal framework of practice" (Hansten & Jackson, 2009). The law itself may appear to be very general, and it usually is. This is why it is important to also be aware of the related rules and regulations, which tell how the law is to be implemented. Every registered nurse needs to know what is in the scope of practice and the legal limits. In addition, every registered nurse needs to know what certified and unlicensed personnel can do. Position descriptions within health care organizations are critical, but they cannot conflict with guidelines developed by the board of nursing. Nurses are responsible for knowing when a job description might conflict with board regulations. One cannot say "I followed the job description" when it does not meet state requirements related to what tasks can be delegated, to whom, and when. The board of nursing is also responsible for clearly describing the principles related to delegation or what is expected of nurses in the state when they delegate.

Nurses can contact their state board of nursing and request a copy of the state's nurse practice act. In addition, the Internet makes it easy to learn more about boards of nursing and related issues. What questions should registered nurses ask when learning about their state laws and regulations pertaining to delegation?

- What activities can be delegated, or what activities cannot be delegated?
- How is delegation defined?
- Does the nurse practice act specify certain tasks for delegation or list any that cannot be delegated?
- Does it authorize delegation based on certain circumstances?
- Does it describe the UAP role?
- What does supervision mean in the state?
- How much supervision must be given when delegation occurs?
- Does the nurse practice act indicate the consequences of inappropriate delegation?
- Does it provide guidelines for reducing delegation risks (Fisher, 2000, p. 58)?

**Standards of practice** are also important documents, although not legal documents. Why would standards be discussed under legal issues related to delegation? When delegation occurs, the tasks performed must meet the standards of practice, as well as the organization's policies and procedures. Nurses are expected to know what these are and how they apply. The RN takes responsibility and accountability for individual nursing practice and determines the appropriate delegation of tasks consistent with the nurse's obligation to provide optimum patient care (Code of Ethics for Nurses with Interpretive Statements, ANA, 2009). Registered nurses may delegate certain nursing tasks to licensed practical/vocational nurses (LPN/LVNs) and UAP. Some states allow LPN/LVNs to delegate certain tasks within their scope of practice to UAP. What happens if the nurse's employer wants tasks delegated when the nurse does not think that this delegation is appropriate (for example, the delegatee is unable to do the task safely)? Using professional judgment through the application of the nursing process and the delegation process, the nurse must act as the patient's advocate by only delegating action that is appropriate for the patient. This also means that the organization cannot just have a list of tasks that can be delegated, because nursing judgment and nursing process must also be applied to the delegation process. If the nurse does not use professional judgment and delegates when it is inappropriate, even if told to do this by supervisors, the nurse is still accountable for errors in delegation. This might result in disciplinary action from the board of nursing and increase liability concerns (American Nurses Association, 2005). Liability means the person/RN is legally responsible for one's own professional practice and for those actions that are delegated. "Nurse managers have a legal duty to know what tasks are within the scope of their state's nurse practice act, the scope of practice of their staff members, and most important of the competency of the staff member to complete the assigned task. In addition, if nurse managers breach the standard of care for either of those duties, the nurse may be held negligent if any harm results from the acts of the subordinate" (Grohar-Murray & DiCroce, 2003, pp. 174–175).

If there is an issue of malpractice, the nurse practice act and standards may be used to support a case or dispute it. One might ask if the organization itself has any liability when there are problems with delegation that is done by its staff? "The legal principle of corporate liability involves an agency's legal duty to provide appropriate facilities, staff, safety, and equipment in the delivery of a service offered to the public" (Grohar-Murray & DiCroce, 2003, p. 175). The organization does have some liability. In addition to this principle, the organization is also responsible based on the principle of **vicarious liability** or *respondeat superior*. This means the organization is responsible for the acts of its employees when they are performing their job. "The failure to delegate and supervise within acceptable standards of professional nursing practice may be seen as malpractice" (Guido, 2001, p. 340). "The degree of knowledge concerning the skills and competencies of those one supervises is of paramount importance. The doctrine of 'knew or should have known' becomes a legal standard in delegating tasks to licensed individuals whom one supervises" (Guido, 2001, p. 340). The delegator does need to determine if the staff member has the ability to do the job or task—known as assessment of competency. However, when staff delegate to UAP or LPN/LVNs, the staff nurse as well as nurse manager need to supervise the work.

Supervision is the "active process of directing, guiding, and influencing the outcome of an individual's performance of an activity" (American Nurses Association, 2005). Supervision may be direct or indirect, with indirect meaning the RN is not present during the performance of the activity and supervision does not include direct observation. Effective supervision strategies with UAP include being clear about what has to be done and when, providing clear directions and asking if the UAP understands what needs to be done, and following up on the performance of the activity to monitor outcomes. The UPA needs to know what should be reported and when. This feedback might include verbal, written, observation, and review of records (Finkelman & Kenner, 2010). Trusting another staff member to complete a task can be difficult, especially for nurses with less experience, but it is important to learn how to do this—to trust others and trust oneself in the delegation decision.

## Critical Delegation Issues: Authority, Responsibility, and Accountability

As was discussed in Chapter 4, organization structure illustrates how work is assigned and describes relationships among staff by identifying authority, responsibility, and accountability. The assignment of work and delegation are closely tied to the organization's structure. The scalar chain that describes the organizational chart with vertical lines and how employees are responsible to one another is an important resource to learn more about authority. "Chief nursing officers are accountable for establishing systems to assess, monitor, verify and communicate ongoing competence requirements in areas related to delegation, both for RNs and delegates" (American Nurses Association, 2005, p. 7). The chief nursing officers include the CNO or Vice President for Nursing Services, to overall administrator for nursing in the organization, and all nurse managers who supervise staff and service units (American Nurses Association, 2009). They all have a connection through accountability and authority when individual nursing staff delegate. **Accountability** identifies who is answerable for what has been done. How is this different from responsibility? A nurse delegates a task to the nursing assistant. The nursing assistant is responsible for his or her performance, and the nurse is accountable for the decision to delegate and to whom to delegate (Hansten & Jackson, 2009). The delegator must take accountability seriously, and this involves identifying the best person for the task or job (American Nurses Association, 2005). Although this is not always easy to determine, it must be done thoughtfully. For example, can a UAP delegate to an RN or LVN? No, this cannot be done. A key question is whether or not the task or job is within the position description of the delegatee and whether the delegator is allowed to delegate the task or job. Overlapping accountability by having more than one person responsible often leads to problems unless this is very clear and both parties are aware of this potential overlap. There are, however, times when shared accountability is appropriate. When this is used, the same principles that are used for individual accountability need to be defined. The American Nurses Association (2005) defines it as "the state of being responsible or answerable. Nurses, as members of a knowledge-based health profession and as licensed health care professionals, must answer to patients, nursing employers, the board of nursing and the civil and criminal court system when the quality of patient care provided is compromised or when allegations of unprofessional, unethical, illegal, unacceptable or inappropriate nursing conduct, actions or responses arise" (p. 4). **Responsibility** is important. It is "the obligation involved when one accepts an assignment" (Kelly-Heidenthal & Marthaler, 2005, p. 9). **Authority** is the "right to act or command the action of others" (Kelly-Heidenthal & Marthaler, 2005, p. 9). A nurse gets authority with his or her job position and is influenced by the state nurse practice act. Concern about autonomy or the right to make a decision and control can best be illustrated in the following two questions:

1. How much authority is the delegatee able to exercise when doing the task/job without referring back to the delegator?
2. How far should the delegator exercise direct influence over the work of the delegatee (Heller, 1998, p. 6)?

Delegation requires thought, and it also requires that the delegator use assessment, critical thinking, and consideration of accountability, authority, and also responsibility. Responsibility can be applied when delegation is assigned. The delegator is responsible for selecting the best person to do the job, explaining the task thoroughly, and validating that the delegatee understands what needs to be done. When authority is given during delegation, knowledge about the job needs to be shared. Others within the organization who need to be informed about which staff members are assigned the delegated task or job should also be told. Resources need to be assigned. Letting the delegatee control the job or task is part of giving the appropriate level of authority. In establishing accountability, the delegator identifies deadlines, feedback time periods, and evaluation criteria, with emphasis on success. If the organization has labor unions, this will affect delegation. Why is this so? Union contracts typically cover issues that are important to delegation such as staffing, safety, work schedules, seniority, and a grievance procedure (Hansten & Jackson, 2009).

The ANA and the NCSBN in a joint statement identify the key delegation principles applicable to all registered nurses (2006, pp. 2–3).

- The RN takes responsibility and accountability for the provision of nursing practice.
- The RN directs care and determines the appropriate utilization of any assistant involved in providing direct patient care.
- The RN may delegate components of care but does not delegate the nursing process itself. Nursing judgment cannot be delegated.
- The decision of whether or not to delegate or assign is based upon the RN's judgment concerning the condition of the patient, the competence of all members of the nursing team, and the degree of supervision that will be required of the RN if a task is delegated.
- The RN delegates only those tasks for which he or she believes the other health care worker has the knowledge and skill to perform, taking into consideration training, cultural competence, experience, and facility/agency policies and procedures.
- The RN individualizes communication regarding delegation to the nursing assistive personnel and patient situation, and the communication should be clear, concise, correct, and complete. The RN verifies comprehension with the nursing assistive personnel and that the assistant accepts the delegation and the responsibility that accompanies it.
- Communication must be a two-way process. Nursing assistive personnel should have the opportunity to ask questions and/or for clarification of expectations.
- The RN uses critical thinking and professional judgment when applying the five rights of delegation.
- Chief Nursing Officers are accountable for establishing systems to assess, monitor, verify, and communicate ongoing comprehensive requirements in areas related to delegation.
- There is both individual accountability and organizational accountability for delegation.
- Organizational accountability for delegation relates to providing sufficient resources.

## Delegation and Unlicensed Assistive Personnel

There is no doubt that UAP are used in many health care organizations; in fact, there are about 65 different job titles for this position, which only confuses the matter more (American Operating Room Nurses, 2005; Oncology Nurses Society, 2007; Zimmerman, 2002). In addition to title differences, there are no universal hiring, training, or job descriptions. Consistency is definitely a problem. As nurses move from setting to setting it is critical that they make sure they understand these differences. There can even be variations from specialty areas or units within the same organization.

With the increasing use of UAP in all types of settings such as acute care, home health care, and long-term care, patients are encountering a variety of staff as they receive care. Patients are also often unsure of the roles even if they know the job title. They are not able to describe the differences between the roles and responsibilities of an RN and UAP. Nursing has a social responsibility and moral mandate to provide care (American Nurses Association, 2009). Uniforms often do not help to clarify differences; even name tags can be unclear and difficult for patients to read.

## The Delegation Process and the NCSBN Guidelines

When delegation is considered, it is important to note that not all tasks or activities should be delegated. How does one determine what might be delegated? Management is involved is setting the health care organization standards and processes, which should reflect the state board of nursing nurse practice act and professional nursing standards. This information should be included in orientation and in staff education on a routine basis to ensure that staff is current in its understanding of delegation. In addition, the following key questions should be asked as the delegation process begins.

1. What is the task or job to be delegated? Consider the complexity and skills that are required for the task or job. Is it clear what needs to be accomplished?
2. To whom should the task or job be delegated? Consider if the delegatee has the skills and time to perform the task or job effectively.
3. How should the task or job be assigned? Consider how much information and explanation needs to be given to the delegatee.
4. How often and in what depth should the delegator follow-up to see that the task or job has been performed effectively?

What activities and tasks can be delegated? Activities and tasks that frequently occur are considered technical by nature, are considered standard and unchanging, have predictable results, and have minimal potential for risks are the typical type of task that is delegated (American Nurses Association, 2005). Box 14-1 identifies the five rights of delegation. Box 14-2 provides some criteria that can be used to determine when to delegate.

Hansten and Jackson (2009) describe delegation as a cyclical process, similar to the nursing process, which includes the following steps:

1. The assessment phase focuses on knowing your world, which includes your practice area and your organization; knowing yourself, your strengths and limitations; and knowing your delegatee. The last element requires that the delegator know the delegatee's competency level and motivation. Neither of these is easy to assess, but both are critical to ensure patient safety and quality of care.
2. The plan requires that you know what needs to be done. If you do not, you will not be able to clearly define the task for the staff member or delegatee. This requires that you have professional and technical skills as well as acknowledge the importance of customer service.
3. Intervention means that you are able to prioritize and match the job to the staff member. Communication, which includes the initial directions and follow-up, plays a critical role. If the delegator does not understand what needs to be done, when, where, to whom, and how, then the task will not be completed as expected. Conflicts and errors may increase during the process, which require collaboration and negotiation.
4. Evaluation is ongoing throughout the delegation process. You need to know how to give constructive feedback as it can be a powerful motivator. Evaluation does require problem solving, particularly if the results or outcomes were not what you expected. Supervision is part of evaluation.

---

**BOX 14-1     FIVE RIGHTS OF DELEGATION**

I. Right Task: One that is delegable for a specific patient or situation.

II. Right Circumstances: Appropriate setting, available resources, and other relevant factors considered.

III. Right Person: Right person is delegating the right task to the right person to be performed by the right person.

IV. Right Direction/Communication: Clear, concise description of the task, including its objective, limits, and expectations.

V. Right Supervision: Appropriate monitoring, evaluation, intervention (as needed), and feedback.

Source: American Nurses Association. (2005). *Principles of delegation.* Silver Spring, MD: Author.

## BOX 14-2  TO DELEGATE OR NOT

The following are some criteria that are used to determine if one should delegate an activity or a task.

- Patient's condition, including complications and stability
- Complexity of the assessment
- Intricacy of the task
- Repetitiveness of the task
- Capabilities of the UAP
- Amount of technology required
- Infection control and safety precautions
- Potential for harm
- Level of supervision that the RN will need to provide
- Predictability of outcome

- Extent of patient interaction
- Environment

Sources: Summarized by author from Yoder-Wise, P. (2007). *Leading and managing in nursing* (4th ed.). St. Louis, MO: Mosby; Zimmerman, P. Delegating to unlicensed assistive personnel. Nursing Spectrum Career Fitness Online Retrieved November 5, 2002, from http://nsweb.nursingspectrum.com/ce/ce124 .htm; American Nurses Association. (2005). *Principles of delegation.* Silver Spring, MD: Author; American Nurses Association & National Council of State Boards of Nursing. (2006). *Joint statement on delegation.* Retrieved from https://www.ncsbn.org/ Joint_statement.pdf; Hansten, R. & Jackson, M. (2009). *Clinical delegation skills.* (4th ed.). Boston: Jones and Bartlett Publishers.

Selection of staff or the delegatee is an important part of the delegation process. Selecting a staff member to do a task who will be honest when they need help or if they have questions or concerns is paramount to successful delegation. Staff that takes initiative can be good choices for some tasks. Staff that is analytical, organized, and able to look at problems carefully will also be more successful. It is easy to fall into the trap of making decisions about delegation too quickly. Sometimes a situation calls for a quick decision; however, whenever possible, it is best to take time and be as objective as possible. Some tasks, activities, or projects may require that the selected staff obtain additional training to do the delegated work. If this is the case, it should be provided; this is an investment, and it will help the organization reach its goals. This training needs to be planned and directed at the needs.

Monitoring progress of a delegable task, activity, or project can be difficult. Too much or too little monitoring may get in the way of success. Heller (1998) identifies some "Do's" and "Don'ts" that can help during the monitoring phase of the delegation process.

### Do's

- Do encourage all delegatees to make their own decisions when appropriate.
- Do move from hands-on to hands-off as soon as possible.
- Do intervene when absolutely necessary, but only at that time.
- Do ask delegatees if they feel thoroughly prepared for the task.

### Don'ts

- Don't say or hint that you doubt the delegatee's ability.
- Don't miss any stage in the briefing process.
- Don't surreptitiously take back a task.
- Don't place seniority above ability.
- Don't deny a delegatee the chance to learn by interfering too much (p. 37).

Monitoring methods that might be used include observation, verbal feedback, written feedback, review of records such as medical records and other standard records, and e-mail. During monitoring it is important to praise and reward delegates. Finding something positive to comment on is important even when progress may not be all that was hoped for. Recognizing effort sometimes goes by the wayside because it is taken for granted. There are times when difficulties are identified during monitoring. How should the delegator handle these difficulties? The first step is to analyze the difficulties before jumping to conclusions. Then talk to the delegatee in a nonthreatening manner. Getting the delegatee engaged in solving the problem can be used to help the delegatee improve and also feel a commitment to assisting in problem solution. There are some circumstances where performance is an issue, and in this case, the organization's procedure for performance evaluation and documentation should be followed. The nurse manager would need to lead this process or whoever is the delegatee's supervisor.

## APPLYING EVIDENCE-BASED PRACTICE

### Evidence for Effective Leadership and Management

**Citation:** Bittner, N., & Gravlin, G. (2009). Critical thinking, delegation, and missed care in nursing practice. *JONA, 39*(3), 142–146.

**Overview:** This qualitative, descriptive study examined how nurses use critical thinking to delegate nursing care. Data were collected from twenty-seven medical-surgical registered nurses who participated in focus groups, which were recorded. The focus group participants were asked to describe clinical situations in which they were involved in delegation. Emphasis was placed on describing the delegation process and a successful and unsuccessful delegation experience and to discuss care omissions. The results indicate that prior to delegating the nurses considered patient condition, competency, experience, and workload of unlicensed assistive personnel (UAP) and the nurses expected unlicensed assistive personnel (UAP) to report significant findings and to have higher level knowledge, including assessment and prioritizing skills. The nurses felt that successful delegation was dependent on the relationship between the RN and the UAP, communication, system support, and nursing leadership. Participants reported frequent instances of missed or omitted routine care.

**Application:** Delegation is a complex process that includes using critical thinking and also clinical reasoning and judgment. More emphasis needs to be placed on understanding the process and also using methods to teach delegation. Ineffective delegation has an impact—on patient outcomes, staff morale, and costs of care. Managers delegate daily, but they also need to help their staff improve their delegation.

**Questions:**

1. *Discuss the relationship of critical thinking to delegation. How does clinical reasoning and judgment fit in?*

2. *What is your opinion of the following result: "…expected unlicensed assistive personnel (UAP) to report significant findings and have higher level knowledge, including assessment and prioritizing skills"? What impact does this have?*

3. *If you were a nurse manager and you recognize that care omission is a serious problem on your unit, what would you do to correct this problem?*

## Effective Delegation

### Assessment of the Delegation Process

The delegation process, like other processes, is fluid and thus must be frequently assessed as to its quality. Are the steps followed? What are the outcomes—for the patient and staff members, the team, unit, and the organization? It is important to understand what effective delegation is. Figure 14-1 provides a description of the delegation process.

### Characteristics of Effective Delegation

Effective delegation requires that the delegator have delegation skills as delegation is not simple. Elements essential for effective delegation include (American Nurses Association, 2005, p. 12):

1. Emphasis on professional nursing practice
2. Definition of delegation, based on the nurse practice act and regulations
3. Review of specific sections of the law and regulations regarding delegation; identification of disciplinary actions related to inappropriate delegation
4. Emphasis on tasks/functions that cannot be delegated nor routinely delegated
5. Focus on RN judgment for task analysis and decision to delegate
6. Determination of the degree of supervision required for delegation
7. Identification of guidelines for lowering risk related to delegation
8. Development of feedback mechanisms to ensure that task is completed and to receive updated data to evaluate the outcome.

**FIGURE 14-1** **National Council of State Boards of Nursing Decision Tree for Delegation to Nursing Assistive Personnel.**

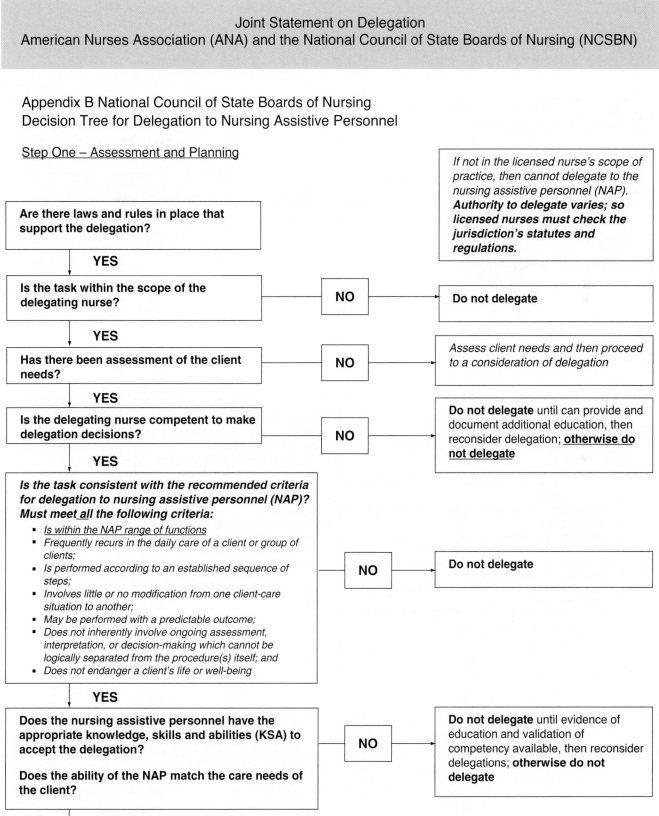

Joint Statement on Delegation
American Nurses Association (ANA) and the National Council of State Boards of Nursing (NCSBN)

Appendix B National Council of State Boards of Nursing
Decision Tree for Delegation to Nursing Assistive Personnel

Step One – Assessment and Planning

*If not in the licensed nurse's scope of practice, then cannot delegate to the nursing assistive personnel (NAP).* **Authority to delegate varies; so licensed nurses must check the jurisdiction's statutes and regulations.**

**Are there laws and rules in place that support the delegation?**

↓ YES

**Is the task within the scope of the delegating nurse?** — **NO** → **Do not delegate**

↓ YES

**Has there been assessment of the client needs?** — **NO** → *Assess client needs and then proceed to a consideration of delegation*

↓ YES

**Is the delegating nurse competent to make delegation decisions?** — **NO** → **Do not delegate** until can provide and document additional education, then reconsider delegation; **otherwise do not delegate**

↓ YES

**Is the task consistent with the recommended criteria for delegation to nursing assistive personnel (NAP)? Must meet all the following criteria:**

- *Is within the NAP range of functions*
- *Frequently recurs in the daily care of a client or group of clients;*
- *Is performed according to an established sequence of steps;*
- *Involves little or no modification from one client-care situation to another;*
- *May be performed with a predictable outcome;*
- *Does not inherently involve ongoing assessment, interpretation, or decision-making which cannot be logically separated from the procedure(s) itself; and*
- *Does not endanger a client's life or well-being*

— **NO** → **Do not delegate**

↓ YES

**Does the nursing assistive personnel have the appropriate knowledge, skills and abilities (KSA) to accept the delegation?**

**Does the ability of the NAP match the care needs of the client?**

— **NO** → **Do not delegate** until evidence of education and validation of competency available, then reconsider delegations; **otherwise do not delegate**

↓ YES

*(continued)*

**FIGURE 14-1**   **National Council of State Boards of Nursing Decision Tree for Delegation to Nursing Assistive Personnel.** *(continued)*

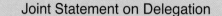

Joint Statement on Delegation
American Nurses Association (ANA) and the National Council of State Boards of Nursing (NCSBN)

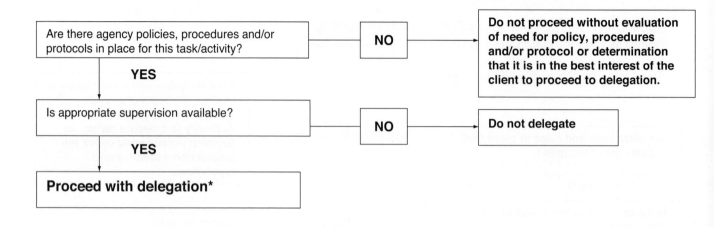

<u>Step Two – Communication</u>

Communication must be a two-way process

| The nurse: | The nursing assistive personnel | Documentation: *Timely, complete and accurate documentation of provided care* |
|---|---|---|
| <ul><li>Assesses the assistant's understanding<ul><li>o How the task is to be accomplished</li><li>o When and what information is to be reported, including<ul><li>✓ Expected observations to report and record</li><li>✓ Specific client concerns that would require prompt reporting.</li></ul></li></ul></li><li>Individualizes for the nursing assistive personnel and client situation</li><li>Addresses any unique client requirements and characteristics, and clear expectations of:</li><li>Assesses the assistant's understanding of expectations, providing clarification if needed.</li><li>Communicates his or her willingness and availability to guide and support assistant.</li><li>Assures appropriate accountability by verifying that the receiving person accepts the delegation and accompanying responsibility</li></ul> | <ul><li>**Ask questions regarding the delegation and seek clarification of expectations if needed**</li><li>Inform the nurse if the assistant has not done a task/function/activity before, or has only done infrequently</li><li>Ask for additional training or supervision</li><li>Affirm understanding of expectations</li><li>Determine the communication method between the nurse and the assistive personnel</li><li>Determine the communication and plan of action in emergency situations.</li></ul> | <ul><li>Facilitates communication with other members of the healthcare team</li><li>Records the nursing care provided.</li></ul> |

**FIGURE 14-1** **National Council of State Boards of Nursing Decision Tree for Delegation to Nursing Assistive Personnel.** *(continued)*

---

### Joint Statement on Delegation
### American Nurses Association (ANA) and the National Council of State Boards of Nursing (NCSBN)

Step Three – Surveillance and Supervision

*The purpose of surveillance and monitoring is related to nurse's responsibility for client care within the context of a client population. The nurse supervises the delegation by mnitoring the performance of the task or function and assures compliance with standards of practice, policies and procedures. Frequency, level and nature of monitoring vary with needs of client and experience of assistant.*

| The nurse considers the: | The nurse determines: | The nurse is responsible for: |
|---|---|---|
| • Client's health care status and stability of condition<br>• Predictability of responses and risks<br>• Setting where care occurs<br>• Availability of resources and support infrastructure.<br>• Complexity of the task being performed. | • The frequency of onsite supervision and assessment based on:<br>  o Needs of the client<br>  o Complexity of the delegated function/task/activity<br>  o Proximity of nurse's location | • Timely intervening and follow-up on problems and concerns. Examples of the need for intervening include:<br>• Alertness to subtle signs and symptoms (which allows nurse and assistant to be proactive, before a client's condition deteriorates significantly).<br>• Awareness of assistant's difficulties in completing delegated activities.<br>• Providing adequate follow-up to problems and/or changing situations is a critical aspect of delegation. |

Step Four – Evaluation and Feedback

*Evaluation is often the forgotten step in delegation.*

In considering the effectiveness of delegation, the nurse addresses the following questions:
- Was the delegation successful?
  - o Was the task/function/activity performed correctly?
  - o Was the client's desired and/or expected outcome achieved?
  - o Was the outcome optimal, satisfactory or unsatisfactory?
  - o Was communication timely and effective?
  - o What went well; what was challenging?
  - o Were there any problems or concerns; if so, how were they addressed?
- Is there a better way to meet the client need?
- Is there a need to adjust the overall plan of care, or should this approach be continued?
- Were there any "learning moments" for the assistant and/or the nurse?
- Was appropriate feedback provided to the assistant regarding the performance of the delegation?
- Was the assistant acknowledged for accomplishing the task/activity/function?

Source: American Nurses Association & National Council of State Boards of Nursing. (2006). *Joint statement on delegation.* Retrieved from https://www.ncsbn.org/Joint_statement.pdf

Effective delegation does not just happen. Every nurse has to learn how to delegate. It takes practice. Even if a nurse has the best intention, delegation may still be difficult. There are also barriers that can interfere with delegation. Effective delegation helps to get work done efficiently and effectively; can reduce budget; meet outcomes; utilize expertise effectively; and facilitate teamwork.

## Barriers to Effective Delegation

Barriers to effective delegation require attention before, during, and after the process. Delegating may mean something different to different staff. Some staff members even think that if they delegate to others this means they are not competent. This clearly indicates that the staff member does not understand delegation. Some staff members may not even be aware of their inner feelings about delegation. The following are some of the typical barriers to effective delegation.

- The attitude of "I would rather do it myself" leads to the question of whether or not this is a good use of time and skills.
- Some staff or managers may think that delegation overburdens the staff that is already overworked. In this case, the delegator is not going through all the delegation process, which requires an assessment of the delegatee's ability to do the job. This involves more than just knowing if the delegatee has the skills, but also if he or she has the time.
- Staff members sometimes have a lack of knowledge and experience about delegation. Realizing they do not know how to do it is sometimes difficult for staff to recognize. There are often few resources for teaching and guiding staff that needs further knowledge and delegation experience.
- Inexperienced delegators will often hesitate to delegate, not knowing what to do. To prevent more problems, they avoid delegating. They try to do everything themselves, which will eventually lead to serious problems.
- Staff members may not even think that delegation is a possibility, or they may use denial (for example, a potential delegator may think that a certain task cannot be delegated when it can be).
- Staff fears loss of control, which is related to lack of trust in others to do the job right, insecurity, and suspiciousness. This interferes with delegation.
- The organization's policies and procedures can be helpful but also these can act as barriers if not updated or applied correctly.
- Position descriptions that do not state clearly responsibilities and accountability are a problem. This applies to both the delegator's and the delegatee's position descriptions.
- Concern about education and training of the delegatee is important. If the delegatee is expected to do a task and the delegatee is not prepared, the delegatee must receive appropriate training and education.
- Sometimes there does not seem to be enough time to consider delegation. Sometimes the situation is so complicated, and must move so quickly, it seems to the delegator that it would be easier and faster to do the task rather than delegate it.
- Some delegators want staff to like them, so delegation is not used in order to lighten workloads.
- The Supernurse syndrome or feeling that others cannot do what you can do so you try to do it all acts as a barrier.
- Lack of organization is always a barrier to effective work. The delegator needs to think through what needs to be done, by whom, when, and so on. This all takes organization.
- Staff turnover does not allow time for developing trust and confidence in staff. Working with the same staff over time allows the delegator to get to know staff and feel more comfortable with delegation.
- Lack of role models to learn how to delegate effectively can be found in most organizations. Student nurses and new graduates need experienced RNs to act as their role models.
- An RN supervising the delegatee may have little contact with the patient. This means the RN must trust the delegatee. It is better for the RN to have some patient contact.
- Poor communication interferes with all steps in the delegation process. Much sharing of information goes on in this process, which requires effective communication.

- If staff have difficulty taking a risk, delegation is difficult. Delegation involves some level of risk. If delegation follows the process, the risk level is less, but it can never be totally eliminated. Much more needs to be done to develop environments where risk taking is valued and not punished.
- Some staff experiences the supermartyr syndrome by refusing to ask others to help. This is particularly important when the delegatee does not ask for help when needed.
- Lack of self-confidence interferes with the delegator's ability to delegate, and when experienced by the delegatee, this can interfere with effective completion of work that has been delegated.
- Fear of criticism is a barrier, both for the delegator and delegatee. More needs to be done to help staff understand evaluation and feedback.
- Poor relationships with staff block effective delegation. Staff may not be motivated to respond appropriately or may not trust the delegator. Lack of respect for staff will be a major barrier, as everyone likes to be respected and appreciated (Kopishke, 2002; Grohar-Murray, & DiCroce, 2003; Hansten & Jackson, 2009).

Additional barriers to effective delegation that need to be considered relate to delegator involvement. Delegators who get too involved in work details (called micromanaging) are not effective. This gets back to earlier comments about the delegator's ability to turn over control and to trust. This does not mean, however, that the delegator does not need feedback at regular intervals to monitor progress because this is an important step in the delegation process. Another barrier is when delegators only delegate the unpleasant or boring activities, keeping tight control over the more interesting activities, or delegate the better tasks to certain staff. Empowering staff, which is done through delegation, requires that staff be given some responsibility for the more interesting activities, not just the boring or less important ones. It is also important to understand the reasons that staff is selected for tasks.

How can barriers be overcome? The most important strategy to remove barriers is for the RN to fully understand why delegation would be used and the delegation process. Following this the RN needs to accept that delegation is part of the job and that the RN cannot do everything. The RN uses experience and judgment to arrive at delegation decisions.

## Supervision and Assignment

It is difficult to discuss delegation without considering supervision and assignment. All three can be confusing, particularly to new graduates. Supervision is defined by the American Nurses Association (2005) as "the active process of directing, guiding and influencing the outcome of an individual's performance of a task. Supervision is generally categorized as on-site (the RN being physically present or immediately available while the task is being performed) or off-site (the RN has the ability to provide direction through various means of written and verbal communications). Individuals engaging in supervision of patient care should not be construed to be managerial supervisors on behalf of the employer" (p. 4). An example of supervision is when a nurse visits all of the team's patients to ensure that the UAP have completed an assigned task. **Assignment** is "the distribution of work that each staff member is responsible for during a given work period" (American Nurses Association, 2005, p. 4). What does this mean in practice? A staff member is assigned to do an activity, which includes the responsibility and accountability for the activity. Assignment must be based on the staff member's skill, knowledge, judgment, and legal scope of practice (Zimmerman, 2002, p. 2). When a nurse is told to care for a group of patients by the nurse manager, this is an assignment. In this example, the nurse manager is accountable only for making the assignment and selecting who will be responsible for the care of the patients. The staff nurse is accountable and responsible for actually providing the care or ensuring that it is provided. In turn, the staff nurse can only delegate work to others, such as UAP, but cannot assign work. "In comparison, delegation is the partial transfer of authority and responsibility regarding care activities, while accountability for completion and outcomes remains with the delegator" (Zimmerman, 2002, p. 2). The nurse manager expects the RN to complete the work assigned. Even if the RN delegates to other staff the RN must still ensure effective completion of the work. The RN as the delegator must analyze and evaluate the outcome of the delegated task or activity.

A key question that now becomes important is what activities can be delegated to the UAP (American Nurses Association & National Council of State Boards of Nursing, 2006; American Nurses Association, 2007). Nursing practice delineates between UAP direct patient care activities and indirect ones by describing them in the following manner.

- **Direct patient care activities:**   These activities assist the patient in meeting basic human needs within the institution, at home, or other health care settings. This includes activities such as assisting the patient with feeding, drinking, ambulating, grooming, toileting, dressing, and socializing. It may also involve the collecting, reporting, and documentation of data related to the previous activities. Data are reported to the RN, who uses the information to make a clinical judgment about patient care.
- **Indirect patient care activities:**   These activities support the patient and their environment, and only incidentally involve direct patient contact. These activities assist in providing a clean, efficient, and safe patient care milieu and typically encompass chore services, companion care, housekeeping, transporting, clerical, stocking, and maintenance tasks.

It is important to note that there are specific types of activities that cannot be delegated to UAP. These include health counseling, teaching, and those activities that require independent, specialized nursing knowledge, skill, or judgment (pp. 2–3).

It may seem clear as to what activities can be delegated and what activities cannot; however, this is a topic that does lead to discussion and debate. Efforts have been made by various groups to change what certain health care providers can or cannot do. This is a great example of when it is important for nurses to become politically active, and many have done this in order to ensure that RNs have a voice in setting these parameters. Glazer (2000) noted that "the profession of nursing needs to develop consensus around what makes a nursing task or activity one that can only be performed by a registered nurse versus what nursing tasks and activities can be shared and delegated" (p. 1). She goes on to identify some key questions that need to be considered: "What is a nursing function? What criteria or logic dictates the functions that are specifically prohibited for unlicensed assistive personnel?" (Glazer, 2000, p. 2). This has become contentious as some nurses are against giving up some activities or concerned about the ability of others such as UAP to do the job safely and provide quality care. Historically, although there are activities that only physicians did, some are now done by RNs. In addition, activities done by RNs are now done by LPN/LVNs or UAP. There is, however, no consensus on this issue other than what is defined by state boards of nursing.

In conclusion, the following key guidelines are important to ensure consistent and effective delegation (Zimmerman, 2002).

- **Start with a positive attitude.**   This includes respecting staff and appreciating the work that they do. Good working relationships go a long way to ensure successful delegation; however, establishing a positive relationship cannot be done at the time of delegation.
- **Clarify availability.**   In some situations, UAP are assigned to several RNs at the same time with each of them delegating activities. This can clearly cause some confusion so it is important to determine what the UAP has time to do based on other activities. The UAP should not be in a position where RNs vie for the UAP.
- **Carefully consider how directions are given during delegation.**   This relates back to respect in that directions should be given in a manner that respects the other staff member—avoiding sharp statements, giving directions on the run, talking down or patronizing, and other ineffective communication approaches.
- **Directions need to be clear.**   Unclear directions can cause more problems for staff and patients. The delegator is responsible for making the directions clear and ensuring that the delegatee understands them. As discussed earlier, directions should include what needs to be done, by whom, how, and when. If the activity is complex, directions should also include

reportable parameters and rationale. An example of this activity would be telling the UAP what blood pressure range should be reported to the RN immediately.

- **Be fair about undesirable activities.**   Nursing is not immune to activities or tasks that are unpleasant or even boring. When these activities are delegated, they should be delegated fairly so that the same person is not always chosen for these activities.

- **Indicate priorities.**   Direction implies that the delegator identifies priorities, what activities are more important, or what should be done first. This should be clear to the delegatee. The RN may work with the UAP to consider all activities that need to be done and prioritize the approaches to be taken.

- **Give and receive feedback.**   The RN gives feedback to the UAP during delegation. This should be ongoing and not just provided when something goes wrong. Feedback needs to be seen as a time for teaching and learning. The RN must also be able to receive and actually seek out feedback from the UAP related to delegation and supervision that the RN provides to ensure that the delegated activity is completed effectively. Is the RN providing clear directions? How does the UAP feel about the activities that are delegated? Is the UAP respected? These are just a few of the questions to consider.

## *CASE STUDY*

### *Getting the Work Done to Reach the Best Outcomes*

A new team leader is struggling with learning a new role and getting the work done. It is like learning on the run. This day is particularly difficult on the surgical unit. There are four new admissions from last night, one is from a serious automobile accident and a second a gunshot wound. Five patients are scheduled for AM surgery. A nursing student is assigned to a patient who is one of the team's patients. This student can only provide basic care as this is the student's first clinical course. The team is composed of the team leader; another RN, who graduated 6 months ago; a licensed practical nurse (LPN); and one unlicensed assistive personnel (UAP), who has worked on the unit for 10 years and must be shared with another team depending upon need. The night shift reported that two patients have elevated temperatures and both are 1-day postop. Today, there are 12 patients assigned to the team; 7 patients have IVs with two to be discontinued. Two patients will be discharged, and three admissions for elective surgery are expected toward the end of the shift. The report has been given, and the team leader is meeting with the team to plan the day.

### Questions:

1. Identify the key team member characteristics that the team leader needs to consider as potential strengths or limitations.

2. What should the team leader remember about delegating to LPNs and to UAP?

3. What should the team leader consider about assignments for the nursing student and working with the student? What are the priorities?

4. Considering the patients assigned to the team and possible tasks and responsibilities, describe how the team leader might delegate to the team.

5. How should the team leader supervise the team members' work?

# APPLYING LEADERSHIP AND MANAGEMENT

## MY HOSPITAL UNIT

You have just reviewed your unit's quality improvement data and the most current staff performance appraisal information. You are concerned about a trend that you identify—delegation is not as effective as it should be. Using the information in this chapter, particularly the NCSBN information and information from the websites, develop a staff education module on delegation. Develop the content, best teaching methods, how staff will access the content, and evaluation methods. Remember evaluation of the educational experience should not just focus on the learning experience but also on its impact on care outcomes. Consider how you need to individualize the content for your unit as you have described your unit over time in this course. Utilize the information found in Figure 14-1. Use the virtual unit site on the textbook website to record the work that you do in the role of nurse manger for your unit.

## Critical Thinking Questions and Activities

1. What are some of the critical aspects of delegation that have been identified by the nursing profession? Visit the site for the National Council of State Boards of Nursing at http://www.ncsbn.org to learn more about the critical issues related to delegation. Explore the following content areas: the delegation decision-making tree, five rights of delegation, and delegation terminology. This is important information to know as you begin to delegate to others. Describe an example of how you might apply the delegation decision-making tree when you delegate a task or activity to a UAP. How is the decision-making grid different from the decision-making tree? You should identify a task or activity and then describe how you would delegate it to a UAP. Respond to each of the questions in the tree found on the website. How might you remember this decision-making tree so that you can apply it in your practice? The decision-making grid provides a scoring mechanism for seven elements. (See Figure 14-1.)

2. How do accountability, authority, and responsibility relate to delegation?

3. Standards for UAP have been a major concern, as noted in this chapter's content. Obtain a copy of a UAP position description from a local health care organization. Working in small teams review the descriptions collected. Summarize your review. What resources might you use to determine the quality of the position description? Your review should consider UAP qualifications, what the UAP may do (tasks and activities), who must supervise the UAP, any restrictions noted, and any information about staff education. Are there any conflicts with the information that you find in your search for information about UAP? Resources that you might use are the organization's standards of care, state board of nursing practice act and other related information, nursing literature, observation, and interviews (nurse managers, team leaders). With sicker patients, shorter lengths of stay, increased use of unlicensed assistive personnel (UAP), and heightened demand for cost-effective care, it is imperative that RNs delegate some aspects of patient care to others.

4. Consider a clinical site where you are for clinical experience. Identify barriers to effective delegation that you observe or experience. For each barrier describe a strategy that might be used to prevent or overcome the barrier.

5. For 1 week in clinical consider the following:
   - What tasks or patient care activities that your patients require could be delegated?
   - Apply the delegation decision-making tree and five rights of delegation. (See Media Links for relevant information about delegation.)
   - Discuss delegation with a team leader.

- When tasks are delegated to UAP, how do they respond?
- If you have an opportunity to observe an RN delegating to a UAP, evaluate the communication, attitude, and response.

6. Find your state's nurse practice act on the Web or in your library. Why is it important for you to be aware of this law? Compare your state's nurse practice act with a UAP position description. Does the law say anything about delegation, and if so, how does it relate to the position description? Is there other information on your state's board of nursing website on delegation, and how might this information be useful?

## Media Links

- **URL: http://www.ncsbn.org/pdfs/delegationtree.pdf**
  NCSBN Delegation Decision-Making Tree
- **URL: http://www.ncsbn.org/pdfs/delegationgrid.pdf**
  NCSBN Delegation Decision-Making Grid
- **URL: http://www.mapnp.org/library/guiding/delegate/basics.htm**
  Basics of Delegation

**Pearson Nursing Student Resources**

Find additional review materials at
**nursing.pearsonhighered.com**

Prepare for success with additional NCLEX®-style practice questions, interactive assignments and activities, Web links, animations and videos, and more!

## References

American Nurses Association. (2005). *Principles of delegation*. Silver Spring, MD: Author.

American Nurses Association & National Council of State Boards of Nursing. (2006). *Joint statement on delegation*. Retrieved from https://www.ncsbn.org/Joint_statement.pdf

American Nurses Association. (2007). Position statement: Registered nurses utilization of nursing assistive personnel in all setting. Silver Spring, MD: Author.

American Nurses Association. (2009). *Guide to the code of ethics for nurses. Interpretation and application*. Silver Spring, MD: Author.

American Operating Room Nurses. (2005). *Standards, recommended practices, and guidelines*. Denver, CO: Author.

Finkelman, A., & Kenner, C. (2010). *Professional nursing concepts. Competencies for quality leadership*. Boston: Jones and Bartlett Publishers.

Fisher, M. (2000). Do you have delegation savvy? *Nursing 2000, 30*(12), 58–59.

Glazer, G. (2000). What makes something a nursing activity or task? *Online Journal of Issues in Nursing*. Retrieved June 23, 2003, from http://www.nursingworld.org

Gordan, S. & Nelson, S. (2005). An end to Angels. *American Journal of Nursing, 105*(5), 62–69.

Grohar-Murray, M., & DiCroce, H. (2003). *Leadership and management in nursing* (3rd ed.). Upper Saddle River, NJ: Prentice Hall.

Guido, G. (2001). *Legal and ethical issues in nursing* (3rd ed.). Upper Saddle River, NJ: Prentice Hall.

Hansten, R., & Jackson, M. (2009). *Clinical delegation skills*. (4th ed.). Boston: Jones and Bartlett Publishers.

Heller, R. (1999). *Learning to lead*. New York: DK Publishing, Inc.

Kopishke, L. (2002). Unlicensed assistive personnel: A dilemma for nurses. *Journal of Legal Nurse Consultant, 13*(1), 3–7.

Oncology Nursing Society. (2002). Position on the role of unlicensed assistive personnel in cancer care. Oncology Nursing Society. Revised October 2007. Retrieved June 4, 2010, from http://www.ons.org/Publications/Positions/Unlicensed

Zimmerman, P. (2002). Delegating to unlicensed assistive personnel. Nursing Spectrum Career Fitness Online. Retrieved November 5, 2002, from http://nsweb.nursingspectrum.com/ce/ce124.html

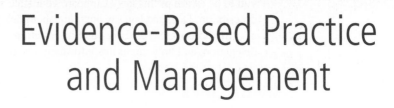

# 15

# Evidence-Based Practice and Management

## LEARNING OUTCOMES

Before you begin, take a moment to familiarize yourself with the learning outcomes for this chapter.

- Describe the nursing research process.
- Discuss the implications of research for nursing leaders and managers.
- Describe the evidence-based practice process.
- Discuss the implications of evidence-based practice for nursing leaders and managers.
- Critique the implications of using evidence-based management.
- Apply the evidence-based management process.
- Explain the importance of evidence-based management to nursing management.
- Compare and contrast research, evidence-based practice, evidence-based management, and quality improvement.

## KEY TERMS

- Applied research
- Basic research
- Evidence-based management
- Evidence-based practice
- Integrative review
- Institutional Review Board
- Meta-analysis
- Meta-synthesis
- Research
- PICO question
- Systematic review

**WHAT'S AHEAD**

The Institute of Medicine (IOM) recommends that health care providers "integrate best research with clinical expertise and patient values for optimum care, and participate in learning and research activities to the extent feasible" (2003, p. 4). This chapter discusses the relationship of research to evidence-based practice (EBP) and the importance of EBP to nursing management. EBP is a topic that is typically covered in nursing research courses and clinical courses; however, nurse managers play a key role in ensuring that EBP is implemented in practice. Evidence-based management (EBM) is a newer term, and it is critical that nurse leaders and managers begin to use EBM to better ensure more effective management decisions.

# Research

## Description of Research

In order to understand evidence-based practice (EBP) and evidence-based management (EBM) it is important to review certain basic information about research. Nursing has an active research initiative that is present in clinical settings and university settings. Nurses are researchers guiding their own research, participating in interprofessional studies with other researchers, managing clinical trials, and guiding patients who are considering participating in clinical trials. The National Institute of Nursing Research (NINR) is the major U.S. nursing research organization. It is part of the National Institutes of Health (NIH) located the Washington, DC, area. According to the NINR, nursing research develops knowledge to (2010):

- Build the scientific foundation for clinical practice
- Prevent disease and disability
- Manage and eliminate symptoms caused by illness
- Enhance end-of-life and palliative care

**Research** is "the systematic inquiry that uses disciplined methods to answer questions or solve problems. The ultimate goal is to develop, refine, and expand a base of knowledge" (Polit & Beck, 2006, p. 4). The two major types of research approaches are basic and applied. **Basic research**'s goal is to broaden the base of knowledge rather than solve an immediate problem. Results from basic research may then be used to develop applied research. **Applied research**'s goal is to find a solution to a practical problem. Nurses typically are involved in more applied research, though some do basic research.

Outcomes research is another type of research, though not as common as the two major types. An outcome is the result of some action. "Nursing outcomes measure states, behaviors, or perceptions of individuals, families, or communities" (Moorehead, Johnson, & Mass, 2004 as cited in Schmidt & Brown, 2009, p. 385). Examples of outcomes are absence of skin ulcers or fluid restriction compliance. The goal of outcomes research is to determine the effectiveness of health care services and patient outcomes, which is critical today if care is to be effective and improved. Nurses play an important role in identifying patient outcomes and intervening to better ensure that outcomes are met, and nurses should be and are involved in outcomes research. Nurse managers and leaders need to take an active role in directing this type of research within their organizations. We need much more knowledge as to how specific nursing actions link to patient outcomes as well as broader nursing delivery issues such as patient classification systems and taxonomies and computerized data sets (Polit & Beck, 2008).

NINR supports clinical or applied research, basic research, and research training that focuses on health and illness across the lifespan (National Institute of Nursing Research, 2010). The Institute's research focus encompasses health promotion and disease prevention, quality of life, health disparities, and end-of-life. NINR sponsors research by outside investigators at colleges, universities, and other research sites (Extramural Research) and conducts its own research at NIH (Intramural Research).

- The Extramural program, managed through the Division of Extramural Activities, accepts unsolicited, investigator-initiated applications, as well as those submitted in response to a published Request for Applications (RFA) or Program Announcement (PA).
- The Intramural program, managed through the Division of Intramural Research, is comprised of the Symptom Management Laboratory, the Pain Research Unit, and the Research Training Section.

"The mission of NINR is to promote and improve the health of individuals, families, communities, and populations. NINR supports and conducts clinical and basic research and research training on health and illness across the lifespan. The Institute's research focus encompasses health promotion and disease prevention, quality of life, health disparities, and end-of-life. NINR seeks to extend nursing science by integrating the biological and behavioral sciences, employing new technologies to research questions, improving research methods, and developing the scientists of the future" (National Institute of Nursing Research, 2010). Appendix C provides more information about NINR and research (see website).

Research design describes the details of a plan for a research project. Content that is typically included is description of the problem, review of literature, type of study (research approach and design), sample description and sample selection method, setting for the study, data collection measurement and instrumentation, data collection process, timeline, data analysis plan, and a description of potential limitations. The research proposal is similar to a nursing care plan or a project plan in that it lays out the steps that will be taken prior to initiating the research project. Typically, the proposal is used to request approval and funding to conduct the research. After approval and funding are received, the study is then conducted. The last part of the research process is data analysis and description of the results and conclusions. This is the important part of the study addressing two key questions: What did the analysis of data demonstrate, and what are the implications of the data?

## Research Barriers and Strategies

Research is not easy to accomplish. The following describes some of the common barriers to research with examples of strategies that might be used to prevent or reduce the barrier (Finkelman & Kenner, 2010, pp. 394, 396).

1. *Lack of funding*: Need to get adequate funding, typically through grants.
2. *Lack of enough time*: Good research takes planning and time to accomplish. The researcher needs blocks of time to work on a study. Some do this full time.
3. *Lack of research competencies*: Research expertise needs to be developed over years. Finding a mentor(s) is important; working with researchers who have been successful can assist a novice researcher.
4. *Lack of participants to be in the sample*: If the study requires participants, it is not always easy to find them and in the number that is required. This takes time and creativity. The study needs to apply ethical principles.
5. *Cannot find the right setting*: Finding and getting a setting to commit to participate in a study can be problematic; it takes contacts and communication.
6. *Lack of statistics expertise*: Using statistical expertise to consult on the study can be very helpful. Researchers work in teams.

Any study conducted in an organization requires support from the organization and management. If this is not present, this will be a major barrier to success.

## Clinical Research: Role of Leaders and Managers

Many health care organizations are involved in conducting research studies, and some of these studies are nursing studies and others may include nurses on the research team, for example in managing a clinical trial. Nurse leaders such as the Chief Nursing Executive may advocate for the organization to have an active nursing research program with nursing staff involvement and support from leadership. Nurse researchers may be hired to lead the program. Depending upon the study, staff may be involved in a study. Nursing staff may initiate a study on a nursing problem of concern. Some of the staff may be qualified to conduct research, and others may need expert assistance. If nursing research is a goal of the organization, staff needs time and resources to ensure that research is conducted effectively. When research is conducted, funding is required. After a study is completed, the staff involved in the study should disseminate the results. This is done by presenting at conferences and publishing articles about the study. Nursing leadership needs to support this phase as much as they support the entire research process. It is the responsibility of the researcher to share results, and this is directly related to EBP. Results must be known before they can be considered in the EBP process. Nurse managers also need to be supportive and encourage staff that has an interest in research.

One approach to increasing nursing research expertise in a health care organization (HCO) is to partner with a college of nursing. Faculty might assist by providing mentoring and staff education about research. Faculty can be invited to consider conducting research in the HCO and also encouraged to include staff. Some HCOs have a designated faculty member or other external nursing expert who acts as their research consultant. Requiring nursing faculty that conducts research in a HCO to present its findings or to ask faculty that may be doing research in another study to share its work with staff are useful methods to emphasize research within a HCO. Some HCOs have annual research days and EBP days where staff members present their work. Encouraging staff members to continue their education also helps to increase research expertise within the organization.

The American Organization of Nurse Executives (AONE) annually identifies research goals on its website (http://www.aone.org) and awards grants for nursing studies and program development. The Magnet Recognition Program recommends active research and evidence-based practice in its Magnet organizations: "Evidence based practice (EBP) is internationally acclaimed as the gold standard for delivering the highest quality care. An essential component of the Forces of Magnetism, EBP characterizes nursing excellence in Magnet organizations. Transforming the nursing work environment to promote and support EBP is an essential process for hospitals embarking on the Magnet journey. In this one-day workshop, participants learn the origins and evolution of EBP in nursing as a professional responsibility" (American Nurses Credentialing Center, 2010). Both initiatives are very supportive of research and EBP and have assisted in increasing nursing research and implementation of EBP within HCOs.

## Ethics, Informed Consent, and Institutional Review Board

History often guides decisions, and the area of research ethics is no exception. There are three examples of past negative experiences with research ethics that have led to major changes in how research is conducted. The Nazi medical experiments conducted during World War II violated basic human rights with little beneficial gain in scientific knowledge (Reich, 1995). After World War II and the Nuremburg trials that focused on physicians who participated in these experiments on innocent people, an important result was the publication of *The Nuremberg Code* (National Institutes of Health, 2010a). This code has provided a prototype for the development of many later codes of research ethics and identified the following rights that must be protected.

- Right to self-determination
- Right to privacy
- Right to anonymity and confidentiality
- Right to fair treatment
- Right to protection from discomfort and harm

The other two examples of serious ethical problems in research studies are the Tuskegee Syphilis Study (1932–1972) and the Willowbrook Study (mid-1950s–1970s) that occurred in the United States. The Tuskegee Study used African-Americans to examine the natural course of syphilis, and the researchers did not give informed consent to participants. Many of them did not even know that they were in a study. This study resulted in participants getting syphilis, complications, and even deaths. Following this study, which lasted for years, the federal government established clearer ethical code for research in the Belmont Report by focusing on "(i) the boundaries between biomedical and behavioral research and the accepted and routine practice of medicine, (ii) the role of assessment of risk-benefit criteria in the determination of the appropriateness of research involving human subjects, (iii) appropriate guidelines for the selection of human subjects for participation in such research and (iv) the nature and definition of informed consent in various research settings" (National Institutes of Health, 2010b). The Willowbrook Study examined hepatitis at an institution for mentally retarded children resulting in major health problems for these children (Krugman, 1986). The parents gave consent but not informed consent as they were told the children were receiving vaccinations when in actuality they were infected with hepatitis.

As a result of these experiences and greater understanding of the need for rights and ethics in research, there are now greater protections for human subjects. The creation of **Institutional Review Boards** (IRB) has contributed to greater protections. The IRB is a committee that reviews research proposals before research is conducted to ensure that the study is conducted ethically. An institution that receives federal funds and conducts research must have an IRB process, and most institutions now have some type of IRB process. All three examples of unethical research behavior mentioned earlier laid the groundwork for major reform in research ethics, particularly involving vulnerable populations. The vulnerable populations that need *extra* protections in research as guided by ethic codes (although all research participants need protections) are as follows:

- Neonates (newborns)
- Children
- Pregnant women and fetuses
- Persons with mental illness
- Persons with cognitive impairment
- Terminally ill
- Persons confined to institutions (e.g., prisons, long-term care hospitals)

To better understand the IRB process one might ask what is the IRB concerned about when research studies are conducted in an organization. Examples of questions that might be considered by the IRB are as follows (Finkelman & Kenner, 2010, pp. 378–379):

1. Are the subjects being deceived, and if so, is this necessary for the integrity of the research?
2. Do the subjects understand the purpose of the project and completely understand his/her role in the project?
3. Are there obvious costs or any hidden costs to people if they participate? Can they withdraw at any time?
4. What are the benefits, if any, to the subjects?
5. What are the risks, immediate and long-term, (if known) to the subjects?
6. How will the researcher protect the subjects' right to confidentiality?
7. Who should the subjects contact with questions?
8. What will be done with the results of the study?

If research is conducted within the organization's patient care areas, nurse leaders and managers have responsibilities related to that research. They need to be knowledgeable about the research process and about the specific research studies. What is the role of the staff? Is staff involved in collecting data, documentation of data, and so on? If studies include patients, staff needs to be informed. Nurse researchers may conduct studies and involve staff. Non-nurses such as physicians and other health care professionals may conduct studies in clinical areas. As mentioned earlier some hospitals have collaborative arrangements with colleges of nursing to provide research consultation to the hospital so that a hospital can conduct effective nursing research. Some hospitals have large nursing research departments and experienced nurse researchers on staff who conduct their own research and also may help staff conduct research. Regardless of the model used, nurse managers need to develop methods for staff to learn about research, attend research conferences, present at conferences, publish its work, and so on. When staff members encounter a clinical question for which they need an answer and there is no available research, then it might mean that the question is appropriate for a research study. However, not all questions lend themselves to a research study and not all staff members are qualified to conduct research as they may have little knowledge or experience in research. In addition, it takes time and funding to conduct studies, and there might not be resources to do this. Figure 15-1 provides a view and comparison of EBP and research.

**FIGURE 15-1  Comparing evidence-based practice and research process.**

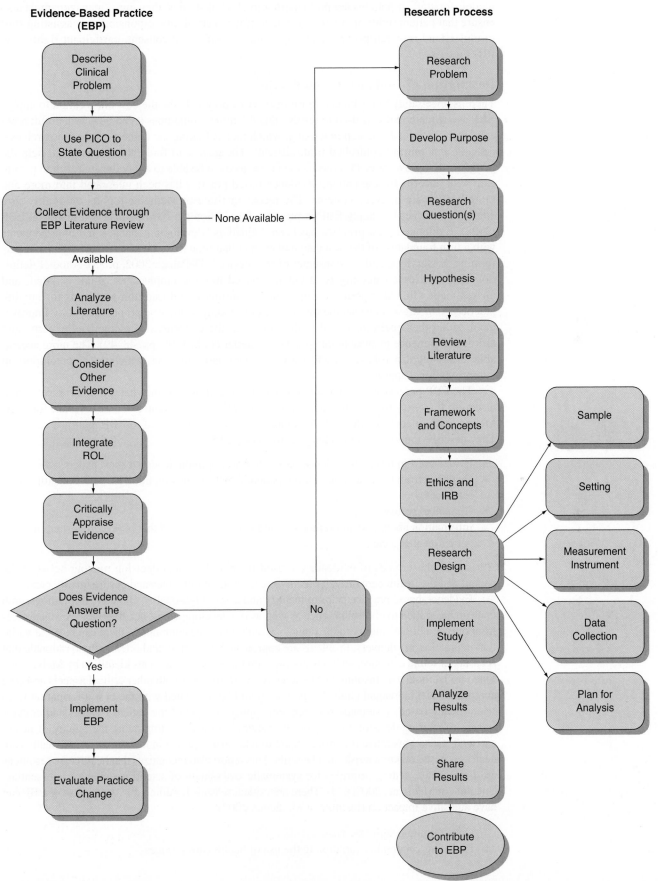

Nurse leaders and managers, who demonstrate a personal interest in research, act as role models for staff. If patients are participating in clinical studies, then nurse managers must also ensure that patient rights are maintained at all times. Part of this responsibility is assisting staff to understand research process and importance of informed consent, participant rights, and IRB process.

## Description of Evidence-Based Practice

There is uncertainty in health care for nurses. How do you know the best intervention to apply? EBP is one method that is used to resolve this dilemma. Sometimes it can be very helpful; however, there is limited research in nursing, which makes finding the highest level of research evidence, a randomized controlled trial, difficult. The goal is to find evidence that will help the patient and improve care. This means the nurse needs to be able to apply the approach to patient care with benefits for the patient. Evidence-based practice has been integrated into more and more health care delivery systems. The recent Institute of Medicine reports on quality care emphasize the need to apply EBP in practice. In addition the IOM published a report on EBP (2008). **Evidence-based practice** has been defined as "developing changes and improvements with a firm foundation of the best data that exist at that time from the science, the individual performing the services, and the consumer of the service" (DePalma, 2002, p. 55). Another definition that focuses on nursing is "Evidence-based nursing emphasizes ritual, isolated, and unsystematic clinical experiences, ungrounded opinions, and tradition as a basis for nursing practices, and stresses instead the use of research findings and, as appropriate, quality improvement data, other operational and evaluation data, the consensus of recognized experts, and affirmed experience to substantiate practice" (Stetler et al., 1998, pp. 48–49). The more acceptable term is evidence-based practice not evidence-based nursing, which does not support an interprofessional approach to care.

The EBP process is a systematic process, but it follows a somewhat different process from research. It is easy to overemphasize research as the only evidence source relevant for EBP. Melnyk and Fineout-Overholt (2005) emphasize that there is more to EBP than just research. They describe the sources of evidence as follows (p. 15):

- Evidence from research evidence-based theories, opinion, leaders/expert panels
- Evidence from the assessment of the patient's history and condition as well as health care resources
- Clinical expertise
- Information about patient preferences and values (something that is very important in patient-centered care)

All four of these types of evidence are used in shared clinical decision making between the patient and the health care provider team to reach patient outcomes and ensure quality care.

Evidence-based practice helps to identify and assess high-quality, clinically relevant research that can be applied to clinical practice as well as the development of health policy. As one travels from one area of the country to the other, or even within one community, there can be great variation in practice and delivery. Problems are approached differently and often with no rationale that is based on sound evidence, which is in sync with the evidence elements identified by Melynk and Fineout-Overholt. The Institute of Medicine ties EBP together with other critical aspects and core competencies. "Individual clinical expertise should be integrated with the best information from scientifically based, systematic research and applied in light of the patient's values and circumstances. Centering decision making on the patient is integral to improving the quality of health care and is also imperative if consumers are to take an active role in making informed health care decisions based on known risks and benefits. This report also recognizes that health care resources are finite. Thus, setting priorities for systematic assessment of scientific evidence is essential" (Institute of Medicine, 2008, p. 3). There are critical reasons for doing this. Active use of EBP can have a positive impact on (Institute of Medicine, 2008):

- Constraining health care costs
- Reducing geographic variation in the use of health care services

- Improving quality
- Consumer-directed health care
- Making health coverage decisions

EBP is particularly concerned with synthesizing results found in professional research so that they can be used to improve care or the delivery of health care services. These **systematic reviews** do the following:

- Estimate the effect of health care interventions.
- Provide generalizable answers, because they are based on a number of studies in different settings and include a variety of participants.
- Identify the individual, clinical, and contextual factors that influence effectiveness.
- Identify uncertainties and gaps in research (Dickson & Entwistle, 1997, p. 3).

Two key goals of evidence-based practice and also evidence-based policy development that are important for organizations to consider are to (a) challenge others to provide evidence for their practice or their policy decisions and (b) critically assess to find and use evidence (Mooney, 2001, 9, 17). Today, patients are more knowledgeable about their illnesses and treatment. Technology has brought much more information to consumers. Information increases control, and now more and more patients want the best. Evidence-based care looks for the best (Cope, 2003). Management needs to keep these two goals in mind. In order to meet these goals, management and staff will need to know how to do the following:

- Frame a clinical question (delivery, or policy question).
- Search for the evidence.
- Evaluate the evidence.
- Implement the evidence (Mooney, 2001, p. 17).

A common method for nurses to use when searching for evidence to improve practice with the goal of asking a searchable and answerable question is to use a PICO question. What is the **PICO question**? This acronym stands for the following (Melnyk & Fineout-Overholt, 2005, p. 30):

1. The "P" needs to be specific—describing the population such as age, gender, diagnosis, ethnicity, other.
2. The "I" can be related to prognostic factors, risk behaviors, exposure to disease, or clinical intervention or treatment.
3. The "C" is comparison with another treatment or no treatment.
4. The "O" is the outcome; what will it be, such as risk of disease or a complication or a side effect, or adverse outcome.

There are different types of PICO questions. Box 15-1 describes the templates that can be used to develop PICO questions. You can fill in the blanks in the template to write your PICO question. For example, using the prevention template: For _____ does the use of _____ reduce the future risk of _____ compared with _____? You might complete this template in this manner: To reduce the development of lung cancer does the use of health education about smoking reduction during the years of 12–18 reduce the future risk developing lung cancer compared with no health education on smoking reduction? The templates simply provide an easy method for writing PICO questions with each template focused on a different issue such as prevention or etiology (cause).

The five steps in the EBP process as described by Melynk and Fineout-Overholt (2005, p. 9) are as follows:

1. Identify a burning clinical issue or question, a PICO question.
2. Collect the best evidence relevant to the question.
3. Critically appraise that evidence before it is used.
4. Integrate the evidence with the other parts of EBP: patient preferences and values, your clinical expertise, assessment information about the patient and patient's history.
5. Evaluate the practice decision or change.

---

**BOX 15-1**    **TEMPLATES FOR PICO QUESTIONS**

**PICO Question Templates:**

**Therapy**: In _____, what is the effect of _____ on _____ compared with _____?

**Etiology**: Are _____ who have _____ at _____ risk for/of _____compared with _____ with/without _____?

**Diagnosis or Diagnostic Test**: Are (is) _____ more accurate in diagnosing _____ compared with _____?

**Prevention**: For _____ does the use of _____ reduce the future risk of _____ compared with _____?

**Prognosis**: Does _____ influence _____ in patients who have _____?

**Meaning**: How do _____ diagnosed with _____ perceive _____?

Source: Melnyk, B. & Fineout-Overholt, E. (2005). *Evidence-based practice in nursing and healthcare.* Philadelphia: Lippincott Williams & Wilkins. Retrieved from http://www.lww.com. Reprinted with permission.

---

Evidence-based practice requires that information is available for specific questions. The research literature is reviewed using explicit scientific methods and includes all relevant research. This valuable information is then available to practitioners and should be helpful in directing their care decisions. An obvious question is how does one get to this information and then how does one know what information is valid and reliable? Evidence-based reviews act as gatekeepers of the knowledge (Evans & Pearson, 2001).

Clearly, criteria need to be used to determine what type of evidence will be useful. The hierarchy of evidence can be described in seven levels with Level I representing the highest or best level (Melnyk & Fineout-Overholt modified from Guyatt & Rennie, 2002 & Harris et al., 2001, p. 10).

- **Level I:** Evidence from a systematic review or meta-analysis of all relevant randomized controlled trials (RCTs) or evidence-based clinical practice guidelines based on systematic reviews of RCTs
- **Level II:** Evidence obtained from at least one well-designed RCT
- **Level III:** Evidence obtained from well-designed controlled trials without randomization
- **Level IV:** Evidence from well-designed case-control and cohort studies
- **Level V:** Evidence from systematic reviews of descriptive and qualitative studies
- **Level VI:** Evidence from a single descriptive or qualitative study
- **Level VII:** Evidence form the opinion of authorities and/or reports of expert committees

Clinicians (nurses, physicians, pharmacists, allied health), health care administrators and nursing administration, health care policy makers, and health care insurers use systematic reviews to find the most current best practice. The highest level of evidence is from systematic reviews, meta-analysis, or EBP-based clinical practice guidelines. These sources provide an overview and rating of quality and strength of evidence from primary research studies, meta-analysis or systematic reviews, published and unpublished, on a specific question. Experts complete these reviews in a systematic manner. Inconsistencies and weaknesses are identified. Most nurses do not develop systematic reviews themselves. EBP experts are best prepared to do these specialized reviews and analysis of research. Clinical nurses do not really have the time to do this type of review. The goal of the search for evidence is to find the evidence in a form that it can be applied to practice based on a PICO question.

The best sources of studies are research journals, and then clinical journals, and they should be peer-reviewed journals. There are several major EBP databases and other sources of EBP literature.

1. *Cochrane Center and Collaboration*: This center develops, maintains, and updates systematic reviews of health care interventions to allow practitioners to make informed decisions.
2. *Joanna Briggs Institute Evidence-Based Practice*: This represents an international collaboration among nursing and allied health centers.

3. *National Clinical Guidelines*: This source is government based though the guidelines on it come from any different sources (http://www.guideline.gov/).
4. Sigma Theta Tau International (STTI) offers EBP resources through its online publication, *Online Journal of Knowledge Synthesis for Nursing (OJKSN)*. This journal provides full-text systematic reviews to guide nursing practice.

There are many advantages for using systematic reviews within the health care delivery system (Academic Center for Evidence-Based Nursing, 2008). They are as follows:

- Reduces large quantities of information into a manageable form
- Establishes generalizability across participants, settings, treatment variations, and study designs
- Assesses consistency and explains inconsistencies of findings across studies
- Increases power in suggesting the cause and effect relationship
- Reduces bias from random and systematic error, improving true reflection of reality
- Integrates existing information for decisions about clinical care, economic decisions, future research design, and policy formation
- Increases efficiency in time between research and clinical implementation
- Provides a basis for continuous updates with new evidence

The IOM report on EBP recommends that effective EBP requires professionals who are able to do the following (Davidoff, 1999; Rosswurm & Larrabee, 1999; Grad, Macaulay, & Warner, 2002 as cited in Institute of Medicine, 2003, p. 57–58):

- Know where and how to find the best possible sources of evidence.
- Formulate clear clinical questions.
- Search for the relevant answers to the questions from the best possible sources of evidence, including those that evaluate or appraise the evidence for its validity and usefulness with respect to a particular patient or population.
- Determine when and how to integrate these new findings into practice.

Mooney (2001) recommends that not only do staff or the reviewers need to evaluate the information based on its scientific merit, as is indicated in the hierarchy described, but also the following must be considered: Have the results been replicated? This helps to establish credibility. Are the results relevant to the practice, policy, or delivery? What are the risks and benefits of incorporating the results into practice, policy, or delivery? Just adopting ideas without considering these factors can be costly. What is the feasibility of incorporating the new evidence? This is tied to the previous question as it can increase costs or limit benefits. Now, what happens after evidence is collected? It could be overwhelming, as the result is often a large amount of information, and some may conflict. Typically, a panel of stakeholders and experts is selected to review the information and come to a consensus about the information (DePalma, 2002).

Participating in evidence-based evaluation of information to arrive at the best view of practice, policy, or delivery requires some skills. The following are some critical skills that are needed to be effective.

- Big-picture thinking
- Critical thinking
- Flexibility/willingness to try new things and be a continuous learner
- Advanced communication and relationship-building skills
- Interdisciplinary (interprofessional) influence and team-building skills
- Outcomes orientation and the ability to demonstrate value added
- Commitment to an evidence-based practice
- Research and data interpretation skills
- Computing and technology skills
- Leadership competency (Mooney, 2001, p. 18)

Mooney (2001) also emphasizes the importance of the knowledge worker, which relates to content in Chapter 1 about knowledge and leadership. "Transitioning to an evidence-based practice requires a different perspective from the traditional role of nurse as 'doer' of treatments and procedures based on institutional policy or personal preference. Rather, the nurse practices as a 'knowledge worker' from an updated and ever-changing knowledge base, contributing to the oncology [or can be any type] health care team as knowledgeable clinical colleague" (Mooney, 2001, p. 17). Others have also commented on the need for nurses to see themselves as knowledge workers. "Clinical scholarship is value-driven—a demonstration of willingness to test creativity, courage, and autonomy because of the love and belief in the work. It is also about intellectual problem solving, activating and disseminating practice innovations, and being collaborative. Acquiring, analyzing, synthesizing, and applying evidence to inform the practice process become key components to being a clinical scholar" (Dickenson-Hazard, 2002, p. 6). Blind acceptance of research results that are then applied to patient care is clearly not what nurses should do. Nurses are able to do more than this. They can play a role in assessing and selecting information to apply to the care. This, however, requires that nurses demonstrate the skills identified by Mooney (2001).

Finding sources of data to support evidence-based practice in nursing may not always be easy. Clearly, well-designed research is the best; however, there may be none available on a particular problem area. The Agency for Health Research and Quality (AHRQ) evaluates research and publishes guidelines based on their reviews. This can be a source of information to support evidence-based practice. "The AHRQ Evidence-Based Practice Center (EPC) Program sponsors and disseminates state of the art systematic reviews on important topics that provide the evidence bases for guidelines, quality improvement projects, quality measures, and insurance coverage decisions. They sponsor both methodological investigations and publications of systematic reviews" (Cronewett, 2002, p. 4). Twelve evidence-based practice centers in the country produce reports that include the critical appraisal of the literature using explicit grading systems (Lohr & Carey, 1999). Cronewett (2002) notes that single discipline scientists typically develop AHRQ EBP reports. They provide one point of view rather than an interprofessional view, which is a disadvantage. Clinicians, patients, and advocacy groups are not usually involved, but when the development of clinical practice guidelines was begun these groups usually did participate. The EBP reports include analyses, evidence tables, references, and search strategies. Cronewett (2002) has some criticisms of the AHRQ evidence-based practice reports due to the incomplete literature, possible database publication biases, and the emphasis on using evidence from randomized controlled trials, which can skew the information, and making the conclusions only relevant to the patient populations included in the studies.

## Advantages and Barriers

The goal is for nurses to make clinically sound and autonomous decisions whenever possible. EBP increases clinical knowledge; the nurse's freedom to act, and impacts the nurse's autonomy, and—make a sound decision with the patient. Implementing EBP is very difficult to accomplish and takes time. What are the barriers to implementing EBP?

- Lack of knowledge about EBP
- Lack of acceptance of the value of EBP—impact on quality and costs
- Nursing shortage limits staff time and energy for change
- View that EBP represents cookbook approach to care
- Lack of knowledge and experience with technology and library searches
- Consider EBP to be research and do not feel can conduct research

This list of barriers can be used by a nurse manager to plan for staff needs when implementing EBP.

One of the major barriers is getting nurses prepared to use EBP. Nurses need to know how to critique a research study. With the average of nurses over 45 years of age this is a challenge since most did not did have content in the formal nursing education The *American Journal of Nursing* estimated that only 35% of nurses subscribe to a professional journal (Mason, 2002); however, with the availability of online access to many journals this may not be an accurate account of the percentage of nurses who have access to professional literature. If nurses need to use an EBP approach, nurses will need to be more aware of the professional literature. Nurse managers need to encourage staff to review the literature, provide training about literature searches, and resources such as computer databases mentioned in this chapter and librarian assistance.

In another study published in 2005 (Pravikoff, Tanner, & Pierce), 760 RNs responded to a 93-item questionnaire about readiness of nurses for EBP. The results from this study indicated that "Although these nurses acknowledge that they frequently need information for practice, they feel much more confident asking colleagues or peers and searching the Internet and World Wide Web than they do using bibliographic databases such as PubMed or CINAHL to find specific information. They don't understand or value research and have received little or no training in the use of tools that would help them find evidence on which to base their practice" (Pravikoff, Tanner, & Pierce, 2005, p. 40).

Schmidt and Brown (2009) recommend strategies to overcome the common barriers to implementing EBP (pp. 9–10).

### Barrier-Time:

- Devote 15 minutes to reading evidence related to a clinical problem.
- Sign up for e-mails that offer summaries of research studies in your area of interest.
- Use a team approach when considering policy changes to distribute the workload among members.
- Bookmark websites having clinical guidelines to promote faster retrieval of information.
- Evaluate available technologies to create time-saving systems that allow quick and convenient retrieval of information at the bedside.
- Negotiate release time from patient care to collect, read, and share information about relevant clinical guidelines.
- Search for already established clinical guidelines because they provide synthesis of existing research.

### Barrier-Research in Practice Not Valued:

- Make a list of reasons why health care providers should value research, and use this list as a springboard for discussions with colleagues.
- Invite nurse researchers to share why they are passionate about their work.
- When disagreements arise about a policy or protocol, find an article (preferably research) that addresses the question.
- When selecting a work environment, ask about the organizational commitment to EBP.
- Link measurement of quality indicators to EBP.
- Participate in EBP activities to demonstrate professionalism that can be rewarded through promotions or merit raises.
- Provide recognition during National Nurses Week for individuals involved in EBP projects.

### Barrier-Lack of Knowledge about EBP and Research:

- Take a course or attend a continuing education offering on EBP.
- Invite a faculty member to a unit meeting to discuss EBP.
- Consult with advance practice nurses about EBP.
- Attend conferences where clinical research is presented and talk with presenters about their studies.
- Volunteer to be on committees that set policies and protocols.
- Create a mentoring program to bring novice and experienced nurses together.

### Barrier-Lack of Technological Skills to Find Evidence:

- Consult with a librarian about how to access databases and retrieve articles.
- Learn to bookmark important websites that are sources of clinical guidelines.
- Commit to acquiring computer skills.

### Barrier-Lack of Resources to Access Evidence:

- Write a proposal for funds to support access to online databases and journals.
- Collaborate with a nursing program for access to resources.
- Investigate funding possibilities from others (i.e. grants, pharmaceutical companies, etc.).

### Barrier-Communication Gap between Researchers and Nursing Staff:

- Identify clinical problems and share them with nurse researchers. (It is easy for staff to confuse research and EBP.)
- Participate in ongoing unit-based studies.

**Barrier-Resistance to Change:**

- Listen to staff concerns about change.
- When considering an EBP project, select one that interests the staff, has a high priority, is likely to be successful, and has baseline data.
- Mobilize talented individuals to act as change agents.
- Create a means to reward individuals who provide leadership during change.

**Barrier Organization Does Not Embrace EBP:**

- Link organizational priorities with EBP to reduce cost and increase efficiency.
- Recruit administrators/managers who value EBP.
- Form coalitions with other health care providers to increase the base of support for EBP.
- Use EBP to meet accreditation standards and gain recognition (i.e., Magnet Recognition).

## Evidence-Based Practice: Role of Nurse Leaders and Managers

How might the evidence-based approach be applied to nursing management or administration? Titler, Cullen, and Ardery (2002) addressed this question, and they emphasized the importance of interprofessional collaboration, which seems to be a key issue with so much of what is happening in health care today. They identify that it must be a continuous process and takes commitment. The key factors in the process are as follows:

1. Incorporating evidence-based practice terminology into the mission, vision, strategic plan, and performance appraisals of staff
2. Integrating the work EBP into the governance structure of nursing departments and the health care system
3. Demonstrating the value of evidence-based practice through administrative behaviors of the chief nurse executive
4. Establishing explicit expectations about EBP for nursing leaders (e.g., nurse managers and advanced practice nurses) who create a culture that values clinical inquiry (Titler, Cullen, & Ardery, 2002, p. 26)

From this description it is clear that to be successful, EBP has to be incorporated into all aspects of the organization structure, culture, and systems. Examples that are given to implement these four factors are integrate EBP in all staff education; monitor and act upon results of key indicators for selected EBPs; select a specific number of EBP examples each year that have been identified from operational or quality improvement data; establish a documentation system that supports EBP and allows for tracking or monitoring of application; provide routine staff education on EBP; incorporate EBP into orientation, and so on. EBP does have much to offer management and the delivery of nursing care to improve care and the way the nurses work, but the organization has to make a commitment to implement it. Box 15-2 describes a tool used by the Johns Hopkins Hospital.

How might EBP evidence be used in practice and how does one go about applying it? One method is through use of protocols that are evidence-based. Protocols may be in the form of "comprehensive plans of care for specified patient populations, procedures for performing clinical actions, bundles of care actions aimed at specific outcomes, standardized order sets, decision algorithms, care maps, and clinical pathways" (Brown, 2009, p. 307). The Institute of Health Improvement (IHI) defines a care bundle as "a group of evidence-based interventions related to a disease process that, when executed together, result in better outcomes than when implemented individually" (2007). How can the evidence be applied in practice?

- Change care for one patient or a population
- Revise or develop a policy or a procedure
- Implement the use of an evidence-based clinical guideline
- Use to revise or develop a clinical pathway or a protocol
- Use in shared governance to improve care
- Educate staff
- Share information through written information, on website, and other materials
- Develop fact sheets and posters to educate staff
- Discuss in staff meetings
- Involve staff in improving care

- Reduce errors; use in root cause analysis
- Educate nursing students

It is always important to note that an organization can have the best written documents such as evidence-based policies and procedures, protocols, and standards; however, if these do not change practice and improve care then they are useless. The nurse manager not only needs to ensure that documents describing care are evidence-based but also ensure that they are applied. This requires monitoring, and this is part of quality improvement. EBP should also have an impact on patient and family education in that patient/family education content and methods used need to be current and effective approaches. Development of infrastructure to better ensure effective EBP integration includes the following (Gawlinski, 2008):

- Discussion of research and EBP
- Engagement of frontline clinicians
- Education of staff by involving them
- Creation of internal expertise for research and EBP
- Adaptation of approaches from the literature that meet needs of the organization
- Improvement of patient care
- Development and maintenance of an individual professional nursing legacy

## Examples of EBP Application in Clinical Settings

Today many health care organizations, particularly acute care hospitals, are trying to implement EBP into nursing practice. It is not easy, takes time, and require a planned effort to resolve the barriers as discussed earlier in this chapter. Two examples of initiatives to implement EBP are briefly described. The nursing literature has many examples to choose from.

One example is the Institute for Johns Hopkins Nursing, which is part of the Johns Hopkins Hospital. The goal for this organization is slightly different as it includes clinical, administration (EBM), and education (The Johns Hopkins Hospital and The Johns Hopkins University School of Nursing). "The goal of EBP is to promote effective nursing interventions, efficient care, and improved outcomes for patients, and to provide the best available evidence for clinical, administrative, and educational decision-making" (Newhouse, Dearholt, Poe, Pugh, & White, 2007, p. xiii). Using EBP provides nurses with more influence in decision making. "Numbering more than 2 million and practicing in most health care settings, nurses make up the largest number of health professionals. Every patient is likely to receive nursing care. Therefore, nurses are in an important position to influence the type, quality, and cost of care provided to patients" (Newhouse, Dearholt, Poe, Pugh, & White, 2007, p. 10). Figure 15-2 describes The Johns Hopkins Nursing Evidence-Based Practice Model and includes consideration of internal and external factors with a 3-prong focus of practice, administration, and education. The model uses a team approach, a team of experts who have experience with the problem and most likely an interprofessional team. The team uses the PICO method during the EBP process as was described in Box 15-2. The EBP project includes 18 steps as shown in Box 15-3 describing project management.

Another example is the Cincinnati Children's Hospital Medical Center. This specialty hospital has integrated EBP in its nursing services by using a mentor program. Box 15-4 describes this program.

## CASE STUDY

### Do We Need Evidence to Improve Care?

A large health care institution has identified errors in medication administration, high rates of falls, and decrease in staff satisfaction. To combat these areas of concern and to decrease the possibility of serious safety events upper administration has mandated that practice will be based on evidence. The way to guarantee that this will happen is to include the infusion of evidence as criteria within the organization's strategic plan. The mission, vision, and specific goals of the organization have been developed to include evidence-based decision making at the point of care.

At the point of care, unit directors are discussing with staff the importance of infusing evidence into care. Discussions include the use of guidelines, protocols, policies, and procedures that are all based on evidence. Nursing staff are discussing how this may occur. Concerns are voiced related to knowledge of evidence-based practice (EBP), time to engage in finding evidence, what to do with the research once identified, and the effect of change. Many staff members are saying, "We have always done it this way"; "It takes too much time to look for and read the evidence"; and "We can't even locate our policies and procedures to help direct us in providing care." In addition, the nursing staff members are verbalizing exhaustion with all the change occurring from quality improvement projects that require multiple tests of change within a short period of time. They ask, "How do you expect me to do any additional work?"

Management involved nursing staff at the point-of-care in collaboration with interprofessional staff to address the areas of concern. The first challenge was to identify a system that will begin to establish a culture based on evidence. Shared governance councils were established to begin to this process. A specific unit actively engaged in identifying a project that would require implementing the EBP process to impact outcomes. The opportunity came with a physician driven research project involving pain control in pediatric patients outside the ICU. The issue for the unit was monitoring parameters and nurse staffing. The unit began its first journey with evidence-based practice on that day in order to meet the needs of the patients and pain team. The process involved staff from all three shifts, the educator for the unit, the unit leadership, and the evidence-based practice mentor.

## Questions:

1. In what ways did nursing leadership begin to establish an evidence-based culture that would lead to improved outcomes?

2. Discuss tools that are needed to facilitate staff in the evidence-based practice process.

3. What additional systems processes are needed to engage staff in the evidence work?

**Contributors:**
Stefanie A. Roberts-Newman RN, MSN, NEA-BC
Chief Nursing Officer
Bethesda North Hospital
Cincinnati, Ohio

Lisa English Long MSN, RN, CNS
Evidence-Based Practice Mentor
Cincinnati Children's Hospital Medical Center
Cincinnati, Ohio

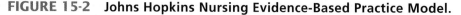

**FIGURE 15-2    Johns Hopkins Nursing Evidence-Based Practice Model.**

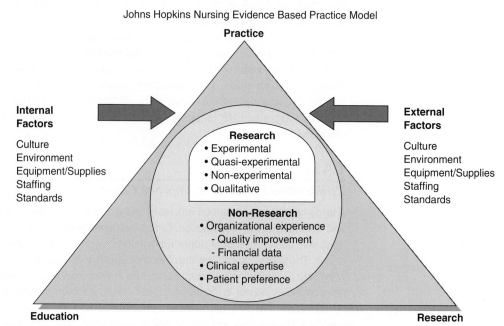

Johns Hopkins Nursing Evidence Based Practice Model

**BOX 15-2   QUESTION DEVELOPMENT TOOL**

# Question Development Tool

**What is the practice issue?**

| | |
|---|---|
| **1.  What is the practice area?** | ☐ Clinical          ☐ Education          ☐ Administration |

**2.  How was the practice issues identified**  (Check all that apply)

- ☐ Safety/risk management concerns
- ☐ Unsatisfactory patient outcomes
- ☐ Wide variations in practice
- ☐ Significant financial concerns
- ☐ Difference between hospital and community practice
- ☐ Clinical practice issue is a concern
- ☐ Procedure or process is a time waster
- ☐ Clinical practice issue has no scientific base

**3.  What is the scope of the problem?**          ☐ Individual
                                                    ☐ Population
                                                    ☐ Institution/system

**4.  What are the PICO Components?**

P – (Patient, Population, or Problem):


I – (Inventory)


C – (Comparison with other treatments, if applicable):


O – (Outcomes)


**5.  What evidence must be gathered?** (Check all that apply)

- ☐ Literature Search
- ☐ Standards (Regulatory, Professional, Community)
- ☐ Guidelines
- ☐ Expert Opinion
- ☐ Patient Preferences
- ☐ Clinical Expertise
- ☐ Financial Analysis

**6.  State the search question in narrow, manageable terms:**

© The Johns Hopkins Hospital/The Johns Hopkins University

Source: Newhouse, R., Dearholt, S., Poe, S., Pugh, L., & White, K. (2007). *Johns Hopkins Nursing Evidence-Based Practice Model and Guidelines*. Indianapolis, IN: Sigma Theta Tau International.  Reprinted with permission from the Institute for Johns Hopkins Nursing, copyright The Johns Hopkins Hospital/The Johns Hopkins University. All Rights Reserved.

| BOX 15-3 | PROJECT MANAGEMENT |
|----------|--------------------|

# Project Management

| Practice Question: | | | | | | |
|---|---|---|---|---|---|---|
| **EBT Team Leader (s):** | | | | | | |
| **EBP Team Members:** | | | | | | |
| **Overall Aim:** | | | | | | |
| | Start Date | Days Required | End Date | Person Assigned | Milestone | Comment / Resources Required |
| **PRACTICE QUESTION:** | | | | | | |
| Step 1: Identify an EBP question | | | | | | |
| Step 2: Define the scope of the practice question | | | | | | |
| Step 3: Assign responsibility for leadership | | | | | | |
| Step 4: Recruit an interdisciplinary team | | | | | | |
| Step 5: Schedule a team conference | | | | | | |
| **EVIDENCE:** | | | | | | |
| Step 6: Conduct an internal and external search for evidence | | | | | | |
| Step 7: Appraise all types of evidence | | | | | | |
| Step 8: Summarize the evidence | | | | | | |
| Step 9: Rate the strength of the evidence | | | | | | |
| Step 10: Develop recommendations for change in systems or processes of care based on the strength of the evidence | | | | | | |
| **TRANSLATION:** | | | | | | |
| Step 11: Determine the appropriateness and feasibility of translating recommendations into the evidence | | | | | | |
| Step 12: Create an action plan | | | | | | |
| Step 13: Implement the change | | | | | | |
| Step 14: Evaluate outcomes | | | | | | |
| Step 15: Report the results of preliminary evaluation to decision makers | | | | | | |
| Step 16: Secure support from decision makers to implement the recommended change internally | | | | | | |
| Step 17: Identify the next steps | | | | | | |
| Step 18: Communicate the findings | | | | | | |

Source: Newhouse, R., Dearholt, S., Poe, S., Pugh, L., & White, K. (2007). *Johns Hopkins Nursing Evidence-Based Practice Model and Guidelines*. Indianapolis, IN: Sigma Theta Tau International. Reprinted with permission from the Institute for Johns Hopkins Nursing, copyright The Johns Hopkins Hospital/The Johns Hopkins University. All Rights Reserved.

| BOX 15-4 | AN EXAMPLE OF AN APPROACH TO EBP INTEGRATION |
|---|---|

Developing systems that support the infusion of evidence into bedside practice is challenging. In a unique role developed at Cincinnati Children's Hospital Medical Center, Evidence-Based Practice Mentors engage health care professionals in the Evidence-Based Practice (EBP) process throughout the entire system. Through the role of mentoring, EBP mentors have identified that the development of processes, resources, and tools is essential to begin and sustain a culture of evidence. A systemwide approach is essential to the development of an evidence program that provides leadership and direction to staff as they address clinical issues. Strategies to support development of a culture of evidence include the organization of an interprofessional team co-led by a nurse and physician. This organizational level team consists of nurses in the role of evidence-based practice mentors, a librarian, nurse educator, and guideline administrators. The team focuses on developing a standardized process for evaluation of evidence. Tools developed to achieve standardization consist of evidence appraisal forms, a process to level and grade evidence, and a guide for forming a recommendation. In addition, an evidence website and evidence summary document has been developed. At the divisional level, a formal evidence-based practice program has been developed. This program is open to all nurses and allied health professionals eligible to apply. Selected participants engage in evidence work for one year that addresses a clinical issue of importance at the point of care. At the unit or point-of-care level staff engages in evidence-based practice through shared governance activities. Council members request consultation services with the EBP mentors to engage in addressing clinical issues through the EBP process. Point-of-care staff, individually or as a member of a project team, can also investigate questionable clinical issues through consultation with an EBP mentor. The mentor provides direction, expertise, and guidance for nurses and allied health professionals to pursue practice changes based on evidence.

Direct outcomes of the systemswide evidence approach include sustained involvement of staff in the formal evidence program, professional development, publications, and presentations. Additional outcomes include development of evidence-based policies and procedures, implementation of safety recommendations related to use of radioisotopes in pediatric patients experiencing seizure activity, and consistent publication of evidence summaries.

**Contributor:**
Lisa English Long MSN, RN, CNS
Evidence-Based Practice Mentor
Cincinnati Children's Hospital Medical Center
Cincinnati, Ohio

There are two other EBP models that are highlighted in this chapter though there are number of EBP implementation models in the nursing literature. The first is the ACE Star model, which was developed at a university, and the second the Iowa model, which was developed at a hospital. Box 15-5 provides web links to learn more about these two models. There are other models in the nursing literature. Most of the models describe similar EBP processes.

## The Federal Government and EBP

Accelerating Change and Transformation in Organizations and Networks (ACTION) is a "model of field-based research designed to promote innovation in health care delivery by accelerating the diffusion of research into practice. The ACTION network includes 15 large partnerships and collaborating organizations that provide health care to more than 100 million Americans" (2009). This five-year plan begun in 2006 is designed to better ensure that research findings are applied in the health care delivery system and not lost. It includes a number of HCOs that have partnered with the Agency for Healthcare Research and Quality. Projects must have "direct relevance to practice, public policy, and/or the organization and management of health care delivery" (Accelerating Change and Transformation in Organizations and Networks, 2009). Initiatives such as this one may help to move EBM into the mainstream of management, including nursing management. (See Media Links for the ACTION website.)

| BOX 15-5 | EXAMPLES OF TWO EVIDENCE-BASED PRACTICE NURSING MODELS |
| --- | --- |

- **ACE Star Model**
  http://www.acestar.uthscsa.edu/Learn_model.htm
- **Iowa Model of Evidence-Based Practice**
  http://www.uihealthcare.com/depts/nursing/rqom/evidencebasedpractice/iowamodel.html

The Agency for Healthcare Research and Quality has in recent years developed Evidence-Based Practice Centers (EPC). "The EPCs develop evidence reports and technology assessments on topics relevant to clinical, social science/behavioral, economic, and other health care organization and delivery issues—specifically those that are common, expensive, and/or significant for the Medicare and Medicaid populations. With this program, AHRQ became a "science partner" with private and public organizations in their efforts to improve the quality, effectiveness, and appropriateness of health care by synthesizing the evidence and facilitating the translation of evidence-based research findings. Topics are nominated by non-federal partners such as professional societies, health plans, insurers, employers, and patient groups." (Agency for Healthcare Research and Quality, 2008). EBP reports can be found on many issues at http://www.ahrq.gov/clinic/epcindex.htm#top.

The National Guideline Clearinghouse provides access to many EBP-based clinical guidelines on its website at http://www.guideline.gov. Its mission "is to provide physicians, nurses, and other health professionals, health care providers, health plans, integrated delivery systems, purchasers and others an accessible mechanism for obtaining objective, detailed information on clinical practice guidelines and to further their dissemination, implementation and use" (2010). Some of the guidelines can be downloaded to personal digital assistants (PDAs).

The health care reform legislation of 2010 also includes evidence-based practice. A non-profit Patient-Centered Outcomes Research Institute is to be established to support comparative effectiveness research. The law also requires that a grant program be established to support delivery of evidence-based and community-based prevention and wellness services to improve prevention activities, reduce chronic disease, and address health disparities; develop a national strategy to improve the nation's health; and to disseminate evidence-based recommendations.

## Evidence-Based Management

"Reports of medical mistakes have splashed across newspapers and magazines in the United States. At the same time, instances of overuse, underuse, and misuse of management tactics and strategies receive far less attention. The sense of urgency associated with improving the quality of medical care does not exist with respect to improving the quality of management decisions making a more evidence-based approach would improve the competence of the decision makers and their motivation to use more scientific methods when making a decision" (Kovner & Rundall, 2009, p. 53). Most nurse managers do not consider evidence such as research on a routine basis when they make management decisions, and many managers are not even familiar with the term management evidence though it is has been highlighted in some nursing professional standards and literature such as the American Organization of Nurse Executives (AONE) 2010–2012 strategic plan. One of the AONE strategic objectives is to "utilize evidence-based management practice and sound research in the development of future patient care delivery systems and practice environments. Explore and support the interrelations of technology, facility design and patient care delivery models" (American Organization of Nurse Executives, 2010).

What is evidence-based management (EBM)? It would seem natural to think that if evidence is important in making clinical or practice decisions it should be important in making management decisions. EBM is the "systematic application of the best available evidence to the evaluation of managerial strategies for improving the performance of health services organizations" (Kovner & Rundall, 2009, p. 56). This definition is not much different from the EBP definition. It is important for nursing leaders and managers to base their decisions on best management evidence whenever possible, preferably management research. The five principles of evidence-based management are as follows (Evidence-Based Management, 2010):

- Face the hard facts, and build a culture in which people are encouraged to tell the truth, even if it is unpleasant.
- Be committed to "fact-based" decision making, which means being committed to getting the best evidence and using it to guide actions.
- Treat your organization as an unfinished prototype; encourage experimentation and learning by doing.
- Look for the risks and drawbacks in what people recommend—even the best medicine has side effects.
- Avoid basing decisions on untested but strongly held beliefs, what you have done in the past, or on uncritical "benchmarking" of what winners do.

### Evidence-Based Management Process

Just as there is an EBP process, there is an EBM process. Both processes are similar. The steps include (Kovner & Rundall, 2009, p. 63):

1. **Formulating the question:**  Formulate the management question so that research studies can be found. This may require a broader question than originally proposed, but if the question is too broad and vague, it will not yield research studies that are helpful. It is best to include clarification of the technique or tool, the setting, and outcome of interest. This is similar to the PICO question used in EBP.
2. **Acquiring research evidence:**  Evidence can be obtained from experts, colleagues, personal experience, and published literature; similar to EBP sources that are more than just research evidence. This requires literature searches similarly done for EBP. The best source is research syntheses of a large number of studies on the question. It is not easy to find this type of evidence, particularly in nursing management. This is not an area that has a large

## APPLYING EVIDENCE-BASED PRACTICE

### Evidence for Effective Leadership and Management

Citation:    Arndt, M. & Bigelow, B. (2009). Evidence-based management in health care organizations: A cautionary note. *Health Care Management Review, 34*(3), 206–213.

Overview:    Evidence-based management (EBM) is a relatively new approach to management, and at this time there is limited research on "the diffusion of evidence-based management or its effectiveness. Instead, advocates make the case for it as a "new" way of decision making that is based on unexpressed assumptions—that decisions based on evidence will yield the anticipated results, with evidence generalizable to other organizations, and that evidence is objective" (p. 206). This article reviews current literature and explores EBM and its current status.

Application:    EBM is important if it can provide evidence to support decisions; however, these authors note that there is a danger in over emphasis on EBM. Management decisions also require creativity and risk taking. Management is too complex with many variables impacting decisions.

Questions:

1. *Why do you think these authors use the term "a cautionary note" in the title of the article?*
2. *Compare EBP and EBM and why they are different from a management perspective.*
3. *Why is creativity and risk taking important in the leadership and management roles?*
4. *How could a manager balance effective use of EBM with some flexibility?*

research library to choose from. Many of the questions that a nurse leader or manager would propose may actually be addressed in health care delivery, business, and organization research, though these areas are also weak in research.

3. **Assessing the quality of the evidence:** Managers should assess the following aspects of the evidence: strength of the research design, study context and setting, sample sizes, control of confounding factors, reliability and validity of measurements, methods and procedures, justification of the conclusions, study sponsorship, and consistency of the findings with other studies. These criteria are very similar to the criteria used to assess EBP evidence.

4. **Presenting the evidence:** This is not a step that is actively considered in EBP, but it is in EBM. When a manager presents evidence to support a decision, the following should be considered in the presentation, whether it is oral or written. It should be timely, brief, easily understood with limited use of jargon, clear description of questions addressed, context of the research, assessment of the quality of the evidence, and the results and the implications for management. This is when the manager "makes the case" for a decision.

5. **Applying the evidence to the decision:** Application of evidence in management is just as difficult as it is to apply evidence in clinical practice. Figure 15-3 provides another description of the decision-making process in relationship to EBM.

Identification of the problem is the description of "the discrepancy between an existing and desired state of affairs" (Kovner & Rundall, 2009, p. 57). Steps 5 and 6 are particularly important as they emphasize the need to analyze alternatives and then select the best alternative based on the evidence on hand. Nurse managers need to take the time to do this. The tendency is to grab at a possible solution with limited consideration of alternatives and analyzing evidence supporting the alternatives.

### Evidence-Based Management: Barriers and Strategies

There are many barriers to implementing EBM; some are similar to the barriers to implementing EBP. Examples of barriers are as follows:

- Lack of leadership support
- Lack of technology and library expertise

### FIGURE 15-3 The Eight-Stage Decision-Making Process.

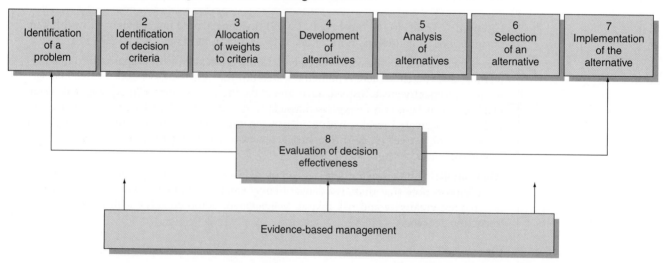

Source: Kovner, A. & Randall, T. (2009). Evidence-based management reconsidered. In A. Kovner, D. Fine, & R. D'Aquila (Eds.), *Evidence-based Management in Healthcare* (pp. 53–57). Adapted by Kovner & Randall from S. Robbins & D. Decenzo. (2004). *Fundamentals of management: Essential concepts and applications*, (4th ed.). Upper Saddle River, NJ: Pearson Prentice Hall. Reprinted with permission. Robbins, Stephen P.; Decenzo, David A., *Fundamentals of management: Essential concepts and applications*, 3rd, ©2001. Printed and electronically reproduced by permission of Pearson Education, Inc., Upper Saddle River, New Jersey.

- Lack of knowledge about EBM and the confusion over the difference between EBM and EBP
- Limited or no recognition of the value of EBM with limited expectation that managers will use EBM
- Limited time
- Restrictions on decision making, e.g., centralized decision making, rigid policies and procedures, and other bureaucratic factors
- Limited relevant research and limited EBM literature such as systematic reviews
- Lack of structure to implement EBM
- Resistance to EBM so that one can make decisions based on personal preferences rather than evidence

What strategies might be used to support the integration of EBM within an HCO? Some examples of implementing systematic processes to make major decisions are provided by Rundall et al. (2009, p. 15):

- Periodically brief managers on recent management research related to the organization's operational and strategic concerns.
- Incorporate research assessments into due diligence reports.
- Train management team members in the steps of evidence-based decision making.
- Establish ties with academic institutions and research centers.

These strategies should be incorporated into nursing management. The last strategy is an important one. Many nursing departments are associated with schools of nursing for EBP implementation. If the school has faculty experienced in leadership and management then using this expertise can assist the HCO and also build stronger bridges with the school of nursing—collaboration will be more evident. D'Aquila (2009) also recommends incorporating EBM into performance evaluation of managers—are they using EBM? This will need to be tracked or monitored. Strategic planning should also demonstrate use of EBM and should include a method for monitoring decision making.

## Research, Evidence-Based Practice, and Quality Improvement

It is easy to get nursing research (NR), evidence-based practice, and quality improvement (QI) confused. Chapters 16 and 17 discuss QI in more detail, but it is important here to clarify similarities and differences in them. Hedges (2006) describe them as a three-legged stool with research, EBP, and QI supporting clinical decisions. Research and EBP have been defined and described earlier in the chapter. Quality improvement involves data collection and analysis "just as they are in research, and herein lies the confusion for many nurses, as the terminology and statistical language is similar with both methods. However, QI has no theoretical underpinnings and does not seek to generate new knowledge or test interventions. It evaluates the work process in a cyclic fashion, benchmarks practice against established indicators, and provides a means to continually evaluate and improve established practice" (Hedges, 2006, p. 457). A key difference in QI from research and EBP is that the data are usually collected and reported internally, within the organization. The purpose is not to generate new knowledge as it is with research. Typically IRB approval is not required nor is participant consent in the same manner as would be done for research; however, there have been recent situations where this has been questioned and this has caused problems. The best approach is to ask the IRB committee if the QI project meets requirements for exemption from IRB requirements (Miller & Emanuel, 2008). The decision as to how to proceed, however, would be decisions made by leadership or management. "By monitoring our practice and patient outcomes (QI), systematically reviewing the evidence (EBP), and conducting scientific studies (NR) when the evidence is lacking, we can strengthen the foundation of our practice. Patients will then be receiving the best care possible by nurses dedicated to the continuous review and revision of their practice" (Hedges, 2006, p. 458).

# APPLYING LEADERSHIP AND MANAGEMENT

## MY HOSPITAL UNIT

You must make a lot of decisions as nurse manager on your unit. Select a problem that you might encounter on a daily basis on your unit and apply the evidence-based management process as described in this chapter to your management question. Include references that you identify as relevant and summarize the key points to answer your management question. Use the virtual unit site from the textbook website to record the work that you do in the role of nurse manager for your unit.

## Critical Thinking Questions and Activities

1. Discuss the barriers to research and strategies that might be used to overcome these barriers. Consider strategies not discussed in the chapter.
2. Discuss the four types of EBP evidence.
3. Develop a PICO question and look for a systematic review or a clinical guideline to answer your question.
4. Discuss the barriers to EBP and strategies that might be used to overcome these barriers. Consider strategies not discussed in the chapter.
5. Why is it important for nurses to use EBP?
6. Describe the EBM process and how it might apply to nursing management.
7. Discuss the barriers to EBM and strategies that might be used to overcome these barriers. Consider strategies not discussed in the chapter.
8. Compare and contrast research, EBP, EBM, and QI. Provide examples for each.

## Media Links

- **URL: http://www.ninr.nih.gov/**
  National Institute of Nursing Research
- **URL: http://ohsr.od.nih.gov/guidelines/nuremberg.html**
  Nuremberg Code (research ethics)
- **URL: http://ohsr.od.nih.gov/guidelines/belmont.html**
  Belmont Report (research ethics)
- **URL: http://www.joannabriggs.edu.au/about/home.php**
  Joanna Briggs Institute (EBP database)
- **URL: http://www.cochrane.org**
  Cochrane Library (EBP database)
- **URL: http://www.acestar.uthscsa.edu/**
  Academic Center for Evidence-Based Practice
- **URL: http://www.ahrq.gov/research/ACTION.htm**
  Accelerating Change and Transformation in Organizations and Networks (ACTION)
- **URL: http://nyu.libguides.com/content.php?pid=27011&sid=234199**
  Evidence-Based Health Care Resources (New York University)
- **URL: http://www.guideline.gov/**
  National Guideline Clearinghouse
- **URL: http://www.ahrq.gov/clinic/epcindex.htm#top**
  AHRQ Evidence-Based Practice Centers Reports

**Pearson Nursing Student Resources**

Find additional review materials at
**nursing.pearsonhighered.com**

Prepare for success with additional NCLEX®-style practice questions, interactive assignments and activities, Web links, animations and videos, and more!

# References

Academic Center for Evidence-Based Nursing. (2008). Star model. Retrieved November 12, 2009, from http://www.acestar.uthscsa.edu

Accelerating Change and Transformation in Organizations and Networks (ACTION) (2009). Retrieved February 14, 2010, from http://www.ahrq.gov/research/ACTION.htm

Agency for Health care Research and Quality. (2008). Evidence-Based Practice Centers. Retrieved February 14, 2010, from http://www.ahrq.gov/clinic/epc

American Nurses Credentialing Center. (2010). Evidence-based practice: Creating a culture of inquiry. Retrieved February 10, 2010, from http://www.nursecredentialing.org/Magnet/MagnetEvents/Magnet-Events-List/RecognitionWorkshops/EBP.aspx

American Organization of Nurse Executives. (2010). 2010–2012 Strategic Plan. Retrieved February 11, 2010, from http://www.aone.org/aone/about/pdfs/2010-2012AONEStratPlanFinal.pdf

Brown, S. (2009). *Evidence-based nursing. The research-practice connection.* Boston: Jones & Bartlett Publishers.

Cope, D. (2003). Evidence-based practice: Making it happen in your clinical setting. *Clinical Journal of Oncology Nursing, 7*(1), 97–98.

Cronewett, L. (2002, February 19). Research, practice and policy: Issues in evidence-based care. *Online Journal of Issues in Nursing.* Retrieved from http://www.nursingworld.org/MainMenuCategories/ANAMarketplace/ANAPeriodicals/OJIN/Columns/KeynotesofNote/EvidenceBasedCare.aspx

Davidoff, E. (1999). In the teeth of evidence. The curious case of evidence-based medicine. *Mount Sinai Journal of Medicine, 66*(2), 75–83.

DePalma, J. (2002). Proposing evidence-based policy process. *Nursing Administration Quarterly, 26*(4), 55–61.

D'Aquila, R. (2009). Application of evidence-based management at an academic medical center: The Yale-New Haven Hospital experience. In A. Kovner, D. Fine, & R. D'Aquila (Eds.), *Evidence-based management in health care* (pp. 17–28). Chicago: Health Administration Press.

Dickson-Hazard, N. (2002). Evidence-based practice, 'the right approach.' *Reflections on Nursing Leadership,* (second quarter), 6.

Dickson-Hazard, N., & Entwistle, V. (1997). Systematic reviews. Keeping up with research evidence. *Systematic Reviews: Examples for nursing, 2,* 3.

Evans, D., & Pearons, A. (2001). Systematic reviews: Gatekeepers of nursing knowledge. *Journal of Clinical Nursing, 10,* 593–599.

Evidence-based management. (2010). Retrieved February 10, 2010, from http://www.evidence-basedmanagement.com/index.html

Finkelman, A., & Kenner, C. (2010). *Professional nursing concepts. Competencies for quality leadership.* Boston: Jones and Bartlett Publishers.

Gawlinski, A. (2008). The power of clinical nursing research: Engage clinicians, improve patients' lives, and forge a professional legacy. *American Journal of Critical Care, 17*(4), 315–326.

Grad, R., Macaulay, A., & Warner, M. (2001). Teaching evidence-based medical care: description and evaluation. *Family Medicine, 33,* 602–606.

Guyatt, G., & Rennie, D. (2002). *Users' guides to the medical literature.* Chicago: AMA Press.

Harris, R. et al. (2001). Current methods of the U.S. Preventive Services task Force: A review of the process. *American Journal of Preventive Medicine, 20,* 303–307.

Hedges, C. (2006). Research, evidence-based practice, and quality improvement. The 3-legged stool. *AACN Advanced Critical Care, 17*(4), 457–459.

Institute of Health Improvement. (2007). What is a bundle? Retrieved May 9, 2007, from http://www.ihi.org/IHI/Topics/CriticalCare

Institute of Medicine. (2003). *Health professions education.* Washington, DC: National Academies Press.

Institute of Medicine. (2008). *Knowing what works in health care.* Washington, DC: National Academies Press.

Kovner, A., Fine, D., & D'Aquila, R. (2009). Introduction. In A. Kovner, D. Fine, & R. D'Aquila (Eds.), *Evidence-based management in health care* (pp. xxi–xxvii). Chicago: Health Administration Press.

Kovner, A., & Rundall, T. (2009). Evidence-based management reconsidered. In A. Kovner, D. Fine, & R. D'Aquila (Eds.). (2009). *Evidence-based management in health care* (pp. 53–78). Chicago: Health Administration Press.

Krugman, S. (1986). The Willowbrook hepatitis studies revisited: Ethical aspects. *Reviews of Infectious Diseases, 8*(1), 157–162.

Lohr, K., & Carey, T. (1999). Assessing "best practice": Issues in grading the quality of studies for systematic reviews. *Joint Commission Journal on Quality Improvement, 25,* 470–479.

Mason, D. (2002). Who says it's best practice? *AJN, 102*(10), 7.

Melnyk, B., & Fineout-Overholt, E. (2005). Making the case for evidence-based practice. In B. Melnyk and E. Fineout-Overholt (Eds.), *Evidence-based practice in nursing and health care* (pp. 3–24). Philadelphia: Lippincott Williams & Wilkins.

Miller, F., & Emanuel, E. (2008). Quality improvement research and informed consent. *New England Journal of Medicine, 358*(8), 765–768.

Mooney, K. (2001). Advocating for quality cancer care: Making evidence-based practice a reality. *ONF28* (2 supplement), 17–21.

Moorehead, S., Johnson, M., & Maas, M. (Eds.). (2004). *Nursing outcomes classification (NOC).* (3rd ed.). St. Louis: Mosby.

National Guideline Clearinghouse. (2010). About NGC. Retrieved February 15, 2010, from http://www.guideline.gov

National Institutes of Health. (2010a). Office of Human Research Subjects: Nuremberg Code. Retrieved March 1, 2010, from http://ohsr.od.nih.gov/guidelines/nuremberg.html

National Institutes of Health. (2010b) Office of Human Research Subjects: Belmont Report. Retrieved March 1, 2010, from http://ohsr.od.nih.gov/guidelines/belmont.html

National Institute of Nursing Research. (2010). Retrieved February 12, 2010, from http://www.ninr.nih.gov

Newhouse, R., Dearholt, S., Poe, S., Pugh, L., & White, K. (2007). *Johns Hopkins nursing evidence-based practice model and guidelines*. Indianapolis, IN: Sigma Theta Tau International.

Polit, D., & Beck, C. (2008). (8th ed.). *Essentials of nursing research*. Philadelphia: Lippincott Williams & Wilkins.

Pravikoff, D., Tanner, A., & Pierce, S. (2005). Readiness for U.S. nurses for evidence-based practice. *American Journal of Nursing, 105*(9), 40–50.

Reich, W. (Ed.). (1995). *Encyclopedia of bioethic*. NY: Simon & Schuster Macmillan.

Rosswurm, M., & Larrabee, J. (1999). A model for change to evidence-based practice. *Image of Nursing Scholarship, 31*, 317–322.

Rundall, T. et al. (2009). Using research evidence when making decisions: Views of health services managers and policymakers. In A. Kovner, D. Fine, & R. D'Aquila (Eds.), *Evidence-based management in health care* (pp. 3–16). Chicago: Health Administration Press.

Rutledge, D., & Grant, M. (2002). Introduction to evidence-based practice in cancer nursing. *Seminars in Oncology Nursing, 18*(2), 1–2.

Schmidt, N. & Brown, J. (2009). What is Evidence-Based Practice. In N. Schmidt & J. Brown (Eds.), *Evidence-based practice for nurses* (pp. 3–33). Boston: Jones & Bartlett Publishers.

Stetler, C. et al. (1998). Utilization-focused integrative reviews in a nursing service. *Applied Nursing Research, 11*(4), 195–206.

Titler, M., Cullen, L., & Ardery, G. (2002). Evidence-based practice: An administrative perspective. *Reflections in Nursing Leadership, 28*(2), 26–27.

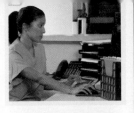
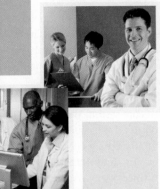

# 16

# Health Care Quality: A Critical Health Policy Issue

## CHAPTER OUTLINE

## LEARNING OUTCOMES

Before you begin, take a moment to familiarize yourself with the learning outcomes for this chapter.

- Analyze the relationship of the Institute of Medicine core competencies to quality improvement.
- Critique critical issues related to defining quality.
- Apply structure, process, and outcomes to quality.
- Identify two factors that support an increased interest in quality care.
- Summarize the recent activity on health care quality of the Institute of Medicine and its importance to health care and nursing.

## KEY TERMS

- Error
- Outcome
- Process
- Quality care
- Safety
- Structure
- System

**WHAT'S AHEAD**

The Institute of Medicine's (IOM) fourth health care profession core competency is to apply quality improvement (QI). The IOM describes this core competency as "identify errors and hazards in care; understand and implement basic safety design principles, such a standardization and simplification; continually understand and measure quality of care in terms of structure, process, and outcomes in relation to patient and community needs; and design and test interventions to change processes an systems of care, with the objective of improving quality" (2003, p. 4). As noted in this report and also the IOM report *To Err Is Human* (1999), the U.S. health care system is dysfunctional and has problems with safety, quality, and inefficiency. Nurses encounter these issues as they try to ensure that patients receive quality, timely care. The health care system is the focus of quality improvement (QI). The system is fragmented and in need of improvement. A **system** "can be defined by the coming together of parts, interconnections, and purpose. While systems can be broken down into parts, which are interesting in and of themselves, the real power lies in the way the parts come together and are interconnected to fulfill some purpose" (Plsek, 2001, p. 309). The health care system is composed of a continuum of services (e.g., medicine, surgery, women's health, pediatrics, etc.), settings (e.g., hospitals, clinics, physician practices, long-term care facilities, home care agencies, hospice, pharmacies, laboratories, etc.), health care professionals (e.g., nurses, physicians, social workers, administrators, etc.), third-party payers/purchasers, and patients/consumers. Ideally, this system should be interconnected and a functioning, effective system for patients to receive effective care (Plsek, 2001). Each patient's care is part of this overall emphasis on health care improvement. Ultimately, the goal is that each patient's outcomes will be met. Quality improvement now emphasizes improvement and describes problem identification as an opportunity to improve. The older term is quality assessment or assurance. QI should be a continuous, active process. How can this be applied to the health care system that is rapidly changing? This chapter discusses the critical issues of quality care and safety in the health care delivery system. With this complex system that is changing daily, the task of determining quality of care and the best way to improve care are difficult to accomplish. It is important to note that prior to the Institute of Medicine quality series the United States had no comprehensive system to monitor health care, judge improvement, or to determine the best strategies to improve health care. The U.S. now has an annual report describing national health care quality data. This chapter focuses on health care quality from a health policy perspective and the history of its expansion, and Chapter 17 continues the discussion by focusing on the implementation of health care quality improvement.

# The Changing View of Quality

Quality is a complex concept, with many factors affecting it. There have recently been some strong influences on the increasing interest in quality, safe care. Assessing and improving care is not a static process. The following discussion includes information about the increased interest in quality of care and the definition of quality care and its critical elements.

## CASE STUDY

### Policy Development Is Not for Us

A local nursing organization is meeting to discuss what the organization's focus should be in the coming year. One member of the executive committee says, "I think we need to consider the IOM quality reports." The treasurer quickly responds, "Those reports have nothing to do with us or health care in our community or state!" The committee is quiet. The president then joins the discussion as he agrees with the suggestion to focus on these reports though he is not sure what to do with the idea.

### Questions:

1. How might the president respond to this discussion in a positive manner?
2. What strategies could the organization use to implement the reports' recommendations? Consider policy development, professional education including continuing education, collaboration with other health care professions, and other professional organizations.
3. How is advocacy connected to this topic?

### The Institute of Medicine Health Care Quality Reports

In the past 10 years there has been increasing interest in the quality of health care, particularly since the publication of the Institute of Medicine report *To Err Is Human* (1999). This report signaled that the system was experiencing frequent and important errors. This result led to the IOM initiative to examine the health care system in more detail. How did this process begin, and where is it today?

President Clinton's Presidential Advisory Commission on Consumer Protection and Quality in the Health Care Industry (1997) was a major reason that the Institute of Medicine took up the issue of quality care. This commission addressed many of the concerns about quality care and the need to make changes to improve care. Three nurse leaders served on the 32-member commission. The purpose of the commission was to advise the president about the impact of health care delivery system changes on quality, consumer protection, and the availability of needed services (Wakefield, 1997). The commission consisted of four subcommittees.

1. The first subcommittee's purpose was to develop a *Consumer Bill of Rights, Protections, and Responsibilities*. Critical issues covered were health care coverage/reimbursement, choice of practitioners, privacy and confidentiality, disclosure of practitioner qualifications, and external appeals processes. Despite the recommendations from this commission, the United States still does not have a Consumer Bill of Rights. This is really the only element of this commission's work that has not been successful.
2. The second subcommittee was created to *identify performance measurement and quality oversight that would improve the validity and reliability of performance measurement data*.
3. The third subcommittee, which was chaired by a nurse, considered the *creation of a quality improvement environment and the internal and external barriers and facilitators of quality improvement*.
4. The fourth subcommittee focused on the *roles of public and private oversight entities, strategies to reach a balance between market-driven quality incentives and regulatory requirements, and the responsibilities of group purchasers to protect quality*.

The final report from the commission, *Quality First: Better Health Care for all Americans*, was published in 1999. This commission and its report stimulated the development of the Quality of Health Care in America project, which resulted in the development of the *Quality Chasm* series of reports initiated by the Institute of Medicine in June, 1998. The purpose of the project was to expand the work of Clinton's commission after it completed its charge and to develop strategies that would improve quality of care over the next 10 years. This has been expanded beyond 10 years. Box 16-1 highlights the key Institute of Medicine reports that are a part of this project.

## BOX 16-1  CURRENT REPORTS ON HEALTH CARE QUALITY

**First report** (Clinton Administration) that stimulated IOM reports.

- Advisory Commission on Consumer Information and Quality in the Health Care Industry. *Quality first: Better health care for all Americans.*

The following reports can be accessed at the websites indicated.

- Institute of Medicine. (1999). *To err is human:* Building a safer health system. Washington, DC: National Academies Press.
  http://www.nap.edu/catalog/9728.html?se_side
- Institute of Medicine. (2001). *Crossing the quality chasm:* A new health system for the 21st century. Washington, DC: National Academies Press.
  http://books.nap.edu/catalog/10027.html?onpi_newsdoc030101
- Institute of Medicine. (2001). *Envisioning the national healthcare quality report.* Washington, DC: National Academies Press.
  http://www.nap.edu/catalog/10073.html?se_side
- Institute of Medicine. (2002). *Leadership by example: Coordinating government roles in improving health care quality.* Washington, DC: National Academies Press.
  http://www.nap.edu/catalog/10537.html?se_side
- Institute of Medicine. (2003). *Who will keep the public healthy?* Educating public health professionals for the 21st century. Washington, DC: National Academies Press.
  http://www.nap.edu/catalog/10542.html?se_side
- Institute of Medicine. (2003). *Health professions education: A bridge to quality.* Washington, DC: National Academies Press.
  http://www.nap.edu/catalog/10681.html?se_side
- Institute of Medicine. (2003). *Priority areas for national action: Transforming health care quality.* (2003). Washington, DC: National Academies Press.
  http://www.nap.edu/catalog/10593.html?onpi_newsdoc010703
- Institute of Medicine. *Keeping patients safe: Transforming the work environment of nurses.* Washington, DC: National Academies Press.
  http://www.nap.edu/catalog/10851.html
- Institute of Medicine. (2003). *Patient safety: Achieving a new standard for care.* Washington, DC: National Academies Press.
  http://www.nap.edu/catalog/10863.html

### Examples of Special Focus IOM Reports

- Institute of Medicine. (2006). *Preventing medication errors.* Washington, DC: National Academies Press.
- Institute of Medicine. (2007). *Hospital-based emergency care: At the breaking point.* Washington, DC: National Academies Press.
- Institute of Medicine. (2007). *Emergency care for children: Growing pains.* Washington, DC: National Academies Press.
- Institute of Medicine. (2005). *Preventing childhood obesity: Health in the balance.* Washington, DC: National Academies Press.
- Institute of Medicine. (2005). *Quality through collaboration: The future of rural health.* Washington, DC: National Academies Press.
- Institute of Medicine. (2006). *Improving the quality of healthcare for mental and substance-use conditions.* Washington, DC: National Academies Press.
- Institute of Medicine. (2006). *From cancer patient to career survivor. Lost in transition.* Washington, DC: National Academies Press.
- Institute of Medicine. (2007). *Preterm birth: Causes, consequences, and prevention.* Washington, DC: National Academies Press.
- Institute of Medicine. (2007). *Cancer care for the whole patient: Meeting psychosocial health needs.* Washington, DC: National Academies Press.

| BOX 16-1 | CURRENT REPORTS ON HEALTH CARE QUALITY (CONTINUED) |
|---|---|

- Institute of Medicine. (2008). *Retooling for an aging America: Building the healthcare workforce.* Washington, DC: National Academies Press.
- Institute of Medicine. (2011). *The future of nursing: Leading, changing, advancing health.* Washigton, DC: National Academies Press.

As indicated by the number of reports and their content, much work has been done since Clinton's advisory commission in 1997. The following discussion provides an overview of the content of these critical reports related to quality health care.

TO ERR IS HUMAN    The first report, *To Err Is Human. Building a Safer Health System* (Institute of Medicine, 1999), focused on safety within the health care delivery system. Data indicated that there have been and continue to be serious safety problems. Examples include the following:

- When data from one study was extrapolated, the result was at least 44,000 Americans die each year as a result of a medication error. Another study indicated the number could be as high as 98,000 (American Hospital Association, 1999; as cited in Institute of Medicine, 1999).
- More people die in a given year as a result of medical errors than from motor vehicle accidents (43,458), breast cancer (42,297), or AIDS (16,516) (Institute of Medicine, 1999).
- Health care costs represent over one-half of total national costs, which include lost income, lost household production, disability, and health care costs (Institute of Medicine, 1999).

There are clear problems, and to date the focus has only been on hospital errors. This, however, does not negate the presence of medical errors in home health care, long-term care, ambulatory care, primary care, and other health care settings. These are settings that require further exploration.

What are some of the outcomes from errors that cause further problems? Cost is certainly a concern, and errors can result in a variety of costs. Complications that result from errors may lead to increased health care costs. Opportunity costs occur when repeat diagnostic tests are required or interventions are needed to counteract adverse drug events. Another critical concern is patients' loss of trust in the health care system and its providers. If a patient experiences an error, this has a direct impact on the patient's trust in the health care system; however, the increase in media coverage of health care quality can also have just as serious an impact on patient trust in the system.

Historically, accrediting and licensing organizations have not focused much on the issue of errors, but this has changed. The decentralized and fragmented health care system certainly has been a factor in contributing to unsafe conditions, and it interferes with improvement (Institute of Medicine, 1999 & 2001a). Multiple providers and ineffective communication also are other problems that affect patient safety. Third-party payers (managed care organizations and other types of insurers) have become more involved in encouraging providers to improve care as they recognize the impact this can have on decreasing costs.

The report on safety clearly states that there is no one answer to solving this problem. This report defines **safety** as "freedom from accidental injury" and defines **error** as "the failure of a planned action to be completed as intended or the use of a wrong plan to achieve an aim" (Institute of Medicine, 1999, p. 3). Errors are directly related to outcomes, which is a significant concern in quality improvement efforts. There are two types of errors: error of planning and error of execution. Errors harm the patient and some errors that do injure the patient may have been preventable adverse events. In 1999, the Institute of Medicine identified three types of quality problems that are used in the measurement of quality.

1. **Misuse:** avoidable complications that prevent patients from receiving full potential benefit of a service
2. **Overuse:** potential for harm from the provision of a service that exceeds the possible benefit
3. **Underuse:** failure to provide a service that would have produced a favorable outcome for the patient

The four key messages from *To Err Is Human* report are "first, the magnitude of harm that results from medical errors is great; second, errors result largely from systems' failures, not individual failures; third, voluntary and mandatory reporting programs are needed now to improve patient safety; and fourth, the IOM committee and others call on health care systems to focus on error reduction as an important part of their operations and to embrace organizational change needed to reorient error-ridden systems and process" (Maddox, Wakefield, & Bull, 2001, p. 9). Nurses must be involved in developing plans to respond to safety problems on the local, state, and national levels. Chapter 17 extends this discussion on quality, focusing on QI implementation.

CROSSING THE QUALITY CHASM    The second major report from the Committee on the Quality of Health Care in America was *Crossing the Quality Chasm* (Institute of Medicine, 2001a), which focused on developing a new health care system for the 21st century, one that improves care. The first conclusion from the report is that the system is in need of repair, one of fundamental change. As this text has emphasized, the report also emphasizes the impact of the rapid change in the health care system: new medical science, new technology, rapid availability of information, and so on. Health care providers cannot keep up and "performance of the health care system varies considerably" (Institute of Medicine, 2001a, p. 3). Content in Chapter 3 on change is relevant to the QI process, which is highly dependent on change for improvement. As was noted in *To Err Is Human*, the system is fragmented and poorly organized, and the system does not make the best use of its resources.

Another conclusion from the report is the impact that the increase of chronic conditions has had on the system. With people living longer, mostly due to advances in medical science and technology, more people are living with chronic conditions. "Chronic conditions, defined as illnesses that last longer than 3 months and are not self-limiting, are now the leading cause of illness, disability, and health problems in this country, and affect almost half of the U.S. population" (Institute of Medicine, 2001a, p. 27). Many of these patients also have co-morbid conditions. They have complicated problems and require collaborative treatment efforts, "involving the definition of clinical problems in terms that both patients and providers understand; joint development of a care plan with goals, targets, and implementations strategies; provision of self-management training and support services; and active, sustained follow-up using visits, telephone calls, e-mail, and Web-based monitoring and decision support programs" (Institute of Medicine, 2001a, p. 27). The complex, fragmented, and disorganized health care system is ineffective in dealing with these problems. Chronic illness is a critical component of patient-centered care as discussed in Chapter 8.

This 2001 report identifies quality as a system property and identifies six aims or goals for improvement, concluding that care should be (Institute of Medicine, 2001a, pp. 5–6)

1. *Safe:*   Avoiding injuries to patients from the care that is intended to help them
2. *Effective:*   Providing services based on scientific knowledge (evidence-based practice) to all who could benefit and reframing from providing services to those not likely to benefit (avoiding underuse and overuse)
3. *Patient-centered:*   Providing care that is respectful of and responsive to individual patient preferences, needs, and values and ensuring that patient values guide all clinical decisions
4. *Timely:*   Reducing waits and harmful delays for both those who receive and those who give care
5. *Efficient:*   Avoiding waste, including waste of equipment, supplies, ideas, and energy
6. *Equitable:*   Providing care that does not vary in quality because of personal characteristics such as gender, ethnicity, geographic location, and socioeconomic status (disparity concern)

These aims or goals are highlighted in Figure 16-1, and all are related to nursing practice and health care management and should be integrated into individual patient care planning and into management.

"Health care has safety and quality problems because it relies on outmoded systems of work. Poor designs set the workforce up to fail, regardless of how hard they try. If we want safer, higher-quality care, we will need to have redesigned systems of care, including the use of information

**FIGURE 16-1   Six aims for improvement of the health care system.**

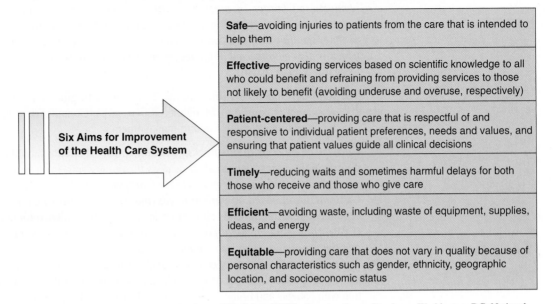

**Six Aims for Improvement of the Health Care System**

**Safe**—avoiding injuries to patients from the care that is intended to help them

**Effective**—providing services based on scientific knowledge to all who could benefit and refraining from providing services to those not likely to benefit (avoiding underuse and overuse, respectively)

**Patient-centered**—providing care that is respectful of and responsive to individual patient preferences, needs and values, and ensuring that patient values guide all clinical decisions

**Timely**—reducing waits and sometimes harmful delays for both those who receive and those who give care

**Efficient**—avoiding waste, including waste of equipment, supplies, ideas, and energy

**Equitable**—providing care that does not vary in quality because of personal characteristics such as gender, ethnicity, geographic location, and socioeconomic status

Source: Author and summarized from Institute of Medicine. (2001). *Crossing the quality chasm.* Washington, DC: National Academy Press, pp. 5–6. Reprinted with permission.

technology to support clinical and administrative processes" (Institute of Medicine, 2001a, p. 4). These identified problems are complex and not easily resolved. Some of them have been addressed, such as redesigning, but the results have not always improved care. How should health care providers resolve them and improve? The report's recommendations that are directly related to nursing care include the following.

- All health care constituents, including policy makers, purchasers, regulators, health professionals, health care trustees and management, and consumers, commit to a national statement of purpose for the health care systems as a whole and to a shared agenda of six aims for improvement that can raise the quality of care to unprecedented levels. *This is related to the six aims identified by the report and described in Figure 16-1. These aims or goals are not easy to accomplish. Each aim is directly related to nursing.*

- Clinicians, patients, and the health care organizations that support care delivery adopt a new set of principles to guide the redesign of care processes. *Identifying critical concerns is important. Often clinicians, managers, patients, health care organizations, and third-party payers do not agree; however, effective QI requires stakeholder collaboration.*

- U.S. Department of Health and Human Services (DHHS) identifies a set of priority conditions to focus initial efforts, provide resources to stimulate innovation, and initiate the change process. *See comments about the report,* Priority Areas for National Action (Institute of Medicine, 2003a), *later in this section. This IOM report identifies specific conditions requiring improvement approaches. This report followed the* Crossing the Quality Chasm *report.*

- Health care organizations design and implement more effective organizational support processes to make change in the delivery of care possible. *As discussed in Chapter 3, change is ever present, and health care organizations and their leaders and staff must learn more effective methods for coping with change to improve and to see change as an opportunity.*

- Purchasers, regulators, health professions, educational institutions, and the DHHS create an environment that fosters and rewards improvement by (a) creating an infrastructure to support evidence-based practice, (b) facilitating the use of information technology (IT), (c) aligning payment incentives, and (d) preparing the workforce to better serve patients in a world of expanding knowledge and rapid change. *There is no doubt that these are key issues, which are discussed throughout this text. DHHS has provided some infrastructure to support evidence-based practice through its website, but more support is needed. As identified in Chapter 18, much has been done to develop information technology. Financial issues and reimbursement are also major areas of deep concern. Nursing education as well as other health care professional education must make changes to meet the new demands, which is also emphasized in the recent report on nursing education* (Benner, Sutphen, Leonard, & Day, 2010).

The IOM developed new rules for the 21st century to guide care delivery and improve the health care system (Institute of Medicine, 2001a, p. 8). Consider how each of the rules might apply to nursing clinical practice and to management.

- **Care based on continuous healing relationships.**  Patients should receive care whenever they need it—access is critical. *How does the nurse assist in ensuring that the patient gets care when needed from the most effective provider?*
- **Customization based on patient needs and values.**  This rule relates directly to patient-centered care. Patient needs and values are sources of evidence for evidence-based practice (EBP). *How can individual patient needs and values be included in the patient care plan and the program or service management plan?*
- **The patient as the source of control.**  Patients need information to make decisions about their own care—patient-centered care. Health care systems and professionals need to share information with patients and bring patients into the decision-making process. *How can the nurse include the patient and patient's family/significant others in the decision-making process?*
- **Shared knowledge and the free flow of information.**  Patients need access to their medical information, and clinicians need access. *What should the nurse do when the patient asks to have access to medical information?*
- **Evidence-based decision making.**  Patients need care that is based on the best possible evidence available. *How can the nurse ensure that care does not vary illogically from clinician to clinician or from place to place?*
- **Safety is a system property.**  Patients need to be safe from harm that may occur within the health care system. There needs to be more attention placed on system errors rather than individual errors. *How does the nurse prevent errors that might impact the patient's care?*
- **The need for transparency.**  The health care system should make information available to patients and their families that allow them to make informed decisions when selecting a health plan, hospital, or clinical practice, or choosing among alternative treatments. *How does the nurse effectively include information describing the system's performance on safety, evidence-based practice, and patient satisfaction in the care planning process?*
- **Anticipation of needs.**  Health care providers and the health system should not just react to events that may occur with patients but rather should anticipate patient needs whenever possible and provide care needed. *How are needs anticipated in the care plan?*
- **Continuous decrease in waste.**  Resources should not be wasted—including patient time. *How does the nurse incorporate effective use of resources in the care planning and implementation process?*
- **Cooperation among clinicians.**  Collaboration and communication are critical among health care professionals and systems (interprofessional teamwork). *How are collaboration and communication critical parts of the care process?*

ENVISIONING THE NATIONAL HEALTHCARE QUALITY REPORT   Following the development of the *Quality Chasm* report, which described the problem and critical concerns, the next question was how do we learn more and how do we monitor the quality of care so that interventions can be taken to improve care. In order to develop a national health quality report and analyze data, there needs to be a new health infrastructure with uniform data standards and computerized clinical data systems. The infrastructure has developed to the point that it can be used to meet this goal. How would a national health care quality report affect efforts to improve quality?

- Supply a common understanding of quality and how to measure it that reflects the best current approaches and practices.
- Identify aspects of the health care system that improve or impede quality.

- Generate data associated with major quality initiatives.
- Educate the public, the media, and other audiences about the importance of health care quality and the current level of quality.
- Identify for policy makers the problem areas in health care quality that most need their attention and action, with the understanding that these priorities may change over time and differ by geographic location.
- Provide policy makers, purchasers, health care providers, and others with realistic benchmarks for quality of care in the form of national, regional, and population comparisons.
- Make it easier to compare the quality of the U.S. health care system with that of other nations.
- Stimulate the refinement of existing measures and the development of new ones.
- Stimulate data collection efforts at the state and local levels (mirroring the national effort) to facilitate targeted quality improvements.
- Incorporate improved measures as they become available and practicable.
- Clarify the many aspects of health care quality and how they affect one another and quality as a whole.
- Encourage data collection efforts needed to refine and develop quality measures and, ultimately, stimulate the development of a health information infrastructure to support quality measurement and reporting (Institute of Medicine, 2001b, p. 31).

*Envisioning the National Healthcare Quality Report* (Institute of Medicine, 2001b) describes a framework that is now used to collect and organize annual data about health care quality, focusing on how the health care delivery system performs in providing personal health care. The framework for the annual report uses a matrix, which is "a tool to visualize possible combinations of the two dimensions of the framework and better understand how various aspects of framework relate to one another" (Institute of Medicine, 2001b, p. 8). The IOM uses two dimensions in the quality matrix to describe quality. *The first dimension focuses on safety, effectiveness, patient centeredness, and timeliness* (Institute of Medicine, 2001b, p. 41).

- *Safety* refers to the avoidance of injury or harm when providing care that is intended to help a person. Subcategories are (1) diagnosis, (2) treatment (e.g. medication, follow-up), and (3) health care environment.
- *Effectiveness* focuses on providing care that is based on scientific knowledge and avoids overuse and underuse. Subcategories are (1) preventive care, (2) acute, (3) chronic and (4) end-of-life care, and (5) appropriateness of procedures.
- *Patient centeredness* focuses on the partnership between the patient (and also as appropriate with families and caregivers) and health care providers. Subcategories are (1) experience of care and (2) effective partnership. This process emphasizes the role of the patients in decision-making about their own care.
- *Timeliness* or receiving care when it is needed with the least amount of delay is part of this dimension. Subcategories are (1) access to the system of care, (2) timeliness in getting to care for a particular problem, and (3) timeliness within and across episodes of care.

*The second dimension of quality care focuses on the consumer perspectives on health care needs and includes* (Institute of Medicine, 2001b, pp. 56–57):

- *Staying healthy* means that the individual needs to get health care to stay well and avoid illness.
- *Getting better* requires care to reach recovery.
- *Living with illness or disability* acknowledges that some health problems cannot be cured, and then the individual needs assistance in learning how to manage and cope long term.
- *Coping with the palliative or end-of-life* requires that individuals need support and care during terminal stages of illness. Families and caregivers are also involved in each of these consumer components of health care.

These components are considered to be key issues for individuals, affected by the individual's age. Across the life span, individuals view these components differently. Health care providers could use this matrix to evaluate an individual patient's care and outcomes. Particularly important and somewhat different is the second dimension in the matrix because this dimension

| TABLE 16-1 | NATIONAL HEALTHCARE QUALITY REPORT MATRIX |
|---|---|

| Consumer Perspectives on Healthcare Needs | Components of Healthcare Quality | | | |
|---|---|---|---|---|
| | Safety | Effectiveness | Patient Centeredness | Timeliness |
| Staying Healthy | | | | |
| Getting Better | | | | |
| Living with Illness or Disability | | | | |
| Coping with the End of Life | | | | |

Source: Institute of Medicine. (IOM). (2001). *Envisioning the National Healthcare Quality Report.* Washington, DC: National Academies Press, p. 61. Reprinted with permission.

expands on the patient or consumer of health care services and personal health issues and perspectives, reinforcing patient-centered care. Both dimensions emphasize quality and patient-centered care. Table 16-1 describes the matrix.

The Agency for Healthcare Resources and Quality (AHRQ), part of the U.S. Department of Health and Human Services, is mandated to collect the data using this quality framework. AHRQ then publishes an annual report describing the results, which is available on the Internet. This health care quality report should "serve as a yardstick or the barometer by which to gauge progress in improving the performance of the health care delivery system in consistently providing high-quality care" (Institute of Medicine, 2001b, p. 2). The report serves as the U.S. annual national report card; however, it does not replace the need for individual health care organizations (HCOs) to monitor their own organization's quality. The information from the national annual report is used by HCOs, insurers, health policy makers, and health professions educators to evaluate services, develop services, and determine health profession education needs. It is also information that nurse managers and nurses can use to increase their awareness of current quality concerns and relate the information to their specific health care organization's services. The report is available through the Internet. (See Media Links at the end of the chapter.)

PRIORITY AREAS FOR NATIONAL ACTION    After identifying the problem in *To Err Is Human* and describing it further in *Crossing the Quality Chasm* (2001a), the IOM concluded that the first step the United States needed to take was to conduct a systematic identification of the priority areas for quality improvement in order to make the necessary changes. In the *Priority Areas for National Action* (Institute of Medicine, 2003a) the IOM identified 20 priority areas. The first two areas are to promote care coordination and self-management/health literacy, both of which affect a broad range of groups and cross all the priority areas of care. The other areas are concerned with the continuum of care across the life span, preventive care, inpatient/surgical care, chronic conditions, end-of-life care, and behavioral care, though it is clear from this list that many are chronic illnesses. The 20 areas are as follows:

- Care coordination
- Self-management/health literacy
- Asthma—appropriate treatment for persons with mild/moderate persistent asthma
- Cancer screening that is evidence-based, with a focus on colorectal and cervical cancer
- Children with special health care needs (who are at increased risk for chronic physical, developmental, and behavioral conditions)
- Diabetes—focus on appropriate management of early disease
- End-of-life with advanced organ system failure—focus on congestive heart failure and chronic obstructive pulmonary disease
- Frailty associated with old age—preventing falls and pressure ulcers, maximizing function, and developing advanced care plans

- Hypertension—focus on appropriate treatment of early disease
- Immunization—children and adult
- Ischemic heart disease—prevention, reduction of recurring events, and optimization of functional capacity
- Major depression—screening and treatment
- Medical management—preventing medication errors and overuse of antibiotics
- Nosocomial infections—prevention and surveillance
- Pain control in advanced cancer
- Pregnancy and childbirth—appropriate prenatal and intrapartum care
- Severe and persistent mental illness—focus on treatment in the public sector
- Stroke—early treatment in the public sector
- Tobacco dependence treatment in adults
- Obesity (Institute of Medicine, 2003a, p. 3)

Using the matrix or framework identified in earlier reports the annual health care report focuses on monitoring these 20 areas. Health care providers should use these priority areas of care as a guide as they develop their QI programs. It is felt that improving care in these 20 areas will make a major difference on quality of care. Over time the list will be revised based on improvement in health care. Communities can also use this list to develop their community health focus and thus improve the quality of life and care of populations in the community. Figure 16-2 provides a summary view of the development of the approach to monitor and assess U.S. health care quality.

**LEADERSHIP BY EXAMPLE**  This report, requested by Congress, examined the federal government's quality enhancement processes (Institute of Medicine, 2003b). It focused on six government programs: Medicare, Medicaid, The State Children's Health Insurance Program (SCHIP), the Department of Defense TRICARE and TRICARE for life programs, the Veteran's Administration program, and the Indian Health Services program. These programs cover more

**FIGURE 16-2  Development of the *Quality Chasm* series.**

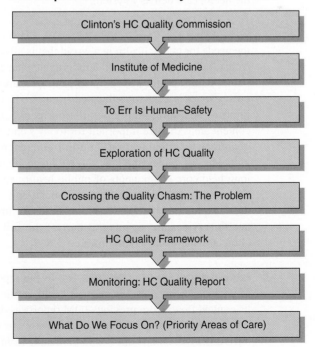

Source: Finkelman, A. & Kenner, C. (2009). *Teaching IOM: Implications of Institute of Medicine Reports for Nursing Education.* Silver Spring, MD: American Nurses Association. © 2009 by American Nurses Association. Reprinted with permission. All rights reserved.

than 100 million people. SCHIP was expanded by legislation signed by President Obama in early 2009. The report's conclusion was that improvement in the government's QI process was particularly needed.

1. There is a lack of consistent performance measurement across and within programs.
2. The usefulness of quality information has been questioned.
3. There is a lack of a conceptual framework to guide the evaluation.
4. There is a lack of computerized clinical data.
5. There is a lack of commitment to guide decisions.
6. There is a lack of a systematic approach for assessing the quality enhancement activities.

Each one of these problems will require substantial changes in the health care delivery system and relate directly to the results of the earlier IOM quality reports.

The report notes that federal leadership is needed because the federal government is in a unique position to assume a lead role to develop a national health care quality improvement initiative. The federal government is a "regulator; purchaser; health care provider; and sponsor of research, education, and training" (Institute of Medicine, 2001b, p. 6). It is the largest purchaser of care, and thus it could have a major impact on many people. It provides direct care to many: military personnel and their families, Native Americans, and veterans. Through these programs the federal government could establish models to improve care. This has already been demonstrated through Medicare and Medicaid. As a regulator the federal government can also affect many health care providers who are not in the federal system; for example, as was noted earlier in this text, health care organizations that accept Medicare or Medicaid funds must comply with federal regulations, which often then impacts all patients, not just Medicare and Medicaid patients. It should be noted that regulation is not the best way to make improvement changes because "the regulatory approach is a blunt tool that generally fails to differentiate among grades of quality" (Institute of Medicine, 2001b, p. 7). Regulation, however, should not be relied on as the only approach to the problem. Through sponsorship of research, education, and training; however, the federal government can have a major impact. The report's conclusions recommended that the federal government lead by example and coordinate government roles in improving health care quality. In doing this, the government will have an impact on all parts of the health care delivery system.

WHO WILL KEEP THE PUBLIC HEALTHY?   This report from the Institute of Medicine addressed the needs for public health in a world that is affected by globalization, rapid travel, scientific and technological advances, and demographic changes. In order to address public health problems, public health professionals need to be prepared to deal with the problems. "A public health professional is a person educated in public health or a related discipline who is employed to improve health through a population focus" (Institute of Medicine, 2003c, p. 4). The eight content areas that are important for today's and future public health professions are informatics, genomics, communication, cultural competence, community-based participatory research, global health, policy and law, and public health ethics. These content areas are in addition to the long held core components of public health: epidemiology, biostatistics, environmental health, health services administration, and social and behavioral science. This report provides an in-depth exploration of the educational needs for improved public health. Public health/community health services are an integral part of the full health care delivery system. Nurses work as clinicians and managers in this area.

HEALTH PROFESSIONS EDUCATION   In the report *Health Professions Education* (Institute of Medicine, 2003d), the education of health professions is viewed as a bridge to quality care, and its content flows from previous IOM reports as described in Figure 16-3.

This report's discussion does not just focus on nursing education, but rather on the need to have qualified, competent health care staff from all health care professional groups in order to improve health care. The report indicates that health professions' education is in need of change to meet the growing demands of the health care system today. "All health professionals should be

**FIGURE 16-3**  **Development of the IOM Healthcare Core Competencies.**

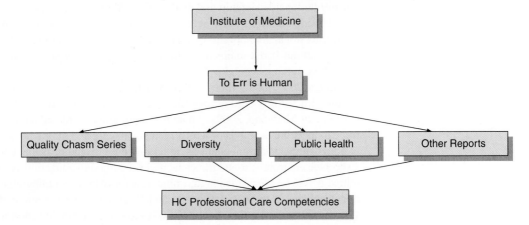

educated to deliver patient-centered care as members of an interprofessional team, emphasizing evidence-based practice, quality improvement approaches, and informatics" (Institute of Medicine, 2003d, p. 3). The five core competencies for all health care professionals (nurses, physicians, pharmacists, health care administrators, allied health and so on) are as follows:

- Provide patient-centered care
- Work in interprofessional teams
- Employ evidence-based practice
- Apply quality improvement
- Utilize informatics

All of these critical areas have been discussed in this text because they are very relevant to nurses, nursing care, and nursing leadership and management. In October 2009, the American Association of Colleges of Nursing (AACN) published a new edition of *The Essentials of Baccalaureate Education for Professional Nursing Practice*, which mentions the five core competencies in the first paragraph. The document specifies the essential content areas and competencies for baccalaureate programs. *Essential II, Basic Organizational and Systems Leadership for Quality Care and Patient Safety*, focuses on knowledge and skills in leadership, quality improvement, and patient safety necessary to provide high quality health care (American Association of Colleges of Nursing, 2009).

**KEEPING PATIENTS SAFE: TRANSFORMING THE WORK ENVIRONMENT OF NURSES**    The IOM report *Keeping Patients Safe: Transforming the Work Environment of Nurses* (Institute of Medicine, 2004) is an important report for nurses in all types of settings. This extensive report addresses critical quality issues with a particular focus on nursing care and nurses and examines these issues from the perspective of the work environment. As the report states, "When we are hospitalized, in a nursing home, or managing a chronic condition in our own homes—at some of our most vulnerable moments—nurses are the health care providers we are most likely to encounter, spend the greatest amount of time with, and be dependent upon for our recovery" (Institute of Medicine, 2004). From the review of the critical work environment the report describes methods for designing the work environment so that nurses may provide safer patient care. The content identifies concerns related to the nursing shortage, health care quality, health care errors, patient safety risk factors, central role of the nurse in patient safety, and work environment threats to patient safety. Recommendations for resolving these concerns include patient safety defenses; evidence-based model for safety defenses; reengineering issues; transformational leadership and evidence-based management; maximizing workforce capability through safe staffing levels, need for knowledge and skills and clinical decision making, and interprofessional collaboration; workspace design; and building and creating a culture of safety. This report has had a major impact on the practice of nursing, health care delivery, and should affect how nursing is taught.

In late 2009, the IOM began a consensus study to examine the future of nursing. The process began with forums held across the country and via the Internet. The study is described as (Institute of Medicine, 2009): An ad hoc committee examined the capacity of the nursing workforce to meet the demands of a reformed health care and public health system. It developed a set of bold national recommendations, including ones that address the delivery of nursing services in a shortage environment and the capacity of the nursing education system. In its report, the committee defined a clear agenda and blueprint for action including changes in public and institutional policies at the national, state, and local levels. Its recommendations address a range of system changes, including innovative ways to solve the nursing shortage in the U.S. The committee examined and produced recommendations related to the following issues, with the goal of identifying vital roles for nurses in designing and implementing a more effective and efficient health care system:

- Reconceptualizing the role of nurses within the context of the entire workforce, the shortage, societal issues, and current and future technology;
- Expanding nursing faculty, increasing the capacity of nursing schools, and redesigning nursing education to assure that it can produce an adequate number of well-prepared nurses able to meet current and future health care demands;
- Examining innovative solutions related to care delivery and health professional education by focusing on nursing and the delivery of nursing services; and
- Attracting and retaining well-prepared nurses in multiple care settings, including acute, ambulatory, primary care, long-term care, community and public health.
- Recommending nurse residency programs.
- Increasing number of baccalaureate prepared nurses to 80% of al RNs by 2020.
- Remove scope of practice barriers for nurse practicioners.

The report, *The Future of Nursing: Leading, Changing, Advancing Health* (2011) is accessible via the IOM website. This is another major report for nursing.

The Institute of Medicine health care quality reports are important sources of information for nurse leaders and managers. Since the publication of the basic reports on quality additional reports has been published that focus on specific problems or specific specialties or health care services such as emergency services, pediatrics, and oncology. All of the reports can be accessed on the Institute of Medicine website.

## Other Indicators of Increased Interest in Health Care Quality

What are factors in the health care delivery environment that indicate there is increased interest in the quality of care? Increased legislation is one indication, which shows a public concern for care. In 2005, the Patient Safety and Quality Improvement Act was signed into law. Box 16-2 describes this legislation.

The Institute of Medicine (IOM) reports from 1999 to 2003 and other related reports that have been published since this time certainly stimulated this legislative activity. The Department of Health and Human Services plays a major role in health care delivery in the United States and in assessing quality care. Box 16-3 highlights some of the activities of DHHS. The DHHS is responsible for developing rules and regulations for most federal health care laws and serves as the administrator for Medicare and Medicaid through the Centers for Medicare and Medicaid Services (CMS).

| BOX 16-2 | THE PATIENT SAFETY AND QUALITY IMPROVEMENT ACT OF 2005 |
|---|---|

The Patient Safety and Quality Improvement Act of 2005 (Public Law 109-41), signed into law on July 29, 2005, was enacted in response to growing concern about patient safety in the United States and the Institute of Medicine's 1999 report, *To Err is Human: Building a Safer Health System.* The law's goal is to improve patient safety by encouraging voluntary and confidential reporting of events that adversely affect patients.

The Patient Safety and Quality Improvement Act signifies the Federal Government's commitment to fostering a culture of patient safety. It creates Patient Safety Organizations (PSOs) to collect, aggregate, and analyze confidential information reported by health care providers. Currently, patient safety improvement efforts are hampered by the fear of discovery of peer deliberations, resulting in under-reporting of events and an inability to aggregate sufficient patient safety event data for analysis. By analyzing patient safety event information, PSOs will be able to identify patterns of failures and propose measures to eliminate patient safety risks and hazards.

Many providers fear that patient safety event reports could be used against them in medical malpractice cases or in disciplinary proceedings. This law addresses these fears by providing Federal legal privilege and confidentiality protections to information that is assembled and reported by providers to a PSO or developed by a PSO ("patient safety work product") for the conduct of patient safety activities. The law also significantly limits the use of this information in criminal, civil, and administrative proceedings and includes provisions for monetary penalties for violations of confidentiality or privilege protections.

The law specifies the role of PSOs and defines "patient safety work product" and "patient safety evaluation systems," which focus on how patient safety event information is collected, developed, analyzed, and maintained. In addition, this law has specific requirements for PSOs, such as the following:

- PSOs are required to work with more than one provider.
- Eligible organizations include public or private entities, profit or not-for-profit entities, provider entities, such as hospital chains, and other entities that establish special components.
- Ineligible organizations include insurance companies or their affiliates.

The law also calls for the establishment of a Network of Patient Safety Databases (NPSD) to provide an interactive, evidence-based management resource for providers, PSOs, and other entities. It will be used to analyze national and regional statistics, including trends and patterns of patient safety events. The NPSD will employ common formats (definitions, data elements, and so on) and will promote interoperability among reporting systems. The Department of Health and Human Services will provide technical assistance to PSOs.

Source: Agency for Healthcare Research and Quality (AHRQ). Retrieved from http://www.ahrq .gov/qual/psoact.htm

| BOX 16-3 | U.S. DEPARTMENT OF HEALTH AND HUMAN SERVICES |
|---|---|

The Department of Health and Human Services (DHHS) is the United States government's principal agency for protecting the health of all Americans and providing essential human services, especially for those who are least able to help themselves.

**The Department includes more than 300 programs** covering a wide spectrum of activities. Some highlights include the following:

- *Health and social science research*
- *Preventing disease, including immunization services*
- *Assuring food and drug safety*

- *Medicare (health insurance for elderly and disabled Americans) and Medicaid (health insurance for low-income people)*
- *Health information technology*
- *Financial assistance and services for low-income families*
- *Improving maternal and infant health*
- *Head Start (pre-school education and services)*
- *Faith-based and community initiatives*
- *Preventing child abuse and domestic violence*
- *Substance abuse treatment and prevention*
- *Services for older Americans, including home-delivered meals*

(continued)

## BOX 16-3  U.S. DEPARTMENT OF HEALTH AND HUMAN SERVICES (CONTINUED)

- *Comprehensive health services for Native Americans*
- *Medical preparedness for emergencies, including potential terrorism.*

**HHS represents almost a quarter of all federal outlays**, and it administers more grant dollars than all other federal agencies combined. DHHS's Medicare program is the nation's largest health insurer, handling more than 1 billion claims per year. Medicare and Medicaid together provide health care insurance for one in four Americans.

**DHHS works closely with state and local governments**, and many DHHS-funded services are provided at the local level by state or county agencies, or through private sector grantees. The Department's programs are administered by 11 operating divisions, including eight agencies in the U.S. Public Health Service and three human services agencies. In addition to the services they deliver, the DHHS programs provide for equitable treatment of beneficiaries nationwide, and they enable the collection of national health and other data. Website: http://www.hhs.gov

**The following are agencies in DHHS:**

*U.S. Public Health Service Agencies*

**National Institutes of Health (NIH)**—NIH is the world's premier medical research organization, supporting over 38,000 research projects nationwide in diseases including cancer, Alzheimer's, diabetes, arthritis, heart ailments and AIDS, and includes 27 separate health institutes and centers. Established: 1887, as the Hygienic Laboratory, Staten Island, N.Y. Headquarters: Bethesda, MD. Website: http://www.nih.gov/

**Food and Drug Administration (FDA)**—FDA assures the safety of foods and cosmetics, and the safety and efficacy of pharmaceuticals, biological products, and medical devices—products that represent almost 25 cents out of every dollar in U.S. consumer spending. Established: 1906, when the Pure Food and Drugs Act gave regulatory authority to the Bureau of Chemistry. Headquarters: Rockville, MD. Website: http://www.fda.gov/

**Centers for Disease Control and Prevention (CDC)**—Working with states and other partners, CDC provides a system of health surveillance to monitor and prevent disease outbreaks (including bioterrorism), implement disease prevention strategies, and maintain national health statistics, and provides for immunization services, workplace safety, and environmental disease prevention. Also guards against international disease transmission, with personnel stationed in more than 25 foreign countries. The CDC director is also administrator of the **Agency for Toxic Substances and Disease Registry**, which helps prevent exposure to hazardous substances from waste sites on the U.S. Environmental Protection Agency's National Priorities List, and develops toxicological profiles of chemicals at these sites. Established: 1946, as the Communicable Disease Center. Headquarters: Atlanta, GA. Website: http://www.cdc.gov/

**Indian Health Service (IHS)**—Working with tribes, IHS provides health services to 1.8 million American Indians and Alaska Natives of more than 560 federally recognized tribes. The Indian health system includes 46 hospitals, 324 health centers, 309 health stations and Alaska Native village clinics, and 34 urban Indian health programs. Established: 1921 (mission transferred from the Interior Department in 1955). Headquarters: Rockville, MD. Website: http://www.ihs.gov/

**Health Resources and Services Administration (HRSA)**—HRSA provides access to essential health care services for people who are low-income, uninsured, or who live in rural areas or urban neighborhoods where health care is scarce. HRSA-funded health centers will provide medical care to nearly 17 million patients at more than 4,000 sites nationwide in FY 2008. The agency maintains the National Health Service Corps and helps build the health care workforce through training and education programs. It administers a variety of programs to improve the health of mothers and children and serves people living with HIV/AIDS through the Ryan White CARE Act programs and also oversees the nation's organ transplantation system. Established: 1982 Headquarters: Rockville, MD. Website: http://www.hrsa.gov/

**Substance Abuse and Mental Health Services Administration (SAMHSA)**—SAMHSA works to improve the quality and availability of substance abuse prevention, addiction treatment and mental health services. It provides funding through block grants to states to support substance abuse and mental health services, including treatment for Americans with serious substance abuse problems or mental health

| BOX 16-3 | U.S. DEPARTMENT OF HEALTH AND HUMAN SERVICES (CONTINUED) |

problems. It also improves substance abuse prevention and treatment services through the identification and dissemination of best practices, and monitors prevalence and incidence of substance abuse. Established: 1992. (A predecessor agency, the Alcohol, Drug Abuse and Mental Health Administration, was established in 1974.) Headquarters: Rockville, MD. Website: http://www.samhsa.gov/

**Agency for Healthcare Research and Quality (AHRQ)**—AHRQ supports research on health care systems, health care quality and cost issues, access to health care, and effectiveness of medical treatments, and also provides evidence-based information on health care outcomes and quality of care. Established: 1989. Headquarters: Rockville, MD. Website: http://www.ahrq.gov/

**Centers for Medicare & Medicaid Services (CMS)**—CMS administers the Medicare and Medicaid programs, which provide health care to almost one in every three Americans. Medicare provides health insurance for more than 44.6 million elderly and disabled Americans. Medicaid, a joint federal-state program, provides health coverage for some 50 million low-income persons, including 24 million children, and nursing home coverage for low-income elderly. CMS also administers the State Children's Health Insurance Program that covers more than 4.4 million children. Established as the Health Care Financing Administration: 1977. Headquarters: Baltimore, MD. Websites: http://www.medicare.gov/ and http://www.cms.hhs.gov/default.asp?

**Administration for Children and Families (ACF)**—ACF is responsible for some 60 programs that promote the economic and social well-being of children, families and communi-

ties. It administers the state-federal welfare program, Temporary Assistance for Needy Families, providing assistance to an estimated 4 million persons, including 3 million children. The AFC administers the national child support enforcement system, collecting nearly $24 billion in FY 2006 in payments from non-custodial parents, based on preliminary data, and also administers the Head Start program, serving nearly 895,000 pre-school children. The AFC provides funds to assist low-income families in paying for child care, and supports state programs to support foster care and provide adoption assistance, and funds programs to prevent child abuse and domestic violence. Established: 1991, bringing together several already-existing programs. Headquarters: Washington, DC Website: http://www.acf.hhs.gov/

**Administration on Aging (AOA)**—AOA supports a nationwide aging network, providing services to the elderly, especially to enable them to remain independent. Supports some 240 million meals for the elderly each year, including home-delivered "meals on wheels." Helps provide transportation and at-home services. Supports ombudsman services for elderly, and provides policy leadership on aging issues. Headquarters: Washington, DC Website: http://www.aoa.dhhs.gov

**THE U.S. PUBLIC HEALTH SERVICE COMMISSIONED CORPS** is a uniformed service of more than 6,000 health professionals who serve in many DHHS and other federal agencies. The Surgeon General is head of the Commissioned Corps.

Source: U.S. Department of Health and Human Services. Retrieved November 17, 2009, from http://www.hhs.gov/about/whatwedo.html

Another indication of interest in health care quality is not governmental but rather focuses on the purchasers of care in the private sector. The Leapfrog Group, a consortium of private and public health care purchasers of health care benefits has developed a clear interest in health care quality (Leapfrog Group, 2009). The group's mission is to "trigger a giant leap forward in quality, customer service, and affordability of health care of all types by (1) supporting informed health care decisions by those who use and pay for health care and (2) by promoting high-value health care through incentives and rewards" (Leapfrog Group, 2009). There is no doubt that businesses want value for the money they spend on health care, and employers are the major purchasers of care because they provide health care coverage for their employees. The development of this type of organization indicates growing interest in collaboration to improve care and control costs.

Health care professional organizations and accrediting organizations have also developed an increased interest in health care quality. The Joint Commission is directly involved with quality and safety issues and has become more concerned with safety due to the recent IOM reports. In 2002, the Joint Commission initiated a program that the American Nurses Association (ANA) supports, "Speak Up: Help Prevent Errors in Your Care" (American Nurses Association, 2002). This initiative urges patients to do the following to help prevent health care errors or to "Speak Up."

- **S**peak up if you have questions or concerns, and if you don't understand, ask again. It's your body, and you have a right to know.
- **P**ay attention to the care you are receiving. Make sure you're getting the right treatments and medications by the right health care professionals. Don't assume anything.
- **E**ducate yourself about your diagnosis, the medical tests you are undergoing, and your treatment plan.
- **A**sk a trusted family member or friend to be your advocate.
- **K**now what medications you take and why you take them. Medication errors are the most common health care errors.
- **U**se a hospital, clinic, surgery center, or other type of health care organization that has undergone a rigorous on-site evaluation against established state-of-the-art quality and safety standards, such as those provided by the Joint Commission.
- **P**articipate in all decisions about your treatment. You are the center of the health care team (Joint Commission, 2003, July 9).

This initiative has expanded into several initiatives that include Help Prevent Errors in Your Care; Help Avoid Mistakes with Your Medicine; Five Things You Can Do to Prevent Infection; Prevent Errors in Your Child's Care; What You Should Know About Pain Management; Help Prevent Medical Test Mistakes; Help Avoid Mistakes in Your Surgery, Planning Your Follow-Up Care; Understanding Your Doctors and Other Caregivers; Know Your Rights; Information for Living Organ Donors; and What You Should Know About Research Studies (Joint Commission, 2009). These brochures are written for patients and are available for use. Looking at the titles there is a definite trend toward emphasizing patient-centered care and quality care.

The Joint Commission also now identifies annual National Patient Safety Goals based on data obtained from accreditation surveys highlighting areas that need improvement. The Joint Commission accredited health care organizations are expected to meet these safety goals. These goals can be found on the Commission's website. (See Media Links in this chapter.) There are also specific goals for ambulatory health care, behavioral health care, hospitals, laboratory, critical access hospitals, long-term care, Medicare-Medicaid long-term care, home care, and office-based surgery.

Health care quality is a topic frequently found in the media today—television, newspapers, and other print media. Stories are presented about complications patients experience due to errors, interventions, or inappropriate care. Examples of this type of media can be found at the local, state, and national levels. Consumers hear these stories and worry about the care that they receive, and this increases interest in health care quality. The Obama administration's initiative to reform health care led to an increase in media stories about the quality of care and consumerism.

Nursing education is also involved, though not as much as it should be (Finkelman & Kenner, 2010). The Quality and Safety Education for Nurses (QSEN) initiative funded by the Robert Wood Johnson Foundation to improve nursing care provides resources and strategies to facilitate learning focused on competency concerns. QSEN focuses on core competencies that are directly related to the IOM five health care professions core competencies, but QSEN increases the number to six competencies and uses slightly different definitions (Quality and Safety Education for Nurses, 2009).

- Patient-centered care
- Teamwork and collaboration
- Evidence-based practice
- Quality improvement
- Safety
- Informatics

The topic of quality improvement is also part of some of the provisions in the health care reform legislation of 2010. A national quality improvement strategy to improve the delivery of health care services, patient health outcomes, and population health will be developed. Multiple stakeholders will participate and measures will be identified. The national strategy is to be presented to Congress by January 1, 2011.

## Quality Improvement: A Growing, Complex Process

The IOM frequently comments on health care complexity and views this as a barrier to understanding safety and quality and to improving health care delivery. Implementing IOM QI approaches "requires that health professionals be clear about what they are trying to accomplish, what changes they can make that will result in an improvement, and how they will know that the improvement occurred" (Institute of Medicine, 2003a, p. 59). Why is health care so complex? Health care is different from other businesses that might have one product or a series of highly related products such as manufacturing. Health care products are determined by the medical problem, the consumer/patient, patient prognosis, the setting, clinical staff expertise, treatment options, current research, reimbursement, health policy, and legislation. Even geographic location can make a difference in health care delivery as there are practice pattern variations from one part of the country to another or rural access compared to urban areas. Specialty areas such as obstetrics, psychiatry, emergency care, intensive care, home health care, behavioral/mental health, and long-term care offer varied services that are influenced by their interventions, roles of the patient and family, patient education needs, prognosis and outcomes, and so on. Patients are very diverse in needs, diagnoses, ethnic and cultural backgrounds, and overall health status and are influenced by genetic background, socioeconomic factors, patient preferences for health care, community differences, and health care coverage/reimbursement concerns. The latter is particularly important when people lose their jobs and health care coverage. For example, if patients put off elective surgery, then there is less surgery to schedule. This leads to financial issues for hospitals that may lead to a change in services or elimination of services that are too expensive to offer.

It is expensive to develop and maintain an effective quality improvement program, but QI programs can lead to improved health care quality and in the long run save money when complications or extended treatment is avoided. Health care organizations want to reduce costs and ensure effective treatment to meet patient outcomes. Developing a QI program that addresses monitoring and improving health care quality is in itself a complex process and should include the IOM matrix describing the two dimensions of quality mentioned earlier in this chapter. There is greater ability today to use informatics for data collection and analysis. Health care organizations are dependent on informatics in the QI monitoring process. By using best practice (EBP) and finding new approaches that are better than current care interventions, health care can be improved. An effective QI program includes the following (Institute of Medicine, 2001a; Institute of Medicine, 2003a, p. 59):

- Continually understand and measure quality of care in terms of structure or the inputs into the system, such as patients, staff, and environments; process, or the interactions between clinicians and patients; and outcomes, or evidence about changes in patients' health status in relation to patient and community needs.
- Assess current practices and compare them with relevant better practices elsewhere as a means of identifying opportunities for improvement.
- Design and test interventions to change the process of care, with the objective of improving quality.
- Identify errors and hazards in care; understand and implement basic safety design principles, such as standardization and simplification and human factors training.
- Both act as an effective member of an interprofessional team and improve the quality of one's own performance through self-assessment and personal change.

Quality is difficult to understand and to monitor. Examples of issues identified by Bodenheimer in 1999 that arise when assessing quality, which are also reemphasized in the IOM reports, are as follows:

1. Health care is not a single product.
2. Different interventions require different measurements.
3. Different groups focus on different issues when considering quality.

4. Overuse, underuse, and misuse are critical in determining quality.
5. Organizations need a culture of quality to improve.
6. Assessment of quality is expensive to do, and this cost is shifted to purchasers and consumers.
7. Patient satisfaction is a questionable measure of the quality of care.

It is not clear how patient satisfaction affects quality or even what it means. For example, if a patient describes quality of care by the saying the staff was friendly and yet expected outcomes were not met (e.g., patient is not able to administer self insulin), did the patient receive quality care? The patient may say "yes" while the health care provider would say "no" (Bodenheimer, 1999, p. 489).

### Definition of Quality

Can **quality care** be defined? This has been a recurring health care question for a long time, and there is no universally accepted definition. The Institute of Medicine (IOM) defines quality as "the degree to which health services for individuals and populations increase the likelihood of desired health outcomes and are consistent with current professional knowledge" (Chassin & Galvin, 1998, p. 1000). This definition is based on three elements that are usually included in a discussion about quality care and monitoring care (Donabedian, 1980). The three accepted elements of quality are **structure**, the environment in which services are provided; *process*, the manner in which services are provided; and *outcome*, the result of services. These elements serve as the framework for the assessment of care. Figure 16-4 describes these elements.

### Measuring and Improving Quality: A Challenge

If quality care can be defined (even though it is complex), measured, and problems identified, can care be improved? Can improvement be achieved for patients at a cost that society can afford? Honest appraisal of the scientific facts suggests that health care can be improved by closing the wide gaps between prevailing practices and the best-known approaches to care and by inventing new forms of care (Berwick & Nolan, 1998). A recommended model for improvement suggested by Berwick and Nolan (1998) focuses on several questions that are important for nurse leaders and managers to consider.

1. What is the organization trying to accomplish?
2. How will the organization know whether a change is an improvement?
3. What change can the organization try that it believes will result in improvement?

These questions aim to arrive at a description of what the organization considers to be quality care. New nurses soon hear about QI when they begin their first jobs. Organizations typically

### FIGURE 16-4   Three elements of quality.

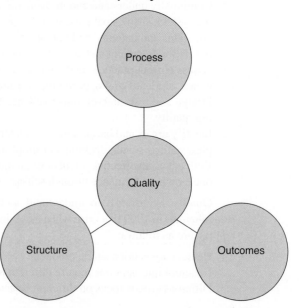

| BOX 16-4 | CUSTOMER AND CONSUMER NEEDS |
|----------|------------------------------|

| Customer | Consumer |
|----------|----------|
| Best value | Services |
| Affordable care | Access |
| Healthy employees | Choice |
| No hassle | Affordability |

have staff that work exclusively on QI and often they are nurses. Committees that focus on QI typically include nurses, physicians, social workers, medical records, laboratory staff, and other staff. Every nurse regardless of position has a responsibility to improve patient care. The American Nurses Association standards of professional performance state, "The registered nurse systematically enhances the quality and effectiveness of nursing practice. Measurement criteria are as follows: Demonstrates quality by documenting the application of the nursing process in a responsible, accountable, and ethical manner; uses the results of quality improvement activities to initiate changes in nursing practice and in the health care delivery system; uses creativity and innovation in nursing practice to improve care delivery; incorporates new knowledge to initiate changes in nursing practice if desired outcomes are not achieved; and participates in quality improvement activities" (American Nurses Association, 2004, p. 33).

Insurers are concerned about value or function of both quality and cost of health care. Both are critical to an insurer's survival. Key questions on quality in the health care reimbursement environment should focus on the needs of the customer or purchaser of the care and the consumer/patient. The customer, typically the employer or government who purchases insurance for employees, wants the best value, affordable care, healthy employees, and no hassle. The consumer or patient wants services, access, choice, and affordability. Sometimes the customer's and the consumer's viewpoints collide. A comparison of these needs is found in Box 16-4.

## Medicare and Quality

The Quality Improvement Organization (QIO) is the federal program that monitors medical necessity and quality for Medicare and Medicaid and their prospective payment systems. What do QIOs do? "By law, the mission of the QIO Program is to improve the effectiveness, efficiency, economy, and quality of services delivered to Medicare beneficiaries" (Centers for Medicare and Medicaid Services, 2009). Based on this statutory requirement, and Centers for Medicare and Medicaid Services (CMS) Program experience, the CMS identifies the core functions of the QIO Program as follows:

- Improving quality of care for beneficiaries;
- Protecting the integrity of the Medicare Trust Fund by ensuring that Medicare pays only for services and goods that are reasonable and necessary and that are provided in the most appropriate setting; and
- Protecting beneficiaries by expeditiously addressing individual complaints, such as beneficiary complaints; provider-based notice appeals; violations of the Emergency Medical Treatment and Labor Act (EMTALA); and other related responsibilities as articulated in QIO-related law.

The CMS relies on QIOs to improve the quality of health care for all Medicare beneficiaries. It views the QIO Program, which is required by law, as an important resource in its effort to improve quality and efficiency of care for Medicare beneficiaries. Throughout its history, the Medicare Program has been instrumental in advancing national efforts to motivate providers in improving quality, and in measuring and improving outcomes of quality (Centers for Medicare and Medicaid Services, 2009).

In the fall of 2007, the CMS made a major change in the Medicare program. The CMS no longer pays for specific complications, or what CMS terms as reasonably preventable medical errors that result in serious consequences for patients that occur in the hospital and could be prevented. These events are referred to as "Never Events." To be included on the list of "Never Events," an event is characterized as (Centers for Medicare and Medicaid, 2007)

- Unambiguous—clearly identifiable and measurable, and thus feasible to include in a reporting system
- Usually preventable—recognizing that some events are not always avoidable, given the complexity of health care
- Serious—resulting in death or loss of a body part, disability, or more than transient loss of a body function
- Any of the following:
  - Adverse
  - Indicative of a problem in a health care facility's safety systems
  - Important for public credibility or public accountability

Current lists of events are available at the CMS website.

What does this change in CMS reimbursement really mean? An example is when a Medicare patient falls and injures him or herself in the hospital; CMS will not pay for the care needed to resolve the injury. The Never Event approach is of great concern to health care providers who wonder if all of these incidents can really be prevented. The second issue for health care providers is who will pay for the care if CMS does not? Hospitals will have to cover the costs not paid by Medicare, and this will have a major impact on hospital budgets. Since there are limits on what the HCO can charge an individual Medicare patient, there is no other source for payment. The purposes of this CMS change are to control Medicare costs and push for greater improvement in care. Since a large percentage of inpatients are Medicare patients, this change has a major impact on the overall status of hospital budgets. With the growing economic problem in general, many hospitals already have financial problems. This policy change only adds to the problems. Following the CMS decision some insurers have now issued their own lists of preventable medical errors by identifying what incidents they will not cover, and the lists are not always the same, meaning hospitals have more events to be concerned about. This expands this type of payment policy to a greater number of patients. In the case of nongovernmental coverage, the patient could be billed for this care, but Medicare patients cannot be billed. Given the growing costs of health care to individuals this approach will only increase the problem. It is hoped that care will be improved, but there may be a heavy price to pay for it.

## Health Resources and Services Administration

The Health Resources and Services Administration (HRSA), a part of the U.S. Department of Health and Human Services, is involved in quality improvement, supporting the recommendations of the IOM Quality Chasm reports. Examples of some of HRSA's key quality improvement programs are as follows (U.S. Department of Health and Human Services, Health Resources and Services Administration, 2010a):

- Health Disparities Collaboration: a national effort to eliminate disparities and improve the care provided by HRSA-supported health care providers, such as health centers, and partners. Includes clinical, financial, operational quality improvement.
- Patient Safety and Clinical Pharmacy Services Collaborative: a national program to improve care delivered by HRSA grantees and other health care providers serving poor, uninsured, and underserved people by replicating leading practices in patient safety and clinical pharmacy services.
- HIV/AIDS Program Quality Care: Ryan White HIV/AIDS Program grantees implement quality management programs that target clinical, administrative, and supportive services.

Details about these programs can be found on the HRSA website.

## APPLYING EVIDENCE-BASED PRACTICE

### Evidence for Effective Leadership and Management

**Citation:** *The Effect of Health Care Working Conditions on Patient Safety.* Summary, Evidence Report/Technology Assessment: Number 74. AHRQ Publication No. 03-E024, March 2003. Agency for Healthcare Research and Quality (AHRQ), Rockville, MD. (Full review available at http://www.ahrq.gov/clinic/epcsums/worksum.htm.

**Overview:** The objective of this systematic review of 115 studies was to identify and summarize evidence from the scientific literature on the effects of health care working conditions on patient safety (medication errors). The researchers developed an analytic framework to define how working conditions are related to patient safety. Antecedent conditions, which are external factors such as personal characteristics of workers and fixed structural characteristics of the system (e.g., geographic location, regulations, and legislation), can affect the impact of working conditions on patient safety. Working conditions are viewed either as resources that improve work quality or act as barriers. The key questions are as follows:

1. Do working conditions affect patient outcomes that are related to patient safety?
2. Do working conditions affect the rate of medical errors?
3. Do working conditions affect the rate of recognition of medical errors after they occur?
4. Do working conditions affect the probability that adverse events will occur following detected or undetected medical errors?
5. Does the complexity of the plan of care influence whether working conditions affect patient outcomes that are related to patient safety?
6. Do working conditions affect measures of service quality in industries other than health care?

Valid evidence was found for all key questions except #4. The largest amount of available evidence was applied to #1. Several different specific working conditions affect outcomes that are related to patient safety. Some working conditions affect rates of medical errors. The report concludes with recommendations of strategies that can be used to improve patient safety.

**Application:** This systematic review evidence provides an example of an extensive systematic review of studies that focused on six important questions related to working conditions and patient safety. The review provides critical information for nurse managers and staff nurses. Working conditions and patient safety are not disconnected topics. Working conditions can be improved, and if this is done, then care can be improved. Tracking patient safety issues prior to implementing strategies and after care is provided can help to determine if care is improved.

### Questions:

1. *Describe a situation you have observed or been involved with where working conditions had an impact on patient safety.*
2. *Would you have added any other questions to this systematic review? Is so, what question(s)?*
3. *Select one of the recommendations from this systematic review and discuss its relevance to nursing.*

HRSA is also committed to improving care for those in the safety net, vulnerable populations. Twelve core measures are used to monitor this care and are particularly important in community and population health. The core measures are as follows (U.S. Department of Health and Human Services, Health Resources and Services Administration, 2010b):

- Medical Condition: Prenatal care; Measure: First trimester care access
- Medical Condition: HIV perinatal prevention; Measure: HIV screening for pregnant women
- Medical Condition: Cancer screening; Measure: Breast cancer screening; Cervical cancer; screening; Colorectal cancer screening
- Medical Condition: Immunizations: Measure: Childhood immunizations; Adult influenza vaccination; Older adult influenza vaccination; Older adult pneumococcal immunization; Hepatitis B vaccine for HIV+ patients
- Medical Condition: Chronic disease management; Measure: Diabetes-HbA1c; Measure: Hypertension control

# APPLYING LEADERSHIP AND MANAGEMENT

## MY HOSPITAL UNIT

Visit the unit you created. Consider the following: What would be an effective approach to integrate the five IOM core competencies into your unit's QI program and your staff education program? Compose your thoughts in a table with a column for each core competency. Clearly describe how the competency would be integrated into the unit's QI initiatives, care delivery, your management, and staff education. Use the virtual unit site from the textbook website to record the work that you do in the role of nurse manger for your unit.

## Critical Thinking Questions and Activities

1. What are two examples that demonstrate the increasing interest in the quality of care?
2. What does "quality" mean to you? How would you apply the concepts of structure, process, and outcomes to your description?
3. How might you apply the quality improvement matrix to your practice?
4. Select one of the IOM *Quality Chasm* reports and go to the IOM website to review the report. The Executive Summary provides an overview of the report. What have you learned from the report? You can divide the reports up and discuss them in teams. What is the key message of the report? Discuss the report's recommendations. How does the report content relate to nursing practice and to nursing management?
5. Describe the U.S. system to monitor care.
6. Visit the site http://www.ahcpr.gov and click on "Quality & Patient Safety." What can you learn about *Americans as Health care Consumers: The Role of Quality Information*?
7. Visit the site http://www.ahcpr.gov and click on "Quality & Patient Safety." Review the Department of Health and Human Services report, *The Challenge and Potential of Assuring Quality Health care for the 21st Century*. What problems does the report identify? What recommendations are suggested for solving these problems?
8. What is the main focus of the site http://www.hcqualitycommission.gov? What has happened to the consumer rights effort? Review information on the report, *Quality First: Better Health care for All Americans*.
9. The site http://www.centerfortransforminghealthcare.org/ is a new Joint Commission program to focus on quality problems, such as hand washing and handoffs.

## Media Links

- **URL: http://www.qsen.org**
  Quality and Safety Education for Nurses
- **URL: http://www.ihi.org**
  Institute of Healthcare Improvement
- **URL: http://www.jointcommission.org/patientsafety/nationalpatientsafetygoals/**
  The Joint Commission National Patient Safety Goals
- **URL: http://nhqrnet.ahrq.gov/nhqrdr/jsp/nhqrdr.jsp#snhere**
  National Healthcare Quality Report
- **URL: http://www.ahrq.gov/research/nursestaffing/nursestaff.htm**
  Agency for Healthcare Research and Quality: Systematic Review of Research on Nursing Staffing and Quality of Care

- **URL: http://www.qualitycheck.org/consumer/searchQCR.aspx**
  Joint Commission Quality Check™
- **URL: http://www.guideline.gov/**
  National Guideline Clearinghouse

**Pearson Nursing Student Resources**

Find additional review materials at
**nursing.pearsonhighered.com**
Prepare for success with additional NCLEX®-style practice questions,
interactive assignments and activities, Web links, animations and
videos, and more!

# References

American Association of Colleges of Nursing. (2009). *The Essentials of Baccalaureate Education for Profession Nursing Practice*. Washington, DC: Author.

American Hospital Association. (1999). *Hospital statistics*. Chicago, IL.

American Nurses Association. (2002, May/June). ANA supports JCAHO prevention program. *The American Nurse*, 5.

American Nurses Association. (2004). *Nursing: Scope and standards of practice*. Silver Spring, MD: American Nurses Association.

Benner, P., Sutphen, M., Leonard, V., & Day, L. (2010). *Educating nurses. A call for radical transformation*. San Francisco: Jossey-Bass.

Berwick, D., & Nolan, T. (1998). Physicians as leaders improving health care. *Annals of Internal Medicine, 128*(4), 289–292.

Bodenheimer, T. (1999). The American health care system: The movement for improved quality in health care. *New England Journal of Medicine, 340*(6), 488–492.

Centers for Medicare and Medicaid Services. (2007). Never Events. Retrieved August 17, 2009, from http://www.cms.hhs .gov/apps/media/press/release.asp? Counter=1863

Centers for Medicare and Medicaid Services. (CMS). (2009). Quality Improvement Organization. Retrieved March 2, 2009, from http://www.cms.gov

Chassin, M., & Galvin, R. (1998). The urgent need to improve health care quality. *Journal of the American Medical Association, 280*(2), 1000–1005.

Donabedian, A. (1980). *Explorations in quality assessment and monitoring*. Vol. I: *The definition of quality and approaches to its assessment*. Ann Arbor, MI: Health Administration Press.

Finkelman, A. & Kenner, C. (2009). *Teaching IOM: Implications of the Institute of Medicine reports for nursing education*. Silver Springs, MD: American Nurses Association.

Institute of Medicine (1999). *To err is human: Building a safer health system*. Washington, DC: National Academies Press.

Institute of Medicine. (2001a). *Crossing the quality chasm: A new health system for the 21st century*. Washington, DC: National Academies Press.

Institute of Medicine. (2001b). *Envisioning the national healthcare quality report*. Washington, DC: National Academies Press.

Institute of Medicine. (2003a). *Priority areas for national action: Transforming health care quality*. Washington, DC: National Academies Press.

Institute of Medicine (2003b). *Leadership by example: Coordinating government roles in improving health care quality*. Washington, DC: National Academies Press.

Institute of Medicine (2003c). *Who will keep the public healthy? Educating public health professionals for the 21st century*. Washington, DC: National Academies Press.

Institute of Medicine. (2003d). *Health professions education: A bridge to quality*. Washington, DC: National Academies Press.

Institute of Medicine. (2004). *Keeping patients safe: Transforming the work environment of nurses*. Washington, DC: The National Academies Press.

Institute of Medicine. (2009). Robert Wood Johnson Foundation Initiative on the Future of Nursing, at the Institute of Medicine. Retrieved November 18, 2009, from http://www.iom.edu/Activities/ Workforce/Nursing.aspx

Joint Commission. (2003). Speak up. Retrieved July 6, 2003, from http://www.jcaho.org

Joint Commission. (2009). Patient safety and speak up. Retrieved November 15, 2009, from http://www.jointcommission.org/ PatientSafety/SpeakUp/

Leapfrog Group. Retrieved November 15, 2009, from http://www.leapfroggroup.org

Maddox, P., Wakefield, M., & Bull, J. (2001). Patient safety and the need for professional and educational change. *Nursing Outlook, 49*(1), 8–13.

Plsek, P. (2001). Redesigning health care with insights from the science of complex adaptive systems. In Institute of Medicine, *Crossing the Quality Chasm* (pp. 309–322).

Quality and Safety Education for Nurses. (2009). Competencies. Retrieved November 15, 2009, from http:// www.qsen.org

U.S. Department of Health and Human Services, Health Resources and Services Administration. (2010a). Quality improvement and safety net providers. Retrieved February 28, 2010, from http:// www.hrsa.gov/quality/

U.S. Department of Health and Human Services, Health Resources and Services Administration. (2010b). HRSA clinical quality performance measures set. Retrieved February 28, 2010, from www .hrsa.gov/quality/coremeasures.htm

Wakefield, M. (1997). Pioneering new ways to ensure quality health care. *Nursing Economics, 15*(4), 225–227.

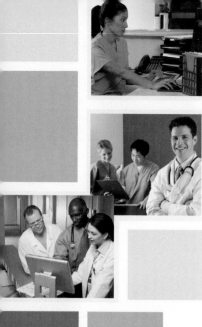

# 17

# Implementing Health Care Quality Improvement

## CHAPTER OUTLINE

## LEARNING OUTCOMES

Before you begin, take a moment to familiarize yourself with the learning outcomes for this chapter.

- Compare and contrast a Blame Culture and a Culture of Safety.
- Describe Joint Commission accreditation and its relevance to quality improvement.
- Compare two methods used to measure and ensure quality, safe care.
- Explain the relevance of quality report cards to quality improvement.
- Discuss the role of nurses in quality improvement and nursing initiatives to improve care.
- Explain the purpose of third-party payer accreditation.
- Discuss the need for interprofessional quality improvement initiatives.

## KEY TERMS

- Access to care
- Accreditation
- Adverse event
- Authorization
- Benchmarking
- Clinical guideline
- Clinical pathway
- Failure modes and effects analysis (FMEA)
- Failure to rescue (FTR)
- Handoff

- Health Plan Employer Data and Information Set (HEDIS)
- Indicator
- Joint Commission
- National Committee for Quality Assurance (NCQA)
- Outcome Assessment Information Set (OASIS)
- Quality report card
- Rapid response team (RRT)

- Risk management
- Root cause analysis
- Sentinel event
- Standards
- Threshold
- Utilization review/ management
- Utilization Review Accreditation Commission (URAC)
- Variances
- Workaround

## WHAT'S AHEAD

This chapter continues the discussion of quality health care by focusing on the implementation of initiatives and strategies to improve patient care. Each nurse plays a role daily in ensuring quality care while care is provided but also is responsible for participating in organizational quality improvement efforts. All health care organizations should have quality improvement (QI) programs, which can be found in hospitals, home health care, long-term care, and so on. Since nursing care represents a major component of all health care, nurses should participate in all levels of QI and also address specific nursing issues related to the quality of care. An understanding of health care quality policy as found in Chapter 16 is necessary to fully understand implementation of QI.

# Quality Care: Measurement and Improvement

As discussed in Chapter 16 the Institute of Medicine (IOM) uses the following definition of quality in its reports: "the degree to which health services for individuals and populations increase the likelihood of desired health outcomes and are consistent with current professional knowledge" (Chassin & Galvin, 1998, p. 1000). Measuring care to determine quality and developing and implementing strategies to improve patient care are critical processes in all types of health care delivery systems, and nurses play an important role in all aspects of quality improvement.

## Placing Blame or Supporting a Culture of Safety

Health care organizations have typically handled errors by identifying the staff member that made the error or asking staff to report errors by completing incident reports to describe the error. Over time this has become a more punitive approach and has not been effective in reducing errors and improving care. Most errors are much more complex than just an error made by an individual, a viewpoint supported by the IOM reports. When an error occurs, the question should not be one of "Who is at fault?" but rather, "Why did our defenses fail?" (Reason, 2000). There are too many people involved in health care, and the health care system is too complex to think that one individual is always the reason for an error. As nurses work with multiple health care providers and teams, it becomes important to understand that errors are more commonly due to system issues. The IOM (1999) reported that the health care system focused on the "blame game" rather than examining causes to improve and limited efforts in focusing on a culture of safety. The IOM reports utilized the work done by Reason to understand errors and the health care environment (Reason, 2000). Staff members are anxious or afraid to report errors, which may prevent them from doing so. Near misses or errors that are caught before they occur are also important to monitor, and this is not being done routinely. However, there is greater movement to change from a blame culture to a culture of safety. This approach sets the stage for greater communication about errors and near misses to improve care. "A fundamental principle of the systems approach to error reduction is the recognition that all humans make mistakes and that errors are to be expected, even in the best organizations" (Reason, 2000, p. 768). Nurse managers and team leaders set the tone for the safety culture on each unit, communicating how errors are handled on a daily basis.

To improve care requires measurement of the status of care delivery, but are there some aspects that cannot be measured? It is not easy to measure quality, and health care organizations struggle to arrive at the best methods. What are some examples of the difficulty of measuring quality? Measuring the quality of the nurse–patient or the physician–patient relationship quantitatively is not easy as there are many variables involved and there are subjective components. Personalities and communication methods also make it difficult (Nadzam, 2009). If knowledge about a specific illness is incomplete, such as with chronic fatigue syndrome, it is difficult to measure quality care for that particular disorder. More research is required before standards and guidelines can be developed to describe the best treatment for many illnesses through the process of evidence-based practice (EBP). Since quality is affected by so many different elements there can be great differences from one experience to another.

## Critical Health Care Safety Issues

Clearly, there are many safety issues in health care; some relate specifically to patients and others to staff. Some of the critical patient issues are medication administration, use of restraints, violence (as patient violence can lead to injuries for the patient, other patients, family members/visitors, and staff), nosocomial infections, and wrong patient receiving treatment or patient receiving the wrong treatment. Each one of these is a complex issue. There are standards related to these safety issues (for example, use of restraints) and the critical steps of medication administration (e.g., right patient, right drug, right dose, right time, and right route). Medication administration, as noted in *To Err Is Human* (Institute of Medicine, 1999), can lead to errors. Some of the reasons for errors in this area are time pressures, fatigue, understaffing, lack of knowledge about the drug and/or the patient, documentation, and systems failure. The American Nurses Association developed documentation principles, which are described in Box 17-1, to assist nurses in their documentation, a critical factor in ensuring safe care.

"Given that nurses comprise the largest component of the health care workforce and are involved with the provision, management, research, and education related to patient care, safety and error reduction in health care are central concerns for the profession and a responsibility for every nurse" (Maddox, Wakefield, & Bull, 2001, p. 8). How should nurses be involved in the CQI (continuous quality improvement) effort? First, nurses need to understand the problem and circumstances related to errors. Contributory factors are important in the analysis of errors or situations when errors could have occurred. These factors can be categorized in the following manner.

- **Institutional:**   regulatory context, medicolegal environment
- **Organization and management:**   financial resources and constraints, policy standards and goals, safety culture and priorities
- **Work environment:**   staffing levels and mix; patterns of workload and shift; design, availability, and maintenance of equipment; administrative and managerial support
- **Team:**   verbal and written communication, supervision and willingness to seek help, team leadership
- **Individual staff member:**   knowledge and skills, motivation and attitude, physical and mental health

## BOX 17-1    PRINCIPLES FOR DOCUMENTATION

- Unique patient identification must be assured within and across paper-based and electronic health care documentation systems.
- Documentation systems must assure the security and confidentiality of patient information.
- Documentation must be accurate and consistent; clear, concise, and complete; reflecting patient response and outcomes related to nursing care; received timely and sequential; retrievable on a permanent basis in a nursing-specific manner; able to be audited.
- Documentation must meet existing standards such as those promulgated by state and federal regulatory agencies (to include HIPAA as enforced through the Department of Justice [DOJ], the Centers for Medicare and Medicaid Services [CMS], and through accrediting organizations such as the Joint Commission and the National Committee for Quality Assurance [NCQA]). Entries into the medical record (including orders) must be legible, complete, and authenticated and dated by the person responsible for ordering,

providing, or evaluating the care provided (Joint Commission).
- Abbreviations, acronyms, and symbols utilized in documentation must be standardized (Joint Commission).
- The nurse must be familiar with organizational policies and/or procedures related to documentation.
- Several terminologies have been recognized by ANA which specify the domain of nursing and contain terms used in the planning, delivery, and evaluation of the nursing care of the patient or client in diverse settings. An ANA-recognized terminology should be employed in documentation so that data can be aggregated. However, in instances where clinicians are using electronic information systems and structured data linked to a reference terminology, the use of an ANA-recognized terminology at the interface may be unnecessary.

Source: American Nurses Association. (2005). *Principles for documentation*. Washington, DC: Author. Reprinted with permission.© 2005 By American Nurses Association. Reprinted with permission. All rights reserved.

- **Task:**   availability and use of protocols, availability and accuracy of test results
- **Patient:**   complexity and seriousness of condition, language and communication, personality and social factors (Vincent, 2003, p. 1050)

It is also important to collect data about possible errors and share the data and its analysis so that prevention strategies can be developed. As the IOM reports indicate, it is important for nurses to recognize that the focus should not be on individual nurses who make errors but rather system characteristics that make errors possible.

Nurse staff-to-patient ratios can impact staff fatigue, consistent staff, communication, teamwork, efficiency, and turnover, all of which can lead to increased errors (American Nurses Association, 2006a; American Nurses Association, 2006b; Christmas, 2008; Hendrich, Chow, Skierczynski, & Zhenqiang, 2008; Benner, Malloch, & Sheets, 2010). The *To Err Is Human* report (Institute of Medicine, 1999) identified five principles that might be helpful in designing safe health care systems. These include (a) providing leadership, (b) respecting human limits in the design process, (c) promoting effective team functioning, (d) anticipating the unexpected, and (e) creating a learning environment. These principles apply to nursing care and staff and are related to what has been discussed in this text about leadership and management. The AHRQ has published a systematic review that addresses the question of the relationship of staffing and quality of care. (See end of chapter activities.)

Additional current QI issues that many hospitals are currently addressing that directly involve nursing management and staff include the following:

- **Failure Modes and Effects Analysis (FMEA):** FMEA focuses on safety in systems and prevention of accidents moving away from the individual focus (Wolf, 2001). It is a "tool that provides a systematic, proactive method for evaluating a process to identify where and how it might fail and to assess the relative impact of different failures in order to identify the parts of the process that are in most need of change" (Institute of Health Improvement, 2008). See Media Links for a website that provides software to use in teaching this method.

- **Failure to Rescue (FTR)**: The "intent of FTR indicator is to measure the hospital's ability to rescue patients that have developed a serious complication" (Manojlovich & Talsma, 2007, p. 504). Surveillance, monitoring patient status, is a key element of FTR (Institute of Medicine, 2004). "FTR has been associated with three complications attributable to nursing care: medication errors, falls, and pressure ulcers. As of fall 2008, these complications are included in the Medicare Never Events" (Finkelman & Kenner, 2009, p. 145). (See Media Links for further information.)
- **Rapid Response Team (RRT)**: RRTs are teams of critical care experts who come to the bedside of patients who are not in intensive care to make rapid decisions when a patient is experiencing life-threatening complications. The Institute of Health Improvement website provides extensive information on RRTs. (See Media Links for further information.)
- **Handoffs**: Handoffs are times in the care process when the patient is moved from one setting to another or from a health care provider or service to another. Examples are transfers from emergency care to inpatient; from one inpatient unit to another; from inpatient unit to operating room; from inpatient unit to radiology; and from hospital to home. These transfers may be for short term or long-term care. These are times of high risk for errors due to decreased sharing of information or confusing communication (Kitch et al., 2008; U.S. Department of Defense, 2010). (See Media Links for further information.)
- **Workarounds**: Work is usually organized around functions; however, it is not always clear who does what, when, and how (Spear & Schmidhofer, 2005). When there is a breakdown or problem, staff often figure out ways to get the work done without really analyzing what is going on. This results in a workaround. Staff may think this saves time, but it often does not. This is often a time of increased risk for errors. (See Media Links for further information.)

## Workplace Safety

Workplace safety has an impact on overall health care quality, staff satisfaction, and staff retention. For staff, some of the key safety issues are needlesticks, ergonomic safety, violence, latex allergies, and infections, such as what occurred with SARS and H1N1 virus when so many health professionals in other countries contracted the disease from patients. Violence in the workplace is also a concern in health care particularly in emergency departments, psychiatric/substance abuse services, and in long-term care. Staff members need to learn how to protect themselves and others without harming the patient who is violent. Concern also exists about the emotional response that follows after staff experiences these incidents. Each one of these safety issues is complex and requires that staff is educated about prevention and that organizations provide support and prevention services as required. The Occupational Safety and Health Administration (OSHA) is the federal agency that is responsible for monitoring safe workplaces. Nurse managers need to consider workplace safety in their planning, staff orientation and training, staff retention and morale, and the impact it has on staff performance and patient care quality. Box 17-2 provides a list of ANA position statements on workplace safety that can be obtained from the ANA website.

## The Accreditation Process

Accreditation of organizations is important to many different types of organizations. For example, schools of nursing are accredited, meaning they receive some type of official approval that they can offer services, which in the case of schools of nursing are courses toward a nursing degree. Hospitals and other types of health care organizations and third-party payer organizations are also accredited. Evaluation is a fact of life; however, it is not simple and can have major ramifications for a health care organization—costs, staff time and energy, and public relations. It may require that the organization institute changes or, in extreme cases, stop providing services. The following discussion offers some information about accreditation in the health care delivery system as a measurement and improvement process.

WHAT IS ACCREDITATION?   **Accreditation** is the process by which organizations are evaluated on their quality, based on established minimum standards and performance. Health care facilities have been accredited for a long time, but the process still has its critics. An important criticism is

| BOX 17-2 | AMERICAN NURSES ASSOCIATION WORKPLACE ADVOCACY POSITION STATEMENTS |

- Assuring Patient Safety: The Employer's Role in Promoting Healthy Nursing Work Hours for Registered Nurses in All Roles and Setting (2006)
- Assuring Patient Safety: Registered Nurses' Responsibility in All Roles and Settings to Guard Against Working When Fatigued (2006)

- Elimination of Manual Patient Handling to Prevent Work-Related Musculoskeletal Disorders (2003)

whether or not quality can be defined. Previous discussion in this chapter identifies a recognized definition for quality of care although there are many other definitions that have been proposed by a number of authorities. Accreditation focuses on quality, and thus the definition of quality is necessary in order to ensure that all who are involved are assessing the same concern, which is quality care. Accreditation has undergone many changes in the last 15 years as it has adjusted to the health care environment and to changes in perspectives of the quality care. The most important change has been the increased focus on continuous quality improvement (CQI or QI) or ongoing efforts to improve care and focusing on systems rather than just focusing on health care provider performance and blame. Accreditation is something that all nurses experience, but the level of that experience varies depending upon the nurse's position. Today, when hospitals are surveyed all staff is expected to be prepared and participate in the process. The goal is to include more direct care providers rather than just management staff. One can conclude that accreditation is not perfect. It has changed over time and now focuses on improvement and performance, requiring understanding and participation from nurses.

THE JOINT COMMISSION    The major organization that accredits health care organizations (HCOs) is the **Joint Commission**. It is a non-profit organization that accredits more than 17,000 health care organizations, including hospitals, long-term care organizations, home care agencies, clinical laboratories, ambulatory care organizations, behavioral health organizations, critical access hospitals, disease-specific care, health care staffing services, and office-based surgery practices. The accreditation process is complex, time consuming, and costly. Participation is voluntary though few HCOs could survive without this accreditation. It is the most important accrediting organization in the United States. Its purpose is to improve the quality of care provided to the public by assessing performance based on the Joint Commission standards. The organization establishes minimum standards and benchmarks for health care organizations to use as they improve care. The Joint Commission emphasizes quality through the CQI process. HCOs go through a survey every three years and may also conduct unscheduled surveys. Periodic Performance Review is also required with submission of specific reports. During the survey and by using updated, periodic reports that accredited HCOs are required to submit, the Joint Commission is trying to find out if the patients are achieving expected outcomes, and if not, why? Examples of some outcomes that the Joint Commission assesses are mortality rates, length-of-stay, adverse incidents, complications, readmission rates, patient/family satisfaction, referrals to specialists, patient adherence to the discharge plan or treatment plan, and prevention adherence (e.g., mammogram, Pap smear, immunizations). All of these outcomes are also of interest to insurers. The Joint Commission standards cover the following areas (Joint Commission, 2009a).

1. Emergency Management
2. Environment of Care
3. Human Resources
4. Information Management
5. Life Safety

6. Medical Staff
7. Medication Management
8. National Patient Safety Goals
9. Performance Improvement
10. Provision of Care, Treatment, and Services
11. Record of Care, Treatment, and Services
12. Rights and Responsibilities of the Individual
13. Waived Testing

With its emphasis on continuous QI throughout the organization the Joint Commission requires its accredited organizations to identify and address sentinel events, defined as "an event that had a negative outcome with a patient that people do not want to happen" (Paolucci, 2001, p. 8). A **root cause analysis** or a systematic review of the event is conducted. The key is to assess the process, not the individual staff that was involved—blame is not the goal but rather prevention of further events. This supports the recommendations from the IOM reports. The QI approach was a major change in the accreditation. Prior to the use of QI standards, accreditation required extensive data collection, and there was a tendency to take a punitive approach. Health care organizations felt that once they met a certain requirement there was nothing else that needed to be done. An analogy would be the student who makes an "A" who then thinks there is nothing else to learn or that there is no risk of the grade going down. Health care organizations did not consistently look for ways to improve but rather just focused on problems. This has now changed as QI has become more acceptable, expected, and continuous.

Related to this effort, the Joint Commission has developed a core measure initiative so that organizations will focus on what matters. The Joint Commission defines core measures as "standardized performance measures, with precisely defined data elements, calculation algorithms, and standardized data-collection protocols" (Nolan, 2004, p. 28). These measures should determine if patients are getting the care that they should receive and also that the data provide benchmarks. The Joint Commission has developed specific rules for collecting and reporting data to ensure better comparison of data from one organization to another. Hospitals must develop strategies to improve care for the core areas, and all of these core areas are highly dependent on nursing care. Nurses need to be directly involved in the core measure initiative.

The Joint Commission surveys its accredited organizations every 3 years for routine accreditation. Health care organizations voluntarily request this accreditation; however, for health care organizations that offer medical training programs, provide clinical experiences for nursing students, and receive federal funding, this accreditation is required. It is thus difficult to view accreditation as truly voluntary. The Joint Commission accreditation process includes unannounced surveys. This change was made due to criticism found in the DHHS report *The External Review of Hospital Quality: A Call for Greater Accountability* (Gallagher & Kany, 2000). The concern was expressed that since hospitals had ample time to prepare for scheduled surveys, the hospitals put all their energy into preparation just prior to a survey and were less involved in maintaining standards between surveys. In addition, surveyors now spend more time on patient units and receive more detailed information about the organization before the actual survey, so that they are better prepared for the survey. The goal is more effective evaluation of health care organizations that are accredited by the Joint Commission.

NURSES AND THE JOINT COMMISSION   All nurses eventually encounter the Joint Commission—through application of its standards, preparation for surveys, and then participation in surveys. Nurses assume leadership roles in all of these phases within health care organizations and also may serve as Joint Commission surveyors. Quality improvement should be continuous with no end. As problems are resolved and care improved, organizations then focus on new concerns and also review past problem areas to determine if improvement continues. Each organization needs to develop plans to ensure that care is assessed and that problems are addressed. The Joint Commission survey should not be the focus, although it usually is; rather, the focus should be on continuous improvement. What usually happens is the survey preparation and process become all consuming. Key steps that organizations complete to meet the improvement goal are as follows:

1. Develop a plan (includes units, services, departments, and the entire organization).
2. Implement the plan.
3. Collect data and analyze the data.
4. Develop reports that summarize the data and analysis so that it can be useful in decision making.
5. Share data and analysis with staff.
6. Develop and implement corrective actions for identified problems.
7. Begin again—with more assessment.

Nursing staff should be involved in all of these steps. As the Joint Commission survey time approaches, organizations begin to prepare for the survey. Staff needs education about the QI program, the Joint Commission, and the survey process. Tension usually increases at the time of a survey. Losing accreditation, although this rarely occurs, is extremely serious. The organization may be required to make changes and report these changes by specific deadlines, which may require additional surveys. All of this is costly and affects the organization's public image.

## Outcomes Management

As health care providers and organizations have become more experienced in assessing quality, they have turned more to performance-based quality care evaluation, which has been strongly supported by the Joint Commission. The critical question in assessing the quality of care is did the patient benefit from the care received? If so, how? If not, why? Quality really cannot be measured until quality is defined and outcomes are identified. These questions are critical to the development of **outcomes**. When outcomes are assessed, there are several aspects to include.

It is necessary to first develop indicators that identify areas of potential problems or improvement of care. This is the content or focus of assessment or evaluation. An **indicator** or measure is a measurable dimension of quality, specifying patient care activities and event occurrences for outcomes that can be monitored.

Indicators must also include a quantity element or **threshold**. This pre-established level indicates the need for more intensive assessment, which can emphasize relative rate or trends that need further investigation. For example, an initial, preoperative, and postoperative pain assessment might include (a) localization of pain, (b) type of pain, (c) duration of pain, (d) time of onset, (e) factors associated with pain, and (f) interventions taken and the outcomes, with a threshold of 92%. The threshold indicates when further evaluation needs to be done—if more than 8% of the patient assessments do not meet this indicator, further investigation is required.

Other indicators focus on **sentinel events** or events that always require investigation (e.g., suicide attempt, cardiac arrest in labor and delivery, lack of referral to specialist, and patient death). The components of quality indicators are described in Box 17-3.

Examples of some outcomes are mortality rates, length-of-stay, adverse incidents, complications, readmission rates, patient/family satisfaction, referrals to specialists, patient adherence to the discharge plan or treatment plan, and prevention adherence (e.g., mammogram, Pap smear, immunizations). Indicators may also focus on process (actual activities done by health care providers) or structure (facilities, equipment, staff, finances). The outcome focus (short-term and long-term results, complications, health status, and functioning) has become more important.

---

**BOX 17-3 COMPONENTS OF QUALITY INDICATORS**

- Accessibility
- Appropriateness
- Continuity
- Effectiveness
- Efficacy

- Efficiency
- Timeliness
- Patient perspective issues
- Safety of care environment

## CASE STUDY

### How Do We Address Poor QI Data?

Four team leaders on a medical unit are meeting with the nurse manager to review QI data for the last quarter. The data concerns medication errors, falls, and nosocomial infections. The QI Department provided data in the form of a graph. The nurse manager expresses concern about the changes in the data compared to the previous quarter. They discuss the impact these changes may have in light of the new CMS Never Events policy. One of the team leaders says that she thinks the problem is staff is not taking this seriously and all of the team leaders need to identify individual staff who make all the errors. Another team leader argues with her saying that this is too narrow a view of the problems. The other two team leaders did not say anything, but they also are confused about how staff responds to errors. Most of the team leaders feel it is their job to focus on individual errors. The nurse manager says they need to come up with a plan to address the changes in unit QI data. She also says, "I think we really need to address our culture of safety."

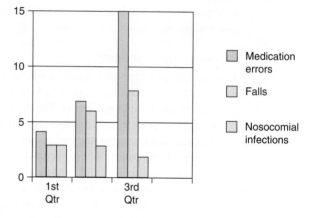

## Questions:

1. Review the data provided in the graph.

2. What does the data tell you?

3. Develop a plan to focus on the problems in the next quarter by identifying goal(s), interventions, and methods to evaluate outcomes. Use the Food and Drug Administration (FDA) Safe Use Initiative information that focuses on collaborating to reduce preventable harm from medications to develop the implementation plan to reduce drug errors and the four stages of the drug system identified by the FDA. (Review http://www.fda.gov/Drugs/DrugSafety/ucm187806.htm.)

4. How would you address the culture of safety on the unit?

---

OUTCOME ASSESSMENT INFORMATION SET (OASIS)   Some health care organizations such as home health care agencies and some insurers are using national evaluation approaches that are not sponsored by the Joint Commission. Home care agencies use a specific outcome-based approach to quality improvement (QI) called **Outcome Assessment Information Set (OASIS)**, which was developed in the 1990s by the U.S. Department of Health and Human Services. This is a standardized, computerized patient-level assessment with items related to the patient's physical and emotional state. The focus is on whether or not the patient benefited from the care—outcomes and performance, which should be the focus of care in all types of settings. The process has two stages.

1. The first is outcome analysis, which includes data collection using the OASIS assessment form, and then processing, editing, and transmitting the data electronically to a central location that collects data from multiple home health agencies. Then each agency receives a risk-adjusted outcomes report, which compares each agency with other agencies providing a quality report card. Data collection occurs at specified intervals in the patient's care process.

2. The second stage is outcome enhancement when each agency that participates in the process selects outcomes for further evaluation—such as identifying problems and strengths, developing best practices that are incorporated in action plans, implementing and monitoring the plans, and evaluating the effect of these actions in subsequent reports (Mosocco, 2001; Centers for Medicare and Medicaid Services, 2010). Home health agencies that receive Medicare reimbursement, which constitutes most of them, are required to participate in OASIS. The data can then be used for benchmarking.

## Methods Used in Establishing Quality Care

Many methods are used in the QI process. Some are used for data collection, while others are used to analyze data or guide health care improvement. The following content describes examples of these methods. Some of these methods have been discussed in more detail in earlier chapters so some of this content is review. It is important to remember that quality care cannot usually be assessed or improved by using only one method.

MONITORING ADVERSE EVENTS    The IOM report on safety *To Err Is Human* (1999) clearly states that there is no single answer to solving this problem. This report defines safety as "freedom from accidental injury" and defines error as "the failure of a planned action to be completed as intended or the use of a wrong plan to achieve an aim" (Institute of Medicine, 1999, p. 3). Errors are directly related to outcomes, which is a significant concern in quality improvement efforts. There are two types of errors: error of planning and error of execution. Errors harm the patient, and some errors that injure the patient may have been preventable adverse events. Box 17-4 identifies some key terms related to errors and quality.

**Adverse events** are now monitored by hospitals to better assess the status of care provided. An adverse event is "an injury resulting from a medical intervention, or in other words, it is not due to the underlying condition of the patient" (Institute of Medicine, 1999, pp. 3–4). Not all adverse events are due to errors and not all are preventable. Analysis is required to determine the relationship of an error to an adverse event. Root cause analysis is used by many HCOs today to better understand these events and improve care, and nurses participate in the root cause analysis process. (See Media Links for more information on the process.) Table 17-1 identifies critical adverse events.

POLICIES AND PROCEDURES    Policies and procedures set standards within a health care organization or insurer that guide decisions and how care is provided and support greater consistency in how care is delivered. This can help to improve care. Policies and procedures should not conflict with regulatory issues in the state such as the Nurse Practice Act and should be in agreement with professional standards. Policies and procedures need to be readily available to staff for review when needed. Many HCOs have put their policies and procedures into their computer systems, reducing the need for hard copy policy and procedure manuals and making it easier to access the information when needed. EBP resources need to be used to develop, review, and update policies and procedures.

STANDARDS OF CARE    A **standard** is an authoritative statement that provides a minimum description of accepted actions expected from a health care organization or an individual health care provider such as a physician, nurse, case manager, and so on and describes expectations about what should be done. Standards of care provide minimum descriptions of accepted actions expected from a health care organization or professional who has specific skill and knowledge levels. They are important in establishing expectations. Standards are developed by professional organizations, legal sources such as nurse practice acts and federal and state laws, regulatory agencies such as accreditation bodies and federal and state agencies, and health care facilities, and are supported by scientific literature and clinical pathways. Two examples are the American Nurses Association's (ANA) *Nursing Administration Scope and Practice* (2009) and *Nursing Scope of Standards of Practice* (2010). Specialty organizations also develop standards such as the *American Society of Clinical Oncology (ASCO) and Oncology Nurses Society (ONS) Chemotherapy Safety Standards* (2009) and *Perioperative Standards and Recommended Practices* (AORN, 2010).

## BOX 17-4    OTHER CRITICAL DEFINITIONS

- *Safety:* Freedom from accidental injury. Example: The patient leaves the hospital after surgery and a 3-day stay with expected outcomes reached and no complications.

- *Error:* The failure of a planned action to be completed as intended or the use of a wrong plan to achieve an aim. Errors are directly related to outcomes. There are two types of errors: *error of planning* and *error of execution.* Errors harm the patient, and some may be *preventable adverse events.*
  Example: The patient is given the wrong medication.

- *Adverse Event:* An injury resulting from a medical intervention, not due to the patient's underlying condition. Not all adverse events are due to errors and not all are preventable. Only investigation and analysis can determine the relationship of an error to an adverse event. When an adverse event is the result of an error, it is considered to be a *preventable adverse event.*
  Example: The patient is given the wrong medication and experiences a seizure. If the patient does not have a seizure disorder then this is most likely is a preventable adverse event, but more needs to be known about the causes. How did the error happen that led to the adverse event? Would this cause a seizure? Examples of causes and types of adverse errors are described in Table 16-1.

- *Misuse:* Avoidable complications that prevent patients from receiving full potential benefit of a service.
  Example: The patient receives a medication that is prescribed but conflicts with the patient's allergies; the patient experiences anaphylaxis and limited benefit from the medication, which should not have been used.

- *Overuse:* Potential for harm that exceeds the possible benefit from a service.
  Example: An older patient is on multiple medications, some of which may interact negatively, and the patient's multiple health care providers are not aware of the medications prescribed by different specialists.

- *Underuse:* Failure to provide a service that would have produced a favorable outcome for the patient.
  Example: The patient is not able to get specialty treatment needed for cancer because of the distance from resources, or the patient's insurer will not reimburse a

medication for arthritis that could make the patient more mobile.

- *Near Miss:* Recognition that an event occurred that might have led to an adverse event. This means that the error *almost* happened. It is important to understand such errors; they provide valuable information for preventing future actual errors.
  Example: The surgical team is preparing the patient's right knee for surgery. The team checks the records only to find out that it is the left knee that requires surgery. An error was prevented, but why was the wrong knee initially prepped?

- *Active Error:* An error that results from noncompliance with a procedure (Reason, 1990). Example: A nurse does not check vital signs to confirm the need for a specific medication, which is required for the medication. The medication is administered when the patient does not need the medication and experiences side effects.

- *Latent Conditions:* Threats not immediately apparent. These indicate problems in the system (Reason, 1990).
  Example: Some staff members are not familiar with a change in policy though it is assumed all are implementing a new policy. An error occurs due to lack of knowledge.

- *Sentinel Event:* An event that has a drastic negative outcome; unexpected death, serious physical or psychological injury, or serious risk. A root cause analysis or a systematic review of the event is conducted to examine the process, not just the individual staff member involved. The goal is not blame but prevention of future events.
  Example: The patient commits suicide while in the hospital for treatment.

- *Root Cause Analysis:* An in-depth analysis of an error to assess the event and identify causes and possible solutions. The Joint Commission root cause analysis matrix includes the following dimensions to be assessed (Joint Commission, 2008a): behavioral assessment process (includes assessment of patient risk to self and to others as appropriate), physical assessment process (includes search for contraband), patient identification process, patient observation procedures, care planning process, continuum of care, staffing levels, orientation and training of staff, competency

---

**BOX 17-4    OTHER CRITICAL DEFINITIONS (CONTINUED)**

assessment and credentialing, supervision of staff (includes supervision of physicians in training), communication with patient or family, communication among staff members, availability of information, adequacy of technological support, equipment maintenance and management, physical environment (includes furnishings, hardware such as bars, hooks, rods, lighting, distractions, security systems and processes, and medication management (includes selection and procurement, storage, ordering and transcribing, preparing and dispensing, administration, and monitoring). Not all of these dimensions apply to every event, but they each need to be considered and then eliminated if not applicable.

Source: Finkelman, A. & Kenner, C. (2009). *Teaching IOM: Implications of the Institute of Medicine Reports for Nursing Education.* Silver Spring, MD: American Nurses Association.

---

**LICENSURE, CREDENTIALING, AND CERTIFICATION**    Professional licensure verification is an important activity in all HCOs. A license means the person has met expected minimal standards set by the state practice act. State laws require that certain health care providers have licenses. Allowing someone to practice without a license means the HCO and the individual are breaking the law. Some states require continuing education credits per licensure renewal cycle with the intent of improving practice. Credentialing is different from checking licensure. It is a more in-depth review process that includes evaluation of licenses, certification if required in a specialty area, evidence of malpractice insurance as required, history of involvement in malpractice suits, and education. Credentialing is not done for all health care staff, but rather primarily used for physicians that practice or admit patients to an HCO. Nurse-midwives and nurse practitioners

---

**TABLE 17-1    ADVERSE EVENTS**

| Causes of Adverse Events | Types of Adverse Events |
|---|---|
| Care planning | Anesthesia events |
| Care process design | Behavioral events |
| Communication | Criminal events |
| Continuum of care | Environment-related events |
| Human factors | Equipment-related events |
| Information management | Infection-related events |
| Organization culture | Medication errors |
| Patient assessment | Medical events |
| Patient identification | Pediatric events |
| Patient involvement & education | Surgical events |
| Physical resources | Transfer-discharge related events |
| — | Other unanticipated events |

Source: WHO Collaborating Centre for Patient Safety Solutions. (2008). Adverse events. Retrieved November 6, 2008, from http://www.ccforpatientsafety.org/. Reprinted with permission.

may also require credentialing. Licensure and credentialing information is kept on file and may be reviewed during Joint Commission surveys or by other accreditors. Specialty certification has also become more important.

UTILIZATION REVIEW/MANAGEMENT     **Utilization review/management** (UR/UM) is the process of evaluating necessity, appropriateness, and efficiency of health care services for specific patients or patient populations. UM or utilization review has been used in acute care settings for a long time; however, it is also very important to third-party payers or insurers. Nurses are frequently hired as UM staff either by health care organizations or by insurers. They have the clinical skills and knowledge necessary to evaluate patient needs and services to determine the necessity, appropriateness, and timeliness of services.

To reduce costs, it is necessary to assess appropriateness of care and timeliness and influence decisions that are made by providers. "Appropriateness" ties UM to QI. UM is not just looking at numbers such as how many days of treatment. It also focuses on what is appropriate care for the patient's problem. Typically, utilization/resource management or review focuses on length-of-stay or treatment, use of services, complications, readmission rates, number of transfers, number and type of prescriptions, number of referrals to specialists, number of procedures, and so forth. Nurses have the necessary skills for utilization/resource management: clinical knowledge; understanding of health care organizations, nursing process, and communication and collaboration within interprofessional teams; and understanding of documentation. This function also requires that the nurse is knowledgeable about health care reimbursement, provider options, benefits, and costs. Case managers are also very involved in resource management, and authorization of services is the key task in resource management. How does UM/UR affect nursing care?

**Authorization**, the major method used in utilization management, is the approval by the third-party payer for a health care provider to provide specific care. The payer or insurer identifies what services or benefits require authorization. This is done at the time the plan is purchased. Plans that have the greatest amount of control have a tight authorization system. To be truly effective in controlling costs, an insurer must be able to influence provider utilization behavior. For example, if an insurer cannot find a way to decrease a provider's number of hospital admissions or the number of referrals to specialists, costs will continue to be a problem. Insurers are particularly active in controlling authorization. The purchaser of the plan, the employer, does not like the idea of health care costs increasing and may decide to drop the insurer and contract with another, more cost-effective insurer.

Who authorizes services is a critical decision. This decision is made in several ways. Probably, the most recognized method is to have authorization done by the primary care provider/physician (PCP). If an enrollee wants to see the PCP, no authorization is required. Some PPOs and managed indemnity plans require that plan staff authorizes services. In this case, the physician or other type of provider would call a plan representative and describe the patient's problems and the need for services. The staff representative compares this information with predetermined criteria. This representative may be a case manager. The nurse case manager discusses the patient's needs with the provider and determines whether authorization can be provided. If the provider does not agree with the decision, the provider is referred to a supervisor or the medical director. Some plans use a different system. They have the enrollee call the plan directly, using a nurse advice line or a case manager. The enrollee does not have to go to the PCP to use a specialist but rather uses the advice line to gain authorization. Predetermined criteria are used to assess the enrollee's needs. Insurers have been trying to find new methods to expedite authorization. Providers have found this to be a time-consuming process and have been particularly insulted that "staff" in the plan is making medical decisions. As insurers have grown more sophisticated, they have moved toward using more nurses in these roles in order to decrease these criticisms. Insurers also recognize the advantages of using health care professionals that can discuss the medical issues with providers and then make clinical decisions, and providers prefer talking with other health care professionals about patients. Predetermined criteria are important; however, it is also important to have professional experience to understand medical problems and needs and the application of the criteria as well as recognize when there might need to be exceptions.

Utilization review and discharge planning (DP) are two functions in hospitals that are interconnected. In some cases the two functions may have been combined. It is becoming more common for UR to be more important than discharge planning. Why is this so? "This predominance of UR over DP evolved partly by the initiative to defend 'medical necessity' and 'appropriateness,' and partly because of the way hospitals contract with—and are paid by—third party payers" (Birmingham, 2007, p. 17). Many of the UR and DP activities are the same such as admission review, continued stay review, and assessment of readiness for discharge. There are, however, some critical components associated with discharge planning that should not be ignored. Some of these are routine monitoring of changes in the plan and counseling the patient and family about the discharge plan and effective patient/family education. Today, with the acuity of patients and staffing shortage, nurses have less and less time to prepare patients for discharge. Patients and their families who are not involved in the discharge planning process are more likely to have problems in the next level of care. This is costly for all concerned.

**CLINICAL GUIDELINES AND CLINICAL PATHWAYS**   Clinical guidelines and clinical pathways are methods or tools that focus on improvement of care. Chapter 7 includes additional information on this topic. The Agency for Healthcare Research and Quality (AHRQ) is the most prominent agency that develops clinical or practice guidelines. Since guidelines identify outcomes and support best practice, they can be useful in determining quality and cost of health care. Professional organizations have also become very active in developing guidelines. How do guidelines and pathways enhance the quality of care? This should improve care, but they also provide a consistent approach to care. Though when a guideline or a pathway is used it needs to be assessed to determine how it applies to a specific patient. These tools can be used to assess care for patient groups (diagnoses, problems, and so on). For example: Was the pathway or the guideline followed? What were the outcomes? HCOs can use these tools to orient staff as to the requirements for care, setting standards.

The AHRQ is an important governmental agency that focuses on health care quality issues. Its mission is "to support research designed to improve the outcomes and quality of health care, reduce its costs, address patient safety and medical errors, and broaden access to effective services" (Agency for Healthcare Research and Quality, 2003, July 9). Its goals are to (a) support improvements in health outcomes, (b) promote patient safety and reduce medication errors, (c) advance the use of information technology for coordinating patient care and conducting quality and outcomes research, and (d) establish an Office of Priority Populations (to ensure that they receive care—low-income groups, minorities, women, children, the elderly, and individuals with special needs). AHRQ has developed quality indicators for inpatient care, safety, and prevention. The AHRQ guidelines website provides examples of guidelines that are evidence-based. (See Media Links for the National Guidelines Clearinghouse.)

**Clinical guidelines** identify outcomes and support best practice, and they can be useful in determining the quality and cost of health care. Professional organizations have also become very active in developing guidelines. How do guidelines enhance the quality of care? Data can help to identify quality problems, particularly problems related to underuse, overuse, or ineffective provision of care. Greater understanding of how patients respond to care for particular problems can help to prevent problems. Patient outcomes and patient satisfaction are important variables to consider as guidelines are implemented and data collected. This should all lead to a more complete view of care required for specific problems and improve guidelines.

**Clinical pathways** can be used in the assessment of quality and cost of health care. Pathways focus on outcomes and the assessment of their achievement. They provide a benchmarking method for individual patients. The promotion of appropriate use of resources in a timely manner is an important component of each pathway, and this promotes cost-effectiveness. When outcomes are not met, then **variance** data are analyzed to determine causes and actions that need to be taken to prevent further problems. This information also provides data that can be used to improve care for other patients who might have similar problems. Variances are analyzed when outcomes are not met to determine causes and actions that need to be taken to prevent further problems. This information also provides data that can be used to improve care for other patients.

BENCHMARKING    **Benchmarking** is a tool that identifies "best practices" (Six Sigma, 2010). It is, however, important to note that it is also a tool that links standards of care, guidelines, documentation, quality improvement programs, and clinical pathways. Benchmarking allows organizations to compare their performance both within the organization and with other organizations. It is a process that uses data to improve. It requires that staff use data-driven, decision-making processes and in so doing makes the organization and its staff aware of options. It begins by identifying the areas of greatest need and those for which there is comparable performance data. Time should not be wasted on correcting problems that will not have an impact or for which it is difficult to obtain data. "The concept of discovering what is the best performance being achieved, whether in your company, by a competitor, or by an entirely different industry. Benchmarking is an improvement tool whereby a company measures its performance or process against other companies' best practices, determines how those companies achieved their performance levels, and uses the information to improve its own performance. Benchmarking is a continuous process whereby an enterprise measures and compares all its functions, systems and practices against strong competitors, identifying quality gaps in the organization, and striving to achieve competitive advantage locally and globally" (Six Sigma, 2008).

Many hospitals, other types of HCOs, and insurers use benchmarking today. One of the popular benchmarking approaches is Six Sigma, which "is a rigorous and a systematic methodology that utilizes information (management by facts) and statistical analysis to measure and improve a company's operational performance, practices, and systems by identifying and preventing 'defects' in manufacturing and service-related processes in order to anticipate and exceed expectations of all stakeholders to accomplish effectiveness" (Six Sigma, 2008).

A key component of benchmarking is sharing, and this has not always been easy for health care organizations. If information is shared, it will benefit others, but this requires some trust. Any organization or insurer that participates in benchmarking will undoubtedly want its legal advisors to review policies and procedures related to this project. Competition has not disappeared; in fact, it has increased. Acknowledging competition and also participating in benchmarking can be a complex endeavor. The report card provided by the National Committee for Quality Assurance (NCQA) is an example of benchmarking, allowing for greater comparison and hopefully improvement of cost and quality of services as changes are made in insurers and with providers (National Committee for Quality Assurance, 2009a). The link to this report is available in the Media Links section at the end of this chapter.

ACCESS TO HEALTH CARE    Access to care is a critical issue in today's health care environment and an integral component of patient-centered care. Assessment of access to care and who is not able to access care is an important measure of the quality of care. Reduced access may result in poorer patient outcomes and can be costly if the patient's condition worsens because the patient was not able to access the right care when needed. How easy is it for a patient to receive care? Economic factors, transportation, and availability of appropriate health care providers may make it difficult for the patient to receive care when it is needed. Access has been greatly affected by the diverse health care delivery and financial arrangements present in the health care environment. There is also an ethical issue interwoven in any discussion of access. Is health care a right? This issue has not been resolved, as there is no state or federal law that says it is a right. The country spends more money on health care than any other service and yet not all citizens receive it. If barriers to coverage and proximity are removed, will the result be equitable access? This is also an unknown. The following are examples of the many elements of access to health care.

1. Ability to get to an appointment (e.g., hours of service for appointments, transportation, time off from work, childcare, and so on)
2. Ability to get specialty care or referral required
3. Ability to pay for care
4. Ability to know when care is needed and seek it
5. Ability to understand health care information and utilize it

6. Ability to access health care facility (e.g., disability access)
7. Ability to choose health care providers
8. Ability to get exams and tests in a timely manner
9. Ability to better ensure patient-centered care
10. Ability to implement evidence-based practice

Access is more than just initial entry into the health care system; it also includes how services are received within the system and the outcomes of that care. As the health care delivery system has changed, greater strain has been put on safety net providers (for example, free-care clinics, public and teaching hospitals, and other health care facilities that provide care to those with limited funds or insurance coverage). These providers are less able to provide uncompensated care without sustaining major financial hardships. In addition, the strain and overload on the health care delivery system affects the quality of the services provided. Given these facts, the improvement of care requires that these problems are addressed to make care more accessible to all who need care. Other factors that are important in considering access are convenience; timeliness; handicap provisions; accommodations for language or sight, health literacy; hours of operation; provider choice; waiting time for urgent and routine care; and timeliness of laboratory tests. Each of these can be used as indicators to determine accessibility of care and thus assist in the evaluation of the quality of care. The Institute of Medicine describes **access to care** as the consumer's ability to access personal health services a person needs when needed to reach the best outcomes (Institute of Medicine, 1993). The major focus today is on accessible primary care, particularly in relation to continuity, time, and provider type. Third-party payers have increased their emphasis on the use of the primary care provider as the gatekeeper or controller of access.

Access for special populations or vulnerable populations has been a major concern. As the health care delivery system has changed, greater strain has been put on safety net providers, for example, free-care clinics, public and teaching hospitals, and other health care facilities that provide care to those with limited funds or insurance coverage. *Healthy People 2010* included access as a critical need for all types of health care needs, and this is also part of the *Healthy People 2020* goals (U.S. Department Health and Human Services, 2010). When a patient does not have access then the patient's health status is at risk and further complications may occur. Vulnerable populations that often have limited access are low-income, children and adolescents, minorities, homeless, mentally ill, uninsured, disabled, elderly veterans, immigrants, and prisoners. These populations are more vulnerable and often less "attractive" to providers and the community. Efforts have been made to resolve some of these concerns, and some of these efforts have been more successful than others. Medicaid has moved to incorporating managed care into its program, but there still are concerns about access for vulnerable populations. Case management can have a positive impact on the health care of vulnerable populations who frequently have complex needs and problems. Health care reform legislation of 2010 should gradually have some impact on this problem.

**RISK MANAGEMENT** **Risk management** (RM) focuses on limiting an organization's financial risk associated with the delivery of care, particularly related to lawsuits, hopefully before incidents occur. The role of a risk manager in an organization is "to maintain a safe and effective health care environment and prevent or reduce loss to the health care organization" (Pike, Janssen, & Brooks, 2002, p. 3). Strategies that health care organizations use include the following:

- Purchasing insurance or self-insuring to protect against financial risk
- Identifying exposures, types, where they occur, frequency, and level of risk
- Implementing medicolegal factors to protect against undue risk
- Implementing organizational programs to prevent occurrence of events that might increase financial risk (e.g., incident report system, staff education about risk and documentation, data collection to assist in identifying potential problems)
- Investigating incidents, which might result in a potential lawsuit, as soon as possible after the incident occurs
- Monitoring strategies for prevention of risk

Risk management staff work closely with QI staff as their responsibilities are interrelated. The key source of information is the organization's occurrence or incident reporting system. Nurses participate in this process by completing the required forms when involved in an incident and following policies and procedures. Most incidents, however, do not result in a lawsuit.

Nurses participate in risk management every day when they ensure patient safety and quality care. Typical areas of high risk include: medication administration, falls, overall patient safety, use of technology and equipment (for example, ensuring that equipment is working correctly before using it in the operating room), assessment and communication of allergies, and any action or intervention that might harm the patient. Health care organizations must also consider the risks to anyone who enters the organization such as visitors, community members, family members, and so on (e.g., a visitor falls in the hallway). Health care organizations and providers also retain legal services to assist them with risk management. Frequently, nurse attorneys are used because they have both the legal and clinical experience to understand the complex problems that arise. These preventive efforts are expensive; however, they are not as expensive as the cost of malpractice suits. Attorneys provide counsel about documentation and actions to be taken if an incident occurs that might put the organization at financial risk. If a nurse is involved in a malpractice suit, the nurse's employer provides legal services; however, the nurse should also consult an attorney who would just represent the nurse. Malpractice insurance, which every nurse should carry, covers most if not all of the legal expenses.

**EVIDENCE-BASED PRACTICE AND EVIDENCE-BASED MANAGEMENT**   Evidence-based practice (EBP) helps to identify and assess high-quality, clinically relevant research that can be applied to clinical practice (Institute of Medicine, 2008). Evidence-based practice is viewed as method to improve the quality of care because basing decisions on evidence can better ensure that the care needs are met in an effective manner. Chapter 15 includes more detailed information about EBP and EBM.

**QUALITY REPORT CARDS**   **Quality report cards** provide specific performance data about an organization. Data that might be found in a HCO report card include admissions, length-of stay per admitting diagnosis, mortality rates per diagnosis, procedures, surgical procedures, qualifications of medical staff, and so on. The organization may then compare these data with data from other similar organizations. The goal is to provide information that is helpful to the purchaser of health care services, the consumer of health care services, and health plans. Employers are primarily interested in differences in quality related to the costs of plans. Patients or consumers are interested in quality comparison among plans and their providers. Health plans also want this performance information for marketing purposes.

Report cards have become more common, and health care professionals and organizations, consumers, and customers are using them more. Changes in report card formats and content rapidly occur as needs change and problems are discovered in the report cards. Third-party payers are interested in data about financial performance, operating performance, membership, changes in service, and the services. Report cards, however, are not perfect. They are costly from the perspective of data collection, data analysis, and data sharing. A report card may indicate improvement in the indicators used to determine the content, but there is no assurance that this affects other aspects of care. If a report card indicates that an insurer plan or HCO has problems the insurer or HCO may not want this information shared. There is, however, no guarantee that releasing this information affects quality or the employer's and the consumer's choices. Many decisions that consumers make about their health care are not always based on quantitative data. Understanding the new data and finding the data may not always be easy. Patients often seek out information and guidance from family members and friends, who have their own personal views and values that may not be based on facts. The National Committee for Quality Assurance provides interactive health care quality reports via the web. (See Media Links to access examples of report cards.)

**NURSING AND QUALITY REPORT CARDS**   Since the mid-1990s nursing has moved more toward using quality reports related to nursing care. In 1994, the ANA initiated an investigation of the impact of workforce restructuring and redesign on the safety and quality of patient care in acute care settings. The purpose of this report was to "explore the nature and strength of the linkages between nursing care and patient outcomes by identifying nursing quality indicators" (Pollard, Mitra, & Mendelson, 1996, p. 1). The result provided a framework for educating nurses, consumers, and policy makers about nursing's contributions within the acute care setting. The project tracked the quality of nursing care provided in acute care settings and considered the current efforts hospitals and health care systems used to track measures of hospital performance with linkages to nursing services (American Nurses Association, 1996).

This was a major step forward for nursing. To ensure quality data, nurses need to develop standardized data reporting processes. There continues to be a need to identify objective measures to assess health care provider performance. Increased insurer influence on outcomes of care through managed care approaches has made this even more important as consumers and providers have become more concerned about the quality of care and provider performance as costs are reduced. Identifying nurse-sensitive quality measures was critical in the 1994 ANA report; however, it must be recognized that outcomes measurement in health care is still a relatively new area. There is much to learn about it. In general, concern exists that databases and report cards that focus on measuring quality have not included nursing-specific quality indicators.

Three types of indicators are used in the report, which are the three critical elements discussed earlier in the chapter and in Chapter 16: patient-focused outcome, process of care, and structure of care-nurse staffing patterns. Outcome indicators focus on how patients and their conditions are affected by their interaction with nursing staff. Process indicators focus on care delivery. The study identified two types of process indicators: (a) how nurses perceive and discharge their roles or nursing satisfaction, and (b) the nature, amount, and quality of care nurses provide to patients. The development of these indicators is part of the ANA's nationwide Nursing Safety and Quality Initiative, a multiphase effort to investigate the impact of health care restructuring on the safety and quality of patient care and on the nursing profession, which includes the indicators for acute care that were previously discussed (Montalvo & Dunton, 2007; Dunton & Montalvo, 2009). Evidence-based methods were used to identify the acute care indicators and were also used to develop the community-based, non-acute care indicators.

In 1998 the ANA established the National Database of Nursing Quality Indicators (NDNQI). As of 2007, over 1000 hospitals participate in this database. This initiative "provides each nurse the opportunity to review the evidence, evaluate their practice, and determine what improvements can be made" (Montalvo & Dunton, 2007, p. 3). The database includes a large number of hospitals, increasing the pool of evaluation data. The indicators are changed based on needs and current data. This initiative is important for the nursing profession and allows nurses to demonstrate their impact on patient outcomes.

## Examples of Nursing Safety Initiatives

TRANSFORMING CARE AT THE BEDSIDE   The Institute for Healthcare Improvement (IHI) is described as "a reliable source of energy, knowledge, and support for a never-ending campaign to improve health care worldwide. Its projects have helped to change health care by focusing on practical solutions that can be used by health care organizations, providers, and health care education" (Institute for Healthcare Improvement, 2009). Its projects and resources focus on safety, effectiveness, patient-centeredness, timeliness, efficiency, and equity, all of which are emphasized in the IOM Quality series. One of IHI's collaborative projects with the Robert Wood Johnson Foundation (RWJF), nursing, and HCOs is Transforming Care at the Bedside (TCAB). This is a "unique innovation initiative that aims to create, test, and implement changes that will dramatically improve care on medical/surgical units, and improve staff satisfaction as well" (Institute for Healthcare Improvement, 2009). Its website provides examples of TCAB pilots and results. TCAB is discussed in other chapters of this textbook.

TAXONOMY OF ERROR, ROOT CAUSE ANALYSIS, AND PRACTICE RESPONSIBILITY (TERCAP)   One of the outcomes from the IOM work (1999) on safety was TERCAP, a new initiative led by the National Council of State Boards of Nursing (NCSBN). TERCAP is a tool that describes nursing practice breakdown. It focuses on (1) safe medication administration, (2) documentation, (3) attentiveness/surveillance (patient monitoring) (4) clinical reasoning (5) prevention (6) intervention (7) interpretation of authorized provider orders (8) professional responsibility/patient

## APPLYING EVIDENCE-BASED PRACTICE

### Evidence for Effective Leadership and Management

**Citation:** Bae, S., Mark, B., & Friend, B. (2009). Impact of nursing unit turnover on patient outcomes in hospitals *Journal of Nursing Scholarship, 42*(1), 40–49.

**Overview:** This secondary analysis study examined how nursing unit turnover impacts workgroup processes. The review also considered how these processes mediate the impact of nurse turnover on patient outcomes. RN and patient data from 268 nursing units at 141 hospitals were used. Researchers examined the turnover rates for six consecutive months; used a questionnaire to gather data about workgroup processes; and data on patient outcomes (unit-level average lengths of stay, patient falls, medication errors, and patient satisfaction). Results indicate that moderate levels of turnover rates have lower workgroup learning levels (how groups learn from their experiences), lower turnover levels have fewer patient falls, and workgroup cohesion and relational coordination have a positive impact on patient satisfaction.

**Application:** Nursing unit turnover is a critical concern throughout the country in all types of health care settings. This study offers an interesting perspective on the interrelationship of nurse unit turnover, workgroup issues, and patient outcomes.

**Questions:**

1. *Why do you think nurse unit turnover impacts patient outcomes and workgroup effectiveness?*
2. *What other factors might impact workgroup cohesion?*
3. *As a chief nurse executive, how might you use the results of this study in your management decisions?*

advocacy (Benner, Malloch, & Sheets, 2010). The goals of studying practice breakdown are to develop a consistent approach to assessing patient safety and reporting errors that will increase knowledge and incentives for error detection, reporting, and prevention while fulfilling the duty to protect the public from unsafe practices" (Benner, Malloch, & Sheets, 2010, p. 2). Using TERCAP, state boards of nursing voluntarily submit data about errors reported to state boards after the boards have completed their review process. This then will provide a database that can be used to meet the goals of the initiative. (See Media Links for further information on TERCAP.)

### Collaborative Initiatives: A Great Need

Nurses are affected by and have valuable opinions about the quality of care and benefit from collaborating with other health care providers such as physicians who have similar views. It is also important to interact with health care professionals who may have different views in order to gain collaboration and arrive at the best solutions. A collaborative effort will have a greater impact on changing health care delivery to improve care. This type of initiative is not common. It needs to happen within individual health care organizations, with individual nurses and other health care professionals, and with health care profession organizations—all joining together in true collaborative efforts to achieve interprofessional quality improvement.

## Program Evaluation

Health care programs or services need to be evaluated on a regular basis, preferably annually. This evaluation needs to include review of the vision and mission statements and goals and objectives. The organizational chart should provide resources to meet the goals. The budget is reviewed. Were outcomes met? Documentation should be reviewed. Staff records are reviewed. Questions that might be included in the program evaluation are as follows:

- What specific activities does staff perform?
- How do managers and staff distribute their time between specific activities and interventions?
- Who is served by the program? Which patients? The community?

- Have staff and managers received sufficient education and training to optimally do their work?
- Is the program meeting the stated programmatic objectives (goals)?
- Is the program cost-effective?
- Are the patients appropriately selected? Does the program target the patients in greatest need of services and those with the best potential for improved outcomes?
- Is the intensity or level of care received by patients appropriate?
- Are patients discharged from services when clinically appropriate? Referred to appropriate follow-up care?
- What does patient satisfaction data indicate?
- Is care patient-centered, and how is it patient-centered?
- How does the interprofessional team function? How do other teams such as management team or the nursing team function? What are the satisfaction levels?
- How is informatics used? How effective are the methods?
- What does the quality data indicate? What the analysis results and implications for improvement?
- How is evidence-based practice and evidence-based management used? How effective is this?
- If the program includes health care professions students, how is the educational program functioning? Include feedback from students, faculty, and staff.

All position descriptions should be reviewed to ensure that they describe the work that is done. Policies and procedures, clinical guidelines, clinical pathways, standards, and so on should be reviewed to ensure that they are evidence-based, current, clear, and effective. Getting feedback from all stakeholders will help to ensure a more comprehensive review.

## Accreditation of Third-Party Payers

Accreditation is also used to evaluate third-party payer organizations or insurers. This process is similar to health care organization accreditation and is based on established minimum standards. There are two major reasons for accrediting insurers. Health care purchasers, who are primarily employers or the government, want objective data to make informed decisions about health plans to support a good return on their investment. Data from accreditation, as well as accreditation status, can supply some objective data. In addition, consumers have become more interested in data about health plans as they make their own decisions about which plan to select from the choices available to them. Purchasers and consumers are interested in two critical elements: cost and quality. They want greater accountability for the quality of services. Report cards describing quality and outcomes data have become more common and accessible through the Internet. Report card data can help patients choose insurers and health care providers such as physicians or hospitals. It is important to note that accreditation is voluntary; however, many purchasers/employers do not contract with insurers that are not accredited. The federal government requires accreditation to award contracts to managed care organization Medicare for beneficiary health care coverage. The following are relevant organizations.

- *National Committee for Quality Assurance* (NCQA): This is an independent, nonprofit organization that began in 1990 but originated from an organization that was founded in 1979 by two managed care trade associations. Its mission is to improve the quality of health care insurance plans. It accredits health plans, wellness and health promotion, managed care organizations, preferred provider organizations, new health plans, disease management programs, and quality plus programs (National Committee for Quality Assurance, 2009b).
- *Health Plan Employer Data and Information Set* (HEDIS): This is a system used by more than 90 percent of U.S. health plans to measure performance (National Committee for Quality Assurance, 2009b). NCQA has continued to develop and use the HEDIS as the NCQA recognizes the need to standardize how health plans calculate and report performance information. HEDIS provides opportunity for benchmarking, comparing similar health plans. Various methods for benchmarking are described at the NCQA website. NCQA describes quality health care as "the extent to which patients get the care they need in a manner that

most effectively protects or restores their health. This means having timely access to care, getting treatment that medical evidence has found to be effective and getting appropriate preventive care. Choosing a high-quality health plan—and a high-quality doctor—plays a significant role in determining whether you'll get high-quality care" (National Committee for Quality Assurance, 2009b). Report cards are also available to assess health plans via the NCQA website.

- *The American Health Care Commission/Utilization Review Accreditation Commission* (**URAC**) is a private, nonprofit, independent accrediting and certification organization for utilization management programs, which began in 1990. Utilization management companies assist third-party payers and health care providers in managing and evaluating the necessity, appropriateness, and efficiency of health care services. The purpose of URAC is to promote quality and preserve patient rights. URAC has 22 accreditation and certification programs. URAC has also developed accreditation standards for case management programs.

## Nurse's Role in Quality Improvement

This chapter has focused on implementation of quality improvement, emphasizing that nurses need to be involved in the process. Leadership is required to be effective in QI. Communication is a critical part of all QI activities. Nurses need to understand the health policy implications of quality as described in Chapters 2 and 16. There are many different roles that nurses may get involved in as they participate in QI in a health care organization. Examples are providing feedback on performance, participation in their own performance appraisal, collecting data, awareness of errors and applying this to their practice, assisting with analysis of data, and using conclusions from quality analysis to improve their practice. Some nurses hold formal positions that focus on QI activities. All nurse managers are directly involved in ensuring quality care and need to be aware of the impact of outcomes. To be effective nurses need an understanding of change and how to plan and implement change, access current literature and critique literature, data collection and analysis (typically staff with statistical expertise are used as a resource to assist with analysis), understanding of QI methods, and ability to work with a team. Most of the competencies discussed in this textbook apply to QI responsibilities including coordination, collaboration, communication, and planning.

## A Review of Past Activities and Future Direction: Nursing and Health Care Quality

Rantz, Bostick, and Riggs (2002) were commissioned by the ANA to conduct the third review of nursing quality measurement. From 1995 to 2000, they identified 315 nursing studies and 7 discussion/process articles on quality of care. It is notable that compared with the second review, 1989–1994, there were 180 more studies in the third review. As has been discussed in this chapter, this is another indication of the growing interest in quality of care, and more than just interest but also action to improve. The Institute of Medicine reports, as noted in Chapter 16, have had a major driving influence on the need for improvement and to take action to improve. The review included studies related to ambulatory care, community health, home health, hospital-based care, Veteran's Affair medical centers, and long-term care; studies across all settings; and quality measurement and nurse-sensitive outcomes. This third review made the following recommendations, which are similar to the recommendations made in the second review.

- Staff should incorporate the NMDS (Nursing Minimum Data Set) elements into all computerized medical record systems and into federal and state databases as they are revised. Collecting these elements should be reviewed as essential data as regulations are promulgated to enforce legislation written to ensure quality of health care services.

- Staff should document nursing hours of care per patient, educational preparation of the nurse provider, and the use of assistive personnel in the delivery of care. Each nurse should have a unique provider identifier. Care delivery hours should be included in all large data sets for all settings.
- A system for determining what constitutes appropriate outcomes for patients in different settings is needed. Data elements for these outcome measures must be included in large data sets for all settings. The system must be sensitive to an individual's potential for self-care or recovery.
- Continued support for research efforts to identify nurse-sensitive outcomes and the relationship among nursing diagnoses, interventions, outcomes, staffing, and staff mix is essential. Support of standardization so that these elements are included in large data sets is also essential.
- Nursing care should provide leadership in quality improvement for health care. Nurses have a long and strong history of quality measurement research that can be invaluable to the outcomes of patients and collaboration with other health care providers (Rantz, Bostick, & Riggs, 2003, p. 7).

Data from studies that address how staffing affects patient outcomes have also increased.

Chapter 9 discussed nurse staffing in more detail; however, it clearly is relevant to this chapter's content. Needleman et al. (2002) reported, based on their study of 1997 data from 799 hospitals in 11 states, which included both medical and surgical patients, that "a higher proportion of hours of nursing care provided by registered nurses and a greater number of hours of care by registered nurses per day are associated with better care for hospitalized patients" (p. 1715). Another study covering 1998 to 1999 and including 210 hospitals in Pennsylvania revealed similar results (Aiken et al., 2002). The objective of this study was to "determine the association between the patient–nurse ratio and patient mortality, failure-to-rescue (deaths associated with complications) (Clarke & Aiken, 2003) among surgical patients, and factors related to nurse retention. The study indicated that hospitals with the highest patient-to-nurse ratios were at considerable risk (twice as likely) to have nurses who experience burnout and job dissatisfaction, factors that can affect quality and safety in health care delivery. Nurses were shown to be important in preventing death given that staffing levels allowed for effective care—surveillance, early detection, and timely interventions that save lives. The study not only considered patients with the risk of death but also those for whom complications could be prevented. Nursing staffing levels also had an effect on these patients. The conclusion from the study is that nurse staffing levels do affect patient outcomes. The DHHS study that was based on 1997 data also supported the conclusion that there is a strong link between patient outcomes and nurse staffing in hospitals (U.S. Department of Health and Human Services, 2001). Lowry (2010) reported on a study that indicated the risk of death among elderly hospitalized with hip fractures increased 20% with the nursing staff was reduced by one full-time nurse each day.

The ANA agrees with the need to recognize the importance of staffing levels and effects on patient outcomes (quality and safety), but the ANA was concerned that the IOM report, *To Err Is Human*, did not address this issue ("Health care errors report sparks major debate, 2000"). However, the later report, *Keeping Patients Safe: Transforming the Work Environment of Nurses*, discusses the staffing issue (Institute of Medicine, 2004). Nursing professional organizations, nurse educators, and nurses in general still must do more to educate and advocate with policy makers, health care leaders, and consumers about this issue. Studies, such as the ones mentioned here, will do much to provide the data that are needed to support greater recognition that improvement of staffing levels and the qualifications of staff can help in major ways to improve the quality and safety of health care, a key concern of health care providers including nurses, consumers, employers, third-party payers, and the government. EBP and EBM are in their infancy stage in nursing. There needs to be more research about quality improvement and nursing, and then the results need to be applied through the EBP and EBM processes. (See Chapter 15.)

In the fall of 2010, the IOM, in collaboration with Robert Wood Johnson Foundation (2011), published a key report on nursing that was influenced by all the preceding *Quality Chasm* reports and the Affordable Care Act of 2010. This landmark report on nursing notes that "Nurses should practice to the full extent of their education and training; nurses achieve higher levels of education and training through an improved education system that promotes seamless academic progression; nurses should be full partners, with physicians and other health professions, in redesigning health care in the United States; and effective workforce planning and policy making require better data collection and an improved information infrastructure" (Institute of Medicine, 2011, p. S-3). How can the nursing profession be transformed so that it can make effective use of current opportunities related to IOM and also health care reform and contribute to "building a health care system that will meet the demand for safe, quality, patient-centered, accessible, and affordable care" (Institute of Medicine, 2011, p. 1-1). The report makes the following recommendations (pp. S-8-S-12):

1. Remove scope of practice barriers. *Advanced practice registered nurses should be able to practice to the full extent of their education and training.*
2. Expand opportunities for nurses to lead and diffuse collaborative improvement efforts. *Private and public funders, health care organizations, nursing education programs, and nursing associations should expand opportunities for nurses to lead and manage collaborative efforts with physicians and other members of the health care team to conduct research and to redesign and improve practice environments and health systems. These entities should also provide opportunities for nurses to diffuse successful practices.*
3. Implement nurse residency programs. *State boards of nursing, accrediting bodies, the federal government, and health care organizations should take actions to support nurses' completion of a transition-to-practice program (nurse residency) after they have completed prelicensure or advanced practice degree program or when they are transitioning into new clinical practice areas.*
4. Increase the proportion of nurses with baccalaureate degree to 80 percent by 2020. *Academic nurse leaders across all schools of nursing should work together to increase the proportion of nurses with baccalaureate degree from 50 to 80 percent by 2020. These leaders should partner with education accrediting bodies, private and public funders, and employers to ensure funding, monitor progress, and increase the diversity of students to create a workforce prepared to meet the demands of diverse populations across the lifespan.*
5. Double the number of nurses with a doctorate by 2020. *Schools of nursing, with support from private and public funders, academic administrators and university trustees, and accrediting bodies, should double the number of nurses with a doctorate by 2020 to add to the cadre of nurse faculty and researchers, with attention to increasing diversity.*
6. Ensure that nurses engage in lifelong learning. *Accrediting bodies, schools of nursing, health care organizations, and continuing competency educators from multiple health professions should collaborate to ensure that nurses and nursing students and faculty continue their education and engage in lifelong learning to gain the competencies needed to provide care for diverse populations across the lifespan.*
7. Prepare and enable nurses to lead change to advance health. *Nurses, nursing education programs, and nursing associations should prepare the nursing workforce to assume leadership positions across all levels, while public, private, and governmental health care decision makers should ensure that leadership positions are available to and filled by nurses.*
8. Build an infrastructure for the collection and analysis of interprofessional health care workforce data. *The National Health Care Workforce Commission, with oversight from the Government Accountability Office and the Health Resources and Services Administration, should lead a collaborative effort to improve research and collection and analysis of data on health care workforce requirements. The Workforce Commission and the Health Resources and Services Administration should collaborate with state licensing boards, state nursing workforce centers, and the Department of Labor in this effort to ensure that the data are timely and publicly accessible.*

This report and its recommendations will have a major impact on nursing, though at this time its full impact is not known.

# APPLYING LEADERSHIP AND MANAGEMENT

## MY HOSPITAL UNIT

You are planning a meeting with your staff to discuss the implementation of the six quality improvement aims that have been identified by the Institute of Medicine. These aims are identified in Chapter 16 and in Figure 16-1, and are important to apply in practice. What will you tell the staff about the aims? How will you get them involved in integrating the six aims in the unit and patient care? Provide specific examples for the staff to get the discussion on track. Consider the content found in this chapter on implementing QI. Use the virtual unit site found on the textbook website to record the work that you do in the role of nurse manager for your unit.

## Critical Thinking Questions and Activities

1. How are outcomes related to the assessment of care and accreditation?
2. Why is accreditation of insurers important?
3. What is the value of quality report cards?
4. Compare and contrast the Blame Culture with the Culture of Safety.
5. Do you think nurses can make an impact on the quality of care? If so, how would this occur (provide examples)? How do nurse managers and team leaders impact quality care?
6. Interview a nurse who works in QI. Develop your interview questions from the chapter content. Share your information with your learning team or class.
7. Identify a safety issue you have concerns about in clinical. Describe the issue, data that you can obtain, and plan to improve care related to the issue.
8. Interview five staff nurses and ask them how they know when quality care has been provided. Summarize the data and then compare with data your classmates collected. What are the trends? Differences?
9. Interview a nurse manager and find out what the manager does to improve care on the manager's assigned unit/service.
10. Go to the Institute for Health Improvement website (http://www.ihi.org) and learn more about FEMA, FTR, RRT, handoffs, and workarounds. How might these apply to the organizations where you are for clinical?
11. Discuss the use of root cause analysis. Review extended content on Media Links that pertain to root cause analysis. What is your opinion of this process? How do you think it could be used by nurses and by the interprofessional team? Would using this process impact care and how?
12. Search the literature to learn more about the impact of the IOM report *The Future of Nursing: Leading Change, Advancing Health* (2011). Discuss in small teams how this report relates to content in this textbook. The full report can be found at http://www.iom.edu/Reports/2010/The-Future-of-Nursing-Leading-Change-Advancing-Health.aspx.

## Media Links

- **URL: http://www.ihi.org**
  Institute of Healthcare Improvement
- **URL: http://www.cms.hhs.gov/OASIS/**
  Centers for Medicare and Medicaid Services/ OASIS Program
- **URL: http://www.jointcommission.org**
  The Joint Commission

- **URL: http://www.qsen.org**
  Quality and Safety Education for Nurses
- **URL: http://www.jointcommission.org/patientsafety/nationalpatientsafetygoals/**
  The Joint Commission National Patient Safety Goals
- **URL: http://nhqrnet.ahrq.gov/nhqrdr/jsp/nhqrdr.jsp#snhere**
  National Healthcare Quality Report
- **URL: http://www.ahrq.gov/research/nursestaffing/nursestaff.htm**
  Agency for Healthcare Research and Quality: Systematic Review of Research on Nursing Staffing and Quality of Care
- **URL: http://www.guideline.gov/**
  National Guideline Clearinghouse
- **URL: http://www.ihi.org/ihßi/workspace/tools/fmea**
  Institute for Health Improvement, Failure Modes and Effects Analysis (FEMA)
- **URL: http://www.ihi.org/IHI/Topics/CriticalCare/IntensiveCare/ImprovementStories/BuildingRapidResponseTeams.htm**
  Institute for Health Improvement, Rapid Response Teams
- **URL: https://www.ncsbn.org/441.htm**
  National Council of State Boards of Nursing: TERCAP
- **URL: http://www.ihi.org/IHI/Topics/CriticalCare/IntensiveCare/ImprovementStories/EarlyNursingInterventionBeyondRapidResponseTeams.htm**
  Institute for Health Improvement: Failure to Rescue
- **URL: http://www.ihi.org/IHI/Topics/PatientSafety/SafetyGeneral/Tools/SBARHandoffReportTool.htm**
  Institute for Health Improvement: Handoffs and Use of SBAR Tool
- **URL: http://www.ihi.org/IHI/Topics/PatientSafety/SafetyGeneral/Literature/AmbiguityandWorkaroundsasContributorstoMedicalError.htm**
  Institute for Health Improvement: Workarounds
- **URL: http://www4.va.gov/ncps/CogAids/RCA/index.html#page=page-1**
  Veteran's Administration, National Center for Patient Safety: Root Cause Analysis
- **URL: http://www.jointcommission.org/Framework_for_Conducting_a_Root_Cause_Analysis_and_Action_Plan/**
  Joint Commission: Facts About Sentinel Events and Root Cause Analysis
- **URL: http://www.ncqa.org/tabid/60/Default.aspx**
  NCQA Quality Report Card
- **URL: https://www.nursingquality.org/**
  National Database of Nursing Quality Indicators

**Pearson Nursing Student Resources**

Find additional review materials at
**nursing.pearsonhighered.com**

Prepare for success with additional NCLEX®-style practice questions, interactive assignments and activities, Web links, animations and videos, and more!

# References

Agency for Healthcare Research and Quality. (2003). Overview. Retrieved July 9, 2003, from http://www.ahrq.gov

Aiken, L., et al. (2002). Hospital nurse staffing and patient mortality, nurse burnout, and job dissatisfaction. *Journal of Medical Association, 288*(16).

American Nurses Association. (1996). *Nursing quality indicators.* Washington, DC: American Nurses Publishing.

American Nurses Association. (2006a). *Assuring patient safety: Registered nurses' responsibility in all roles and setting to guard against working when fatigued.* Silver Spring, MD: Author.

American Nurses Association. (2006b). *Assuring patient safety: The employers' role in promoting healthy nursing work hours for registered nurses in all roles and settings.* Silver Spring, MD: Author.

Birmingham, J. (2007). Case management: Two regulations with coexisting functions (utilization review + discharge planning = case management). *Professional Case Management, 12*(1), 16–24.

Centers for Medicare and Medicaid Services. (2010). OASIS. Retrieved April 15, 2010, from http://www.cms.gov/OASIS/

Chassin, M., & Galvin, R. (1998). The urgent need to improve health care quality. *Journal of the American Medical Association, 280*(2), 1000–1005.

Christmas, K. (2008). How work environment impacts retention. *Nursing Economics, 26*(5), 316–318.

Clarke, S., & Aiken, L. (2003). Failure to rescue. *American Journal of Nursing, 103*(1), 42–48.

Dunton, N. & Montalvo, I. (2009). *Sustained improvements in nursing quality hospital performance on NDNQI indicators 2007–2008.* Silver Spring, MD: American Nurses Association.

Finkelman, A. & Kenner, C. (2009). *Teaching IOM: Implications of the Institute of Medicine reports for nursing education.*

Finkelman, A. & Kenner, C. (2010). *Professional nursing concepts. Competencies for quality leadership.* Boston: Jones and Bartlett Publishers.

Gallagher, R., & Kany, K. (2000). Does JCAHO see the truth? *American Journal of Nursing, 100*(4), 74.

Hendrich, A., Chow, M., Skierczynski, & Zhenqiang, L. (2008). A 36-hospital time and motion study. How do medical-surgical nurses spend their time? *Permanente Journal, 12*(3).

Institute for Health Care Improvement. (2008). Medication reconciliation review. Retrieved October 2, 2009, from http://www.ihi.org/IHI/Topics/PatientSafety/MedicationSystems/Tools/Medication+Reconciliation+Review.htm

Institute of Medicine. (1993). *Access to health care in America.* Washington, DC: National Academies Press.

Institute of Medicine (1999). *To err is human: Building a safer health system.* Washington, DC: National Academies Press.

Institute of Medicine. (2004). *Keeping patients safe: Transforming the work environment of nurses.* Washington, DC: The National Academies Press.

Institute of Medicine. (2008). *Knowing what works in health care. A roadmap for the nation.* Washington, DC: The National Academies Press.

Institute of Medicine. (2011). *The future of nursing: Leading change, advancing health.* Washington, DC: The National Academies Press.

Joint Commission. (2009a). 2009 Standards. Retrieved August 19, 2009, from http://www.jointcommission.org/AccreditationPrograms/Hospitals/Standards/09_FAQs/default.htm

Joint Commission. (2009b). Patient Safety and Speak Up. Retrieved November 15, 2009, from http://www.jointcommission.org/PatientSafety/SpeakUp/

Kitch, B. et al. (2008). Handoffs causing patient harm: A survey of medical and surgical house staff. *The Joint Commission Journal of Quality and Patient Safety, 34*(10), 563–570.

Lowry, F. (March 10, 2010). Shortage of nurses means death after hip fractures. Abstract 125, American Association of Orthopedic Surgeons, 2010 conference, New Orleans.

Maddox, P., Wakefield, M., & Bull, J. (2001). Patient safety and the need for professional and educational change. *Nursing Outlook, 49*(1), 8–13.

Manojilovich, M. & Talsma, A. (2007). Identifying nursing processes to reduce failure to rescue. *Journal of Nursing Administration, 37*(11), 504–509.

Montalvo, I., & Dunton, N. (2007). *Transforming nursing data into quality care: Profiles of quality improvement in U.S. health care facilities.* Silver Spring, MD: American Nurses Association.

Mosocco, D. (2001). Data management using outcomes-based quality improvement. *Home Care Provider, 6*(12), 205–211.

Nadzam, D. (2009). Nurses' role in communication and patient safety. *Journal of Nursing Care Quality, 24*(3), 184–188.

National Committee for Quality Assurance. (2009a). Report Cards. Retrieved May 2, 2009, from http://www.ncqa.org/tabid/60/Default.aspx

National Committee for Quality Assurance. (2009b). Health Plan Accreditation. Retrieved August 19, 2009, from http://www.ncqa.org/tabid/689/Default.aspx

National Guideline Clearinghouse. (2009). Guidelines. Retrieved December 2, 2009, from http://www.guideline.gov/

Nolan, E. (2004). Quality at the core of JCAHO initiative. *Nursing Spectrum/Midwestern Edition, 5*(6), 28.

Paolucci, M. (2001). The Joint Commission gains an RN perspective. *Nurse Week Great Lakes, 1*(5), 8.

Pike, J., Janssen, R., & Brooks, P. (2002). Role and function of a hospital risk manager. *Journal of Legal Nurse Consultants, 13*(2), 3–13.

Pollard, P., Mitra, K., & Mendelson, D. (1996). *Nursing report card for acute care.* Washington, DC: American Nurses Publishing, Inc.

Rantz, M., Bostick, J., & Riggs, C. (2002). *Nursing quality measurement: A review of nursing studies 1995–2000.* Washington, DC: American Nursing Publishing, Inc.

Reason, J. (2000). Human error: Models and management. *British Medical Journal, 320*(7237), 768–770.

Six Sigma. (2008). Overview Retrieved February 27, 2008, from http://www.isixsigma.com

Six Sigma. (2010). Understanding the purpose of benchmarking. Retrieved May 30, 2010, from http://www.isixsigma.com/index.php?option=com_k2&view=item&id=225&Itemid=1&Itemid=1

Spear, J. & Schmidhofer, M. (2005). Ambiguity and workarounds as contributors to medical error. *Annals of Internal Medicine, 142*(8), 627–630.

U.S. Department of Defense. (2010). *Patient safety program. Healthcare communications toolkit to improve transitions in care.* Retrieved May 10, 2010, from http://health.mil/dodpatientsafety

U.S. Department of Health and Human Services. (2010). *Healthy people 2020.* Retrieved April 30, 2010, from http://www.healthypeople.gov

U.S. Department of Health and Human Services. (2001). *Nurse staffing and patient outcomes in hospitals.* Washington, DC: Author and the Health Resources and Services Research and Quality, Agency for Healthcare Research and Quality, Centers for Medicare and Medicaid Services (formerly Health Care Financing Administration), and the National Institute of Nursing Research.

Vincent, C. (2003). Understanding and responding to adverse events. *New England Journal of Nursing, 348*(11), 1051–1056.

Wolf, Z. (2007). Caring for the whole patient: The Institute of Medicine proposes a new standard of care. *Community Oncology, 4*(12), 748–751.

# 18

# Health Care Informatics and Technology

## CHAPTER OUTLINE

## LEARNING OUTCOMES

Before you begin, take a moment to familiarize yourself with the learning outcomes for this chapter.

- Describe the Institute of Medicine informatics core competency.
- Discuss the importance of information and clinical technology to nursing.
- Examine critical issues related to privacy and confidentiality and informatics.
- Analyze the current status of the electronic medical record and other associated information technology methods.
- Critique the implications of telehealth to nursing practice and health care.

## KEY TERMS

- Algorithms
- E-health
- Protocols
- Telehealth
- Telenursing
- Telepresence
- Videoconferencing

**WHAT'S AHEAD**

The continued expansion of health care information technology offers important opportunities for nursing education, practice, research, and administration. For nurses to participate in the technology revolution, whether a staff nurse or in a management position, they need to be knowledgeable about health care technology, appreciate the implications of its use, develop the required skills, and apply them to practice and management. This chapter discusses critical technology issues and their implications for health care practice and management.

# Importance of Information and Clinical Technology

The explosion of information and technology has brought the health care delivery system into a new era, which has allowed health care to expand into new areas and to improve others. Information and technology have affected clinical practice, communication, structure of organizations, consumers, workforce issues, quality care issues and outcomes, costs and reimbursement, and ethical and legal concerns. In July 2002, the American Nurses Association (ANA) sponsored an important conference, "Using Innovative Technology to Enhance Patient Care Delivery." This conference focused on the following seven issues that reflected the broad impact of technology in the health care environment, all of which have an impact on nurses and continue to be relevant today.

- Improve patient safety and quality
- Improve operational efficiency and effectiveness in interprofessional practice
- Improve medication use processes to decrease errors
- Improve health technologies that empower patients and enhance patient care
- Create future care environments that improve efficiencies, clinical outcomes, and the healing experience
- Improve practice environments through simulation
- Improve workforce productivity through automation

Since the ANA conference, information technology has greatly expanded in all sectors including health care. There is much known and unknown about the implications of a technologically driven environment. At the same time that technology and information are surging forward, health care is confronted with a growing nursing shortage as well as shortages of other health care providers. Information technology (IT) might be seen as a possible method for helping to cope with the shortage such as by utilizing more effective documentation methods. Many examples are described in this chapter that may make a difference, or at least make health care delivery more efficient and effective. Technology may be one of these factors. "Clinical information systems can be one of those immediate actions that can help nurses feel more confident about the care they are delivering. In addition to preventing medical errors, streamlining workflow and communications, and reducing redundant data entry, these systems can have a lasting and positive effect on overall job satisfaction, providing significant influence on retaining our invaluable nursing resources" (Meadows, 2002, p. 48).

The American Nurses Association published "standards for nursing informatics, which is a nursing specialty that integrates nursing science, computer science, and information science to manage and communicate data, information, knowledge, and wisdom in nursing practice" (2008, p. 1). The first edition of these standards was published in 2001. Nurses in this specialty may function in any of the following areas (American Nurses Association, 2008):

- Administration, leadership, and management
- Analysis
- Compliance and integrity management
- Consultation
- Coordination, facilitation, and integration

- Development of informatic solutions
- Educational and professional development
- Policy development and advocacy
- Telehealth and **telenursing**
- Research and evaluation

The Institute of Medicine (IOM) reports about the health care system recognize the critical role that IT has in the health care delivery system and will have in the future. The clearest indication of its importance is the inclusion of IT in the five health care professions core competencies. This competency is described as "Utilize informatics to communicate, manage knowledge, mitigate error, and support decision making using information technology" (2003, p. 4). Every health care professional should meet the following requirements (Institute of Medicine, 2003, p. 63):

- Employ word processing, presentation, and data analysis software.
- Search, retrieve, manage, and make decisions using electronic data from internal information databases and external online databases and the Internet.
- Communicate using e-mail, instant messaging, listservs, and file transfers.
- Understand security protections such as access control, data security, and data encryption, and directly address ethical and legal issues related to the use of information technology in practice.
- Enhance education and access to reliable health information for patients.

The report discusses the use of informatics to reduce errors and thus improve care. Some of the methods used to do this are discussed later in this chapter. Health care providers can more easily manage knowledge and information needed to provide evidence-based practice, allowing them to access professional literature. Computerized databases provide greater collection of data, analysis of data, and leads to more effective use of data in practice and research. The IOM also notes that computerized decision-making support systems are effective in improving care. Clearly, communication can be more effective and timely by using e-mail, accessing electronic medical records (EMR), organization Internet sites, Internet, and by other electronic means of communication (Institute of Medicine, 2003). Health care reform of 2010 included provisions about health informatics.

## Technology and Caring

Even though there are many positive aspects of information technology, some drawbacks exist that need to be considered as health care organizations incorporated more IT. "Connectivity is the buzzword of the new millennium. We are connected to the Internet, to local area networks, and to paging systems and voice mailboxes. But are we forgetting the goal of emotional connectivity" (Simpson & Keegan, 2002, p. 80)? It is particularly important for health care providers to consider the total impact of technology on practice and organizations. Emotional Intelligence leadership, which was discussed in Chapter 1, has become more important in organizations with staff members tuning in more to their emotions and reactions, how these emotions and reactions affect others, and making changes in behavior to improve relationships and communications. Technology may interfere with this process. Talking through "machines" limits real observations and emotional connections. Does it increase isolation? Does it prevent honest communication? If it does, then it is important to try to figure out ways to prevent these problems. Advancement of technologies is not going away so it is important to use it effectively. Patients need providers who are connected to them, understand the emotional side of health care, and use the power of the human interaction. The goal should not be to throw out or ignore information technology but rather to be aware of potential problems and build in methods to maintain personal connection with patients. It is also important to note that this feeling of isolationism can occur with staff. Despite these concerns, health care requires the use of IT. Information technology cannot be separated from knowledge expansion—with so much increasing knowledge how can one keep up? Health care organizations now need clinical decision-support tools and information systems more than ever. This is very costly, but no organization can afford not to invest in the technology to keep current to improve care. In addition, insurers and accrediting organizations demand more and more data to demonstrate outcomes. The nursing profession needs to appreciate the importance of data and how best to use data. IT provides much data about health care including nursing, and tapping into these data to better understand both the impact of nursing care on patient outcomes and the cost of care can benefit nursing.

## Informatics: Terminology and Standardized Language

Computer literacy or the knowledge and skills needed to use basic computer applications and computer technology is a required competency today. For most people this is not a major issue anymore since so many people have integrated computers and other associated technology into their daily lives. Information literacy is the ability to recognize when information is needed and to locate, evaluate, and effectively use that information (American Nurses Association, 2008). Nurses do need more information and experience doing this. With the explosion of information—data, literature, research results, evidence-based practice—information literacy is critical. Some of the informatic terms that may be new to nurses are as follows:

- *Data*: Discrete entities described objectively without interpretation.
- *Databank*: A large store of information; may include several databases.
- *Database*: Systematically arranged data in a computer; can be retrieved and manipulated often for analysis purposes.
- *Data Mining*: Locating and identifying unknown patterns and relationships within data.
- *Data Analysis Software*: Computer software that can analyze data.
- *Software*: Computer programs and applications.
- *Security protections* (access control, data security, and data encryption): Methods used to ensure that information is not read or taken by persons not authorized to access the information.
- *Clinical Information System (CIS)*: Clinical information systems support the acquisition, storage, manipulation, and distribution of clinical information throughout a health care organization with a focus on electronic communication, e.g., electronic medical records, clinical data repositories, decision support programs (such as application of clinical guidelines and drug interaction checking), handheld devices for collecting data and viewing reference material, imaging modalities, and communication tools such as electronic messaging systems.
- *Clinical Data Repository*: This type of system "provides longitudinal clinical data storage of patient information fed from all of the other clinical information systems, including patient demographic data" (Meadows, 2002, p. 48). Data can be used to improve patient care, in research, for education purposes, and assist with clinical decision making.
- *Decision Support Systems*: Computer applications designed to facilitate human decision making. Decision support systems are typically rule-based. They use a knowledge base and a set of rules to analyze data and information and provide recommendations (American Nurses Association, 2008).

Standardized Language is a collection of terms with definitions for use in informational systems databases. This enables comparisons to be made because the same term is used to denote the same condition. Standardized language is necessary for documentation in electronic health records (American Nurses Association, 2008). This is a difficult issue today as health care providers often use terminology that is specific to their profession. Nursing has persisted in doing this with the emphasis on the *North America Nursing Diagnosis Association (NANDA®)*, *Nursing Intervention Classification (NIC®)*, *and Nursing Outcome Classification (NOC®)*, which are terminology systems that focus on nursing diagnoses, interventions, and outcomes. They are commonly used in nursing education and yet there is not widespread use in clinical practice. This is confusing for nursing students who might learn this terminology and then enter the workplace where it may or may not be used. When it is used in practice other health care professionals, particularly physicians, have no idea what it means. "Creating a common language is no small task. Developing and adhering to distinct profession-specific terms may be a manifestation of professionals' desire to preserve identity, status or control" (Institute of Medicine, 2003, p. 123). All of the IOM core competencies are related to communication, and if there is a problem such as with terminology then patient care is affected. The IOM recommended that an interprofessional group, created by the Department of

Health and Human Services (DHHS), develop a common language across health disciplines "on a core set of competencies that includes patient-centered care, interprofessional teams, evidence-based practice, quality improvement, and informatics" (2003, p. 124). This will not be easy to achieve and to this date has not been done. It requires compromises among health care providers. This also has an impact on EMR use—standardized terminology is required.

The American Nurses Association notes that "The data element sets and terminologies are foundational to standardization of nursing documentation and verbal communication that will lead to a reduction in errors and an increase in the quality and continuity of care. It is through standardization of nurse documentation and communication of a patient's care that the many nurses caring for a patient develop a shared understanding of that care. Moreover, the process generates the nursing data needed to develop increasingly more sophisticated decision support tools in the electronic record and to identify and disseminate best nursing practices" (2006). The statements are nursing focused and examples are provided; however, for this type of data to be fully understood and utilized by all health care providers standardization of terminology is required. A minimum data set is the minimum categories of data with uniform definitions and categories, concerning a specific aspect or dimension of the health care system that meets the basic needs of multiple data users. Examples are the nursing minimum data set (NMDS) and the Nursing Management Minimum Data Set (NMMDS) (American Nurses Association, 2008).

The NMDS describes patient problems across health care settings, different populations, geographic areas, and time. These clinical data also assist in identifying nursing diagnoses, nursing interventions, and nurse-sensitive patient outcomes. This is also useful in assessing resources used in the provision of nursing care. The goal is to be able to link data between health care organizations and providers. Data can also be used for research and health care policy. The NMMDS focuses on nursing administrative data elements in all types of settings.

There are some other data sets. The International Classification of Nursing Practice (ICNP®) is a unified nursing language system applicable to all types of nursing care. It includes nursing diagnoses, nursing interventions, and nursing outcomes (International Council of Nurses, 2008). The Omaha System is a comprehensive and standardized taxonomy designed to improve practice, documentation, and information management in home health care, community and public health (Omaha System, 2005). The Perioperative Nursing Data Set (PNDS) is a standardized nursing vocabulary that addresses the perioperative patient experience from pre-admission until discharge including nursing diagnoses, interventions, and outcomes (Association of Perioperative Registered Nurses, 2008). There are some terminology systems that cross multiple health care professions, something we need more of, such as the Systematic Nomenclature of Medicine Clinical Terms (SNOMED CT®). This is a comprehensive clinical terminology recognized by the Federal Government systems for the electronic exchange of clinical health information (National Library of Medicine, 2008).

## Information Technology: Critical Issues

As information explodes and staff members try to cope with it and want information to be helpful to them, several issues become important, particularly privacy and confidentiality, nursing informatics specialty, and nursing administration and informatics.

PRIVACY AND CONFIDENTIALITY    The 1996 Health Insurance Portability and Accountability Act (HIPAA) has had major effects on IT. First, the law mandates that there be a standardized method for insurance companies and physicians to reduce overhead and increase the payment time for patient care, but this must be done in a manner that ensures patient privacy. Privacy and confidentiality have long been issues in health care, and IT developed with little control related to privacy and confidentiality. This law, however, has had an effect on IT. Chapter 2 contains additional content about this law and recent changes. The law identifies steps that must be taken by health care providers to protect this privacy. Today, health care organizations of all types are required to meet certain requirements to better ensure patient privacy and confidentiality.

DEVELOPMENT, IMPLEMENTATION, AND EVALUATION OF THE CLINICAL INFORMATION SYSTEM   "The ability of health care delivery networks to effectively manage and leverage clinical information to meet strategic clinical goals is a cornerstone of their transformation and survival as integrated information-based clinical enterprises. Successful health care delivery networks will be those that can apply emerging clinical information technologies to meet strategic clinical goals" (Snyder-Halpern & Chervany, 2000, p. 591). It is difficult to find a health care organization that is not using or evaluating for use some type of clinical information system. Some systems have been more effective than others. Making decisions about these clinical information systems is a complex process requiring input from many staff throughout an organization. Selecting the right system is not easy. It is also a very costly decision. After the selection, staff requires training and needs time to adjust. What is needed to develop a clinical information system strategic plan?

1. A clinical vision should be developed that describes the organization's future view of itself. What does the organization believe about the role of IT in its services? This will provide guidelines for how invested the organization will be and at what cost.
2. Clinical strategy should include the general organizational activities that support the organization's vision. This needs to include external influences. How will or could IT affect this strategy?
3. Strategic clinical goals are then developed that are important for the organization and its work. What needs to be included in the goals to support IT?
4. Strategic clinical vital signs are used to evaluate whether or not goals are obtained. How can IT be used to collect data, analyze data, and perform decision making? These goals are then used in the evaluation of IT to assist in determining needed improvements (Snyder-Halpern & Chervany, 2000, pp. 585–586).

As these issues are considered, the organization needs to review such factors as the role of nurses. Will nurses be able to access the IT system for documentation, to obtain clinical resource information, e-mail, and so on? Will physician orders be covered by the system, which has an impact on nursing? Will the IT system become integral to all aspects of the organization? How will staff have input into the system? These are only a few of the considerations that have an impact on health care IT systems.

## Nursing Informatics Specialty

There is a nursing specialty that focuses on IT. "Nursing informatics (NI) is a specialty that integrates nursing science, computer science, and information science to manage and communicate data, information, knowledge, and wisdom in nursing practice. NI supports consumers, patients, nurses, and other providers in their decision making in all roles and settings. This support is accomplished through the use of information structures, information processes, and information technology. The goal of NI is to improve the health of populations, communities, families, and individuals by optimizing information management and communication" (American Nurses Association, 2008, p. 1). It is important for all nurses to understand the importance of data collection and data analysis; then know how to apply data and knowledge to improve patient care. NI specialty certification is available through the American Nurses Credentialing Center (ANCC). What does an informatics nurse do? This specialty focuses on the (American Nurses Association, 2007):

- Methods and technologies of information handling in nursing
- Development, support, and evaluation of applications, tools, processes, and structures that help nurses to manage data in direct care of patients
- Theory formulation, design, development, marketing, selection, testing, implementation, training, maintenance, evaluation, and enhancement of IT for nursing care

These nurses hold positions in clinical practice, education, consultation, research, administration, and informatic businesses.

## Nursing Administration and Informatics

All levels of nursing administration need to play a major role in all aspects of IT within a health care organization. The American Association of Nurse Executives (AONE) states, "Technology is recognized as a key lever within the system of health care delivery. It has the unique capacity to either reduce or increase workload demand. Creating appropriate balance and/or impact is a critical role for leadership (2009). The chief nurse executive (CNE) must take the leadership in the selection and implementation of information systems for the health care organization. It is not easy to acquire information systems (American Association of Nurse Executives, 2007). If nursing leadership is not actively involved, the result can be a very negative impact on patient care and nurses. Nurse managers are directly involved daily in IT particularly in HCOs that use an EMR. Active nurse participation in reviewing EMR systems, evaluation of process and implementation, staff training, and long-term evaluation of the EMR is critical to successful transition to the EMR. A transition to an EMR will inevitably encounter some problems. If nurses are not actively involved the problems will be greater. In addition, as noted in the chapter on change, staff that is involved in the change process will have more buy in and the change will be more effective.

# Technology: Implications on Health Care Delivery

Technology is more than just IT. It also includes technology that can be applied in clinical care, education, and research. The following discussion provides some information about the impact that technology has had and will continue to have on various aspects of health care delivery.

The IOM recommendations indicate that informatics can lead to safe quality care, and it can but there can also be problems (Institute of Medicine, 2003). "There is a perception that technology will lead to fewer errors than strategies that focus on staff performance; however, technology may in some circumstances lead to more errors. This is particularly true when the technology fails to take into account end users, increases in staff time, replicates an already bad process or is implemented with insufficient training. The best approach is not always clear, and most approaches have advantages and disadvantages" (Finkelman & Kenner, 2009, p. 164). Patient-centered care requires collaboration and coordination and interprofessional care is part of this process (Institute of Medicine, 2001; 2003). Information is critical to this process. How it is communicated and maintained impacts the quality of care and control of errors. Ideally, the best system is one that can share information from HCOs to individual providers and vice versa. The United States does not have this system and to get this system will be very expensive and difficult. There is a recognition that more must be done to achieve it, but it will take time. Most HCOs do not have the same EMR systems, making sharing very difficult. Many HCOs have had problems with their EMRs, and this has led to problems, and costly ones. Though there has been a push to move to EMRs, a study published in 2008 (Furukawa, Raghu, Spaulding, & Avinze) included evaluation of 5,082 health care facilities focused on eight health care IT applications to reduce medication errors such as EMRs, clinical decision support, and computerized physician order entry. In 2006 only 2.24 of the eight applications had been adapted, and one-quarter used none of the applications. The size of the hospital made a difference, with larger hospitals adopting more applications. States that had an active state program to reduce errors or had regulations about safety more health care facilities used the IT applications (48 percent higher). This study indicates that much more will have to be done to improve. With passage of health care reform legislation there is hope that there will be improvement. The health care reform legislation of 2010 includes a provision that health plans must implement uniform standards for electronic exchange of health information to reduce paperwork and administrative costs.

## Telehealth

**Telehealth** is the use of telecommunications equipment and communications networks for transferring health care information between participants at different locations. This technology offers opportunities to provide care when face-to-face interaction is impossible. Telehealth applies telecommunication and computer technologies to the broad spectrum of public health and medicine (U.S. Department of Health and Human Services, 2000). In addition, it provides many opportunities for consumer health informatics. (See Chapter 10.) The future holds more opportunity for telehealth with the following changes occurring in telehealth.

- A shift from a predominately rural focus to the provision of home health care and school-based health care in the inner city
- The movement from a preoccupation with acquisition and transport of information to an emphasis on the quality of the information being transmitted
- A switch from a practitioner-based health care system to a patient-empowered and preventive health care system, and in turn, from a patient-based system to a consumer-oriented system (Dakins, 2002, p. 14)

"The most successful telehealth systems employ a variety of telecommunication modalities including two-way interactive video consultations, teleradiology, and telepathology that link primary care providers in rural areas or inner city clinics to experts in large, tertiary centers. Virtual environments for health care delivery and education have been made possible by the same advances in technology that have given us lifelike, computerized video games, and military robotic medics" (Predko, 2001). The critical factor with effective telehealth is the ability of health care providers such as the nurse to envision innovative and practical ways to apply the technology to clinical practice and health care management. When it is applied, safety and quality must always be addressed and monitored.

Standards have been developed for most nursing specialties, and telehealth nursing is no exception. The American Academy of Ambulatory Care Nursing (AAACN) has developed some of these standards because "Telehealth nursing has been identified as one of the new and exciting areas of interest and specialty in ambulatory care nursing" (American Academy of Ambulatory Care Nursing, 2001, p. 7). The AAACN recognizes that telehealth nursing is an evolving specialty that requires standards. As has been stated by many experts, this area of health care directly affects consumers/patients and the organization's effectiveness. The AAACN definition of telehealth nursing practice describes it as "Nursing practice using the nursing process to provide care for individual patients or defined patient populations through telecommunications media. Telehealth nursing practice occurs in many different health care settings" (American Academy of Ambulatory Care Nursing, 2001, p. 1). Critical criteria for telehealth nursing practice include the following:

- Using protocols, algorithms, or guidelines to systematically assess and address patient needs.
- Prioritizing the urgency of patient needs.
- Developing a collaborative plan of care with the patient and his/her support systems. The plan of care may include: wellness promotion, prevention education, advice for care counseling, disease state management, and care coordination.
- Evaluating outcomes of practice and care.

Prioritizing, developing plans of care, and outcome evaluation are typical concerns for nurses, but protocols, algorithms, and guidelines may be new concepts for some nurses. Benefits from using these tools include consistency, accuracy, quality, completeness, ease, and (some) legal protection. These three tools are often used interchangeably; however, they are somewhat different as can be seen in the following definitions.

The nurse who provides telenursing uses a variety of tools such as protocols, algorithms, and guidelines to guide clinical decisions (American Academy of Ambulatory Care Nursing, 2001). For example, patients who call a nurse telephone advice line that is offered to insurance plan members would consult specific protocols, algorithms, or guidelines for questions regarding cardiac, diabetes, or obstetrical concerns. All of these represent standards related to providing care by using technology. **Protocols** define the ongoing care or management of a broad problem or issue in six areas: (a) assessment/data collection/caller interview process; (b) classification/determination of acuity; (c) nature/type/degree of advice/intervention/direction to the caller; (d) information/education of caller; (e) validation of patient understanding/verbal contracting; and (f) evaluation/follow-up/effectiveness of advice or intervention. A protocol directs the advice/triage/education/counseling process, assisting in the organization of large amounts of significant information in priority order. It helps show the interrelationship of data, forcing consideration of all possible or likely decision choices and by so doing directs decision making to be based upon data. **Algorithms** are written clinical questions using branch chain logic (flowchart). An algorithm prescribes what steps to take given particular circumstances or characteristics. Some algorithms also include designated points in the decision-making process where physicians and other caregivers need to discuss with patients or families their preferences for particular options. Algorithms rely on the nurse's ability to analyze and interpret patient responses to clinical questions. Guidelines are typically a more narrative description of assessment steps that includes education and counseling text to support the nurse during the call.

Costs need to be considered for all changes in health care, and the use of technology is no exception. There needs to be careful cost-benefit analysis when decisions are made to use technology. Telehealth is less costly than more traditional methods of practice if one considers staffing and time required and can be a cost-effective means of delivering health care. It is clear that there needs to be more research about this topic. Individual health care providers such as physician offices, clinics, hospitals, home health care agencies, and long-term care facilities should all be doing their own cost-benefit analysis before decisions are made about using information technology and telehealth technologies and monitoring cost-benefit factions when these are implemented. It is important to avoid jumping on the bandwagon when a strategy appears new and exciting. It may offer much, but this needs careful analysis. If there is to be effective use of technology, barriers need to be assessed. The most critical barrier is a lack of reimbursement or limited reimbursement for these services. The inclusion of this content in nursing education, continuing education, and nursing research focused on this area of practice would help to lower the barriers and increase understanding of its use.

## Implications for Clinical Practice

The following are examples of clinical applications of new technology.

**Automated medication administration:** With increased data indicating that medication errors are an important factor in patient complications and deaths, there is more interest in medication administration methods that might decrease this risk (Institute of Medicine, 1999). Bar coding is also useful in collecting data about medication administration that can be used to improve care. "Point-of-service bar coding during medication administration helps caregivers ensure medication safety through automated verification that all of the "five rights" have been met: the right patient, medication, time, dose, and route" (Meadows, 2002, p. 47). The Institute for Safe Medication Practices (ISMP) strongly supports bar coding, and the FDA proposed legislation that required bar codes (Roark, 2004).

**Unit-dose systems:** This system provides individual prepackaged doses. This improves patient care by allowing the nurse to safely identify dose and medication without using multiple dose systems. The medication is prepared in single doses for the patient. When this is combined with the bar coding system the nurse can check the bar code on the unit dose with the nurse's name and the patient's identification. As with any system, for it to work effectively, the nurse needs to follow the required procedure.

**Point-of-care clinical documentation systems:** This system brings documentation to the patient where care is provided thus reducing errors and increasing timely documentation and is directly connected to patient-centered care. There is less chance that the nurse will forget to document an activity or to document it incompletely. Using an EMR with point-of-care capability also saves time and improves coordination of care.

**Professional order entry system (POES):** This type of system is often found in health care organizations today. Physicians and other health care professionals enter their orders into the computer rather than on a hard copy of the medical record. This has much to offer patient care and nurses. Orders are legible, which helps, as illegibility is a major problem with medical records. Most computer systems alert providers to errors, conflicts such as drug incompatibilities, and allergies. Some systems are "eliminating errors by addressing the 'golden second'—the point between clinical decision and action" (Meadows, 2002, p. 47). Providers can be notified when orders need to be reviewed or renewed. This also decreases the need for the nurse to be the "policeman" and remind providers about orders. How does this help nurses? Time is saved when less time is spent following up on orders setting up possible interprofessional conflicts. Nurses can feel more confident that the orders are correct. Errors can be decreased—errors made by physicians when orders are incorrect, and nurse errors when orders are not transcribed correctly as is required in a paper record and when orders are followed incorrectly because the orders are not clear and so on. The medical records become interactive due to these alerts, communicating when something might be wrong or something needs to be done.

**Electronic medical record (EMR):** Documenting in a paperless system has many advantages, for example, decreased time; reduced transcription, storage, copying, and labor costs; improved access for providers; less loss of record material; and improved access for audits (Kerfoot & Simpson, 2002). Data are available when needed with less dependence on memory, which improves clinical decision making. The record is easier to read. Access to the record by staff can occur with more ease. The problem of lost records will be a thing of the past; however, when a computer system goes down this is a major crisis. EMRs require back-up systems.

**"Smart" administration pump:** This technology offers a method to administer fluids and medications and at the same time monitor the patient at the bedside for errors (Kerfoot & Simpson, 2002). As time is always important in direct care, it is critical that the equipment maintenance and repair are monitored to ensure safe care.

**Pharmacy system:** This system provides computerized pharmacy orders, checking, and dispensing, as well as online documentation. (Bar coding may be part of the system.) Online reference systems are also included in this type of system, allowing for application of evidence-based knowledge (Kerfoot & Simpson, 2002).

**Remote telemetry monitoring:** This technology allows nurses to receive pages or provides a page alarm that notifies the nurse of the patient's identification, heart rate, and a readout of rhythm (Donnelly, 2000). The nurse can then evaluate the patient's condition and take appropriate action. Some examples where it might be used are EKG monitoring and fetal monitoring.

## APPLYING EVIDENCE-BASED PRACTICE

### Evidence for Effective Leadership and Management

**Citation:** Thompson, D., Johnston, P., & Spurr, C. (2009). The impact of electronic medical records on nursing efficiency. *JONA, 39*(10), 444–451.

**Overview:** This systematic review evaluated 11 studies on quantifying the impact of the electronic medical record (EMR) technology focusing "on the time required to complete one or more non-patient care-related nursing activities" (p. 445). The researchers classified the studies results as successes or failures. "Successes were defined as those studies that quantified a reduction in the amount of time spent by nurses on indirect and non-patient care activities as a result of using electronic documentation and other EMR tools. Failures were defined as those studies that quantified an increase or no change in the amount of nursing time spent on indirect and non-patient care activities" (p. 445). The results identify EMR features that can reduce time, and those that do not. Utilizing what is learned from the systematic review, this article then describes a case study which describes how benefit, proactive planning in implementing EMR can improve efficiency.

**Application:** Using EMRs is now highly recommended, though as these researchers note, there is limited research to date on its impact. Decision making about EMRs and implementing them are not simple processes. Much needs to be factored in, and also we do not know enough to always make the best decisions. Nurses who use EMRs often describe their frustrations with this new documentation and technology.

**Questions:**

1. *In reviewing the EMR features that lead to success and those that lead to failure, what is your opinion of the features?*
2. *Why do you think there has been limited research on the use of EMRs even though hospitals began to actively implement them in 2000?*
3. *Why is benefit, proactive planning critical when a health care organization implements an EMR?*

**Medical e-mail:** Physicians are using e-mail more and more to communicate with their patients (Hafner, 2002). However, careful attention has to be paid to patient privacy issues. Advanced practice nurses may also find this to be a useful communication tool. There may, however, be concern that some patients may abuse this communication method, and they may also expect providers to respond quickly. In reality, this concern does not seem to be an actual problem. Some providers are using this method for select patients who send the provider daily monitoring data so that the provider can get a better picture of a problem. Messages need to be clear as misinterpretation or misunderstandings are risks. E-mail does offer a paper trail, documenting what has been told to patients, which can be helpful and decreases communication confusion. E-mail guidelines that have been developed for physicians include the following: (a) inform patient if anyone else will be reading the messages, (b) limit sending group e-mail that lists other recipients, (c) ask patients what type of communication they prefer, and (d) archive the messages (sent and received to patients) (Hafner, 2002). All of these suggestions seem reasonable. Whether or not the system has a Web-based, secure message system is of critical concern, and this should be noted on all messages. Since some people in a family share the same e-mail address, this has a direct implication for confidentiality.

**Handheld communication systems:** There is more and more software for handheld devices such as personal digital assistants (PDAs) that allow staff to get information quickly when they need it. Now some of this is available through smartphones so that the person only has to carry one device. Staff can document and search for medical information, search the current *Physician Desk Reference* for drugs or nursing software on drugs, communicate with others, monitor patient information, and make work-planning notes. These systems are gradually replacing small note pads and index cards. Some systems have photograph options, which could be used to document visual data. At this time, some of these systems can be expensive, although prices will probably decrease. Most organizations do not provide them for their staff.

**Internet prescription:** A patient can now go on the Internet and obtain prescribed drugs. There are great safety and legal risks with this practice as these companies may "operate as if they were outside the scope of traditional state and federal laws and regulations" (Waters, 2002, p. 12). Consumers need to get their drugs through reliable Internet sites.

**Home health and IT:** What is happening in this health care setting? Web-based programs for patient monitoring and interactive video-based programs are expanding. Congestive heart disease, diabetes, and coronary disease are the three conditions that have been focused on when these services have been developed. They are chronic illnesses that if managed well can reduce health care costs. Many personal monitoring devices related to many chronic diseases are either available or in development. Examples of these devices include "a monitor in the bathroom shower that scans for signs of melanoma; a wristwatch-like device that constantly checks pulse, respiration, and temperature; computerized eyeglasses that jog a failing memory with whispered cues; and a 'smart badge' that senses a developing infection and identifies the antibiotic need" (Predko, 2001, p. 79). There has been an expansion of disease management for chronic illnesses and with this comes the need for greater patient education, self-management, and also monitoring methods. Telehealth offers many options to meet these requirements. Home health also is increasing its use of IT for documentation, with many agencies providing nurses with computers that can be used in the home and on the road. Cellular telephones are clearly a major benefit to home health nurses to keep in touch with patients, home office, and for emergencies.

## CASE STUDY

### EMR: Can It Improve Care and Work?

Your hospital implemented an electronic medical record (EMR) six months ago. An interprofessional committee composed of representatives and management from nursing, medicine, informatics, hospital administration, finance, quality improvement, admissions, policy and procedure committee, and case management has been formed. The purpose of the committee is to assess the current status of the project and to determine interventions that might be needed at this point. A nursing staff survey indicates that 60% are satisfied, and a physician survey indicates that 48% are satisfied. These percentages need to increase. QI reports indicate that documentation is still not complete; the alert systems are not always effective; staff is keeping back-up hard copies and there is no control on these copies; and there is an insufficient number of computers on some units. The staff and physicians do not feel that they are prepared to use the system. The "talk" in the hallways is that this project will fail.

## Questions:

1. What are the problems?
2. Is more information needed to fully understand the problems, and if so, what information?
3. What needs to be done to resolve the problems?
4. What could have been done to prevent these problems when the project was initially planned and implemented?
5. How would you plan further evaluation (including timeline)?

---

# Implications for Nursing Education

Information technology and telehealth certainly have implications for nursing education. Students expect greater use of IT as they use it more in their personal lives. iPods, PDAs, Internet tools such as Facebook® and MySpace®, and mobile telephones can provide instant information and can also be very interactive. These methods can be used to increase student-faculty communication and have the potential to provide different methods for student-faculty supervision in the clinical area. This is particularly true in areas like community health when students are in multiple sites with faculty moving from site to site to see students. If faculty does not make the changes to incorporate more information technology, students will push for it more and more. This whole era is changing the face of learning and education at all levels. Teaching is moving more and more to facilitation of learning. "There is a shift away from traditional pedagogy to the creation of learning partnerships and learning cultures. Pedagogy has to do with optimizing the transmission of information. The children (and young adults) do not want augmented, predigested information. They want to learn by doing, where they synthesize their own understanding, usually based on experimentation. Learning, therefore, becomes experimental" (Richards, 2001, p. 7). This movement can be seen in the rapid and solid growth of online courses and degree programs, e-books, increased use of the Web to post course documents, use of e-mail to communicate with students, and video access via university websites. IT also means that there are more and more opportunities for learning to be a continuous, lifelong process, as more and more nurses can easily access it. To attract the Net Generation, schools of nursing will have to turn to these new strategies and adapt their philosophies of learning and teaching, which should focus more on facilitation of learning with faculty in the role of facilitator. This is not only important to attract students into nursing but also to prepare nurses who can function and contribute in a highly technological health care environment. Nurses returning to school for BSN degrees or graduate degrees may have to play catch-up in this new learning environment, and faculty has to be prepared to assist them or lose them. "Baby Boomers lived in a slow-motion world compared to the Net Generation. The children of the digital age expect things to happen fast, because in their world, things do happen fast, including learning" (Richards, 2001, p. 8).

Distance education, or education provided in such a way that the student and instructor are either separated by time or distance, has become an important method for providing continuing education, additional academic degrees, and certification. Benefits of this method are flexibility for the student; decreased cost for students such as less travel, parking, and so on; fewer campus buildings needed at schools; increased opportunity to include faculty, such as experts, for short-term teaching; broader mix of students from different geographic areas with different perspectives; opportunity to develop different and innovative teaching strategies; and flexibility for faculty that can travel, teach, and work from home while teaching. Technology can also be used to bring courses to staff within health care organizations and allow organizations with multiple sites to conduct education and training programs without staff travel by using computers, **videoconferencing**, and other new technology.

# Implications for Patient Education

E-health is now commonplace in many health care organizations. Consumers use the Internet to find health information, store personal health information, communicate with health care providers, and in many other ways. This allows the patient or consumer to be in more control of his or her health. This technology is not perfect, and there are concerns about the quality of health material posted on the Web. Much of the information, however, is of good quality and helpful to health care providers and patients/consumers. **E-health** is "the use of emerging information and communication technology, especially the Internet, to improve or enable health and health care" (Eng, 2001, p. 3). Connectivity is one of the key factors in today's personal and work environment, which includes the health care environment. Consumers and providers expect more and more information to be quickly available, but they also want credible information. "Wireless access to data potentially increases that effectiveness by giving caregivers remote access to clinical data anywhere, anytime through web-enabled telephones, wireless personal digital assistants (PDAs), or e-mails containing clinical alerts that require intervention. The combined effect of mobility and instant alerts enables faster, more accurate decision making, and ultimately better outcomes" (Meadows, 2002, p. 295). What do consumers want? They want to be able to get to their health care information quickly and easily. Many are also interested in communicating with their health care providers via many of the possible technologies (for example, e-mail and voice mail).

Many health care organizations have developed their own websites. A key purpose of these sites is marketing and public relations. Nursing needs to be featured on these sites. For acute care sites the answer is simple. Nurses provide most of the care in hospitals, and consumers should see nursing featured on these sites. Nursing leadership in health care organizations needs to step up and insist that nurses are featured on the website, and nurses also need to be involved in developing the site, with nurse leaders involved in major decisions related to e-health. Nurse leaders also need to develop their own technological skills and those of the nursing staff to improve technical IQ (TIQ) (Kerfoot, 2000). These websites can also assist with the organization's recruitment and retention (advertising jobs, recognizing expertise, sharing what nurses are contributing); patient education and consumer guidelines; nursing continuing education; linking the nursing staff with resources via the Web; communication of nursing activities such as committees, and so on. Some of this information must be available via pin number or some sort of privacy system, and other parts should be open to the public. The following are some consumer- or patient-oriented materials that could help nurses in the management of care if they were made available to patients on the organization's website.

- Preoperative instructions
- Patient education guides for common problems (for example, diabetes, cardiac, and so on)
- Description of postoperative experience
- Description of admission process
- Description of discharge process
- Description of discharge planning and role of the patient
- Family visiting guidelines
- Patient rights
- Intensive care guidelines for family members
- Helping your child with hospitalization
- Hospital diets
- Helping your child cope with a parent/grandparent in the hospital
- Appropriate flowers and plants to send to ensure safety
- Reimbursement issues and procedures
- Talking with your doctor
- Talking with your nurse
- Who is who? Finding your way around our staff
- Patient satisfaction and patient advocacy

These are only a few examples. Any educational content and information also needs to be individualized when patients receive care, and patients would then need to have contact with staff for questions and discussion.

## Implications for Nursing Research

Informatics has had and will continue to have an effect on nursing research. This effect is felt both in the use of informatics as a tool to facilitate research and as a focus of research—application in the clinical practice and administration. There is a greater need to understand informatics and its implications for the profession. Many health care organizations, with their increasing ability to access technology, will probably increase their research activity. There is greater ability to communicate across organizations and to seek information and consultation. Databases can maintain data for use in research and through various searching capabilities data can be mined to get a clearer picture of an issue. Nurse researchers need to understand the possibilities and work with IT experts. It is easier now to apply statistics with the various computer-based statistical software packages.

## Technology and Health Care Reimbursement

With the rapid growth of information technology, the management and provision of health care have been radically changed. Information is available today via many different types of technology giving health care providers the opportunity to track patient information across health care settings and virtually anywhere in the world to analyze the data effectively. Insurers are finding that telephone patient advice is an excellent triage method that allows patients to speak directly with a health care professional, who is often a nurse. This method can be used for triage, counseling, disease management, education, self-care support, and appointment and referral services (Greenberg & Schultz, 2002). Questions can be answered, which may prevent the need for an office visit. Patients can also be assessed and referred to the best resource for service. Patient education and guidance can also be provided. Assessment over the phone requires a highly skilled practitioner who can identify critical information that may be communicated in subtle ways. Nurses with their assessment skills and ability to collaborate with physicians are particularly effective in this role. Patient advice systems via telephone require clear documentation policies and guidelines that include content related to whom is called, when, for what reason, and required assessment data and interventions. Follow-up is a critical topic as it should be part of the services and the documentation of those services. This form of communication between nurses and patients must take into consideration the importance of trust, establishing a good relationship, and the need to individualize care. The latter is important because many organizations that use patient advice systems follow very specific protocols, algorithms, and guidelines. If, however, this care is not individualized, it could have serious consequences. "Cookbook" care must be avoided. The assessment is the key to successful telephone nursing—providing the interventions for needs that should be addressed, which may or may not be found in the guidelines. There are four typical interventions used by nurses in this practice arena: telephone consultation, telephone follow-up, surveillance via telephone, and triage via telephone (Androwich & Haas, 2001). The easiest and probably the most common of the four typical interventions used in patient advice systems is using the telephone for patient follow-up. Day surgery unit/ambulatory staff might call patients before surgery to discuss preoperative requirements and after discharge to determine their status and whether they are following discharge advice. Many health care providers are using the telephone to contact patients and remind them of appointments to decrease the number of patients who do not show up for appointments. Missed appointments are expensive for providers because this time could have been used to see other patients. Health care providers, particularly hospitals, are using the telephone to obtain initial intake information and thus reduce admission time, while at the same time providing the patient with pertinent information. Insurers call patients who have failed to keep appointments or to obtain satisfaction data. The telephone is certainly not new; however, health care providers are now using this technology to their advantage. The use of the telephone for these purposes does take staff time, and this does affect costs; however, it usually is less time than would be required for an in-person encounter— it saves time for the provider and the patient. Staff members that make the calls need training, policies, and guidelines related to the purposes of the calls, privacy issues, whom to call and what to say, and documentation.

# APPLYING LEADERSHIP AND MANAGEMENT

## MY HOSPITAL UNIT

Your hospital is implementing an EMR system. In order to be proactive, each nurse manager is required to identify issues and problems that might occur on his or her unit. You need to consider your unit, patients, staff, documentation issues that might be special, ability of staff to respond to change, educational needs regarding documentation and EMR and IT, and so on. You are sitting down at your office desk to begin this huge task. How will you portray your response? In narrative form, table, and so on? You want to be clear to your director. Prepare the response that you will send to the director. It should be specific to your unit, and past decisions you have made in other chapters about your unit need to be considered. Use the virtual unit site on the textbook website to record the work that you do in the role of nurse manager for your unit.

## Critical Thinking Questions and Activities

1. Use of technology in health care varies from community to community. You have probably noticed that some health care organizations use technology more than others. Use of the computer has become very common although some organizations still have a long way to go in how the computer is used. What is used in your community? The class might want to develop a list of health care organizations and a survey that would include the common types of technology that might be used today. Then find out what is used in the health care organizations: What type of technology is used, by whom, why, what is the patient population, and what is the value of its use? Ask nurses in some of the health care organizations what they think about the organization's computer documentation system (if they have one). What do they see as the pros and cons to using it? You might also ask fellow students to rate different computer documentation systems that they have used in different health care settings. Your responses will depend on your local health care organizations, but it will probably include use of computers, technology in treatment such as in surgery and other specialties, use of telephone, videoconferencing, telehealth, and other methods. Criteria that might be used to assess effectiveness would be initial cost, maintenance cost, training costs, error rate, safety issues, need for back-up systems, staff reaction, and so on.
2. How do you think the increasing use of technology in health care both for medical and nursing interventions and communication has impacted the caring part of nursing? Discuss this question with your classmates.
3. Working in teams develop a list of potential problems that might lead to errors when using an EMR. Identify strategies that might be implemented to prevent these problems.
4. Working in teams, discuss how telehealth might be used in the future—use your imagination.

## Media Links

- **URL: http://www.atmeda.org/**
  Alliance for Nursing Informatics
- **URL: http://www.ania-caring.org/**
  American Nursing Informatics Association (ANIA)
- **URL: http://www.atmeda.org/**
  American Telemedicine Association
- **URL: http://www.himss.org/asp/topics_nursingInformatics.asp**
  Healthcare Information and Management Systems Society (HIMSS)

- **URL: http://www.tigersummit.com/**
  Technology Informatics Guiding Educational Reform
- **URL: http://www.nursing-informatics.com/sitemap.html**
  Online source for articles, lessons, tutorials, and discussions about computers in nursing

**Pearson Nursing Student Resources**

Find additional review materials at
**nursing.pearsonhighered.com**
Prepare for success with additional NCLEX®-style practice questions, interactive assignments and activities, Web links, animations and videos, and more!

# References

American Academy of Ambulatory Care Nursing, Telehealth Nursing Practice Standards Task Force. (2001). *AAACN telehealth nursing practice administration and practice standards.* Pittman, NJ: Author.

American Nurses Association. (2002) Using innovative technology to enhance patient care delivery. Washington, DC: Author.

American Nurses Association (ANA). (2006). Nursing Practice Information Infrastructure: Glossary. Retrieved March 5, 2008, from http://www.nursingworld.org/npii/glossary.htm

American Nurses Association (ANA). (2008). *Nursing informatics: Scope and standards of practice.* Washington, DC: Author.

American Organization of Nurse Executives. (2007). *AONE guiding principles: For defining the role of the nurse executive in technology acquisition and implementation.* Chicago, IL: Author.

American Organization of Nurse Executives. (2009). *AONE guiding principles: For the nurse executive to enhance clinical outcomes by leveraging technology.* Chicago, IL: Author.

Association of Perioperative Registered Nurses (APRN). (2008). Retrieved March 7, 2008, from http://www.aorn.org/PracticeResources/PNDS/

Androwich, I., & Haas, S. (2001). Ambulatory care nursing. In J. Dochterman & H. Grace (Eds.), *Current issues in nursing* (6th ed., pp. 150–158). St. Louis: Mosby, Inc.

Dakins, D. (2002). Home is where the health care is. *Telemedicine Today, 9*(2), 18–21.

Eng, T. (2001). *The health landscape: A terrain map of emerging information and communication technologies in health and health care.* Princeton, NJ: Robert Wood Johnson.

Finkelman, A., & Kenner, C. (2009). *Teaching IOM.* Silver Spring, MD: American Nurses Association Publishing.

Furukawa, M., Raghu, T., Spaulding, T., & Avinze, J. (2008). Hospitals slow to adopt health IT applications targeting medication safety, study says. *Health Affairs, 27*(3), 865–875.

Greenberg, M., & Schultz, C. (2002). Telephone nursing: Client experiences and perceptions. *Nursing Economics, 20*(4), 181–187.

Hafner, K. (2002, June 6). 'Dear doctor' meets 'return to sender.' *New York Times,* E1, E6.

Institute of Medicine. (1999). *Crossing the quality chasm: A new health system for the 21st century.* Washington, DC: National Academies Press.

Institute of Medicine (IOM). (1999). *To err is human.* Washington, DC: National Academies Press.

Institute of Medicine (IOM). (2001). *Crossing the quality chasm.* Washington, DC: National Academies Press.

Institute of Medicine (IOM). (2003). *Health professions education.* Washington, DC: National Academies Press.

International Council of Nurses. (ICN). (2008). International Classification for Nursing Practice (ICNP®). Retrieved October 17, 2010, from http://www.icn.ch/publications/classification-of-nursing-practice/classification-of-nursing-practice.html

Kerfoot, K. (2000). TIQ (Technical IQ)—A survival skill for the new millennium. *Nursing Economics, 18*(1), 29–31.

Kerfoot, K., & Simpson, R. (2002). Knowledge-driven care: Powerful medicine. *Reflections on Nursing LEADERSHIP* (third quarter), 22–24, 44.

Kosko, B. (1999). *Fuzzy future.* New York: Harmony Books.

Meadows, G. (2002). The nursing shortage: Can information technology help? *Nursing Economics, 20*(1), 46–48.

National Library of Medicine (NLM). (2008). Retrieved March 12, 2008, from http://www.nlm.nih.gov/research/umls/Snomed/snomed_main.html

Omaha System. (2005). The Omaha System: Solving the clinical data-information puzzle. Retrieved from http://www.omahasystem.org/

Predko, J. (2001). Use of distance technology for education, practice, and research. In J. Dochterman & H. Grace (Eds.), *Current issues in nursing* (6th ed., pp. 75–81). St. Louis: Mosby.

Richards, J. (2001). Nursing in a digital age. *Nursing Economics, 19*(1), 6–10, 34.

Roark, D. (2004). Bar codes & drug administration. *AJN, 104*(1), 63–66.

Simpson, R., & Keegan, A. (2002). How connected are you? Employing emotional intelligence in a high-tech world. (Nursing informatics). *Nursing Administration Quarterly, 26*(2), 80–87.

Snyder-Halpern, R., & Chervany, N. (2000). A clinical information system strategic planning model for integrated health care delivery networks. *Journal of Nursing Administration, 30*(12), 583–591.

U.S. Department of Health and Human Services. (2000). *Healthy People 2010.* Washington, DC: Author.

Waters, R. (2002). Thinking outside the box helps break through barriers. *Telemedicine Today, 9*(2), 9–17.

# A

# Nurse Executive Competencies

## I. Communication and Relationship-Building

a. Effective Communication
- Make oral presentations to diverse audiences on nursing, health care, and organizational issues
- Produce cogent and persuasive written materials to address nursing, health care, and organizational issues appropriate to the audience
- Resolve and manage conflict

b. Relationship Management
- Build trusting, collaborative relationships with
  - Staff
  - Peers
  - Other disciplines and ancillary services
  - Physicians
  - Vendors
  - Community leaders
  - Legislators
  - Nursing and other educational programs
- Deliver "bad news" in such a way as to maintain credibility
- Follow through on promises and concerns
- Provide service recovery to dissatisfied customers
- Care about people as individuals and demonstrate empathy and concern while ensuring that organizational goals and objectives are met
- Accomplish objectives through persuasion, celebrate successes and accomplishments, and communicate a shared vision
- Assert views in non-threatening, non-judgmental ways

c. Influencing Behaviors
- Create and communicate a shared vision
- Reward appropriate behaviors and confront and manage inappropriate behaviors
- Develop, communicate and monitor behavior expectations

d. Diversity
- Create an environment which recognizes and values differences in staff, physicians, patients, and communities
- Assess current environment and establish indicators of progress toward cultural competency
- Define diversity in terms of gender, race, religion, ethnicity, sexual orientation, age, etc.
- Analyze population data to identify cultural clusters
- Define cultural competency and permeate principles throughout the organization
- Confront inappropriate behaviors and attitudes toward diverse group
- Develop processes to incorporate cultural beliefs into care

e. Shared Decision Making
- Engage staff and others in decision making
- Promote decisions that are patient-centered
- Provide an environment conducive to opinion sharing

f. Community Involvement
- Represent the organization to non–health care constituents within the community
- Provide consultation to community and business leaders regarding nursing and health care
- Be an effective board member for community and/or professional organizations

g. Medical Staff Relationships
- Build credibility with physicians as a champion for patient care, quality, and nursing professionalism
- Confront and address inappropriate behavior towards patients and staff
- Represent nursing at medical executive committee and other medical staff committees
- Collaborate with medical staff leaders in determining needed patient care services
- Collaborate with physicians to develop patient care protocols, policies, and procedures
- Collaborate with physicians to determine patient care equipment and facility needs
- Utilize medical staff mechanisms to address physician clinical performance issues
- Facilitate disputes involving physicians and nurses or other disciplines

h. Academic Relationships
- Determine current and future supply and demand for nursing care
- Identify educational needs of existing and potential nursing staff
- Collaborate with nursing programs to provide required resources
- Collaborate with nursing programs in evaluating quality of graduating clinicians and develop mechanisms to enhance this quality
- Serve on academic advisory councils
- Collaborate with nursing faculty in nursing research and incorporate nursing research into practice

# II. Knowledge of the Health Care Environment

a. Clinical Practice Knowledge
- Maintain knowledge of current nursing practice and the roles and functions of patient care team members
- Articulate patient care standards as published by JCAHO [Joint Commission], CMS, and professional nursing literature
- Understand, articulate, and ensure compliance with the State Nurse Practice Act, State Board of Nursing regulations, regulatory agency standards, and policies of the organization
- Ensure that written organization clinical policies and procedures are reviewed and updated in accordance with evidence-based practice
- Role model lifelong learning, including clinical subjects such as disease processes, pharmaceuticals, and clinical technology

b. Delivery Models/Work Design
- Maintain current knowledge of patient care delivery systems and innovations
- Articulate various delivery systems and patient care models and the advantages/disadvantages of each
- Serve as change agent when patient care work/workflow is redesigned
- Determine when new delivery models are appropriate, and then envision and develop them

c. Health Care Economics
- Articulate federal and state payment systems and regulations, as well as private insurance issues, which affect organization's finances
- Understand and articulate individual organization's payer mix, CMI, and benchmark database

d. Health Care Policy
- Articulate federal and state laws and regulations that affect the provision of patient care e.g., tort reform, malpractice/negligence, reimbursement

## EFFECTIVE 2010 (CONTINUED)

| Provision | Health Care Delivery and Possible Nursing Implications |
|---|---|
| Improve access to care by increasing funding by $11 billion for school-based health centers (effective 2010); nurse-managed health clinics (effective 2010), and community health centers and National Health Service Corps (over 5 years—effective 2011); | This provision provides opportunities for nurses to expand practice into new areas or improve areas already active. |
| Insurance plans may not place lifetime limits on benefits and restrictive annual limits. | This provision is important for all insured to limit costs. |
| Insurers may not rescind policies to avoid paying medical bills when a person becomes ill. | This provision protects patients to ensure payment of medical bills covered by the patient's insurance plan. |

## EFFECTIVE 2011

| Provision | Health Care Delivery and Possible Nursing Implications |
|---|---|
| A 50% discount will be provided on brand-name drugs for Prescription Drug Plan or Medicare Advantage enrollees. Additional discounts on brand-name and generic drugs will be phased in to completely close the "doughnut hole" by 2020. | This provision addresses further the problems with Medicare Part D-Prescription coverage. |
| Cover only proven preventive services and eliminate cost-sharing for preventive services in Medicare and Medicaid. | This provision further addresses preventive services and also emphasizes need for evidence-based preventive services. |
| The Medicare payroll tax will increase from 1.45% to 2.35% for individuals earning more than $200,000 and married filing jointly above $250,000. | This type of provision impacts Medicare beneficiaries in that some employees will have to contribute more the Medicare fund; based on income levels. |
| States can offer home- and community-based services to the disabled through Medicaid rather than institutional care beginning October 1. | This provision impacts home care and other community-based services; impacting nurses and nursing care for disabled and providing more services outside of institutions. |
| Medicare will provide free annual wellness visits and personalized prevention plans. New plans will be required to cover preventive services with no co-pay. | This provision further supports wellness and prevention. Nurses may be involved in providing these services and developing programs. |
| Pharmaceutical companies will provide a 50% discount on brand name prescription drugs for seniors; additional discounts phased in over the next ten years. | This provision reduces costs of prescriptions for seniors increasing use of prescribed medications. |
| A plan to provide a vehicle for small businesses to offer tax-free benefits will be created. This would ease the small employer's administrative burden of sponsoring a cafeteria plan. | This provision increases insurance coverage to employees who often do not get insurance coverage option. |
| Develop a national quality improvement strategy to improve delivery of health care services, patient health outcomes, and population health with multiple stakeholders; include measures. The national strategy needs to be submitted to Congress by January 1, 2011. | This provision is directly related to the Institute of Medicine reports on health quality. Nurses should be involved in this initiative. |
| Community Living Assistance Services and Supports (CLASS), a voluntary long-term care program, will be created. When employees contribute to the program for five years they will be entitled to a $50 per day cast benefit to pay for long-term care. CLASS does not cover all long-term care expenses. This is the first national government-run long-term care insurance program, primarily offered through employers. | This provision is a significant step toward addressing the needs of the people who need long-term care. This will impact nurses and nursing in long-term care. |

## EFFECTIVE 2011 (CONTINUED)

| Provision | Health Care Delivery and Possible Nursing Implications |
|---|---|
| Develop a Medicaid plan option for enrollees with at least two chronic illnesses, one condition and risk of developing another, or at least one serious and persistent mental health conditions to designate a provider as a health home. | This provision relates to information in the Institute of Medicine reports on the need for better care for chronic illness. Nurses are involved daily in caring for these patients. The focus here is on better care planning. |
| Develop the Community-based Collaborative Care Network Program, which would provide support to consortiums of health care providers to coordinate and integrate health services targeted at low-income uninsured and underinsured. Funds for this are appropriated for five years beginning FY2011. | This provision relates to the Institute of Medicine recommendations to better coordinate care. Nurses who work in community health will need to be involved in this program. |
| Provide access to comprehensive health risk assessment and a personalized prevention plan for Medicare beneficiaries. Health risk assessment model to be developed with 18 months after law's effective date. | This provision relates to nursing; increasing the emphasis on health risk assessment and a personalized prevention plan, which could be done by nurses. |
| Provide incentives to Medicare and Medicaid beneficiaries to complete behavior modification programs (criteria need to be developed). | There is need to increase effective completion of behavior modification programs for problems such as substance abuse, obesity, smoking, and other similar problems. Nurses frequently direct these programs and also refer patients to these programs. |
| Five-year grants provided to small employers that establish wellness programs. | Nurses in occupational health may be involved in developing and implementing these programs. |
| Establish a new trauma center program to increase emergency capacity; fund research; develop demonstration programs to design, implement, and evaluate innovative emergency care models. | This provision is relevant to nurses who work in emergency and trauma care. Nurses should be involved in all aspects of this provision. This is an opportunity to address emergency nursing care issues. More effective emergency services also impacts acute care in that capacity or ability to admit patients should be improved. |
| Provide resources to evaluate employer-based wellness programs and conduct a national worksite survey to assess employer-based health policies and programs. (Study to be completed by 2012.) | Nurses in occupational health may be involved in developing and implementing these programs. |
| Chain restaurants and food vending machines must disclose nutritional content of each item. | This provision is relevant to nurses who work in community health. |
| Community First Choice Option for Medicaid beneficiaries with disabilities to receive community-based attendant services and supports rather than institutional care. | This is a new program that improves care for patients with disabilities and has implications for nurses who work in home health care. |
| Address the nursing shortage and retention of nurses: increase capacity for education, support training programs, provide loan repayment and retention grants, and create a career ladder to nursing. | This provision is important for all nurses and has a direct impact on the quality of nursing care. |
| Provide grants (up to 3 years) to employ and provide training for family nurse practitioners who provide primary care in federally qualified health centers and nurse-managed health clinics. (See http://www.cms.hhs.gov/MLNProducts/downloads/fqhcfactsheet.pdf for information on federally qualified health centers.) | This provision focuses on nurses and advanced practice nurses. It recognizes the important role nurses have in these delivery services. |

## EFFECTIVE 2012

| Provision | Health Care Delivery and Possible Nursing Implications |
| --- | --- |
| Create the Independence in Home demonstration program; providing primary care services in the home for high-need Medicare beneficiaries with goal of reducing preventable hospitalization, readmissions, improve health outcomes, improve efficiency of care, reduce costs, and achieve patient satisfaction. | This provision emphasizes need for greater in home services, and area that has strong nursing presence. |
| Improve collection and reporting of data on race, ethnicity, sex, primary language, disability status, underserved rural and frontier populations; include data on access and treatment for people with disabilities; data should be analyzed to identify trends in disparities. | The Institute of Medicine reports on disparities are reflected in this provision. The annual disparities report is one method for collecting data. Data need to be analyzed and then results applied to improve care. This has a direct impact on nurses and nursing care, and nurses should be involved in this initiative. |
| Required mental health parity, which means deductibles, co-payments, and limits on the number of visits or days of coverage for mental health and substance abuse treatment must be no more restrictive then for medical and surgical needs. | This provision has implications for nurses who work in mental health. This is an area of care that has struggled with parity problems and discrimination. |
| Establish more training for behavioral health professionals. | This provision should provide more funding for training, for example for advanced practice nurses or nurse clinical specialists in mental health. |
| Develop nongovernmental research centers to investigate effective treatment for mental illness. | This provision may provide greater opportunity for nurse researchers in area of mental health. |

## EFFECTIVE 2013

| Provision | Health Care Delivery and Possible Nursing Implications |
| --- | --- |
| Health plans must implement uniform standards for electronic exchange of health information to reduce paperwork and administrative costs. | This provision is an important on in setting standards for electronic information and to reduce costs. |
| Increase Medicaid payments for fee-for-service and managed care primary care services provided by primary care physicians (family medicine, general internal medicine, or pediatric medicine). | This provision will provide greater access to providers for Medicaid beneficiaries who are often limited in providers who will accept Medicaid payment rates. |

## EFFECTIVE 2014

| Provision | Health Care Delivery and Possible Nursing Implications |
| --- | --- |
| Citizens will be required to have acceptable coverage or pay a penalty of $95 in 2014, $325 in 2015, $695 (or up to 2.5% of income) in 2016. Families will pay half the amount for children, up to a cap of $2,250 per family. After 2016, penalties are indexed to Consumer Price Index. | This provision is a major change. It requires people to have health care insurance, and if they do not, fees must be paid. This will pressure people to get coverage, increasing patients, and increasing need for more staff. |

## EFFECTIVE 2014 (CONTINUED)

| Provision | Health Care Delivery and Possible Nursing Implications |
| --- | --- |
| Companies with 50 or more employees must offer coverage to employees or pay a $2,000 penalty per employee after their first 30 if at least one of their employees receives a tax credit. Waiting periods before insurance takes effect is limited to 90 days. Employers who offer coverage but whose employees receive tax credits will pay $3,000 for each worker receiving a tax credit. | Increases coverage to people who in the past may have not had offer of insurance coverage. Leads to more patients and need for more staff. |
| Health plans will be prohibited from imposing annual limits on coverage. | This provision provides for greater coverage since limits are decreased and reduces costs for enrollees. |
| Insurers can no longer refuse to sell or renew policies because of an individual's health status. Health plans can no longer exclude coverage for pre-existing conditions. Insurers can't charge higher rates because of health status, gender, or other factors. | This eliminates exclusions and discrimination in health care coverage. |
| Health insurance exchanges will open in each state to individuals and small employers to comparison shop for standardized health packages. | This provision will provide more consumer information to make informed decisions about health care coverage. |
| Medicaid eligibility will increase to 133% of federal poverty level for all nonelderly individuals to ensure that people obtain affordable health care in the most efficient and appropriate manner. States will receive increased federal funding to cover these new populations. | This provision will increase the number of insured people, requiring more staff at time of shortage. |

Sources: Health Care and Education Reconciliation Act of 2010 (P.L. 111-152); Health Reform http://www .healthreform.gov/; White House Health Reform http://www.whitehouse.gov/healthreform; The Henry Kaiser Family Foundation http://www.kff.org; *New York Times* (March 24, 2010), How people will be affected by the overhaul, p. A18; Wolf, R. & Young, A. (March 23, 2010). Bill spreads the pain, benefits. *USA Today*, pp. 4A–3A; Span, P. (March 30, 2010). Options expand for affordable long-term care. *New York Times*, p. D5.

# C

# National Institute of Nursing Research Areas of Research Emphasis (2006–2010)

## Promoting Health and Preventing Disease

The interplay of biology and behavior is especially apparent in health promotion and disease prevention. As our understanding of the role that lifestyle plays in disease increases, so does the need for predictors and strategies that target long-term behavior change. The development of interventions based on well-defined underlying mechanisms is critical to advancing health promotion and disease prevention.

Environmental and genetic factors, as well as emerging diseases, interact with behavior to create new challenges. Socioeconomic factors influencing health include housing, population density, and other factors related to geographic location. Many potential interventions must be studied, and perhaps modified, to take into account differences among urban, suburban, rural, and remote environments. NINR seeks to support research that will do the following:

- Develop biomarkers to assess disease risk and response to treatment, identify susceptibility genes for at-risk individuals, and design interventions to moderate risk (e.g., neurohumoral markers for differential response to intervention).
- Develop or improve bio-behavioral methods, measures, and intervention strategies to optimize health.
- Identify factors that influence decision making that results in behavioral changes that promote health and prevent disease and disability.
- Identify and develop individual and family interventions designed to sustain health-promoting behaviors over time (e.g., prevention of obesity; prevention of HIV/AIDS transmission).
- Design intervention studies using community-based approaches to facilitate health promotion/ risk reduction behaviors (e.g., families with special needs, such as parents or caregivers of persons with chronic illness or developmental disabilities).
- Investigate opportunities to identify and ameliorate the long-term consequences of prematurity, including near-term infants at risk for complications.

## Improving Quality of Life

Prevention and treatment of disease are the principal goals of clinical research. Attainment of these goals is constrained by many factors, including the complexity of diseases and disorders for which the underlying mechanisms and pathways to intervention are not fully understood. Moreover, even successful treatment and survival of disease often leave patients facing many challenges in daily living. Our science offers many opportunities for research that will improve quality of life by enhancing the individual's role in managing disease, relieving symptoms of disease and disability, and improving outcomes.

# Self-Management

Our science brings a unique perspective to the interactions among healthy persons, patients and their families, and health practitioners. Self-management incorporates facets of both symptom management and the adoption of health-promoting behaviors. It is particularly important that persons at risk for disease, long-term survivors of disease, and persons with chronic disabilities succeed in modifying behavior in order to manage their own health. This focus on self-management research was in response to the desire of many people to take more responsibility for their own health, and to the increasing imperative of controlling the costs of health care.

As technology advances, new opportunities for the development of self-management strategies will emerge. In turn, improved tools for self-management will further stimulate the research agendas for technology development and research methods. NINR seeks to support research that will do the following:

- Develop technologies to facilitate early self-identification and self-reporting of symptoms.
- Design self-management decision-making strategies that promote healthy lifestyle choices such as diet, exercise, and primary health care practices.
- Define the behaviors that support adherence to treatment for complex acute and chronic illnesses.
- Evaluate factors that impact independence and self-care in long-term care settings.
- Identify strategies for self-management and promotion of personal health among long-term survivors of disease and persons with chronic disabilities, including routine health monitoring and attention to co-morbid conditions.

# Symptom Management

For the patient, a symptom may represent a minor annoyance, a disturbing portent, or a terrible burden. To the clinician or scientist, the same symptom may serve as a diagnostic aid, an indicator of disease severity, or an outcome that shows the success or failure of an intervention. Symptoms may appear or change at multiple points in the trajectory of illness and intervention, causing patients to seek relief or reassurance, or interrupting the course of treatment because of concerns about unpleasant or dangerous side effects. NINR seeks to support research that will

- Delineate causative mechanisms underlying symptoms and improve recognition of symptoms by patients, their caregivers, and health care providers.
- Develop interventions that improve patient response and adaptation to symptoms and symptom clusters in discrete and co-morbid conditions.
- Design strategies to improve management of symptoms over disease trajectories, including the transition from acute to chronic illness and periods of long-term survivorship of formerly life-threatening illnesses.
- Develop strategies for assessment and intervention to improve health-related quality of life in persons with chronic or life-threatening illnesses.

# Caregiving

The Institute seeks to provide a scientific foundation for improving outcomes for care providers and recipients across diverse settings. Recent trends show that an increased number of our population lives to an advanced age, and children who in earlier times might have succumbed to premature birth, childhood illness or injury, now survive. Informal families and networks of peers augment or replace the traditional family as providers of informal care. Changes in the incidence and prevalence of acute and chronic illnesses combined with the proliferation of diverse health care settings (e.g., assisted living facilities, nursing homes, and home care provided by professionals or family members) are opening up new lines of research inquiry. NINR seeks to support research that will

- Design interventions aimed at improving physiological and cognitive function in residents of long-term care facilities.
- Develop interventions to improve the quality of caregiving.
- Evaluate factors that impact the health and quality of life of informal caregivers and recipients.
- Identify factors that improve the transition from one care setting to another.
- Develop models for first responders in events such as natural disasters, environmental hazards, and other emergency situations.

# Eliminating Health Disparities

NINR's commitment to eliminating health disparities dovetails with a period of growing national and international recognition of the impact of race, gender, socioeconomic status, ethnic origin, geography, and culture on the health of individuals and groups.

A greater understanding is needed of predisposing factors for many diseases and disorders. Socioeconomic factors, including living conditions, interact with biology and behavior to influence health outcomes. Culturally based practices can affect either risk or protective factors for many conditions. Inequities in access to treatment and differences in response to treatment present challenges to the well-being of individuals, families and communities.

NINR's focus on health promotion and disease prevention, and its consistent commitment to cultural sensitivity, position the Institute for leadership in NIH and Department of Health and Human Services (HHS) efforts to eliminate disparities in health and quality of life. NINR is a regular contributor to strategic planning related to health disparities at NIH and HHS. The success of NIH efforts to develop research infrastructure in minority-serving institutions has laid the groundwork for making research findings, tools, and methods more widely accessible.

Focusing on the integration of biology and behavior is critical to health disparities research. Gender differences, for example, reflect biological factors based on sex and the behavioral and cultural differences between the male and female in society. Research involving "underserved populations" may incorporate many variables—age, minority status, geographic location, economic status, disability, and unrecognized co-morbid conditions, to name just a few. NINR will continue to develop and refine strategies to promote institutional and individual capacity for expanded research in this field. The Institute will support research that will

- Elucidate mechanisms underlying disparities and design interventions to eliminate them, with particular attention to issues of geography (rural and remote settings), minority status, underserved populations, and persons whose chronic or temporary disabilities limit their access to care.
- Design culturally appropriate interventions to communicate risks and susceptibility to at-risk populations.
- Apply findings from bio-behavioral, descriptive, and intervention studies to factors influencing health disparities among youth and adolescents.
- Identify strategies that will reduce the long-term adverse consequences of poor maternal and reproductive health in minorities and underserved populations.
- Evaluate and modify partnership and training programs to build capacity in minority-serving institutions and expand the pool of investigators from underrepresented groups.

# Setting Directions for End-of-Life Research

The end of life has long been a focus of our science, given the importance of palliative care and respect for dying persons. Many factors have recently converged to increase public and professional interest in topics relevant to the end of life.

Advances in medicine and public health have altered the prospects for survival in every age group, but particularly in the very young and the very old. Many premature and low birth-weight infants benefit from perinatal advances, while others face protracted courses of decline involving difficult decisions about appropriate interventions and quality of life. Cancer is no longer a death sentence for many children, but families whose children do not respond to treatment or are born with lethal genetic diseases often find themselves faced with choices no parent envisions having to make on behalf of a child. Almost everyone will confront similar decisions as their parents and other elders survive chronic and acute illnesses and live long enough to suffer from dementia, frailty, and organ failure. Only through research can one ensure that dying patients will receive adequate management of their symptoms of pain, fatigue, and depression, particularly if they are cognitively impaired or suffer from psychological impairments. Ironically, the medical and technological advances that extend life also set the stage for a prolonged process of dying, and generate new questions about the dying process itself.

The urgency of issues at the end of life has created important research opportunities. NIH has a broad interest in these research questions, given the number of diseases and conditions at the end of life. NINR has issued a number of research solicitations in response to the 1997 Institute of Medicine report, "Approaching Death: Improving Care at the End of Life." Because of NINR's emphasis on integrating biological and behavioral science in this area, the Institute has been designated the lead Institute for end-of-life research at NIH. This represents an important opportunity for nursing science to shape future directions in an emerging field and to lead the way in addressing some of the most critical questions in clinical care today.

Source: National Institute of Nursing Research. (2006–2010). *Strategic Plan*. Retrieved February 10, 2010, from http://www.ninr.nih.gov/AboutNINR/NINRMissionandStrategicPlan/

# INDEX